BIOMEDICAL PHYSICS
IN RADIOTHERAPY
FOR CANCER

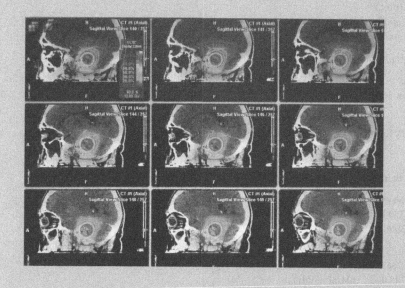

Loredana Marcu, Royal Adelaide Hospital

Eva Bezak, Royal Adelaide Hospital

Barry Allen, University of NSW

CSIRO
PUBLISHING

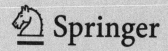

Springer

National Library of Australia Cataloguing-in-Publication entry

Marcu, Loredana.

Biomedical physics in radiotherapy for cancer/by Loredana Marcu, Eva Bezak and Barry Allen.

9780643094048 (pbk.)
9780643103306 (epdf)
9780643103313 (epub)

Includes bibliographical references and index.

Medical physics.
Cancer – Radiotherapy.

Bezak, Eva.
Allen, B. J. (Barry John)

616.9940642

Published exclusively in Australia and New Zealand by

CSIRO PUBLISHING
150 Oxford Street (PO Box 1139)
Collingwood VIC 3066
Australia

Telephone:	+61 3 9662 7666
Local call:	1300 788 000 (Australia only)
Fax:	+61 3 9662 7555
Email:	publishing.sales@csiro.au
Web site:	www.publish.csiro.au

Published in the Americas, Europe and Rest of the World (excluding Australia and New Zealand) by
Springer Science + Business Media B.V., with ISBN 978-0-85729-732-7
springer.com

Front cover: Image sequences of stereotactic radiotherapy planning for brain lesion (courtesy Royal Adelaide Hospital)

Set in 10/13 Adobe Minion Pro and ITC Stone Sans
Cover and text design by James Kelly
Typeset by Desktop Concepts Pty Ltd, Melbourne
Index by Bruce Gillespie
Printed in China by 1010 Printing International Ltd

CSIRO PUBLISHING publishes and distributes scientific, technical and health science books, magazines and journals from Australia to a worldwide audience and conducts these activities autonomously from the research activities of the Commonwealth Scientific and Industrial Research Organisation (CSIRO). The views expressed in this publication are those of the author(s) and do not necessarily represent those of, and should not be attributed to, the publisher or CSIRO.

Foreword

Biomedical Physics in Radiotherapy for Cancer provides an overview of the rapid technological advances in the planning and delivery of radiation therapy for the treatment of cancer which has occurred in the last 15 years or so and how these have transformed the practice of clinical radiotherapy. Each of the current widely available radiation treatment modalities is covered and highly specialised treatment techniques such as stereotactic radiotherapy, brachytherapy and heavy ion therapy are also included. In the closing chapters of the book, the evolving fields of targeted radiotherapy and continuing refinements in predictive assays converge to bring the ultimate goal of individualising patient treatments or personalised medicine a reality in the near future.

It is written by Medical Physicists involved in the provision of comprehensive radiation therapy services in one of the largest Radiation Oncology departments in Australia. Unlike most Medical Physics textbooks, this book does not dwell unduly on technical detail and complicated formulae but gives a refreshing perspective of the radiobiological basis of each technological advance for Radiotherapy for Cancer. In addition, examples of clinical applications are provided in each chapter as well as evidence of therapeutic gains of the various technological advances from long term clinical trial data where available.

As many of the discernable patient benefits from the technological advances are based mainly on short-term data from studies in a number of malignant disease sites, the authors are right in reserving judgement on the success of the treatment approaches until several more years follow-up have elapsed to ensure that any long term advantages in tumour control through radiation dose escalation are not negated by increased late normal tissue radiation effects resulting in worse treatment related morbidity. The authors also correctly emphasise the importance of radiobiological considerations in radiation therapy of cancer in order to maximise the potential gains of recent technological advances in radiotherapy in terms of local cure whilst minimising late normal tissue effects and treatment related complications.

I would commend this book to all involved in Radiotherapy for Cancer but in particular to trainees in Medical Physics, Radiation Therapy, Radiation Oncology and Radiation Nursing. The authors are cognisant of the varying needs of the different trainee groups and refer each to sources of further information other than the up to date list of references in each chapter.

Professor Eric Yeoh
MD, FRCP (EDIN), FRCR, FRANZCR
Professor in Discipline of Medicine
University of Adelaide
Adjunct Professor in Division of Health Sciences
University of South Australia
Director
Radiation Oncology Department
Royal Adelaide Hospital

Contents

Acknowledgements

The journey of writing a book is an exhaustive one and it would not have happened without support of many kind people we met along the way.

The authors would like to express immense gratitude to the CSIRO Publishing staff, Mr John Manger, Ms Tracey Millen and Ms Deepa Travers for their ongoing support and work on editing the chapters and figures as well as for their trust in this project.

The authors would like to kindly thank Mr John Lawson, Ms Raelene Nelligan, Dr Justin Shepherd, Mr Scott Penfold, Mr David Horsman, Mr Michael Douglass, Mr Alex Santos, Mr Richard Vidanage and Miss Christine Robinson for their assistance in proof reading chapters of this book, it is greatly appreciated.

Lastly, the authors would like to thank their families and friends for their understanding and encouragement during preparation of this manuscript.

The Authors

Introduction

The aim of this book is to bring together three major scientific foundations of radiation oncology: radiotherapy physics, radiobiology and clinical trials. All three disciplines are closely intertwined and co-dependent when providing and developing new radiotherapy treatment techniques for cancer patients. While physics provides well established theories and understanding of the interaction of radiation with matter, radiobiology applies this knowledge to the biological environment. Here, due to the high degree of complexity of biological systems, rigorous theories derived from first principles cannot be established and empirical data based on laboratory experiments and clinical trials with patients are required to develop semi-empirical models/concepts. The radiation and nuclear physics and technology together with the results of clinical trials are thus at the base of modern radiobiology. On the other hand, understanding of the response of biological systems to irradiation has a direct impact on development of new radiotherapy treatment techniques utilising current physics/engineering know-how.

While there are books on both physics and radiobiology applied in radiotherapy published before, the scientific literature lacks books presenting the two aspects of cancer treatment with radiation (as supported by clinical trials) in a single volume. In addition, the books currently available on the market do not generally provide summaries or evaluation of major clinical trials.

Radiobiology is the science behind radiotherapy, therefore this book presents the rationale for using radiation in various modalities and schedules for a diversity of tumours. Starting with an introduction to both radiotherapy and radiobiology the book continues with the major aspects of radiotherapy (types of radiation, apparatus used in the treatment process, conventional treatment modalities, unconventional treatment methods, dosimetry) and radiobiology (biological effects of radiation, tumour characteristics and behaviour during treatment, normal tissue toxicity, models in radiobiology). Each chapter is designed with the three disciplines in mind, illustrating their relationship, explaining the basic science, showing the role of radiobiology in the development of radiotherapy and discussing the evidence provided by clinical trials. Modern radiotherapy strongly relies on physics and technology when delivering radiation as well as on cell biology when assessing tumour and normal tissue response to radiation. The book is topical with the current trends of translational research in radiation oncology. While radiotherapy has been mostly technology driven in the past, it is now recognised that input from biological disciplines should be increased and physics, biology based on clinical trials outcomes need to be combined to provide best cancer treatment.

Some of the key benefits the book will provide to the reader:

- updated information on radiotherapy physics, technology and radiobiology and clinical trials
- explanation of the rationale in using radiation in the treatment of cancer
- presentation of three major disciplines in one book
- easy accessibility to information for both under- and postgraduate students to use in their courses
- textbook for oncology medical registrars in their preparation for specialist exams
- comprehensive overview of the major aspect of treatment with radiotherapy: useful tool for all novices in the area (doctors, physicists, radiation therapists, nurses, and any scientists with interest in radiation oncology).
- inclusion, summary and findings of major clinical trials conducted recently in relation to specific topics.

The Authors

1 Interactions of radiation with matter

1.1 IONISING RADIATION

Radiation (i.e. energy that is radiated and propagated in the form of rays or waves or particles) is classified into two main groups: *non-ionising* and *ionising*, depending on its ability to ionise matter. Ionising radiation is radiation with enough energy to be able to remove tightly bound electrons from the orbit of an atom, causing the atom to become charged or ionised. Some examples of ionising and non-ionising radiation are listed in Table 1.1.

Atoms and molecules are electrically neutral. This means the number of negatively charged electrons is exactly equal to the number of positively charged protons. Most of the matter around us is electrically neutral. However, when there is an ionising radiation source available, atoms or molecules can gain or lose electrons and acquire a net electrical charge. This process is called ionisation. The minimum energy required to ionise an atom, ranges from a few electron Volts (eV) for alkali elements to 24.5 eV for helium (noble gas). Specific forms of ionising radiation include: a) particulate radiation, consisting of atomic or subatomic particles (electrons, protons, etc.) which carry energy in the form of kinetic energy or mass in motion and b) electromagnetic radiation, in which energy is carried by oscillating electrical and magnetic fields propagating at the speed of light. The medium traversed by radiation can be ionised directly or indirectly.

Directly ionising radiation deposits energy in the medium through direct Coulomb inter-actions

Table 1.1. Examples of ionising and non-ionising radiation.

Non-ionising radiation (cannot ionise matter)	Ionising radiation (can ionise matter either directly or indirectly)	
	Directly ionising radiation (charged particles)	Indirectly ionising radiation (neutral particles)
Radio waves ranging from long waves to the broadcast band	electrons, protons, alpha particles, heavy ions	photons (ultra violet radiation), X-rays, gamma
Infrared radiations		neutrons
Visible light		

L. Marcu et al., *Biomedical Physics in Radiotherapy for Cancer*,
DOI 10.1007/978-0-85729-733-4_1, © CSIRO 2012

between the directly ionising charged particle (e.g. an alpha particle) and orbital electrons of atoms in the medium. Indirectly ionising radiation (photons or neutrons) deposits energy in the medium through a two step process: I) a charged particle is released in the medium (photons liberate atomic electrons or generate positrons, neutrons release protons or heavier ions), II) the released charged particles deposit energy to the medium through direct Coulomb interactions with orbital electrons of the atoms in the medium.

Photon radiation is further classified as below:

- *Characteristic X-rays*: result from electron transitions between atomic shells
- *Bremsstrahlung X-rays*: result from electron-nucleus Coulomb interactions
- *Gamma rays*: result from nuclear transitions
- *Annihilation quanta*: result from positron-electron annihilation

Both directly and indirectly ionising radiations are used in treatment of cancer. In some cases non-cancerous tumours are also treated. The branch of medicine that uses radiation in the treatment of disease is called radiotherapy or radiation oncology.

1.2 X-RAYS

X-rays were discovered by Roentgen in 1895 in Germany during his study of ultraviolet light in the discharge tube (stream of electrons). BaPt cyanide filter paper placed in the vicinity of the discharge tube started glowing due to fluorescence. Roentgen concluded that another type of radiation must have been produced, presumably during the interaction of electrons with the tube's glass walls. This radiation could be detected outside the tube and also caused exposure of photographic plates and ionised a gas. He named this new radiation X-rays. They were subsequently extensively investigated and eventually classified as one form of electromagnetic radiation. Within months they began to be used for medical purposes.

The main properties of X-rays are listed below. X-rays:

- Are electromagnetic waves of short wavelengths, e.g. X-ray energy of 1 MeV corresponds to wave-

length, λ, of about 1.24 pm. Short wavelengths are used for studies of diffraction of X-rays from crystalline structures, known as X-ray crystallography.
- Travel at or near the velocity of light.
- Travel in straight lines and are unaffected by electric and magnetic fields (as they have zero electric charge).
- Various normally opaque materials are transparent to X-rays. The degree of transparency depends on their atomic number, Z, and photon energy. High Z materials are more absorbing than low Z and any material is more transparent to higher energy photons.
- Obey inverse square law (i.e. their intensity reduces as the square of the distance from the source).
- Are generated by high voltages in X-ray tubes in which an electron beam in vacuum is stopped by a metal anode.
- Do not readily reflect or refract.
- Discharge electrified bodies and ionise gases (make them conductive).
- Have energy and momentum and undergo interactions with electrons and nuclei of the medium (absorption, scatter), e.g. photoelectric effect, Compton scatter (incoherent), Thomson scatter (coherent) and pair production.
- Main sources of X-rays are bremsstrahlung radiation of continuous energy distribution and characteristic atomic radiation of discrete energy.
- May follow α and β decay.
- Can be polarised by scattering, e.g. two carbon blocks behave as polariser and analyser (i.e. they show properties of electromagnetic waves).
- Reflect very little except at low energies and off smooth metal surfaces at grazing incidence.
- In diagnostic radiology (imaging) peak voltages of ~50–150 kV are used to produce X-rays, while in radiation therapy corresponding voltages are in the range of 4–25 MV.

X-ray photons typically have the wavelengths of the same size or less than the diameter of a single atom, about 0.1 nm (or 0.1×10^{-9} m). X-rays can penetrate through soft material such as flesh. Much of the X-ray spectrum overlaps with gamma rays. X-rays and

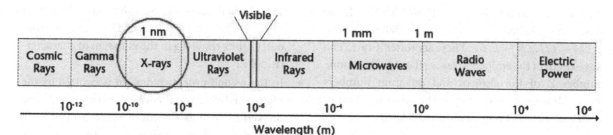

Figure 1.1. Wavelengths of various types of electromagnetic radiation.

gamma rays mainly differ only in the manner of their production. X-rays are produced by electrons whilst gamma rays are produced by nuclei (see Figure 1.1).

1.2.1 Characteristic X-rays

Characteristic X-rays are the characteristic atomic line spectra. An electron with kinetic energy, E_e, passing through a medium will interact with atoms of the material. In most cases it will cause ionisation, i.e. the ejection of the outer shell electrons. Occasionally, the electron may also eject an electron from the lower atomic shell (mostly K, L and M). The hole created in the shell will be filled with electrons from outer atomic orbits and characteristic radiation will be emitted (see Figure 1.2).

Characteristic X-rays have discrete energies as they correspond to discrete atomic energy levels. The energy of the photon (similar to γ decay of the nucleus) will be equal to the energy difference between the two atomic levels involved in transition.

If a gap in the K shell is filled with an electron from the L shell, then the energy of the emitted characteristic X-ray is:

$$E_{X\text{-}ray} = h\nu = E_K - E_L \qquad (1.1)$$

where E_K and E_L are electron binding energies on these levels, h is the Planck constant and ν is the frequency of the X-ray electromagnetic radiation.

As the atomic energy levels are specific for a particular element, particular X-ray energies will belong to a certain atomic species only, hence the name characteristic X-rays. If an electron is ejected from a K shell, so-called K X-ray series are emitted, also known as Lyman series: K_a: $L \rightarrow K$, K_p: $M \rightarrow K$, etc. These are hard

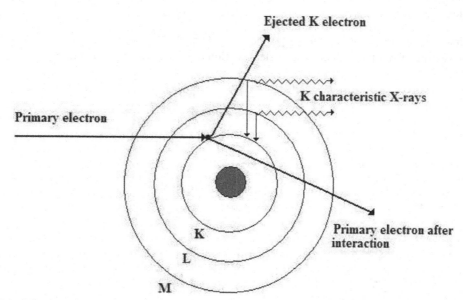

Figure 1.2. Principle of production of characteristic radiation.

X-rays. If an electron is ejected from L shell, L X-ray series are emitted, also known as Balmer series: L_a: $M \to L$, L_p: $N \to L$, etc. These are softer X-rays. The wavelength of the emitted X-ray is related to the atomic number Z of the element and quantum numbers (energy level numbers), n, m, of the orbits involved in transition as (also known as Moseley's law):

$$\frac{1}{\lambda} = R(Z - 0.3)^2 \left(\frac{1}{n^2} - \frac{1}{m^2} \right) \qquad (1.2)$$

where R is the Rydberg constant.

L, M and higher orbital levels correspond to electron angular momentum larger than 0, (i.e. the orbital quantum number is non-zero) and therefore are degenerated (i.e. have non-zero magnetic quantum number). In the electromagnetic field these levels will split to sublevels belonging to individual magnetic numbers. Consequently, X-rays of slightly different energies ($K_{\alpha 1}$, $K_{\alpha 2}$) will be emitted, depending on which sublevel the transition has occurred from. This phenomenon is known as fine structure of characteristic X-rays.

1.2.2 Bremsstrahlung radiation

When a high voltage is applied between electrodes, streams of electrons (cathode rays) are accelerated from the cathode to the anode, producing X-rays as they strike the anode. Two different processes give rise to radiation of X-ray frequency:

- In the first process radiation is emitted when incoming electrons from the cathode knock electrons from inner orbits (near the anode nuclei) out of orbit. They are then replaced by electrons from outer orbits resulting in the emission of characteristic X-rays.

- In the second process radiation is emitted by the high-speed electrons themselves as they are slowed or even stopped as a result of attractive Coulomb interaction when passing near the positively charged nuclei of the anode material. This radiation is called *bremsstrahlung* (German for braking radiation), see Figure 1.3.

The strong attractive force of the positively charged nucleus will deflect the electron from its initial trajectory and decelerate it. The lost energy will be carried away by a photon of energy hν. Only very rarely will the electron loose all of its energy in one interaction with the nucleus. In this case all of its energy will be converted into electromagnetic radiation, $E_e = E_{X\text{-}ray} = h\nu$.

The spectrum of bremsstrahlung radiation is continuous, as an electron may lose any amount of energy during its interaction with the nucleus. The end-point (maximum energy of the radiated X-rays, or in other words the smallest wavelength of emitted X-rays, λ_{min}), will correspond to the initial kinetic energy of the electron:

$$h\nu = \frac{hc}{\lambda_{min}} = E_e \qquad (1.3)$$

The energy distribution of bremsstrahlung radiation is given by Kramer's relation:

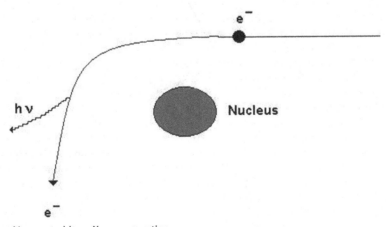

Figure 1.3. Principle of bremsstrahlung X-ray generation.

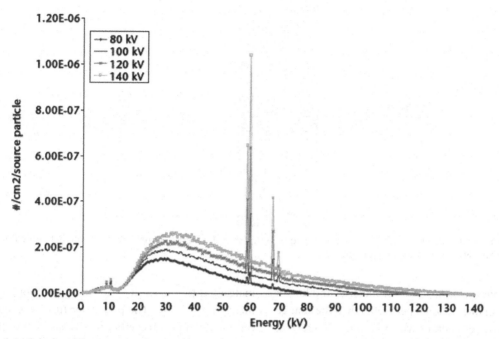

Figure 1.4. Calculated X-ray spectra from an X-ray tube, using tungsten target and Al filter. (Reprinted from Taleei and Shahriari 2009. Copyright (2009), with permission from Elsevier)

$$I_E \sim KZ(E_e - E) \qquad (1.4)$$

where I_E is the intensity (number) of X-rays with energy E, E_e is the electron kinetic energy and K is a constant. As the intensity is proportional to the atomic number, Z, bremsstrahlung X-rays will be produced more intensively in heavier elements (e.g. tungsten).

As the two X-ray generation processes cannot be separated, the distribution of X-ray frequencies emitted from any particular anode material will consist of a continuous range of frequencies emitted in the bremsstrahlung process, with superimposed sharp peaks corresponding to discrete X-ray frequencies. The sharp peaks constitute the X-ray line spectrum for the particular anode material and will vary for different materials (see Figure 1.4).

The graph above shows filtrated X-ray spectra with the X-rays of small energies missing, even though, according to the equation 1.4, they are produced with large intensity. Very soft X-rays are not useful for the majority of applications and are therefore for practical purposes filtered out of the spectrum (absorbed by a layer of material placed in its path). Filtering is the

removal of soft radiation by absorption in the glass envelope of the tube, metal filter (Al, Cu) and the anode material itself.

The bremsstrahlung rate of electron energy loss is inversely proportional to the square of electron mass (strictly speaking, other charged particles will also undergo bremsstrahlung processes, but due to their large mass, the effect is negligible) and to the square of the atomic number of the nucleus involved in the interaction:

$$\frac{dE}{dt} \propto \frac{Z^2 e^2}{m_e^2} \qquad (1.5)$$

1.3 INTERACTION OF X-RAYS WITH MATTER

1.3.1 Linear attenuation coefficient

When a beam of X-ray photons passes through an object, interactions occur that result in a decrease of the number of transmitted (non-interacting) photons. There are a number of factors that can affect the attenuation of X-ray photons. Consider a thin slab of uniform material with thickness dx as shown in Figure 1.5.

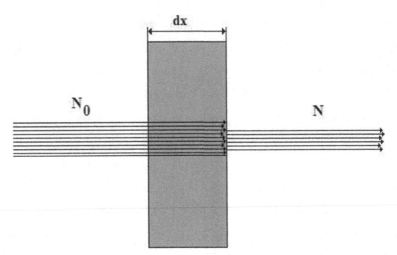

Figure 1.5. Schematic showing X-ray photons impinging on a thin slab of material. Some X-rays will interact inside the material and only N photons will pass through.

If N X-rays are *incident* on the material and have a probability of interaction μ per meter, then the change in the number of photons which have not interacted, dN is given by:

$$dN = -\mu N dx \qquad (1.6)$$

After integration over the total thickness of the slab, T, we get:

$$N = N_0 e^{-\mu T} \qquad (1.7)$$

where N is the number of photons which emerge from the slab without having interacted in the slab and N_0 is the number of photons entering the slab. The coefficient μ is referred to as the **linear attenuation coefficient** and the equation (1.7) is known as the Lambert-Beers law. It is common to define the units of the linear attenuation coefficient as cm^{-1}, assuming the thickness of the material is measured in cm. The thickness of a given material that will attenuate (reduce) the intensity of the incident beam to half is called half value layer (HVL). It is related to the linear attenuation coefficient, μ, as:

$$HVL = \frac{0.693}{\mu} \qquad (1.8)$$

The linear attenuation coefficient changes in proportion to the density, ρ, of the material. As a result, it would be beneficial to have a factor that does not change. An example of this is water, where the linear attenuation in vapour is much lower than for ice. Nor-

malising μ to the density will be constant for any element ($\mu/\rho = const$). The parameter (μ/ρ) is known as the mass attenuation coefficient and has units of cm^2/g.

The mass attenuation coefficient, μ/ρ, gives the probability that the X-rays will interact with the material through various processes. In short, it can be considered a function of the following parameters:

$$\mu/\rho = \tau + \sigma_R + \sigma + \kappa_p + \kappa_t \qquad (1.9)$$

The individual symbols represent different types of possible interactions. τ is the attenuation coefficient due to the photoelectric effect, σ_R is the Rayleigh scatter attenuation coefficient, σ is the Compton scatter effect coefficient, κ_p corresponds to pair-production, and κ_t is the triplet attenuation coefficient.

It is likely that the attenuating material does not consist of a pure element. Furthermore, most available attenuation tables provide the mass attenuation coefficients for elements or simple compounds only. In order to account for the elemental composition of the attenuator, one must take the percentage average by weight of each element:

$$(\mu/\rho)_{compound} = \sum w_i (\mu/\rho)_i \qquad (1.10)$$

where w_i is the weight fraction of element i, and $(\mu/\rho)_i$ is the mass attenuation coefficient of element i. Apart from linear and mass attenuation coefficients, corresponding atomic and electronic attenuation coefficients are used as well (Johns and Cunningham 1983).

The attenuation coefficient, μ, is a macroscopic coefficient that is related to the atomic microscopic cross-section (~ size of the atom), σ, as follows:

$$\mu = n\sigma \qquad (1.11)$$

where n is the number of target atoms per unit area.

1.3.2 Photoelectric effect

Photoelectric (PE) absorption was first observed with ultraviolet light on metal surfaces. A correct explanation of the photo-effect was given by Einstein; triggering the onset of quantum physics. Photoelectron absorption is the dominant process for X-ray absorption for photon energies up to about 300–500 keV (depending on the Z of the absorber) and is more dominant for elements of higher atomic numbers. The process of photoelectric absorption is shown in Figure 1.6. The incident photon is *completely absorbed* by an atom of the absorbing material, and one of the atomic electrons (from inner K, L, M, N shells) is ejected. This ejected electron is called a photoelectron. As the electron is bound to the atom, for its energy and momentum to be conserved, the kinetic energy, E_e, of the ejected photoelectron is given by Einstein equation:

$$E_e = h\nu - B_e \qquad (1.12)$$

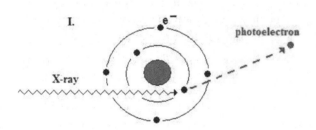

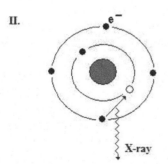

Figure 1.6. Schematics explaining the principle of the photoelectric effect.

where B_e is the binding energy of the atomic electron. The vacancy left in the atomic structure by the ejected electron is filled by one of the electrons from a higher shell. This transition is consequently accompanied by an emission of a characteristic X-ray.

Photoelectric process is characterised by the linear (and corresponding mass) absorption coefficient, τ. The interaction is dependent on the atomic number Z of the absorbing material and on the energy of the impinging X-rays. An approximate expression for the absorption probability is:

$$\tau/\rho \propto \frac{Z^n}{E^3} \qquad (1.13)$$

where n is normally between 3 (for high Z) and 3.8 (for low Z) depending on the elemental composition of the absorber. This dependence on the atomic number explains the choice of high Z materials such as lead for shielding purposes.

The reason for the above relation can be explained by quantum mechanics. The electron carries away more momentum than the photon of zero mass brought in. To conserve momentum, the electron must be bound to a nucleus. The recoil back to the nucleus is carried by the electric field which is much stronger for K shell than L shell, i.e.: the recoil increases greatly with photon energy.

Figure 1.7 shows the mass photoelectric effect coefficients for water and lead (on a log-log scale). The ratio of the atomic numbers for water (Z=7.2) and lead (Z= 82) is about 11. The ratio of corresponding mass photoelectric coefficients though (above B_K), is ~1000; i.e. for the same X-ray energy, lead will attenuate 1000 times more than water (in the photoelectric range of energies only).

Absorption edges, the distinct peaks on the lead cross-section function, correspond to binding energies of electrons on K, L, ... levels; i.e. if the photon energy matches the binding energy, B, of an electron, the probability of photoelectric absorption increases markedly (for example, the electron binding energy on the K atomic level, B_K, for lead is ~88 keV and for water ~0.6 keV).

Since photoelectric absorption occurs at low X-ray energies, the photoelectrons will have low kinetic energies as well and radiation losses due to bremsstrahlung

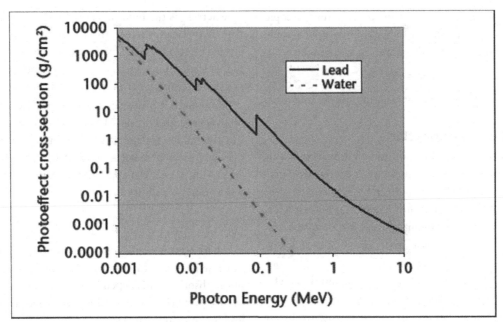

Figure 1.7. Mass photoelectric effect cross-sections, τ/ρ, for water and lead displayed as a function of interacting photon energy.

will be minimal. Correspondingly, in the case of photoelectric effect, the energy transferred from X-rays is equal to the energy absorbed in the medium. The angular distribution of emitted photoelectrons depends on the X-ray energy. For UV and soft X-rays, electrons follow a dipole pattern as expected for electromagnetic waves (i.e. they will be ejected in a direction perpendicular to the photon trajectory). For harder X-rays, the electrons are projected into the forward hemisphere. Photoelectric effect can be associated with the emission of Auger electrons instead of emitting a characteristic photon. This process mostly occurs for lighter elements. As photoelectric interaction is so highly dependent on the Z of the absorbing material, 'photoeffect' X-ray energies are suitable for imaging as good differentiation (contrast) of structures with different Z is possible.

1.3.3 Compton scattering

Compton Scattering (CS), also known as incoherent scattering, occurs when the incident X-ray photon ejects an outer shell electron from an atom and a photon of lower energy (greater wavelength) is scattered from the atom (see Figure 1.8). Compton Scattering was discovered by Compton in 1922 and the

relativistic quantum theory was developed by Klein and Nishina by 1928. Relativistic energy and momentum are conserved in this process. Compton Scattering is important for materials with a low atomic number. At energies of 300 keV–10 MeV the absorption of radiation is mainly due to the Compton effect.

The change in the wavelengths between the incoming, λ, and the scattered, λ' photons is given by:

$$\lambda' - \lambda = \frac{h}{m_0 c}(1 - \cos\theta) \qquad (1.14)$$

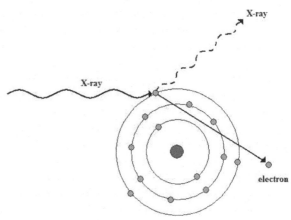

Figure 1.8. Schematics explaining the principle of Compton scattering.

where θ is the scattering angle between the trajectory of the scattered photon and trajectory of the incident photon, h is the Planck constant and m_0 the electron mass. Correspondingly, the energy of the scattered photon, E'_γ is:

$$E'_\gamma = \frac{E_\gamma}{1 + (E_\gamma/m_0c^2)(1 - \cos\theta)} \qquad (1.15)$$

where E_γ is the energy of the incident photon. The kinetic energy of the electron is equal to the difference in energies between the incident and scattered photons (binding energy of an outer e⁻ is small compared to kinetic energy and can be neglected):

$$E_e = E_\gamma - E'_\gamma = \frac{E_\gamma^2(1 - \cos\theta)}{m_0c^2 + E_\gamma(1 - \cos\theta)} \qquad (1.16)$$

It can be seen that, since all photon scattering angles are possible, the electron energy ranges from zero for 0° scattering angle to $2E'_\gamma/(m_0c^2 + 2E_\gamma)$ for 180° scattering angle (backscattering), and that the photon never loses the whole of its energy in one collision. The scattered photon will then propagate through the attenuator/medium and may undergo an interaction with other atomic electrons or may escape out of the medium completely. This process, where the scattered photon escapes, is very important for X-ray spectroscopy. If the full energy of the incident photon is not absorbed in the X-ray detector, then there is a continuous background in the energy spectrum, known as the Compton continuum. This continuum extends up to an energy corresponding to the maximum energy transfer, where there is a sharp cut-off point, known as the Compton edge (see Figure 1.9). Compton scattering is the most probable process for photons in the intermediate energy range (few hundred keV to a few MeV) and the probability

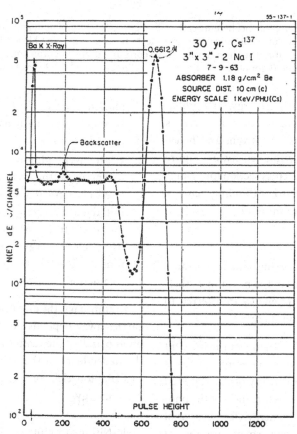

Figure 1.9. Typical spectrum measured with an X-ray detector. Photoabsorption peak and Compton continuum are clearly distinguishable. (Courtesy Royal Adelaide Hospital)

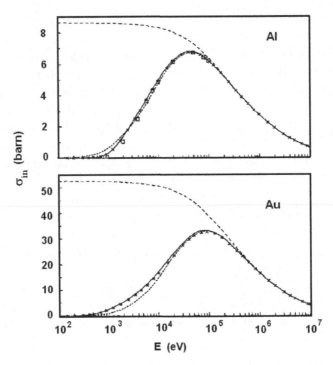

Figure 1.10. Cross sections for Compton incoherent scattering of photons by aluminium and gold atoms as functions of the photon energy E. The long dashed curve corresponds to cross-section calculation using Klein-Nishina formula, assuming photon interaction with a free electron. The short dashed curve corresponds to Compton cross-section taking the binding energy of the electron into account. (Reprinted from Brusa *et al.* 1996. Copyright (1996), with permission from Elsevier)

decreases rapidly with increasing energy. The probability is also dependent on the number of electrons available for the photon to scatter from, and hence increases with increasing electron density, N_e. Figure 1.10 shows the total electronic cross section for Compton process for free electron (binding energy neglected) and for gold and aluminium.

Energy transfer

In incoherent Compton scattering energy is transferred by photons to electrons of the medium as their kinetic energy. The amount of energy transferred to an electron depends on photon energy:

1. **Low energy photons.** If the energy of the incident photon is 88 keV, the maximum electron energy is 23 keV and the minimum energy of the scattered photon is 65 keV. This means that most of the photons are scattered with an energy close to that of the incident X-ray and only small amounts of energy are transferred to electrons. Numerous interactions are required to transfer all of the

photon energy. As $E_\gamma \to 0$, Compton scattering becomes indistinguishable from Thomson (elastic) scattering.

2. **High energy photons.** The photon loses most of its energy to the scattered electron and the scattered photon carries away only a fraction of the initial energy: e.g. if E_γ is 5.1 MeV, then the maximum electron energy is 4.87 MeV and only 0.23 MeV of energy is scattered. High energy photons can lose most of their kinetic energy in one interaction.

In summary, the amount of energy that an electron carries away depends on the energy of the incident photon and on the scattering angle. Figure 1.11 shows the dependence of the maximum energy transferred to Compton electrons as a function of the incident X-ray energy.

Klein-Nishina formula

At higher energies, the relative intensity of scattered radiation as predicted by classical Thompson scatter-

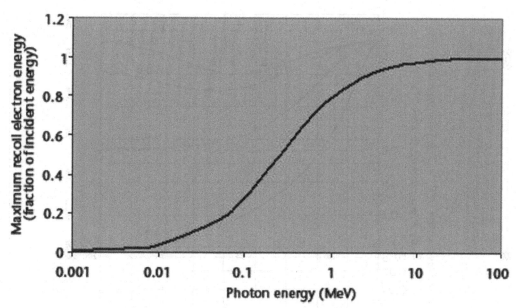

Figure 1.11. The dependence of the maximum energy transferred to electrons in Compton scattering interaction as a function of the incident X-ray energy.

ing is incorrect. The formula corrected for scattered radiation that incorporates the Breit-Dirac recoil factor, R, also known as radiation pressure, and that takes into account relativistic quantum mechanics and the interaction of the spin and magnetic moment of the electron with electromagnetic radiation is known as the Klein-Nishina formula. In simpler terms, the Klein-Nishina formula gives a more exact angular distribution of Compton scattered X-rays. The formula is derived for an interaction of a photon with a free electron; the electron binding energies are neglected. The Klein-Nishina formula allows the calculation of a differential cross-section per unit solid angle, $d\Omega$, due to Compton scattering; i.e. it gives the probability for a scattered X-ray to be emitted in a certain direction relative to the incident photon. It is equal to the classical Thomson cross-section, $\frac{d\sigma_0}{d\Omega}$, (valid for photons of zero energy) multiplied by a factor F_{KN}:

$$\frac{d\sigma}{d\Omega} = \frac{d\sigma_0}{d\Omega}F_{KN} = \frac{r_o^2}{2}(1 + \cos^2\theta)F_{KN} \quad (1.17)$$

where

$$F_{KN} = \left\{\frac{1}{1 + \alpha(1 - \cos\theta)}\right\}^2 \times$$
$$\left\{1 + \frac{\alpha^2(1 - \cos\theta)^2}{[1 + \alpha(1 - \cos\theta)](1 + \cos^2\theta)}\right\} \quad (1.18)$$

and

$$\alpha = \frac{E_\gamma}{m_o c^2}$$

and $r_o = 2.81794 \times 10^{-15}$ m, is the classical electron radius.

The F_{KN} factor is always smaller then 1 and decreases with increasing photon energy. Figure 1.12 (Johns and Cunningham 1983) shows the dependence of the differential Compton cross-section per unit solid angle as a function of photon scattering angle for different photon energies. The higher the energy of the incident photon, the bigger the deviation from the classical cross-section. The total cross-section can be achieved by integration of the above coefficient over the solid angle. The total cross-section expresses the overall probability that the photon will interact with a free electron in the Compton process (regardless of where they are scattered into). At low photon energies, the binding energy of the electron has to be taken into account for correct probability calculation.

Dependence of Compton effect on the atomic number

The attenuation coefficient for the Compton effect is equal to the product of the electron cross-section, σ_e, and the number of electrons per unit volume. As there

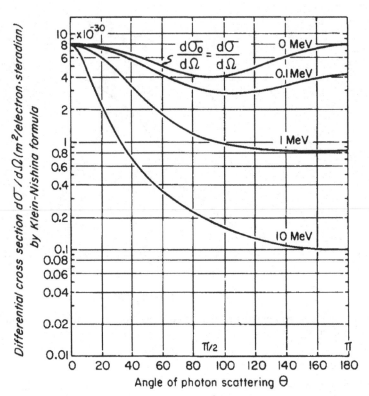

Figure 1.12. The dependence of the differential Compton cross-section per unit solid angle as a function of photon scattering angle for different photon energies. (Reprinted from Johns and Cunningham 1983. Copyright (1983), with permission from Charles C Thomas, Publisher, Ltd.)

are Z electrons per each atom of atomic number Z, the Compton mass attenuation coefficient per unit mass therefore will be:

$$\frac{\sigma}{\rho} = \frac{N}{A}(Z\sigma_e) \propto \frac{Z}{A} \approx 1 \rightarrow 1/2\,(Hydrogen \rightarrow Uranium)$$

where N is the number of atoms per unit volume. As a result of Z/A dependence, the mass attenuation coefficient changes very little across the periodic table. If the radiation beam energy is in the range where Compton scatter dominates, the attenuation is approximately the same for equal masses of material per unit area.

Angular distribution of emitted electrons

Most of the photons are scattered around the 90 degree angle, as the differential cross-section per unit scattering angle, $\frac{d\sigma}{d\theta}$, is proportional to $\sim \sin(\theta)$. The electron scattering angle, ϕ, is then related to the photon scattering angle (from the conservation of momentum) as:

$$\cos\phi = (1 + \alpha)\tan(\theta/2) \qquad (1.19)$$

Consequently, electrons can never be scattered backwards ($\phi \leq 90°$), but will be ejected in a forward direction with maximum around 45 degrees.

In summary, Compton scattering is an inelastic process between a photon and a quasi-free electron (neglecting binding energy). It is almost independent of Z of the material but depends on the total mass (density) of the absorber. The probability of interaction decreases with increasing photon energy. The fraction of incident energy absorbed and transferred also increases with photon energy. It is a dominant interaction process for photon energies between 200 keV and 10 MeV.

1.3.4 Pair production

The third important X-ray interaction process is pair production, illustrated in Figure 1.13. If the incident photon energy is greater than 1.022 MeV (twice the electron rest mass), then in the presence of an atomic nucleus: an electron/positron pair can be generated. Any residual energy is distributed between the electron and positron as kinetic energy. Once the positron

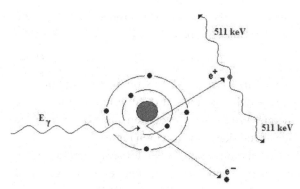

Figure 1.13. Schematics of the physical principle of the pair production process.

slows down to thermal energies through interactions with the absorbing medium, it will annihilate with one the atomic electrons producing two photons of 511 keV energies.

The process of pair production only becomes important at high X-ray energies (from 2 to 10 MeV). Pair production can be expressed by an equation which represents the conservation of total energy (or mass-energy):

$$h\nu = 2(m_0 c^2) + E_{e^-} + E_{e^+} \qquad (1.20)$$

Here, $m_0 c^2 = 0.511$ MeV represents the rest energy of an electron, which is equal to that of the positron, (the factor of 2 in the equation). E_{e^-} and E_{e^+} represent kinetic energies of the electron and positron immediately after their formation. For photon energies below $2m_0 c^2$, the process cannot occur; in other words, 1.02 MeV is the threshold energy for pair production. As the momentum must be conserved, the process cannot take place in empty space; something must absorb the momentum, p, ($p = h/\lambda = h\nu/c$) of the initial photon. In the threshold situation, the particles have to be created at rest and cannot themselves absorb any momentum. The photon momentum can be absorbed by an atomic nucleus, which has mass thousands of times larger than that of an electron or positron and can therefore absorb momentum without absorbing much energy. As a result the energy-conservation equation 1.20 remains approximately valid. More precisely, the threshold energy for production of an electron-positron pair in the Coulomb field of a nucleus of mass, M_{nuc}, is:

$$E_\gamma \geq 2m_0 c^2 + \frac{2m_0^2 c^2}{M_{nuc}} \qquad (1.21)$$

Since for all practical cases $M_{nuc} \gg m_0$, the equation can be reduced to: $E_\gamma \geq 2m_0 c$.

The probability of pair production can be calculated from quantum mechanics. Heitler (Heitler 1944) showed that pair production is nearly the inverse process of bremsstrahlung process. The corresponding differential cross-section, $\frac{d\kappa}{d\Omega}$, for formation of e^+ and e^- pair is:

$$\frac{d\kappa}{d\Omega} = \frac{Z^2}{137}\frac{r_0}{2\pi}m_0^2 c^4 F_{pair} \qquad (1.22)$$

where F_{pair} is a function of momentum and energy of an electron-positron pair.

The total cross-section also depends on screening of the nucleus by electrons (as the process happens in the electromagnetic field of the nucleus), another expression for atomic cross-section that accounts for screening and that you may find in literature (Evans 1995) is:

$$\kappa_p = 4\alpha r_0^2 Z^2 \left(\frac{7}{9}\ln\frac{183}{Z^{1/3}} - \frac{1}{54} \right) [cm^2/atom] \qquad (1.23)$$

$$\alpha = \frac{h\nu}{m_0 c^2}$$

This expression is valid for energies ~10 MeV and above, where full screening is achieved.

The cross-section per atom increases as a function of ~Z^2, the cross-section per mass increases with Z. The coefficients also increase rapidly with the energy of the photon. At high energies the photons can be more easily stopped (compared to lower energies) due to pair production process, i.e. the high energy beam is less penetrating. This behaviour is in contrast to photoelectric absorption and Compton scattering, for which the cross-sections decrease with energy. Pair production cross-section as a function of X-ray energy is shown for various materials in the figure below note the dependence on Z of the attenuator.

Angular distribution of produced particles: the electron–positron pairs tend to come out in a forward cone with angle $\theta \sim 1/\gamma$ where:

$$\gamma = \frac{E_\gamma}{m_0 c^2}$$

The kinetic energies of e^+ and e^- are not necessarily equal. The distribution is a function of E_γ and Z, but usually results in a fairly flat behaviour (i.e. energy can be shared with equal probability for all possible

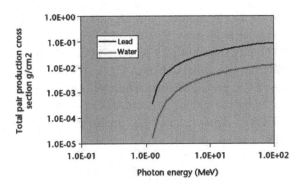

Figure 1.14. Total mass pair production cross-sections for water and lead as a function of photon energy.

combinations) that is reducing rapidly to zero for the extreme case when one particle only receives all photon energy (minus 1.022 MeV).

An inverse process to pair production is called pair annihilation, in which a particle and its antiparticle collide and annihilate each other, with the total energy of the two particles appearing as electromagnetic radiation. In the case of an electron and positron, the energy balance can be written as:

$$2(m_0 c^2) + E_{e^-} + E_{e^+} = 2h\nu \qquad (1.24)$$

The first term represents the rest energy of both particles, the second and third terms are the kinetic energies just before the collision, and the term on the right-hand side of the equation represents the creating of two photons, each having a the same frequency ν and energy $h\nu$. If the kinetic energies of the two initial particles were both small ($\ll m_0 c^2$), the total momentum before the collision would be close to zero. From conservation of momentum, the momentum after annihilation must also be approximately zero, and the only way that this can happen is for the two photons to be emitted in opposite directions such that their individual momenta cancel.

Triplet production is also possible. It occurs when the recoil particle is an electron, which gets a lot of recoil energy compared to the nucleus. The energy

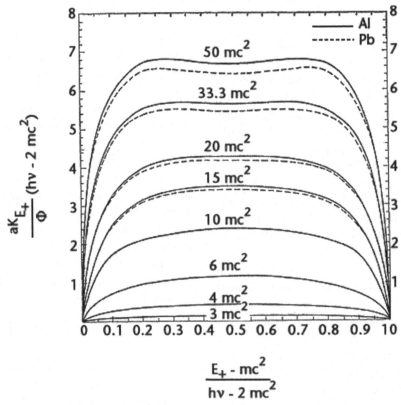

Figure 1.15. Energy Distribution of electron-positron pairs. The graph gives the probability that a particle with energy between $E+dE$ will be generated in the pair production process in Al and Pb. (Reprinted figure with permission from: Meaker Davisson C and Evans RD (1952) Gamma ray absorption coefficients. Figure 24, *Rev. Mod. Phys.* **24**: 79–107. Copyright (1952) by the American Physical Society)

threshold is $4\,m_0c^2$ and its probability is much smaller compared to pair production.

1.3.5   Coherent scattering

Coherent scattering is a process in which no energy is converted into kinetic energy (e.g. of electrons) but all energy is scattered. It is an elastic process, which involves an atom as a whole. It occurs for low X-ray energies, for which corresponding wavelengths are much larger than the size of an atom. Since the mass of the atom is very large compared to massless photon, the scattered photon loses no energy; it only changes its direction:

$$E_{scat} = E_{incident} \qquad (1.25)$$

This is an important process for interactions of blue light in the sky, ultraviolet and soft X-rays. It forms the basis of X-ray diffraction, where coherence involves many atoms in a crystal lattice.

Using classical physics, it can be explained by a 'radio-transmitter' effect, where the photon represents an oscillating electromagnetic (EM) field. It sets atomic electrons into vibration (oscillation). As a result of oscillating charge, an electromagnetic field will be generated (emitted). Electrons will oscillate with the same frequency, ν_{e^-}, as that of the interacting photon, ν_γ:

$$\nu_{e^-} = \nu_\gamma \qquad (1.26)$$

The generated electromagnetic field will have the same frequency as electron vibrations:

$$\nu_\gamma = \nu_{e^-} = \nu_{\gamma'} \Rightarrow E_\gamma = E_{\gamma'}$$

As all the electrons radiate in phase, the cross-section, σ, for coherent scattering will be proportional to Z^2 of the interacting atoms. For very soft X-ray energies, the cross-section is constant but it decreases rapidly at higher X-ray energies. The cross-section becomes negligible for $E_\gamma >100$ keV. The scattered X-rays are mostly emitted in the forward direction.

A special case of coherent scattering involving a single free electron is known as **Thomson** (classical) scattering. The cross-section for Thomson scattering can be derived from classical electrodynamics, with the incoming photon representing an electromagnetic field with two perpendicular electric and magnetic components ($\vec{E} \perp \vec{B}$). The scattered photon is also described by an electromagnetic vector. The ratio of electric field intensities for both incoming and scattered photons represents the probability that the radiation will be scattered and can be therefore written as cross-section:

$$\frac{d\sigma}{d\Omega} = \frac{1}{2}r_0^2(1 + \cos^2\theta) \qquad (1.27)$$

where θ is the scattering angle. This expression is called the Thomson coefficient or classical scattering coefficient. It correctly gives the amount of energy scattered (or a fractional number of photons scattered) into a unit solid angle for zero energy photons. After integration over all scattering angles, the total cross-section for Thomson scattering is obtained:

$$\sigma_{TS} = \frac{8}{3}\pi r_0^2 \qquad (1.28)$$

Scattering involving all atomic electrons (and therefore more realistic) is known as Rayleigh scattering. It is a cooperative phenomenon involving all electrons in the atom. Incident photons are scattered by bound electrons without any ionisation or excitation of the atom. The process occurs for low photon energies and large Z (where electron binding energies will not allow photoelectric absorption). The cross-section for Rayleigh scattering (RS) is equal to that of Thomson scattering multiplied by the square of the atomic form factor $F(x,Z)$:

$$\sigma_{RS} = \sigma_{TS}[F(x,Z)]^2 \qquad (1.29)$$

or:

$$\frac{d\sigma_{RS}}{d\theta} = \frac{r_0^2}{2}(1 + \cos^2\theta)[F(x,Z)]^2 2\pi\sin\theta \quad (1.30)$$

where Z is the atomic number and the parameter x is related to the scattering angle, θ, and photon wavelength, λ, as:

$$x = \frac{(\sin\frac{\theta}{2})}{\lambda} \qquad (1.31)$$

The atomic form factor is proportional to Z of the attenuator for small scattering angles and close to zero for large scattering angles. As a result, Rayleigh scattering will be most probable in the forward direction.

1.3.6   Total interaction coefficient

The total attenuation coefficient (cross-section) is the sum of probabilities corresponding to individual interactions: $\mu/\rho = \tau + \sigma_R + \sigma + \kappa_p + \kappa_t$. The dependence of the total attenuation coefficient as a function

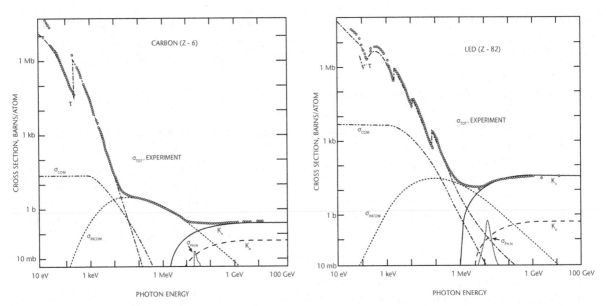

Figure 1.16. Total interaction cross-section, σ_{TOT} in carbon and lead over the photon energy range 10 eV to 100 GeV. Contributions of atomic photoeffect, τ, coherent scattering, σ_{COH}, incoherent (Compton) scattering, σ_{INCOH}, nuclear-field pair production, κ_n, electron-field pair production (triplet), κ_e, and nuclear photoabsorption, $\sigma_{PH.N}$, are displayed as well. (Reproduced from Hubbell *et al.* 1977. Copyright (1977), with permission from IOP Publishing Ltd.)

of energy is shown in the Figure 1.16. The individual interaction coefficients are displayed as well.

Total photon cross sections in carbon and lead, as a function of energy, show the contributions of different processes: atomic photo-effect (photon absorption and electron ejection), coherent scattering (Rayleigh scattering; atom is neither ionised nor excited), incoherent scattering (Compton scattering off an outer shell electron), pair production, photonuclear absorption (nuclear absorption, usually followed by emission of a neutron or other particle). The graph shows clearly the dominance of the photo-electric effect for low energy X-rays, above 100 keV, Compton scattering is the dominant process. At energies above 10 MeV, the cross-section (attenuation coefficient) increases as a function of energy due to pair production. The differences in cross-sections between interactions in carbon and lead reflect the Z^n dependence of photo-effect and pair production.

1.4 INTERACTIONS OF HEAVY CHARGED PARTICLES WITH MATTER

In the previous sections the interactions of photons with matter have been discussed. During their interactions X-rays produce energetic electrons, i.e.

charged particles with mass. Their interactions with the material are different to that of photons and this will be the topic of the current section. X-rays, γ-rays, but also neutrons and neutrinos all have zero net electric charge. In order to detect them they must interact with matter and produce an energetic charged particle. In the case of gamma and X-rays, a photo-electron or Compton electrons are mostly produced. In the case of neutrons, a proton is given kinetic energy in a billiard ball collision (elastic collision).

Charged particles can be divided into two groups:

1) **electrons** and **positrons** (originated e.g. from radioactive decay, Auger electrons, internal conversion electrons, delta electrons, Compton electrons, …)

2) **heavy charged particles** such as the alpha particle, fission fragments, protons, deuterons, tritons, and μ and π mesons.

Charged particles interact with matter primarily through the Coulomb interaction. Differences in the energy deposition trails between the two types of charged particles are due to their mass differences. The maximum energy that can be transferred from a charged particle to an electron in a single collision is about 1/500 of the particle energy per nucleon for heavy particles. Due to this small energy transfer and the fact that at any time the particle is interacting with more than one electron, the heavy particles appear to continuously slow down, gradually losing their kinetic energy along an unaltered linear path (this is also known as **Continuous Slowing Down Approximation**). However, occasional nuclear collision will cause large energy loss and deflection in the trajectory.

On the other hand, energy losses and changes in directions can be quite large for electrons after the collisions with other electrons and the electron trajectory can be altered significantly during stopping in matter (also known as **Energy and Range Straggling**).

Charged particles lose their energy primarily through two types of interactions: collisional (electronic and nuclear) and radiative:

1. **Collisional** interactions.
   (a) **Electronic**
   These are inelastic collisions with atomic electrons, resulting in excitation or ionisation. These processes ultimately end with the heating of the absorber (through atomic and molecular vibrations) unless the ions and electrons can be separated using an electric field as is done in radiation detectors.
   (b) **Nuclear**
   These are elastic collisions with atomic nuclei; e.g. Rutherford backscattering, nuclear reactions (rare), Moth and Moller scatterings.

2. **Radiative** interactions.
   These are type of inelastic collisions where a charged particle undergoes an electromagnetic (Coulomb) interaction with positively charged nuclei. As a result, the particle's momentum is altered and electromagnetic radiation is emitted (a photon). However, this interaction is important for electrons only. Radiative energy loss is mostly due to bremsstrahlung as the probability of nuclear excitation is quite low.

1.4.1 Bragg peak

Charged particles interacting in the absorbing material will leave along their trajectory a trail of ionised matter, electrons and ions (this is actually the basic principle of detecting particles in radiation detectors). Ionised tracks created in a cloud chamber by two protons and some electrons are shown in Figure 1.17. It

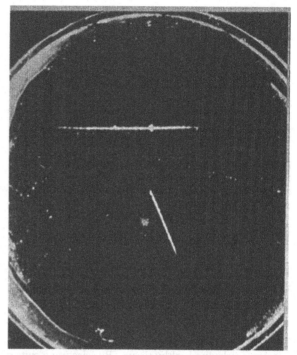

Figure 1.17. Ionisation tracks generated by two protons and two electrons in a cloud chamber. (Reprinted figure from: Blackett PMS and Occhialini GPS: *Proceedings of the Royal Society of London. Series A, Containing Papers of a Mathematical and Physical Character*, Photograph 14, Vol. 139, No. 839. Copyright (1933), with permission from the Royal Society)

can be seen that heavier protons have generated a much more densely ionised tracks compared to those resulting from passage of lighter electrons.

If the absorber is thick enough, particles will interact with the material until they lose all their energy; i.e. are completely stopped. The average energy loss per ion pair is independent of particle type and is specific for a given absorber (~33.85 eV in air, 3.3 eV in Ge). The plot of specific energy loss (which can be related to specific ionisation or number of generated ion pairs) along the track of a charged particle is called a Bragg curve. A typical Bragg curve is displayed in Figure 1.18 for a proton beam with initial energy of 200 MeV. As the energy falls, the specific energy loss increases according to the so-called Bethe-Bloch formula, describing the energy loss of charged particles. This increase in energy loss as the particle is slowing down results in the high number of ions formed near the end of particle's track. This is represented by a sharp peak (Bragg peak) on the Bragg curve. Up to 80% of particle energy is lost within the

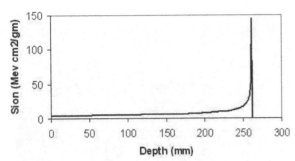

Figure 1.18. Energy loss of 200 MeV protons in water as a function of depth, calculated using SRIM Monte Carlo code (Ziegler 1999). The energy loss, characterised by stopping power S_{ion}, increases as the protons come to a complete stop giving rise to a Bragg peak at the end of the proton trajectory.

Bragg peak. Deposition of energy by charged particles is thus very different to that of X-rays, which deposit energy exponentially. This is of important consequence for radiotherapy, as the use of charged particles makes it possible to deposit most of the energy at depth while sparing overlaying healthy tissues. By selecting a suitable initial particle beam energy, the depth of Bragg peak (energy deposition) can be controlled appropriately to match the tumour position in tissue.

In the case of electrons, the energy deposition increases only slowly with penetration depth due to the fact that their direction is changed drastically (energy and range straggling). In fact, multiple changes in direction completely smear out the Bragg peak which is then not observed for electrons stopping in matter. For electrons, the energy deposition is spread in the transverse direction as it progresses forward in the initial direction, until approximately the last 1 keV which is deposited in the forward direction.

1.4.2   Linear energy transfer (LET)

Linear energy transfer is a quantity describing the quality of radiation. It is the rate at which an ionising particle deposits energy along its track (the energy decrement lost in the infinitesimal material thickness, dx). If only the energy transferred to the material in the vicinity of the particle track is considered, and secondary electrons with energies larger than a certain value, Δ, are excluded (ICRU 60), then the restricted linear energy transfer, LET, is:

$$LET = \frac{dE}{dx} \, [\text{keV/}\mu\text{m}] \qquad (1.32)$$

Since electrons of high energy have a large range, the energy limit, Δ, effectively excludes electrons that travel far from the primary particle. Heavy particles (protons, α–particles, neutrons (indirect ionisation only by neutrons)) have high LET and produce dense highly ionised tracks. The higher the LET, the shorter the range into the material the particle can penetrate. LET is also referred to as *specific energy loss* and is inversely proportional to the square of particle velocity (reason for the Bragg peak):

$$\frac{dE}{dx} \sim \frac{1}{v^2} \qquad (1.33)$$

As the kinetic energy of a particle is proportional to the product of mass and square of the velocity, for the same kinetic energy electrons will have much larger velocity compared to heavier counterparts, that means that LET for electrons will be much smaller. For 1 MeV of kinetic energy, electron LET is about 0.2 keV/µm compared to 200 keV/µm for an α-particle.

The LET is related to biological damage of cells. The degree of severity and permanence of biological transformation are directly linked to the local rate of energy deposition and ionisation along the particle track. The higher the LET, the higher the so-called radiation quality factor in determining dose equivalent (see Section 1.6).

1.4.3   Stopping power (mass stopping power)

Mass stopping power is the energy loss per unit thickness of the attenuator, measured in g/cm² (thickness):

$$S_{ion} = \frac{1}{\rho}\left(\frac{dE}{dx}\right)\left[\frac{\text{MeV}}{\text{g/cm}^2}\right] \qquad (1.34)$$

where the subscript 'ion' means the energy loss by ionisation (i.e. collisions of the particle with the electrons of the absorber) only, and ρ is the density of the absorbing material. This is to differentiate this mechanism of energy loss from energy loss due to radiative processes. S_{ion} can be calculated from semi-empirical Bethe-Bloch formula, but is often determined experimentally.

Similarly, radiative stopping power, S_{rad}, can be defined for radiation losses (i.e. bremsstrahlung for electrons). The fraction of energy lost to electromagnetic radiation is inversely proportional to the charged particle's mass. Bremsstrahlung probability will therefore be extremely low for heavy charged particles (compared to electrons). Even at 100 MeV, for example, heavy particles dissipate most of their energy through the collisional processes. The total stopping power is the sum of stopping powers corresponding to two interaction processes:

$$S_{TOT} = S_{ion} + S_{rad} \qquad (1.35)$$

Both radiative and ionisation losses are proportional to the density of electrons of the absorber ($\sim ZN_e$), which is largest for hydrogen. As mentioned above, the stopping of charged particles in matter is by collisional and radiative processes occurring in frequencies given by their individual interaction cross sections (or probabilities). The experimentally observed stopping is a statistical average of the two processes occurring as the particle slows down.

Energy straggling

Energy loss in a material is a statistical or stochastic process. Therefore, a spread of energies always results when an initially monoenergetic beam of particles enters the absorber. This produces an energy distribution curve of a finite width known as the energy straggling peak. The straggling peak is approximately Gaussian shaped, with a width that increases with the ratio Z/A; i.e. for lower atomic numbers (where the Z/A ratio is higher) the widths are larger. This is due to the fact that shielding (screening) of inner electrons is less in the lower Z elements, i.e. there is more stopping effect per electron. In general, particles lose energy in collisions involving small energy transfers/losses only. However, there are also less frequent large energy losses due to nuclear interactions. For electrons, there is also more straggling due to radiative energy loss than due to collision energy loss due to $1/h\nu$ dependence of the radiative cross-section. Also the energy loss on average is greater for radiative losses.

1.4.4   Range of charged particles

The range of a charged particle is the finite distance beyond which there will be no particles in the material; i.e. all particles will come to stop at this and before this distance into the attenuator. This is quite different from photons, which are only exponentially attenuated and can never be stopped completely.

Range can be derived from the stopping power formula:

$$R = \int_E^0 dx = \int_E^0 \frac{dE}{dE} dx = - \int_0^E \frac{1}{dE/dx} dE = \int_0^E \frac{dE}{S_{tot}(E)}$$
$$(1.36)$$

Figure 1.19 of ionisation tracks produced by monoenergetic alpha particles from ^{212}Po in a cloud chamber shows that most of the particles will reach the same distance into the absorber. This is however not the case for electrons, that change direction rapidly. The mean range is the range at which the number of electrons detected is one-half the original value. The rule of thumb for the range of electrons in water is:

$$R(cm) = \frac{E(MeV)}{2} \qquad (1.37)$$

and for other materials:

$$R(cm) = \frac{E(MeV)}{2} \frac{1}{\rho} \qquad (1.38)$$

If the range of electrons is expressed in terms of g/cm^2, it is independent of the absorbing material and only depends upon energy.

Factors affecting range R:

Energy: Range is approximately linear with energy since the Bethe-Bloch equation for stopping power is inversely proportional to E.

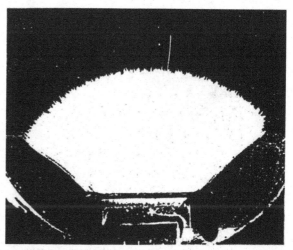

Figure 1.19. Ionisation tracks produced by monoenergetic alpha particles from ^{212}Po decay in a cloud chamber. Most of the particles will reach the same distance into the absorber; i.e. have the same range. (Courtesy University of Adelaide)

Mass: for the same kinetic energy, the electron is much faster than the alpha due to its smaller mass, and therefore the electron has less time to spend near orbital electrons. This reduces the effect of Coulomb interactions (hence stopping power) and increases range.

Charge: the larger the charge, the larger the stopping power and therefore shorter the range. Range is inversely proportional to the square of the charge of the particle.

For example, a tritium particle with $Z=1$ will have ¼ of the stopping power of a He-3 particle with $Z=2$.

Density: The stopping power increases with increasing density. The range is inversely proportional to the density of the absorbing medium.

Range straggling

The same statistical factors that cause energy straggling result in straggling of range: the total path of energy loss is different for each initially monoenergetic particle in the beam. For protons or alpha particles, straggling results in variation of only a few percent about the mean range. However, range straggling is significant for electrons. Figure 1.20 displays the result of a Monte Carlo calculation for stopping of 3 MeV

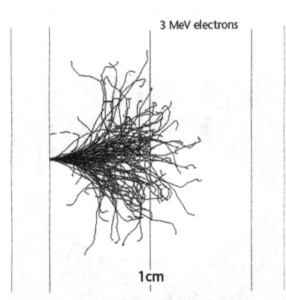

3 MeV electrons

1cm

Figure 1.20. Stopping of 3 MeV electrons in water, displaying the complex trajectories of electrons as a result of collisions with electrons of the absorber. (Calculated using EGS4 Monte Carlo code, courtesy the Royal Adelaide Hospital)

electrons in water (100 histories) demonstrating the range straggling. Notice that the range is ~1.5 cm.

1.4.5   Bethe-Bloch formula

The ionisational energy losses of heavy charged particles in matter are described by the semi empirical Bethe-Bloch formula (Bethe and Ashkin 1953). In derivation of the formula, a particle of charge ze and mass, M, is considered to be moving with velocity, v, passing near a light electron of charge, e, and mass, m_0, at an impact parameter, b (see Figure 1.21).

The transverse momentum transfer to the light electron due to Coulomb interaction between the charged particle and an electron, written in terms of the angle, θ, is:

$$\Delta p = \frac{zke^2}{bv} \int_{-\pi/2}^{\pi/2} (\cos\theta)\, d\theta = \frac{2zr_0 m_0 c^2}{bv} \quad (1.39)$$

where ke^2 was substituted by $r_0 m_0 c^2$ from the expression for the classical radius of the electron. The impact parameter, b, represents the shortest distance between the particle trajectory and the electron.

Consequently, the energy transferred to the electron (or energy lost by the particle) is:

$$\Delta E(b) = \frac{\Delta p^2}{2m_0} = \frac{z^2 r_0^2 m_0 c^4}{b^2} \frac{M}{E} \quad (1.40)$$

It should be noted that the energy loss is inversely proportional to the particle's energy, E, and inversely

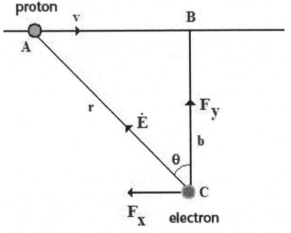

Figure 1.21. Schematic geometry for Bethe-Bloch formula derivation. Heavy particle (proton) of velocity, v, interacts with an atomic electron at point C.

proportional to the square of the impact parameter; i.e close collisions will involve large energy transfers compared to more distant interactions. In order to determine the total energy transferred from the particle to all electrons it has interacted with, the number of interacting electrons must be determined first. The number of electrons present in a cylindrical sheath between b and db surrounding the particle's trajectory of length Δx is given by:

$$\Delta n = (N_e 2\pi\rho b)\, db\Delta x \qquad (1.41)$$

where N_e is the electron density per gram of the material of density, ρ. As the number of electrons is proportional to b, the number of collisions resulting in large energy transfers will be small as fewer electrons are involved (and vice versa). The total energy loss, dE, over the distance, dx, is then obtained by the product of energy loss per interaction multiplied by the number of electrons and integrated over all impact parameters:

$$\frac{dE}{dx} = 4\pi N_e \rho \frac{z^2 r_0^2 m_0 c^2}{\beta^2} \ln\frac{b_{max}}{b_{min}} \qquad (1.42)$$

where β was used to substitute v/c in the above expression. The quantity dE/dx is the linear energy transfer introduced in Section 1.4.2. There will be some limit to the maximum possible impact parameter, as at some distance the energy transfer will not be large enough to overcome the electron binding energy. Linear energy transfer expressed in terms of mass thickness, known as the stopping power is then (relativistic corrections are included):

$$S_{ion} = \frac{1}{\rho}\left(\frac{dE}{dx}\right)$$
$$= 4\pi r_0^2 N_e \frac{z^2 m_0 c^2}{\beta^2}\left(\ln\frac{2m_0 c^2 \beta^2}{I(1-\beta^2)} - \beta^2 - \sum_i \frac{c_i}{Z}\right)$$

$$(1.42)$$

where I is **the mean excitation potential** for all Z atomic electrons. It is an element dependent parameter, which is determined experimentally and can be estimated roughly as: $I = 16(Z)^{0.9}$ (for $Z > 2$). I for copper is 322 eV and for muscle 75.9 eV (Johns and Cunningham 1983). General behaviour of the ionisational stopping power as a function of kinetic energy relative to the rest mass of the particle is displayed in Figure

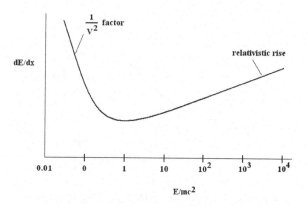

Figure 1.22. General dependence of the ionisational stopping power, S_{ion}, of a heavy charged particle moving in a medium, as a function of the particle energy.

1.22. Note the rapid increase in stopping power at energies below the rest mass and a slower rising at high energies due to relativistic effects.

1.4.6 Rutherford scattering

The most common form of particle nuclear stopping (i.e. energy loss) is due to elastic scattering (collision) of the particle from the nuclei of the absorber known as Rutherford scattering. There is no particle or nuclear excitation involved and the process is essentially governed by conservation of momentum and energy. The cross section can be derived both from classical mechanics as well as quantum mechanics. In the classical approach it is assumed that the only acting force is the Coulomb force and both the particle and the nucleus represent point like charges. It is also assumed that no recoil energy is given to the nucleus (due to mass difference). If the particle has charge ze and that of nucleus is Ze, then the Coulomb potential between them is:

$$V(r) = \frac{Zze^2}{4\pi\varepsilon_0 r} \qquad (1.43)$$

The schematic of the scattering event is shown in Figure 1.23. The impact parameter, b, is the distance between the particle and the nucleus, if undeflected by the interaction (original trajectory). The cross-section for Rutherford scattering, $d\sigma$, in terms of number of particles scattered into the solid angle, $d\Omega$, is:

$$\frac{d\sigma}{d\Omega} \approx \frac{1}{\sin^4(\theta/2)} \qquad (1.44)$$

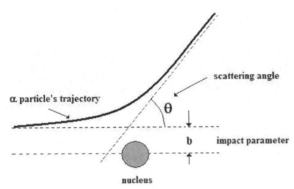

Figure 1.23. Schematic geometry for Rutherford scattering cross-section derivation.

Derivation of the Rutheford scattering can be found in many textbooks (e.g. Williams 1991). Rutherford scattering is used as an important analytical method in solid state physics, used to identify material composition or crystal orientation of samples.

1.4.7   Interactions of electrons with matter

The basic interactions of electrons with matter are: ionisation, excitation, bremsstrahlung, nuclear and electron scattering, Cerenkov radiation, molecular bond breakage and heat (at low energies). Interactions of electrons are thus very similar to those of heavy particles. There are though 3 major differences and all of them are related to the small mass of electron:

1. Relativistic effects
    These are important even at low energies (β (v/c) → 1 for E_{kin} of 100 keV)
2. Energy and range straggling
    Energy losses and changes in directions can be quite large after the collisions with other electrons.
3. Radiative losses
    Energy losses due to bremsstrahlung radiation process are significant.

In clinical radiotherapy, for both photon and electron beams, it is electrons that deposit energy and give rise to absorbed dose. In order to calculate/determine the dose distribution in the medium, the energy loss rate (or the rate of ionisation) and electron trajectories must be known. These can be calculated by knowing the differential interaction cross-sections, σ, that give the probability that an electron incident on a unit

volume of an absorber will interact with a particle in the medium and will lose a certain amount of its kinetic energy, dE, and be scattered through a certain angle, θ.

Collisions with electrons of the medium resulting in ionisation and excitation are the most likely process of electron stopping in matter. The energy loss is described by the Bethe Bloch formula derived in the previous section. However, the Bethe-Bloch formula for electrons must take into account the following: 1) the small electron mass; 2) the electron is identical to the particles with which it interacts, thus giving the possibility to the 'exchange of identity', i.e. the incoming particle has a probability of becoming the atomic electron with the atomic electron becoming the outgoing particle; 3) relativistic effects. In electron-electron interactions, as the both particles are identical, the question arises as to which one of the scattered particles after the interaction is the original electron. By convention, the electron that comes out of the collision with larger energy is considered to be the original incident electron. Consequently, the maximum energy transferred in the interaction is half of the kinetic energy, E_{kin}, of the primary electron.

It is important to note that S_{ion} is proportional to Z/A and therefore to the number of electrons per unit mass. Water has a high effective Z/A (0.56) due to its hydrogen content; as a result, the collisional (ionisation) mass stopping power, S_{ion}, will be relatively high as well. For body tissues, Z/A is relatively constant and therefore they will have similar S_{ion} values. High atomic number absorbers have lower S_{ion} values compared to lower Z materials, because Z/A is less (0.40 for Pb).

Positrons behave nearly the same as electrons as they lose their energy in the absorber. Additionally, the 511 keV annihilation photons will be emitted from the point where a positron has reached thermal equilibrium with the absorber (i.e. the point where it stopped).

Radiative energy loss

As mentioned in Section 1.2, when the high energy electrons pass near positively charged nuclei, they are slowed down as a result of the attractive Coulomb interaction. The energy lost in the deceleration is emitted in the form of a bremsstrahlung photon with energy $h\nu$. The cross section for radiative energy loss for electrons is (Koch and Motz 1959):

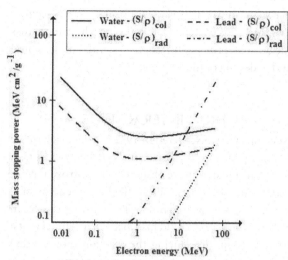

Figure 1.24. Dependence of electron collisional and radiative mass stopping powers in water and lead as a function of electron energy.

$$\frac{d\sigma}{dh\nu} = \frac{1}{137}\left(\frac{e^2}{m_0 c^2}\right)BZ^2\left(\frac{E + m_0 c^2}{E}\right)\frac{1}{h\nu} \quad (1.45)$$

where B is a function of Z and E. Mass radiative stopping power, S_{rad}, of an electron in a material of atomic number Z and mass number A, with N_A atoms per unit volume then is:

$$S_{rad} = \frac{4N_A Z^2}{A}r_0^2 E\frac{183}{Z^{1/3}} \quad (1.46)$$

The importance of radiative stopping power compared to ionisational stopping power increases with electron energy, E. The ratio of S_{rad} to S_{ion} is approximately:

$$\frac{S_{rad}}{S_{ion}} = \frac{E(Z + 1.2)}{800} \quad (1.47)$$

Critical energy, E_c, is the energy for which the two stopping powers are equal. For water E_c is 93 MeV and for lead 6.9 MeV. The value is lower for lead due to the dependence of the radiative stopping power on Z.

Figure 1.24 shows the dependence of collisional (ionisational) and radiative electron stopping powers in water and lead. Radiative losses are present in lead even for electron energies below 1 MeV; at about 7 MeV radiative losses are more significant than collisional.

Figure 1.25 shows the results of Monte Carlo calculations of 12 MeV electrons stopping in water and lead (horizontal scale is 1 cm between two vertical lines). Note that bremsstrahlung production is more significant for lead.

Bremsstrahlung yield

Bremsstrahlung yield is a physical quantity describing the fraction of electron energy lost in radiative (bremsstrahlung) processes. It is a useful quantity and is tabulated for different media (e.g. bone, muscle,

12 MeV electrons in water

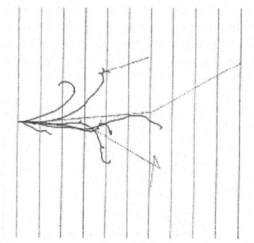

12 MeV electrons in lead

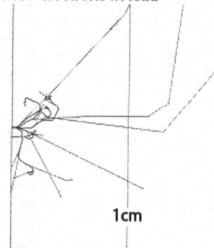

1cm

Figure 1.25. Monte Carlo calculated electron trajectories of 12 MeV electrons stopping in water and lead (horizontal scale is 1 cm between two vertical lines). Bremsstrahlung production is more significant for lead. (Courtesy Royal Adelaide Hospital)

water, lead) for a quick estimate of losses due to radiation processes. It is given by:

$$B = \frac{1}{E_0} \int_0^{E_0} \frac{S_{rad}(E)}{S_{tot}(E)} dE$$

$$= \frac{1}{E_0} \int_0^{E_0} \frac{S_{rad}(E)}{S_{rad}(E) + S_{coll}(E)} dE \qquad (1.48)$$

where the expression under the integral is the total energy radiated by the electron

Scattering power

In the case of electrons, due to significant range straggling, a third stopping power is defined, known as the mass scattering power, giving the probability for scattering through an angle θ, after traversing material (density ρ) of thickness dx. It is approximately proportional to Z of the absorber and decreases with the square of the energy (at relativistic energies):

$$\frac{d\overline{\theta}^2}{\rho dx} \approx \frac{Z}{E^2} \qquad (1.49)$$

When passing through the absorber, the electrons will undergo many small angle scatterings, a process known as multiple scattering. In radiotherapy, it is used to produce electron beams of useful size for treatment purposes, as accelerators produce pencil beams of electrons only, with dimensions of a few mm. This size is not clinically useful. Consequently, thin metal foils (usually a combination of Sn, Au or Pb foil) are used to broaden the electron beam to sizes of up to 30×30 cm^2. A dual foil system is usually applied. The first foil is designed to widen the beam by multiple scattering, while the second foil is designed to make the beam intensity uniform in cross-section. The thickness of the second foil is not the same across the beam to provide the required amount of flattening and widening of the beam.

1.5 NEUTRON INTERACTIONS

Neutrons were discovered in 1932 by Chadwick in the following reaction ^{11}B(α, n)^{14}N (Chadwick 1932). Neutron collisions were observed with nitrogen in air, using a cloud chamber. From the known energy of α particles and measured range of unknown particles in a cloud chamber, it could have been determined that a particle is emitted during the reaction (not a γ-ray) with mass of $\oplus$1.008 atomic mass units (amu).

Neutrons have no charge; therefore they can easily penetrate into the area of nuclear forces and interact with the nucleus (scattering or absorption). There is no Coulomb Barrier present, so neutrons can interact with nuclei at very low kinetic energies: $E_n \approx 0$ eV. If a compound nucleus is formed during reaction (i.e. absorption of the neutron by a nucleus), the energy brought in by the neutron is:

$$E = E_n + E_{BE} \qquad (1.50)$$

Where binding energy, E_{BE}, is around 6–8 MeV; i.e. the compound nucleus will be in a highly excited state and will decay. Nuclear interactions with neutrons are very energy dependent and at small energies wave properties of neutrons become important.

As properties and interactions of neutrons vary with their kinetic energy it is customary to classify neutrons according to their energies (see Table 1.2), which can range from hundreds of MeV down to

Table 1.2. Energy classification of neutrons.

Name	Energy (eV)	Wavelength (m)
Ultracold neutrons	10^{-6}	2.8×10^{-8}
Cold	10^{-6}–0.005	2.8×10^{-8}–4×10^{-10}
Thermal	0.005–0.5	4×10^{-10}–4×10^{-11}
Resonant	0.5–1000	4×10^{-11}–9×10^{-13}
Medium	1000–5×10^5	9×10^{-13}–4×10^{-14}
Fast	5×10^5–20×10^6	4×10^{-14}–6.4×10^{-14}
High Energy	Above 20×10^6	Less than 6.4×10^{-14}

fractions of an eV. Neutrons are uncharged particles and do not interact with atomic electrons in the matter through which they traverse, but they do interact with the nuclei of these atoms. The nuclear force, which leads to these interactions, is very short ranged, meaning that the neutrons have to pass close to a nucleus for an interaction to take place.

1.5.1   Nuclear reactions with neutrons

The most common nuclear reactions involving neutrons, n, with nuclei, A, are:

1. *A(n, n)A* reaction: a neutron is emitted after the reaction; this is a neutron scattering event:
   a) If after the scattering event, the nucleus is left in its ground state, the scattering was **elastic**
   b) If after the scattering event, the nucleus is left in its excited state, the scattering was **inelastic**

   In both cases of scattering, the target nucleus involved will be recoiled. Inelastic scattering occurs for higher neutron energies >10 MeV. Examples of inelastic scattering include: *(n ,n'), (n, n, γ), (n, 2n)* and the nucleus is left in the excited state.

2. *(n,γ)* reaction. This is a very common radiative capture reaction (i.e. neutron is captured and a gamma ray, γ, is emitted), which occurs for slow neutrons for almost any element. It is utilised in a technique known as neutron activation analysis. If a nucleus captures a high-energy neutron with a big probability, the reaction is called resonant capture.

3. *(n,p), (n,d)* reactions (capture of neutron followed by emission of a proton or a deuteron). These reactions happen more often for fast neutrons and lighter nuclei, for example:
   $n + {}^{35}Cl \rightarrow {}^{35}S + p + 0.65\ MeV$.

4. *(n, α)* reaction. This is an important reaction used for neutron detection. It has high cross-section for thermal neutrons interacting with Boron:
   $n + {}^{10}B \rightarrow {}^{3}H + \alpha + 2.791\ MeV$.

5. *(n, fission)* reaction occurs for fast and slow neutrons on heavy elements.

For fast neutrons, scatter is more probable than capture. Fast neutrons are first slowed down in inelastic collisions and then captured. The cross section for neutron reactions at very low energies follows a

'**1/v law**', meaning that the probability of nuclear reactions (and neutron capture) increases with lower neutron energy (and therefore velocity, v). This also explains why it is important to slow down (moderate) neutrons in nuclear reactors. The slower the neutron, the larger the probability that it will be captured and cause fission.

Neutrons ionise the environment they traverse indirectly. Elastic scattering of the neutrons with the nuclei of the material and with the hydrogen (and other lighter elements) nuclei in particular, will result in proton recoil. Protons will then move through the absorber causing ionisation. Because the mass of protons and the other recoiling nuclei is much greater than that of electrons, they generate a much denser ionisation path. Once neutrons have been slowed down by collisions to thermal energy, 0.025 eV, they are readily captured by some of the reactions described above. A very common reaction is the *(n, γ)* reaction. The gamma photons produced in this reaction will cause indirect ionisation.

1.6   RADIOACTIVITY
1.6.1   Basic definitions

Atoms consist of a cloud of electrons (e-) and a nucleus containing protons (p) and neutrons (n). The collective name for protons and neutrons is nucleons. Properties of these elementary particles are summarised in Table 1.3.

Neutrons are 2.5 electron masses heavier than protons, which makes them unstable. The mean life, τ, of a neutron is 898 s and it decays as:

$$n \rightarrow p + e^- + \tilde{v}_e + 0.782\ MeV \quad (1.51)$$
$$\text{(released as kinetic energy)}$$

where $\tilde{v}_e$ is an antineutrino.

Nuclear force

Protons and neutrons are bound in the nucleus by the nuclear force, which is a strong interaction (there are four types of interaction in nature: strong, electromagnetic, weak and gravitational). The nuclear force is the strongest force in nature (gravity is ~10^{39} times weaker) and has the following properties:

• it is short ranged (less than 2 fermi (fm); i.e. 10^{-15} m)

Table 1.3. Basic properties of elementary particles constituting atoms.

Particle	Mass (kg)	Mass (MeV)	Charge (C)	Spin	Stability
e-	9.1×10^{-31}	0.511	1.6×10^{-19}	$\pm 1/2\ \hbar$	stable
p	1.6726×10^{-27}	938.27	1.6×10^{-19}	$\pm 1/2\ \hbar$	stable
n	1.6749×10^{-27}	939.57	0	$\pm 1/2\ \hbar$	unstable

Where:
1 eV (electron volt) = 1.6×10^{-19} J
$h = 1.054 \times 10^{-34}$ Js (Planck's constant)
Mass (kg) can be related to energy using Einstein's formula. Strictly speaking kg ~MeV/c^2, but in the universal unit system $c^2 = 1$, therefore mass is expressed in MeV only.

- saturates (i.e. does not increase indefinitely at shorter distances or with increasing number of nucleons
- there is a repulsive force present at distances of less than 0.5 fm)
- is charge independent (exists between p-p, n-p and n-n pairs).

Nuclear potential reflects forces that act upon nucleons as a function of distance between the nucleons (protons and neutrons). The correct nuclear potential should contain:

- potential well (strong interaction) that will keep the nucleons together inside the nucleus and that acts only between 0.5–2 fm.
- high barrier at very short distances (repulsive force) for distances of less than 0.5 fm
- Coulomb interaction barrier – reflecting Coulomb repulsive interaction between protons for distances larger than 2 fm (when the protons are outside the range of strong interaction).

System of elements

In 1868 Mendeleev developed the Periodic Table of Elements, reflecting the atomic nature of the elements. The notation used for describing elements is:

$$_Z^A Chemical\ Symbol_N$$

Where:

Z is the atomic number of the element and is equal to the number of protons in the nucleus and number of electrons in the atomic shell. It is also the sequential number of the element in the periodic table.

A is the mass number of the nucleus and is equal to the total number of nucleons (sum of protons and neutrons) in the nucleus.

N is the neutron number and is equal to A − Z.

Isotopes: $_8^{15}O, _8^{16}O, _8^{17}O$, are nuclei with the same Z (the same element) but different A (same chemical properties but different nuclear characteristics)

Isotones: $_8^{15}O, _7^{14}N$, are nuclei with same neutron number N

Isobars: $_8^{15}O, _7^{15}N$, are nuclei with same A (same mass) but different Z (different elements)

Mirror nuclei: $_6^4He, _4^6Be$, are pair of isobaric nuclei, where one nucleus has the same number of protons as the number of neutrons in the other nucleus: $Z_1 = N_2$ and $N_1 = Z_2$

More than 110 elements are currently known, of which 90 are naturally occurring from $_1^1H$ to $_{92}U$. Up to lead (Pb), all naturally occurring elements are stable and lie on or near a line in the N-Z plane (line of stability). Initially the number of protons matches quite closely the number of neutrons in the nucleus (up to mass A=35). Then the number of neutrons, N, increases faster than number of protons, Z, to compensate the Coulomb repulsion between protons: $N \sim 1.5Z$. After mass A >209 there are no naturally occurring stable nuclei.

Stable nuclei will always remain the same (will not change); unless interfered with (e.g. bombarded by energetic particles).

Unstable nuclei will at some time after their formation undergo a transformation and will change into another element. This transformation is called nuclear decay. As particles and gamma rays are emitted (in most cases) during nuclear decay, the unstable nuclei are also called **radioactive nuclei** and the associated processes (nuclear decay and particle emission) are known as radioactivity.

Nuclei of the Earth's elements were formed in nucleosynthesis process during an explosion of super-nova some 4.5 billion years ago. Until now only about 300 isotopes have remained on Earth. Most of these isotopes are stable or practically stable (have half lives comparable to the age of the Earth). Many of the isotopes originally formed were unstable and have since all decayed. If any of these isotopes are needed today (e.g. for a medical application) they have to be made artificially (man-made).

The known types of nuclear decays are: α, β^-, β^+, γ (associated with internal conversion and Auger electrons), electron capture and fission.

Conditions for nuclear decay

Energy, E, of the decay must be positive: $E > 0$; i.e. Energy must be released during the process and the final system (the new nucleus) is in a state of lower energy. Conservation laws are observed (mostly!) in nuclear decay, including energy, charge, baryon number, parity, spin and others. Various selection rules defining the probabilities of individual decay modes apply.

Alpha decay

Alpha decay is a strong interaction (nuclear) process. The following transformation of the parent nucleus with atomic number Z and mass A occurs:

$$(Z, A) \rightarrow (Z - 2, A - 4) + \alpha \quad (1.52)$$

Parent nucleus   Daughter nucleus   Emitted particle

where an α particle is a nucleus of ^4_2He. The energy released in α decay satisfies the following condition:

$$E_\alpha = M(Z,A) - M(Z - 2, A - 4) - M(2,4) > 0 \quad (1.53)$$

This is fulfilled only when $M_P - M_D > M_\alpha$; i.e. the mass difference between parent and daughter nuclei is larger than the mass of an α particle. The energy of the decay, E_α, is released as kinetic energy of the α particle (energy of the recoiling nucleus can be neglected). The energy spectra of emitted α particles are discrete, as they correspond to nuclear transitions between discrete nuclear energy levels. It occurs for heavier nuclei only (Z >82, A~144–206).

Beta decay

Beta decay is a weak interaction process. Two processes are possible:

a) $\beta^-: n \rightarrow p + e^- + \tilde{v}_e \quad (1.54)$

in β^- decay, a neutron transforms into a proton with the emission of an electron and an antineutrino. The corresponding isotope transformation is:

$$(Z,A) \rightarrow (Z + 1, A) + e^- + \tilde{v}_e \quad (1.55)$$

And the corresponding energy condition for β^- decay is:

$$E_{\beta^-} = M(Z,A) - M(Z + 1, A) > 0 \quad (1.56)$$

b) $\beta^+: p \rightarrow n + e^+ + v_e \quad (1.57)$

in β^+ decay, a proton transforms into a neutron with the emission of a positron and a neutrino. The corresponding isotope transformation is:

$$(Z,A) \rightarrow (Z - 1, A) + e^+ + v_e \quad (1.58$$

and the corresponding energy condition for β^+ decay is:

$$Q_{\beta^+} = M(Z,A) - M(Z - 1, A) - m_{e^+} - m_e > 0$$

i.e. $M_P - M_D > 2m_e$

$$(1.59)$$

The energy spectra of emitted electrons or positrons are continuous. Beta decay occurs for lighter nuclei and is governed by selection rules explained by quantum mechanics.

Electron capture

Electron capture is a weak interaction process (it is really a form of β decay):

$$e^- + p \rightarrow n + v_e \quad (1.60)$$

In electron capture decay, a proton interacts with an atomic electron (from a lower shell) to transform into a neutron. A neutrino is emitted from the nucleus as a result of the process. The corresponding isotope transformation is:

$$e^- + (Z,A) \rightarrow (Z - 1, A) + v_e \quad (1.61)$$

and the corresponding energy condition for electron capture decay is:

$$E_{EC} = m_e + M(Z,A) - M(Z - 1, A) > 0$$

i.e. $M_P - M_D > 0$

$$(1.62)$$

Consequently, depending on the mass difference, ΔM, between the parent and daughter isotope the following decay scenarios can occur:

i)   If $0 < \Delta M < 2m_e$; Only electron capture is possible
ii)   If $\Delta M > 2m_e$; Both β^+ and electron capture are possible (competing processes)

During the electron capture process, a vacancy will be created in the atomic electron shell. This electron hole will be filled by electrons from higher shells. As a result, X-ray radiation will be emitted during decay by electron capture.

Gamma transition (decay)

Gamma decay is an electromagnetic interaction. It is an accompanying process. After any decay the daughter nucleus is often left in the excited state (not in the ground state). As the excited state is not the state with the lowest energy, a transition to a lower state will occur. Consequently, γ rays will be emitted with the energy equal to the energy difference, ΔE, between the two nuclear levels involved in the transition:

$$E_\gamma = h\nu = \Delta E = E_2 - E_1 \qquad (1.63)$$

Conservation laws and selection rules apply in gamma transition. The energy spectra of emitted γ rays are discrete. It can also be associated with atomic processes: Internal conversion and Auger electrons.

Internal conversion

When a nucleus makes a transition to a lower nuclear level, the excitation energy is not emitted in the form of γ quantum, but it is given to an atomic electron from the shell close to the nucleus. The electron will then have enough energy to leave the atom; i.e. instead of a γ-ray an atomic electron will be emitted. The electron will be subsequently filled with e- from higher shells and X-rays will be emitted.

Auger electrons

When an electron hole is filled, the energy of accompanying X-ray radiation may be given to an electron on the outer atomic shells; i.e. no X-rays will be emitted but the outer shell electron will leave the atom. These electrons are called Auger electrons.

1.6.2   Quantities and units of radioactivity

Activity

Activity represents the number of nuclear disintegrations (decays) per second:

$$A = \frac{dN}{dt}; \text{unit: s}^{-1} = \text{Bq (Becquerel)} \qquad (1.64)$$

where N is the number of radioactive nuclei in the sample. The old unit of activity is Curie (Ci), measured as the number of disintegrations per second of 1 gram of Radium source in equilibrium with daughter products. Its conversion to Becquerel is given by:

$$1Ci = 3.70 \times 10^{10} \text{ Bq} \qquad (1.65)$$

Mean life

If the radioactive sample contains initially N_0 radioactive nuclei then after time, t, there will be N nuclei left in the sample:

$$N(t) = N_0 e^{-\frac{t}{\tau}} \qquad (1.66)$$

where τ is the mean life of the isotope. The value of τ can vary from 10^{-21} s to billions of years.

Half-life

This is the time after which one half of the initial number of nuclei will be decayed. It is related to the mean life of the isotope as:

$$T_{1/2} = \tau \ln 2 \qquad (1.67)$$

Decay probability

The probability that a nucleus will decay is expressed by the constant λ. This is related to the mean life of the nucleus:

$$\lambda = \frac{1}{\tau} \qquad (1.68)$$

Branching ratio

Some isotopes can decay by one decay mode only and some can decay by more modes, e.g. α or β, β^+ or electron captures (competing decay modes). In the latter case, the branching ratio of a particular decay mode can be calculated. This is the probability that expresses the likelihood of one particular form of transition. It is expressed in %:

$$BR = \frac{\sum\limits_n D_1}{\sum\limits_i \sum\limits_n D_i} \qquad (1.69)$$

where

$$\sum_n D_1$$

is the number of decays for 1 decay mode and

$$\sum_i \sum_n D_i$$

is the total number of all decays.

Mean life, half life and decay probability are the properties of a given isotope. All the nuclei of the same isotope will have the same value of $T_{1/2}, \tau, \lambda$. But these values will vary from isotope to isotope.

In medical physics the removal of the isotope from the body is not only given by its physical decay, but also by the removal of the isotope through biological processes (e.g. urine, sweat, breath). Biological processes can be characterised by their own half life. The total effective half life then is:

$$\frac{1}{T_{1/2effective}} = \frac{1}{T_{1/2Physical}} + \frac{1}{T_{1/2Biological}} \quad (1.70)$$

Decay chains; Bateman equations

Consider a situation when a daughter product, B, is not a stable isotope but also decays (into an isotope C). Thus a chain of decay processes takes place:

$$A \xrightarrow{\lambda_1} B \xrightarrow{\lambda_2} C$$

At time t, there will be N_A nuclei of isotope A in the sample:

$$N_A = N_{Ao} e^{-\lambda_1 t} \quad (1.71)$$

Activity of the isotope A is then:

$$A_A = -\frac{dN_A}{dt} = \lambda_1 N_A \quad (1.72)$$

Daughter B is produced with the same rate as the parent A decays. The amount of B isotope in the sample decreases in the sample at the same time due to decay to isotope C:

$$\frac{dN_B}{dt} = \lambda_1 N_A - \lambda_2 N_B = \lambda_1 N_{Ao} e^{-\lambda_1 t} - \lambda_2 N_B$$

(i.e. formation − decay)

$$(1.73)$$

This equation is called Bateman's equation (Leo 1994). The solution of this differential equation is:

$$N_B(t) = \left(\frac{\lambda_1}{\lambda_2 - \lambda_1}\right) N_{Ao} (e^{-\lambda_1 t} - e^{-\lambda_2 t}) \quad (1.74)$$

The activity of daughter B is: $A_B = \lambda_2 N_B$. Using the above solution for N_B, the activity of B then is:

$$A_B = A_A \left(\frac{\lambda_2}{\lambda_2 - \lambda_1}\right)(1 - \exp\{-(\lambda_2 - \lambda_1)\})$$

$$(1.75)$$

Knowing the activity of isotopes A and B, we can calculate when the maximum amount of isotope B is produced in the sample. The isotope B reaches maximum when

$$\frac{dN_B}{dt} = 0.$$

For this condition, the solution of equation 1.73 is: $\lambda_1 N_A = \lambda_2 N_B$. This means that that B maximises when the activity of the daughter isotope B is equal to the activity of the parent isotope A!

For more extensive decay chains, the Bateman's equations are complicated. A simplification can be though used in the case where the parent is a long lived isotope and daughters short lived, i.e. $T_2 \ll T_1$ or $\lambda_2 \gg \lambda_1$; in this case: $\lambda_2 - \lambda_1 \sim \lambda_2$. The equation for activity of isotope B will simplify to:

$$A_B = A_A \frac{\lambda_2}{\lambda_2}(1 - e^{-\lambda_2 t}) \quad (1.76)$$

After a few half lives the exponential expression in the brackets will approximate to 0, and then: $A_B = A_A$. This means that initially, the activity of the daughter isotope will be increasing, and after several half lives the activity of the daughter will be the same as the activity of the parent. After that the daughter will continue decaying with the half life of the parent. This situation is called *secular equilibrium*. Secular equilibrium is observed in natural decay chains. If there is no leaching (for example removal of isotopes by mining) of decay products, all daughters will be in equilibrium with the parent isotope (e.g. uranium), as the parents are long lived (billions of years). The practical consequence of Bateman's equation and secular equilibrium is the timing of 'leaching' of isotope products in isotope generators. These generators are used to artificially make radioactive isotopes that are not available in nature but are required e.g. for medical purposes (nuclear medicine). The daughter isotope will be removed from the sample only when its maximum concentration has been reached. After the removal,

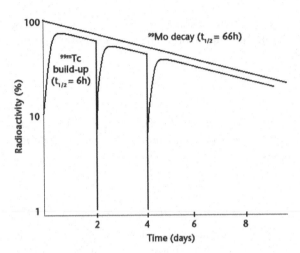

Figure 1.26. The decay growth of ^{99}Mo/^{99}mTC generator. Radioactive decay of parent ^{99}Mo and ^{99}mTC activity build-up prior to elution (leaching).

1.6.3   Sources of radionuclides and ionising radiation

Radioactive isotopes originate from two sources: natural and anthropogenic (man-made). The naturally occurring radioisotopes are cosmogenic or terrestrial. The cosmogenic radioisotopes are produced in nuclear reactions of cosmic rays with elements in the atmosphere and as a result ^{14}C, ^{22}Ne, ^{10}Be are constantly being generated. The terrestrial isotopes are the original primordial long-half-life isotopes generated at the time of the Earth's formation, these include ^{40}K, ^{87}Rb and radioactive series that produce a number of secondary radioisotopes through their decay (e.g. ^{238}U, ^{234}U, ^{230}Th, ^{232}Th, ^{224}Ra, ^{228}Ra, ^{220}Rn, ^{214}Po, ^{210}Po, ^{210}Pb, ^{208}Tl). The man-made isotopes are produced either in nuclear reactors or accelerators.

the sample will be left alone for the activity of the daughter to build up again to a maximum level (see Figure 1.26).

They are primarily used for medical and scientific purposes. Additional sources of man-made radiation products result from nuclear weapon testing and from nuclear power plants.

Both the natural and man-made sources contribute to the radiation exposure of mankind. Radon and medical use of radiations are the biggest contributors. Irradiation by natural sources is further increased by industry, mining in particular, as the radioactive elements are brought up to the surface.

Natural radioactive series are long decay chains (series) of radioisotopes occurring in nature. They are based on α decay ($\Delta Z = -2, \Delta A = -4$) and β⁻ decay ($\Delta Z = +1, \Delta A = 0$). The parent isotopes have extremely long half lives (this is the reason why the series are still present). There are four decay series possible, with three of them still occurring. Table 1.4 summarises the properties of these four natural radioactive series. The activities of all daughters are approximately equal (result of secular equilibrium), however mining and escape of radon gas disturbs the equilibrium.

1.7   RADIATION QUANTITIES AND UNITS

The most commonly used radiation protection quantities are absorbed dose, equivalent dose and effective dose.

Absorbed dose is a very broad nomenclature when dealing with radiation quantities since it expresses the energy absorbed per unit mass without taking into consideration the type of the radiation involved. It was shown in the previous sections that different types of ionising radiation interact differently with matter. Therefore, to illustrate the effectiveness (or the damaging power) of various ionising radiations it is crucial to define a more comprehensive quantity that includes the weighting factor for each radiation type. This new quantity is called *equivalent dose*.

Table 1.4.   Characteristics of the four natural decay series.

Series name	4n	4n + 1	4n + 2	4n +3
Parent	$^{232}_{90}$Th	$^{237}_{93}$Np	$^{238}_{92}$U	$^{235}_{92}$U
Stable daughter (end of decay chain)	$^{208}_{82}$Pb	$^{209}_{83}$Bi	$^{206}_{82}$Pb	$^{207}_{82}$Pb
Parent half-life	1.4×10^{10}y	2.3×10^6y	4.5×10^9y	7.1×10^8y
Occurs at present	Yes	No	Yes	Yes

Furthermore, since various tissues and organs have different structural architectures and radiosensitivities, tissue-related weighting factors have been determined, leading to a more complex element named *effective dose*.

Absorbed dose is defined as the energy absorbed per unit mass, and measures the amount of ionising radiation. In SI the unit for the absorbed dose is Gray (Gy). Therefore, 1 Gy = 1 J/kg. The old unit (non-SI) for absorbed dose is *rad*, where 1 Gy = 100 rad.

If an amount of energy dε is absorbed by a material of mass dm, the absorbed dose D is defined as:

$$D = \frac{d\varepsilon}{dm} \qquad (1.77)$$

In radiobiology and for radiation protection purposes the average dose, D_T, over a given organ or tissue, T, is defined:

$$D_T = \frac{\varepsilon_T}{m_T} \qquad (1.78)$$

where m_T is the organ/tissue mass and ε_T represents the total energy absorbed by the tissue T.

1.7.1 Radiation weighting factors and equivalent dose

Since the biological effects of radiation depend not only on dose but also on the type of ionising radiation, another quantity shall be defined, which incorporates, besides the amount of radiation, also the quality of radiation. The radiation weighting factor, w_R, quantifies the effectiveness (or damaging power) of various types of ionising radiation. The radiation weighting factor has been determined from radiobiological experiments and the values of w_R corresponding to various types of radiation are tabulated in the ICRP100 report. Based on their damaging power, the w_R values for different types of radiation are listed in Table 1.5.

The *equivalent dose*, H_T can now be defined as the absorbed dose, D, averaged over a tissue or organ and weighted for the radiation quality of interest. The SI unit for equivalent dose is Sievert (Sv), and 1 Sv = 1 J/kg, since the weighting factor is non-dimensional.

As a given tissue/organ T may be subject to more than one type of radiation, H_T is generally defined as a sum of weighted average doses, $D_{T,R}$, due to all types of radiation incident on T:

$$H_T = \sum_R w_R D_{T,R} \qquad (1.79)$$

where R is an index illustrating the type of radiation.

To exemplify the equivalence between various types of radiation, one can state that 2 Gy absorbed dose from α-particle interaction produces the same damage as 40 Gy due to X-rays (w_R for α-particles is 20), since in both situations the equivalent dose is 40 Sv.

1.7.2 Tissue weighting factors and effective dose

Dose equivalents for various tissues and organs may differ substantially due to variations in tissue radiosensitivity. Therefore the need arises to define a tissue weighting factor, w_T, to consider tissue response to radiation damage.

Table 1.5. Radiation weighting factors (ICRP report).

Radiation category	Type of radiation	Energy	w_R
Sparsely ionising radiation	Photons	all energies	1
	Electrons	all energies	1
	Muons	all energies	1
Densely ionising radiation	Neutrons	E <10 keV	5
		10 keV to 100 keV	10
		>100 keV to 2 MeV	20
		>2 MeV to 20 MeV	10
		>20 MeV	5
	Protons, other than recoil protons	E >2 MeV	5
	α-particles, heavy nuclei	all energies	20

Table 1.6. Tissue weighting factors (ICRP report).

Organ	Tissue weighting factor (w_T)
Gonads	0.20
Colon, stomach, bone marrow, lung	0.12
Chest, liver, bladder, thyroid, esophagus, adrenals, brain, small intestine, kidney, muscle, pancreas, spleen, thymus, uterus	0.05
Skin, bone surface	0.01

The most complex radiation quantity can now be defined, which considers both the type of radiation and the response of particular tissue to the damaging effect of ionising radiation. This quantity is called *effective dose*, and represents the sum of the weighted equivalent doses in all the tissues and organs within the body, exposed to ionising radiation. Similarly to the equivalent dose, the SI unit for the effective dose is Sievert.

Mathematically, the effective dose H is defined as:

$$H = \sum_T w_T H_T \qquad (1.80)$$

The latest tissue weighting factors are reported in the ICRP 100. Table 1.6 presents a list with the most important ones.

The most important role of the above described quantities is in radiation protection. While epidemiological data on tissue-specific risk after radiation exposure is scarce, data on whole body irradiation and risk is better documented due to retrospective studies on the A-bomb survivors and also on the population exposed after the Chernobyl accident. Therefore, the effective dose is a useful radiobiological tool in assessing the organ-specific risk of developing radiation-induced side effects after radiation exposure, while knowing the risks after total body exposure.

1.8   THE INTERACTION OF RADIATION WITH CELLS

The process of interaction between the ionising radiation and the cell can be broken down into four main stages: the physical, the physicochemical, the chemical and finally – the biological stage.

1. **The physical stage** – lasts only a small fraction of a second ($\sim 10^{-16}$) in which energy is deposited in the cell and causes ionisation. In water the process is the following:

$$H_2O \xrightarrow{\text{radiation}} H_2O^+ + e^-$$

2. **The physicochemical stage** – lasts about 10^{-6} s, in which the ions interact with other water molecules resulting in a number of new products:

$$H_2O^+ \longrightarrow H^+ + OH$$

The negative ion attaches to a neutral water molecule, which then dissociates:

$$H_2O + e^- \longrightarrow H_2O^-$$
$$H_2O^- \longrightarrow H + OH^-$$

Thus the products of the reactions are H^+, OH^-, H and OH. The two former ions (H^+, OH^-) take no part in subsequent reactions. The other two products (H, OH) are called *free radicals* (they have an unpaired electron) and are chemically highly reactive.

Another reaction product is hydrogen peroxide, H_2O_2, which is a strong oxidising agent and is formed by the reaction:

$$OH + OH \longrightarrow H_2O_2$$

3. **The chemical stage** – lasts a few seconds, in which the reaction products interact with the important organic molecules of the cell. The free radicals and oxidising agents may attack the complex molecules which form the chromosomes. They may, for example, attach themselves to a molecule or cause links in long chain molecules to be broken.

The effects of radiation on biological macromolecules (proteins) can be classified in terms of those in:

- aqueous solution
- solid state.

The most important reactions in aqueous solutions are produced by the indirect attack of hydroxyl radicals, hydrogen peroxide and hydrated electrons.

Irradiation in the solid state produces direct cleavage of bonds.

Both direct and indirect effects are significant. When radiation acts indirectly, the radiation effect produced by a given dose is independent of the concentration of the solute (or organism). For direct action the effect increases proportionately with concentration.

Radiation damage has different effects on different types of macromolecules:

- Hydrogen is abstracted from simple sugars by hydroxyl radicals;
- The enzymatic activity (the main biological interest in the radiation chemistry of proteins) decreases exponentially with the radiation dose;
- Nucleic acids suffer major damage including chain scission and cross-linking to the complementary strand or to another nucleic acid molecule.

4. **The biological stage** – the time scale varies from tens of minutes to tens of years (early and late effects). The chemical changes may result in:

- the early death of the cell or the prevention or delay of cell division (results in the depletion of the cell population within organs of the body: deterministic effects);
- a permanent modification which is passed on to daughter cells (can result in cancer of the exposed individual or, if the modification is to a germ cell, the damage may be transmitted to later generations (hereditary effects): stochastic effects).

1.9 DNA – THE TARGET

DNA (deoxyribonucleic acid) is known to be the critical cellular target for the damaging effects of ionising radiation. DNA is the molecule which encodes the genetic material. The DNA molecule comprises a chain built from four building blocks (A, G, C, T) that are assembled to form a double helix and held together by week hydrogen bonds between base pairs of nucleotides.

A nucleotide consists of:

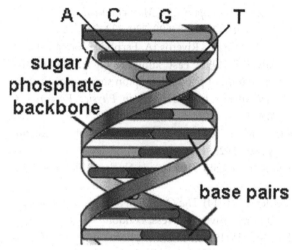

Figure 1.27. Graphic representation of the DNA.

- a pentose sugar (deoxyribose)
- a phosphate group
- a nitrogenous base, which can be a:
  - purine base (adenine (A), guanine (G)
  - pyrimidine base (cytosine (C), thymine (T).

The helix consists of two strands, each with a sugar-phosphate backbone, held together by hydrogen bonds between the bases A-T and C-G (Figure 1.27). The sequence of these bases along the chain forms the genetic code.

Radiation damage to DNA can be initiated by both direct and indirect effects. Direct effects involve the formation of ionic, radical and excited intermediates as a result of the deposition of energy within the DNA. Indirect effects involve the interaction of the DNA with water radiolysis products such as OH radicals, H-atoms or hydrated electrons.

Cellular damage and repair are discussed in more details in Chapter 2 (Section 2.4) and also in Chapter 5 (Section 5.2).

1.10 REFERENCES

Bethe H and Ashkin J (1953) Passage of radiations through matter. In: *Experimental Nuclear Physics*. (Ed. E Segré) p. 253. J. Wiley, New York.

Blackett PMS and Occhialini GPS (1933) Some photographs of the tracks of penetrating radiation source. *Proceedings of the Royal Society of London. Series A,*

Containing Papers of a Mathematical and Physical Character **139** (839): 699, 720, 722, 724, 726.

Brusa D, Stutz G, Riveros JA, Fernbdez-Varea JM and Salvat F (1996) Fast sampling algorithm for the simulation of photon Compton scattering. *Nuclear Instruments and Methods in Physics Research A* **379**: 167–175.

Chadwick J (1932) Possible existence of a neutron. *Nature* **192**: 312.

Evans RD (1955) *The Atomic Nucleus.* McGraw-Hill, New York.

Heitler W (1944) *The Quantum Theory of Radiation.* Oxford University Press, London.

Hubbell JH (1999) Review of photon interaction cross section data in the medical and biological context. *Physics in Medicine and Biology* **44**: R1–R22.

Hubbell JH, Veigele WJ, Briggs EA, Brown RT, Cromer DT and Howerton RJ (1975) Atomic form factors, incoherent scattering functions, and photon scattering cross sections. *Journal of Physical Chemistry* Ref. Data **4**: 471–538; erratum in **6**: 615–616 (1977).

International Commission on Radiation Units and Measurements (ICRU) (1998) 'Fundamental quantities and units for ionizing radiation'. Report 60. International Commission on Radiation Units and Measurements, Bethesda, Maryland, USA.

International Commission on Radiological Protection (2007) 'Human alimentary tract model for radiological protection'. ICRP Publication 100. (Ed. CH Clement). Elsevier.

Johns HE and Cunningham JR (1983) *The Physics of Radiology.* 4th edn. Thomas, Springfield, Illinois.

Koch HW and Motz JW (1959) Bremsstrahlung cross-section formulas and related data. *Reviews of Modern Physics* **31**: 920–955.

Leo RW (1994) *Techniques for Nuclear and Particle Physics Experiments: A How-to Approach.* 2nd edn. Springer Verlag, Germany.

Meaker Davisson C and Evans RD (1952) Gamma ray absorption coefficients. *Reviews of Modern Physics* **24**: 79–107.

Taleei R and Shahriari M (2009) Monte Carlo simulation of X-ray spectra and evaluation of filter effect using MCNP4C and FLUKA code. *Applied Radiation and Isotopes* **67**: 266–271.

Williams WSC (1991) *Nuclear and Particle Physics.* Oxford Science Publications, UK.

Ziegler F (1999) Stopping of energetic light ions in elemental matter. *Journal of Applied Physics/ Applied Physics Reviews* **85**: 1249–1272.

Zolle I (Ed.) (2007) *Technetium-99m Pharmaceuticals: Preparation and Quality Control in Nuclear Medicine.* Springer, Berlin.

2 Elements of radiobiology

Radiation biology is the science that studies the interaction of ionising radiation with the living cell, the damage created to the cell, and also the ability of the cell to repair the radiation-produced damage. Models of cellular response to ionising radiation have evolved from the very simplistic ones to more complex models, incorporating more and more radiobiological parameters.

2.1 TARGET THEORY

Target theory in radiation biology refers to the theoretical modelling that attempts to predict quantitatively the response of cells to radiation. Targets are entities (like the DNA of a cell or the cell itself) that may be affected by radiation. In target theory, radiation may hit or miss a target. Two main postulates underlying the theory are that:

1. the number of targets affected by radiation determines the extent of the resulting biological effect
2. the response of a target to radiation is stochastic (random) in nature.

The aim of the target theory is therefore to establish a relationship between the number of targets affected and the characteristics of the ionising radiation hitting the targets.

2.1.1 Single hit single target theory

The simplest version of target theory is the 'single hit single target' model, which assumes that each cell contains one single target. In this theory, a single hit to a target affects the cell. Targets are then assumed to be in constant exposure to radiation for a period of time t. Assuming the probability that no more than one hit will affect a target and that the event is independent of the situation in other targets, one can model the single hit single target theory in terms of Poisson statistics.

Let δt be a time interval which is sufficiently small that only one hit can occur, and suppose that k denotes a probability per unit time of a target being hit. Then $k\delta t$ is the probability that a target is hit during δt. The larger the number of potential targets N_0 in a volume, the greater the probability that there will be a hit. Also, the occurrence of a hit will depend on the cell's properties and the characteristics of radiation. Consequently $k = \kappa N_0$, where κ is a parameter which characterises the likelihood of a target being hit. While the probability of one target (out of N_0) being hit is, therefore, $p \equiv \kappa N_0 \delta t$, the probability that no targets are hit is $q \equiv 1 - \kappa N_0 \delta t$.

In order to find the number of cells which are likely to survive after t, one has to obtain the probability that there will be zero hits ($N = 0$) during that time period. This is expressed as q^s, where $s = \delta t / T$ repre-

L. Marcu et al., *Biomedical Physics in Radiotherapy for Cancer*,
DOI 10.1007/978-0-85729-733-4_2, © CSIRO 2012

sents the number of time intervals. By considering the limit $s \to \infty$ (or equivalently $\delta t \to 0$):

$$P(0) = \lim_{s \to \infty} q^s \qquad (2.1)$$

$$\lim_{s \to \infty} \left(1 - \frac{\lambda}{s}\right)^s = e^{-\lambda} \qquad (2.2)$$

where $\lambda = \kappa N_0 t$, the probability $P(0) = e^{-\lambda}$ is obtained.

Therefore, based on single hit target theory, the surviving fraction of cells N/N_0 after irradiation for a time interval t is $e^{-\lambda}$.

If λ is defined as a ratio of a radiation dose D to the reference dose that will affect $1/e$ cells, D_0, then $\lambda \equiv D/D_0$. Finally, $N/N_0 = \exp(-D/D_0)$.

2.1.2   Single hit multiple target theory

When a target is considered to be a DNA base of a cell, each cell contains multiple targets. In this case, one hit may affect a target, however the cell will be affected only when several targets within the cell are hit. This is the principle of single hit multiple target theory, in which it is still assumed that one hit will affect a target, but more than one target needs to be hit in order to damage the cell. This principle is also more biologically realistic, knowing that double strand breaks within the DNA rather than single strand breaks are needed for irreparable cellular damage.

Suppose that n targets in a cell need to be hit to affect the integrity of the cell. It was shown before that the probability that one target will be hit is $1 - e^{-\lambda}$. Therefore, the probability that n targets will be hit is $(1 - e^{-\lambda})^n$. Consequently, the probability that a cell will survive is:

$$S = 1 - \left(1 - e^{-\lambda}\right)^n = 1 - \left(1 - e^{-D/D_0}\right)^n \qquad (2.3)$$

S is the survival curve corresponding to the single hit multiple target theory.

In both of the above target theories it is assumed that surviving fractions are dose-rate independent, which means they depend on the overall dose delivered but not on the period of time over which the radiation is delivered. This assumption relates purely to the theory, since this is not occurring in reality. In addition, since application of Poisson statistics assumes that the hits are statistically independent of

one another, the theories may not apply to the situations for densely ionising radiations.

2.1.3   Linear quadratic model

The linear quadratic model, introduced by Douglas and Fowler in the seventies (Douglas and Fowler 1976), is a combination of single hit single target and double hit single target theories. In *multiple hit single target* theory, each cell is assumed to contain a single target but more than one hit is necessary to impair or inactivate the cell (the target). Double hit single target theory leads to the surviving fraction whose logarithm is quadratic as a function of dose, D. Since the linear quadratic model is a combination of single hit single target and double hit single target theories, the survival curve is represented by the following equation:

$$\log S = \log S_1 + \log S_2 \text{ (i.e. } S = S_1 S_2) \qquad (2.4)$$

where $\log S_1$ is linear in D and $\log S_2$ is quadratic in D. This leads to the equation:

$$\log S = -\alpha D - \beta D^2 \qquad (2.5)$$

where α and β are constants.

The expression $S = S_1 S_2$ implies that the two types of events are statistically independent of each other. Therefore, in the linear quadratic model, a cell can be affected by a single lethal event or by two events which are not lethal individually but may become lethal when accumulated. Thus, the linear quadratic formalism describes dose-response relations, which result from acute or protracted dose delivery regimens, taking into consideration lethal lesions resulting from one (for example, a lethal point mutation in a vital gene is a one-track event) or two independent radiation events (leading to chromosome aberration).

The dose at which the α and β components are equal is referred to as the α/β ratio (Figure 2.1).

When radiotherapy is fractionated in 'n' number of fractions each delivering a dose 'd', then the linear quadratic equation becomes:

$$S = \exp\left[-n(\alpha d + \beta d^2)\right] = \exp\left[-nd(\alpha + \beta d)\right] \qquad (2.6)$$

The initial slope of the survival curve in Figure 2.1 is determined by the linear component α (single-hit killing) which dominates the radiation response at low doses and the shoulder is given by the quadratic

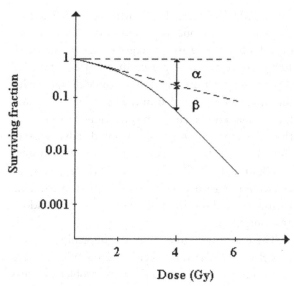

Figure 2.1. The α and β components of the Linear Quadratic model.

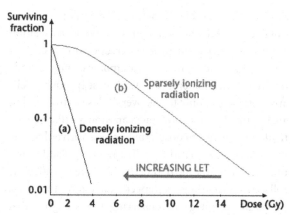

Figure 2.2. Survival curves as a function of LET.

component β (multiple-hit killing) which causes the curve to bend at higher doses.

As already presented above, LET is a measure of the energy deposition along the track of an ionising particle. Thus, heavy particles (neutrons, protons, alpha particles) have a high LET and produce greater biological damage than electrons and photons which have a low LET. Figure 2.2 illustrates the fact that the higher the LET the steeper the survival curve. This means that for high LET radiation the α/β ratio is high (β very small) while for low LET radiation α/β has a low value (β is high). Curve (a) is typical for densely ionising radiation when the dose-response curve is a straight line. In this situation the survival curve can be described by just one parameter, which is the linear parameter, α. Curve (b) is representative for sparsely ionising radiation (X-rays, electrons) and the dose-response curve presents with a shoulder, due to cell repair processes, characterised by the quadratic parameter, β.

It has been shown that most tumours have an α/β ratio around 10 Gy (with $\alpha = 0.35\,\text{Gy}^{-1}$ and $\beta = 0.035\,\text{Gy}^{-2}$). These values apply to the early responding normal tissues. However, late responding tissues present with a much lower α/β ratio, of 3 Gy, with $\alpha = 0.15\,\text{Gy}^{-1}$ and $\beta = 0.05\,\text{Gy}^{-1}$ (see Table 2.1 for some examples).

There are, however, exceptions from the rule, since one of the most controversial α/β ratio in the literature is α/β for prostate. Unlike the vast majority of tumours, prostate cancers may have a very low α/β ratio, around 1.5 Gy (Overgaard 1985; King and Fowler 2001). The implications of these findings on prostate treatment are

Table 2.1. α/β ratios for early and late responding tissues for various end-points (Overgaard 1985; Steel 2002).

Tissue	End-point	α/β (Gy)
Skin	Erythema	10.5–11.3
	Moist desquamation	10.0
	Late fibrosis	1.9–2.3
	Telangiectasia	5.7
Lung	Pneumonitis	4.4–6.9
	Late fibrosis	3.0–3.6
Bone	Rib fracture	1.8–2.5
Spinal cord	Myelopathy	<3.3

significant, since hyperfractation is not the most suitable schedule. Just the opposite, hypofractation (high doses delivered in fewer fractions) is the treatment choice for prostate carcinomas, due to the uniquely slow proliferation rate of these tumours. Cells are sensitive not only to the overall dose delivered, but also to the dose rate. Prostate carcinoma cells are particularly sensitive to dose-rate, more sensitive than the surrounding normal tissues like rectum, bladder and urethra (the lower the α/β ratio, the more sensitive the cells are to the dose-rate effect). Therefore, there is a potential advantage in delivering doses higher that 2 Gy/fraction in a smaller number of fractions than in conventionally fractionated treatment regimen.

The LQ model presented so far incorporates two major assumptions:

1. There is full repair between subsequent fractions (the fractions are far enough apart to consider the incomplete repair negligible) and
2. There is no proliferation of tumour cells (there is no time factor taken into account. However overall treatment time plays a crucial role for tumours with high cell turnover).

To account for the highly proliferative tumours, the LQ model has been extended by considering the time factor, through overall treatment time, tumour kick-off time and potential doubling time. A more complex formulation of the linear quadratic model can be presented as:

$$S = \exp\left[-nd(\alpha + \beta d) + \frac{\ln 2\,(T - T_k)}{T_p}\right] \quad (2.7)$$

where:

T_p is the potential doubling time and represents the time to double the cell population considering that no cell death has occurred.

T_k is the kick-off time. It was shown that for certain tumour types (especially highly proliferating ones, like head & neck) in a short period of time after the start of radiotherapy the tumour begins to grow more rapidly than before irradiation. This time is called kick-off time.

T is the overall treatment time.

The extended LQ model for repopulation was first suggested by Travis and Tucker (1987) and afterwards

developed by several others. There were trials to further extend the model to account for cell redistribution along the cycle and reoxygenation (Brenner *et al.* 1995). However, since the accuracy of equation 2.7 was not demonstrated, and some would disagree with the time factors included in the equation, the 'plain' linear quadratic formalism (equation 2.6) remains the accepted one. Also, the main disadvantage of equation 2.7 is the number of the unknown parameters (four: α/β, T, T_k, T_p), therefore there is need for cell kinetic measurements (proliferation rate during treatment, radioresistance) before any calculations are completed.

There are some uncertainties concerning the LQ model in the low dose region (below 1.5 Gy) thus imposing some limitations. This problem occurs because of scarcity of clinical data for doses less than 2 Gy.

Currently the linear quadratic formalism is widely used for analysing cell survival *in vitro,* for comparing radiotherapy regimens, and for studying various radiobiological endpoints. Although it has significant limitations, the LQ model is still the best tool currently available for drawing sensible conclusions based on fundamental information on radiobiological damage.

2.2   CELL SURVIVAL CURVES

Many molecules in aqueous solutions exist in an ionised state due to dissociation into positively and negatively charged ions that coexist in a stable equilibrium (Nias 2000). However, when interacting with the living tissue, ionising radiation is known to produce ions that are not in stable equilibrium. These ions are highly reactive (abnormal species) called free radicals. Free radical ions disrupt normal molecular structures and damage the biological target, the deoxyribonucleic acid (DNA). Radiation deposition results in DNA damage manifested by single- and double-strand breaks in the sugar phosphate backbone of the molecule.

Radiation damage is largely manifested by the loss of cellular reproductive integrity. Some cells undergo apoptosis (programmed death) while others show no morphologic evidence of radiation damage until they attempt to divide.

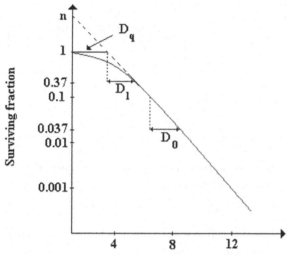

Figure 2.3. Survival curve parameters.

As illustrated in Figure 2.3, both D_1 and D_0 are doses required to reduce the fraction of surviving cells to 37% of its previous value. If the initial number of cells is N_0 (for zero dose) and the number of cells for a given dose D is N, $N = N_0 e^{-D/D_0}$ represents the single hit survival curve; for $D = D_0$, $N = N_0 e^{-1}$, thus $N = 0.37 N_0$.

The presence of the shoulder in the survival curve for sparsely ionising radiation is possibly due to repair processes. The shoulder region is quantified by extrapolation of the exponential portion of the curve to the y-axis intercept. This point is referred to as the extrapolation number n, while the dose in between the 100% survival point and the extrapolation line is called quasi-threshold dose D_q.

When evaluating survival curves from various cell lines it is useful to define a quantity which relates to the differences in radiosensitivity between the specific populations. Based on observations of survival curve parameters from several cell populations originating from mice, the D_0 values show a narrow range (100–200 cGy) compared with significantly larger variations in values for D_q (65–900 cGy) (Nias 2000). There is also evidence for a wide variation in the extrapolation numbers of the curves derived from human cell lines (1.1–163 cGy) (see Table 2.3).

Therefore, it was suggested, that a more relevant radiosensitivity parameter should be introduced, which would account for the variation in the size of the shoulder of survival curves. The parameter that has been defined for this is SF_2 (Surviving Fraction at

Cell survival curves describe the relationship between the radiation dose and the proportion of cells that survive:

- For differentiated cells (nonproliferating), cell death means loss of a specific function.
- For proliferating cells, death represents loss of reproductive integrity (reproductive death).

The graph in Figure 2.3 shows a survival curve of a cell population hit by sparsely ionising radiation. The fraction of cell survival is plotted on a logarithmic scale against dose on a linear scale.

The main elements of a cell survival curve and their interpretation are illustrated in Table 2.2.

Table 2.2. The main elements of a cell survival curve.

Element of cell survival curve	Symbol	Interpretation
The initial slope of the curve	D_1	Characterises the initial slope of the curve due to single event killing. It is the dose required to reduce the fraction of surviving cells to 37% of its previous value.
The final slope of the curve	D_0	Characterises the final slope of the curve due to multiple event killing. It is the dose required to reduce the fraction of surviving cells to 37% of its previous value.
The extrapolation number	n	The intersection point between the y axis and the extrapolated exponential part of the curve. It is a quantification of the shoulder region of the survival curve.
The quasi-threshold dose	D_q	Represents the dose in between the 100% survival point and the extrapolation line.

Table 2.3.   Human tumour cell survival parameters (Nias 2000).

Tumour type	D_0 (Gy)	n	Survival after 2 Gy (SF_2)
Melanoma	1	40	0.77
Colon	1	5.5	0.40
Rectum	0.7	163	0.54
Cervix	1.3	3.8	0.48
Burkitt lymphoma	1.25	1.1	0.18

the 2 Gy level). Data from human tumour cell survival show a variation in SF_2 from 0.18 (Burkitt lymphoma) to 0.77 (melanoma) (Nias 2000).

The steepness of the initial slope is an important determinant of the success of fractionated radiotherapy. Fractionated radiotherapy is more representative of clinical radiotherapy than the single dose irradiation experiments in the laboratory. For a fractionated treatment regimen the survival curve (called **effective dose survival curve**) becomes an exponential function of dose. Therefore, the shoulder of the survival curve is repeated many times (depending on the number of fractions) (see Figure 2.4).

In this situation, D_0 of the effective survival curve also represents the reciprocal of the slope, defined as the dose required to reduce the fraction of surviving cells to 37%. For calculation purposes it is useful to define the dose required to kill 90% of the population (D_{10}) resulting in 10% survival. Considering all of the above, the relationship between D_0 and D_{10} can be written as:

$$D_{10} = \ln 10 \times D_0 = 2.3 \times D_0 \qquad (2.8)$$

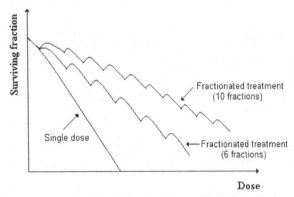

Figure 2.4. The effect of fractionation on the cell survival curve.

Survival curves are useful tools for dose calculations when D_0 and D_q are known:

$$D = D_q + T \times D_{10} = D_q + T \times 2.3 D_0 \qquad (2.9)$$

where T is the power of 10 by which the surviving fraction is to be reduced.

2.3   THE CELL CYCLE AND CELLULAR RADIOSENSITIVITY

Cellular growth and functioning is governed by a biologic clock named the cell cycle. The cell cycle clock controls cellular division and DNA replication, checks for possible misrepair or mutations, arrests cells for repair and orders apoptosis when needed.

Cell division is a basic biological process that results in an increase in somatic cell numbers over time. Mitosis (cell division) is common in both normal cells and tumour cells, however cancer cells grow uncontrollably. In normal tissues there is a balance between cell proliferation, differentiation and cell loss. Conversely, tumours grow because the homeostatic control mechanisms that maintain the appropriate number of cells in normal tissue are defective, leading to an imbalance between cell proliferation and death, which results in an expansion of the cell population.

Cells propagate through an orderly sequence represented by the four phases constituting the cell cycle (Figure 2.5). These are: mitosis (M) when the cell divides in two daughter cells, the postmitotic phase or first 'gap' (G_1) during which the cell prepares for DNA synthesis, the synthetic phase (S) when the DNA is duplicated and the postsynthetic phase or second gap (G_2) when the cell prepares for division. Some cellular types, after mitosis, enter a resting phase called G_0. This phase is out of the cell cycle, and the resting (quiescent) cells may remain in G_0 indefinitely or re-enter

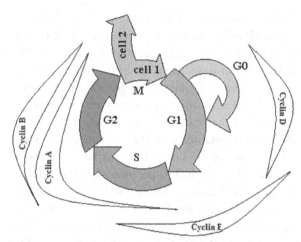

Figure 2.5. Schematic representation of the cell cycle and of the fluctuating concentrations of cyclins.

the cell cycle in response to an external stimulus. Progression through the cell cycle is restricted at particular checkpoints which are set at various stages of the division cycle: G_1, S, and G_2/M phases (Hartwell and Weinert 1989). These checkpoints can arrest damaged cells for repair, redirect cells to G_0 or trigger apoptosis (programmed cell death). The control molecules which dictate the pace of events in the cell cycle are the cyclins and the cyclin-dependent-kinases (cdk) (Nurse 2000). They represent the cell cycle clock. Cyclins are proteins found along the cell cycle in fluctuating concentrations. The main role of the cyclins is to activate another protein, the kinase, which drives the checkpoints by allowing cells to pass or to be arrested at a certain stage. This control mechanism between cyclins and cyclin-dependent kinases creates the ordered progression of cells along the mitotic cycle.

The lengths of the various phases of the cycle have been determined by flow cytometric measurements (Hall 2000). The only consistent phase-length for different cell lines is the S phase, which represents one third of the whole cell cycle time while mitosis is the shortest (1–2 hours), G_1 is the most variable, but also usually the longest.

Mammalian cell populations usually proliferate asynchronously. Therefore cells will be distributed throughout the cell cycle phases, although unevenly. The most probable distribution is supposed to be the exponential one, with the largest population in G_1 and smallest in mitosis (Hall 2000).

Depending on their position in the mitotic cycle, cells respond differently to radiation. It was found that, cells are most radiosensitive during and close to M phase, and most resistant in late S phase (Sinclair 1969). Cells with longer G_1 phases also have a resistant peak early in G_1. The quiescent cells situated in G_0 are also known to be relatively radioresistant (Nias 2000).

Cells in the S phase have high radioresistance due to the existence of natural sulfhydryl compounds in the cell. Sulfhydryl compounds are radioprotectors because they are scavengers of free radicals present at the highest levels in S phase of the cell cycle and lowest in mitosis.

2.4 CHARACTERISATION OF RADIATION DAMAGE

Radiation damage to the living cell can be either lethal (irreparable) or reparable under certain circumstances. Repairable damage can be classified into: sublethal damage and potentially lethal damage, as described in the paragraphs below.

2.4.1 Lethal damage

By definition, any damage where there is no possibility for cellular repair is lethal because it leads irreversibly to cell death. Cell death can affect the functionality of a tissue or organ depending on the extent of cell loss. Therefore, radiation-produced cell loss is deterministic in nature. A small radiation dose can lead to cell loss without affecting the exposed tissue or organ. However, if the dose is greater than a certain threshold dose, the probability of causing damage increases with the dose since higher dose implies more cell loss.

2.4.2 Sublethal damage (SLD)

Sublethal damage is damage caused by radiation, which under normal circumstances is repaired, unless a subsequent radiation dose is delivered to the cell before the damage can be repaired thus transforming it into lethal damage. Repair of sublethal damage (SLDR) is encouraged by a fractionated radiotherapy schedule, since there is time for repairable damage to be fixed between two consecutive radiation doses. Even in the case of hyperfractionated radiotherapy when two or more radiation fractions are given in a single day, keeping at least 6 hours in between fractions, allows sublethal damage in normal tissues to be repaired. Consequently, if a radiation dose is split into fractions separated by several hours, an increase in cell survival can be observed due to the repair of sublethal damage.

Example: In a split-dose experiment with cultured Chinese hamster cells (Elkind *et al.* 1965) it was shown that while a single dose of 15.58 Gy leads to a surviving fraction of 0.005, the same total dose administered in two fractions separated by a 30 minute time interval led to a surviving fraction of 0.02. In the experiment the cells were incubated at room temperature between the two fractions (for various time intervals) (see Figure 2.6 A). Keeping the cells at 24°C aimed to prevent the process of redistribution of cells in the cell cycle. Thus the cells were kept in the same phase of the cell cycle they were during the first irradiation. Since after the first dose of radiation most of the hamster cells would be in the S phase (which is the most radioresistant), it would be possible to assess repair capacity of sublethal damage without the confounding effect of cell-cycle redistribution.

A parallel experiment, with cells incubated between two fractions at their growing temperature of 37°C, has allowed the natural progression of cells in the cycle (see Figure 2.6 B). However, this time, the effect of variability of cellular radioresistance in the cell cycle can be shown in the cell survival curve. Partial synchronisation of the cells results from differentiated cell kill as cells in the more sensitive phases of the cell cycle are more affected than those cells which, at the time of irradiation, are in the more resistant phases of the cycle. After the significant increase in cell survival when the two fractions are less than 2.5 hours apart (*sublethal damage repair*), instead of a plateau area obtained with the previous experiment, there is a decrease in survival that reaches a minimum at about 6 hours, which is the time when the cells hit by the second dose are in the most sensitive period (G_2/M) (*redistribution of cells in the cycle*). The surviving cells also suffer division delay (discussed later in this Chapter) after the first dose of radiation. Finally, there is an increase in the cell survival curve due to mitosis, as cells reaching the M phase undergo division (*repopulation*). It is also to be noted that the cell cycle time of Chinese hamster cells in culture is as short as 10 hours. Therefore, this experimental set-up is representative of rapidly proliferating cells, populations such as head & neck tumours, since slowly growing ones would need correspondingly longer times to undergo the above described events.

Consequently, the cell survival curve indicates an interplay between three major radiobiological processes: repair, redistribution of cells in the cell cycle and repopulation.

Although the above results have been obtained for studies done on cultured hamster cells, the repair of

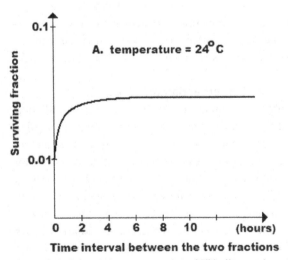

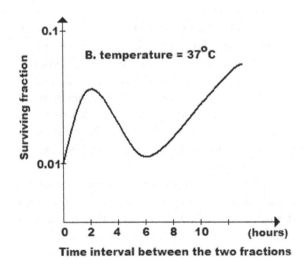

Figure 2.6. Schematic representation of Elkind's experiment.

sublethal damage has been shown for other mammalian cells, both *in vitro* and *in vivo*. One of the differences between the two categories is in regards to repair time being longer in late-responding *in vivo* normal tissue than *in vitro* cell cultures. The repair (recovery) of sublethal damage is also known as split-dose recovery, or Elkind recovery (in honour of M.M. Elkind who experimentally evidenced the SLDR of hamster cells in culture).

Radiation *dose-rate* also affects the cellular response to sublethal damage. By decreasing the dose-rate and prolonging the exposure time to radiation, the damage created to the tissue is also reduced. This outcome is explained by the ability of the tissue to repair the sublethal damage that occurs during an extended radiation exposure. During fractionated radiotherapy, given that there is enough time for the tissue to repair the sublethal damage between two consecutive fractions, the survival curve is represented by multiply-repeating shoulders. Continuous low dose-rate irradiation may be considered as consisting of an infinite number of small fractions, having similar effect on cell survival as fractionated irradiation. The dose-rate effect caused by SLDR is predominant between 0.01 and 1 Gy/min (Hall 2000).

It is important to mention that the dose-rate effect is strongly cell line dependent. For a large number of human cells cultured *in vitro*, because of the variation in repair time, the survival curves are usually shallow and show a great variation in slope after low-dose rate irradiation. On the contrary at high dose rates, the lack of sublethal damage repair time leads to steep survival curves. There are some notable exceptions among cell lines which respond to the *inverse dose-rate effect* such as HeLa cells. In other words, there is a range of dose rates for which lowering the dose rate in such cells results in less cell survival. This counterintuitive phenomenon is explained by the cell arrest in the radiosensitive G_2 phase caused by low dose rates. As a consequence, under continuous low dose rate irradiation, an asynchronous cell population turns into partially synchronised population, located mainly in the radiosensitive phase of the cycle (G_2) becoming, therefore, vulnerable to subsequent radiation doses. At higher dose rates, cells are held up ('frozen') at the phase of the cycle they were located in at the start of irradiation thus having, on average, higher radioresistance than the cells blocked in G_2 by low dose rates.

2.4.3   Potentially lethal damage (PLD)

This type of radiation cell damage is potentially lethal, because it normally leads to cell death unless the postirradiation environment is changed. PLD caused by radiation has been shown to be repaired if postirradiation conditions are kept suboptimal for growth. In such an environment the irradiated cells do not undergo mitosis and are prevented from expressing cell lethality due to chromosomal damage. The delay in mitosis provides time for the damaged chromosomal DNA to be repaired. Evidence of PLD has been demonstrated in cell culture experiments, two examples of which are quoted below:

Experimental example 1: Cells in culture were left to grow until the colonies became confluent, at which stage they stopped proliferating because they have outgrown the medium. After irradiation, part of the cell culture was plated in fresh growth medium, and the other part left in the confluent phase, in the old growth medium. Comparison of cell survival curves for the two situations revealed that cells kept in their pre-irradiation environment had higher survival than the cells which were re-plated in fresh medium. The non-proliferating cells were presumably able to repair the potentially lethal damage because of mitotic arrest, while cells in the fresh medium regained their proliferative ability thus undergoing mitosis with damaged chromosomes.

Experimental example 2: Cell cultures growing under normal conditions (37°C) before irradiation are left to grow, at the same temperature, post irradiation. Since cells are still able to proliferate at this temperature, the radiation-induced potentially lethal damage is transformed into a lethal damage within a few minutes. However, if the same cells post irradiation are cooled down to 20°C, cell proliferation ceases, allowing time for repair of PLD.

Recovery from potentially lethal damage is a characteristic of tissues with non-proliferating cells and also of tissues with very small growth fraction. Quiescent cells out of the mitotic cycle in the G_0 phase have been shown to be radioresistant. This has been attributed to their ability to repair any potentially lethal damage in contrast to cycling cells which are more prone to this type of damage.

Division delay can also be considered as a type of radiation-induced repairable damage (although some chemicals can cause division delay as well). Division delay is the process whereby cells are held up ('arrested') in various transition points along the cell cycle (usually at the G_1/S, or G_2/M transition points), either because of inhibition of DNA synthesis (G_1/S) or of mitosis (G_2/M).

Division delay produced by radiation depends both on the dose of radiation delivered and on the point in the cell cycle when the dose to the cell is delivered. For synchronised HeLa cells, studies have shown that, on average, the duration of delay for a full cell cycle is 1 min/cGy (Nias 2000).

As mentioned above, cells have well-defined molecular mechanisms which control progression through the cell cycle to ensure that DNA replication and/or mitosis can be completed. These control mechanisms are guided by cell-cycle checkpoints. For instance, the G_2/M checkpoint prevents cells from initiating mitosis when they experience DNA damage during G_2, or when they progress into G_2 with unrepaired damage. G_1 checkpoints can sense DNA damage through protein assemblies whose active components are the protein kinases ATM (ataxia telangiectasia mutated) and ATR (ATM-related). ATM recognises double-strand breaks produced by ionising radiation, while ATR is activated by ultraviolet irradiation expressed by DNA-base damage.

Cells with an intact DNA-damage response either arrest or die in response to DNA damage. However, cells with mutated or nonexistent checkpoint enzymes (kinases) progress through the cycle with damaged or misrepaired DNA, process that usually ends up in transformation to a malignant phenotype. One of the most important players in triggering the process of elimination of damaged cells from the mitotic cycle is the tumour suppressor gene, p53. p53 is a gene, encoding a protein that regulates cell growth. It is called tumour suppressor gene because of its ability to cause potentially cancerous cells to destroy themselves.

Mutations in p53 are found in most tumour types. Additionally, there is a rare condition known as Li-Fraumeni syndrome, when a person inherits only one functional copy of the p53 gene from the parents. The affected person is predisposed to cancer and usually develops several independent tumours in various tissues in early adulthood.

2.5 LOSS OF REPRODUCTIVE ABILITY IN CELLS

Cell survival is a determinant of tissue function, whether healthy or malignant. Tissue functionality is dictated by the number of the constituent cells that have the ability to renew the cell population when damaged. The biological effect of a radiation dose is usually measured *in vitro* by cell survival assay. Cell survival assay measures the clonogenic capacity of individual cells. The clonogenic capacity or colony forming ability of cells relates to cells which are able to form cell colonies, each of which is defined as a progeny of at least 50 cells. Cells which after irradiation are capable of undergoing about 6 consecutive mitoses are considered to have retained their clonogenic capacity.

The first assay of clonogenic capacity or colony forming ability in mammalian cells was reported by Puck and Markus in 1956. Single cells from Chinese hamsters were plated in Petri dishes, in a growth medium to allow the cells to grow into colonies. After irradiating the cells, the ability of the cells to form colonies was reduced. The irradiated cells were therefore considered to have suffered loss of colony-forming ability (see Figure 2.7).

2.5.1 Clonogenic assay

Clonogenic assays constitute the foundation for cellular response to radiation. The principle of the assay consists of the comparison of the clonogenic capacity

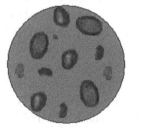 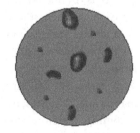

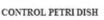
CONTROL PETRI DISH   IRRADIATED PETRI DISH

Figure 2.7. Illustration of the loss of colony-forming ability after irradiation.

between unirradiated (control) and an irradiated cell culture, using the same single-cell suspension plated under identical conditions. The number of cells plated, for both the control and the irradiated cultures are counted. Let us consider that the control Petri dish contains 100 cells, and the irradiated has 500 cells (a larger number is plated, since it is expected that radiation will have killed a certain amount of cells). After an incubation period, the colonies from both dishes are determined. If, for example, the number of colonies in the control dish is 25 and there are only 10 in the irradiated dish, the plating efficiency (PE) can be calculated, by dividing the number of colonies which have formed by the number of plated cells in each dish separately:

$$PE_{control} = \frac{25}{100} = 0.25$$

$$PE_{irradiated} = \frac{10}{500} = 0.02$$

The surviving fraction (SF) is calculated as the ratio between the plating efficiencies:

$$SF = \frac{PE_{irradiated}}{PE_{control}} = \frac{0.02}{0.25} = 0.08$$

Therefore, the surviving fraction of cells resulting from this experiment is only 8%.

It is expected to obtain a variation in colony counts when the number of the plated cells differs. The question arising is whether this dependence of colony counts on the initial number of plated cells is linear. Unless this is the case, cell survival curves would be erroneous.

A number of assays are available to assess the proliferative ability of both normal and malignant cells. One of the first *in vivo* assays was developed by Hewitt and Wilson by means of *endpoint-dilution technique*. The assay consisted of implantation into mammals of various concentrations of diluted cells originating from irradiated mice liver (infiltrated with lymphocytic leukemia cells). In the new environment the mice subsequently developed leukemias. The percent of tumours was then plotted against the number of cells implanted and TD_{50} determined (where TD_{50} is the number of cells required to create 50% tumours, or to provoke tumours in 50% of the animals). Cell survival was given by the ratio between TD_{50} obtained for the control (unirradiated) tumours and TD_{50} obtained for the irradiated tumours. Although requir-

ing a large number of animals and all together time consuming, the endpoint-dilution technique has been adapted for radiosensitivity studies of normal tissues. A faster alternative of the above described technique is the *lung colony assay.* This technique, developed by Hill and Bush assesses the clonogenic ability of solid tumour cells (sarcoma) irradiated *in situ*. Once removed from donor mice, the tumours were prepared into single-cell suspensions and injected into recipient mice. A certain percentage of cells proliferated in the lungs and created colonies in about 3 weeks after inoculation. The lung colonies were then counted and the dose-response curves derived.

The most common *in situ* clonogenic assay is the **spleen-colony assay** employed by Till and McCulloch to assess radiosensitivity of bone marrow cells. This assay is similar to the above described dilution technique, excepting the fact that the spleen-colony assay uses normal bone marrow cells rather then leukemia cells, and the colonies form in the spleen. In the experiment conducted by Till and McCulloch bone marrow cells (in known quantity) from mice irradiated with various doses of radiation were injected into recipient mice, that had received whole body irradiation to suppress endogenous hemopoiesis. In about 10 days after injecting the bone marrow cells the recipient mice started to develop colonies in the spleen. The spleens were then removed and the colonies counted. With this assay, Till and McCulloch obtained the first survival curve for bone marrow cells, which being very steep, showed high sensitivity to radiation.

The *crypt cell assay* is one of the most representative clonogenic assays for normal tissue and has been perfected by Withers and Elkind. Crypt cells are renewing stem cells in the intestinal epithelium, therefore constantly dividing. Mice are exposed to a sufficiently high whole-body dose (11–16 Gy) to reduce the number of surviving crypt cells to a low level. Due to their proliferative ability, the surviving cells regenerate rapidly the crypt population. Histologic sections are made 3–4 days after irradiation and the fraction of crypt cells capable of repopulation are counted. This fraction of renewing cells is plotted against the radiation dose delivered and the survival curve for intestinal crypt cells is obtained.

Clonogenic assays remain to be useful tools in assessing normal tissue sensitivity and tumour response to various therapeutic agents. As the aim of cancer treatment is to kill clonogenic (stem) cells which otherwise would be able to repopulate the tumour, colony-forming assays can give indications upon the effectiveness of cancer treatment and predict the outcome of the therapy.

2.5.2   Main quantifying factors in radiation biology: LET, RBE, OER

Radiation can cure cancer but can also provoke it. Therefore, it is important to understand the ways that ionising radiation interacts with the matter and how the result is quantified (LET), to know about the effect that different types of radiation can have on both normal and cancerous tissue and how their toxicity compares (RBE) and also to learn about the role of tissue oxygenation in radiotherapy and how radiobiology can assist in counteracting the impediment induced by the lack of oxygen (OER).

2.6   LINEAR ENERGY TRANSFER (LET)

The previous chapter demonstrated that different types of ionising radiation interact differently with the living tissue, and result in different levels of damage. The variation in the biological effects induced by various ionising radiations is given by the intensity of the ionisation, quantified in terms of the *linear energy transfer* (LET).

Linear energy transfer is the energy transferred to tissue per unit length of track traversed by the ionising radiation particle under consideration. More exactly, LET is the rate of energy loss per unit path length of the ionising radiation particle in which the energy from interaction with the medium is locally absorbed. The attribute 'locally' postulates that only that fraction of energy is considered which leads to ionisations and/or excitations within the considered site. The remaining kinetic energy of particles leaving the site is excluded.

Since the energy per unit length of track varies over a wide range, one should define LET as the average energy, dE, locally transferred to the medium by a charged particle traversing a distance dl. Mathematically, LET is expressed as:

$$LET = \frac{dE}{dl} \qquad (2.10)$$

The unit for LET is keV/μm.

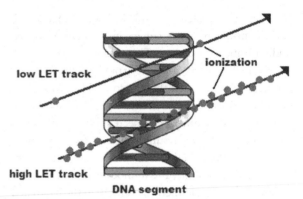

Figure 2.8. Ionisation tracks produced by low LET and high LET particles when interacting with the DNA.

Radiation as a function of LET can be classified into (Figure 2.8):

- sparsely ionising (photons, electrons) [low LET]
- densely ionising (neutrons, alpha particles, low energy protons) [high LET].

Some uncharged particles, as for instance neutrons, are categorised as high LET radiation although they are not able to produce direct ionisations. Neutrons interact with atomic nuclei resulting in the release of protons. Protons, therefore, are secondary products of the neutron-matter interaction and they are densely ionising particles, producing a high number of ionisations along their track. Depending also on their initial energy, neutrons can produce, indirectly, biological damage to various degrees as indicated by the radiation weighting factors.

2.6.1   Energy dependence of LET

The average LET value is given in Table 2.4. This is because of the energy dependence of LET. For example, the LET varies with the attenuation of Co-60 radiation in matter, ranging from ~0.2 to ~2 keV/μm; 80% of the dose is delivered with LET <0.3 keV/μm.

In the case of neutrons, the LET spectrum varies markedly with energy, ranging from 1 to 50 keV/μm for 0.1 MeV neutrons and from 5 to 500 keV/μm for 14 MeV neutrons. The average LET value peaks at 200–400 keV neutrons.

High energy charged particles from accelerators have quite low LET values, except in the region of the Bragg peak where the particle energy reduces quickly, and the LET increases in value.

Table 2.4. Typical LET values for a range of radiations and energies.

Radiation type and energy	LET$_{av}$ (keV/μm)	LET$_{max}$ (keV/μm)
Gamma Co-60 – 1.17, 1.33 MeV	0.22	
X-ray – 200 kV	1.7	
Beta Tritium – 18.6 keV	4.7	
X-ray – 50 kV	6.3	
Alpha Tb-149 – 4.0 MeV		143
Alpha accelerator – 5.3 MeV	43	
Alpha At-211 – 6.7 MeV		104
Alpha Bi-213 – 8.35 MeV		102

2.7 RELATIVE BIOLOGICAL EFFECTIVENESS (RBE)

The concept of 'relative biological effectiveness' (RBE) has been introduced to quantitatively express the quality of radiation. By definition, RBE is the ratio of the dose of a reference 250 kV X-ray and the dose of the test radiation, which produces the same amount of biological damage for the same endpoint or isoeffect. Mathematically RBE can be expressed as:

$$RBE = \frac{D(250 \text{ kV Xray})}{D(test\ radiation)}\bigg|_{ISOEFFECT} \quad (2.11)$$

The following example is presented in order to show the variation of RBE with radiation dose. The graph in Figure 2.9 shows typical survival curves of mammalian cell lines irradiated with low energy (kV) X-rays (considered as a reference radiation) and high energy (MeV) neutrons (test radiation), respectively. Using the above definition, RBE can be calculated for both high surviving fraction (due to low dose irradiation) and low surviving fraction (due to high dose irradiation).

The ratio of X-ray dose to neutron dose that would lead to the same endpoint, in this case a surviving fraction of 0.75 is approximately:

$$RBE_{LD} = \frac{250cGy}{50cGy} = 5 \quad (2.12)$$

while the ratio of X-ray dose to neutron dose which would give a surviving fraction of 0.1 is:

$$RBE_{HD} = \frac{500cGy}{200cGy} = 2.5 \quad (2.13)$$

The results show that RBE is larger for lower doses of radiation (RBE$_{LD}$) and smaller for higher doses of

radiation (RBE$_{HD}$). The rationale behind this observation is based on the differences in cellular repair capacity of the same cell line when irradiated with X-rays and neutrons, respectively. When irradiated with low doses of X-rays, cells are able to repair the resulting sublethal damage as reflected by the broad shoulder of the X-ray survival curve. On the contrary, lesions in cells caused by high LET radiation such as neutrons are less repairable, as reflected by the steep cell survival curve, with no discernable shoulder. As the doses are increased, in both cases the repair of damage is less successful, the X-ray survival curve becomes steeper (reflecting exponential killing), and therefore RBE is smaller.

To illustrate the effect of dose/fraction on RBE, the above experiment is reconsidered for fractionated

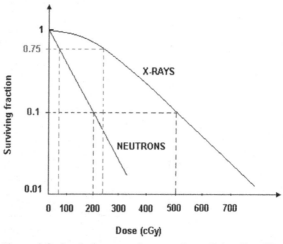

Figure 2.9. Survival curves of mammalian cells irradiated by X-rays and neutrons in a single-dose experiment.

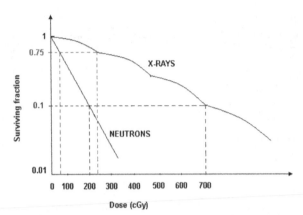

Figure 2.10. Survival curves of mammalian cells irradiated by X-rays and neutrons in a fractionated dose experiment.

irradiation to produce the same level of survival as in the single-dose experiment (Figure 2.10). While for neutrons fractionation does not significantly influence the outcome, fractionated X-ray irradiation expands the shoulder of X-ray cell survival curve increasing the RBE.

In the fractionated irradiation experiment the ratio of X-ray dose to neutron dose which would give a surviving fraction of 0.1 is:

$$RBE_{HDfX} = \frac{700cGy}{200cGy} = 3.5 \qquad (2.14)$$

meaning that $RBE_{HDsingle} < RBE_{HDfractionated}$.

From the above examples one can conclude that RBE depends on the extent of biological damage and, consequently, on the amount of dose administered. RBE also depends on the dose rate, since the slope of the survival curve (obtained for sparsely ionising radiation) varies in accordance with dose rate. Because of variations in the capacity to repair sublethal damage among tissues, RBE will be higher for tissues with high repair capability, and lower for tissues with poor repair ability.

2.7.1 RBE as a function of LET

To quantitatively illustrate the dependence of RBE on the quality of radiation, the relative biological effectiveness has been plotted as a function of linear energy transfer (LET) (see Figure 2.11).

An increasing dependence of RBE with LET might be expected, since higher LET particles have a more damaging effect on tissues. However, Figure 2.11 shows that while this intuitive behaviour does occur up to ~100 keV, RBE starts to decrease with increasing LET above 100 keV/μm. Sparsely ionising radiation (low LET) has a low RBE since the distance between two consecutive ionisations from the same incident particle (single track) is too long to produce double strand breaks, and single strand breaks can be easily repaired. Therefore, low-LET radiation is inefficient because more than one particle has to hit the cell in order to

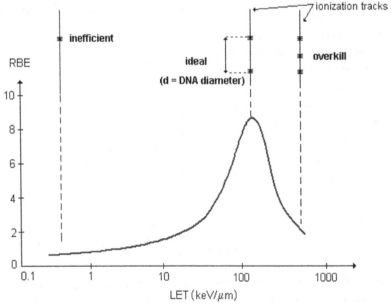

Figure 2.11. Plot of RBE versus LET.

produce irreparable damage. With increasing LET, the probability of causing double strand breaks during the same ionisation track increases. The optimum LET, and therefore the highest RBE is reached for 100 keV/μ, since the distance between two consecutive ionisation events resulting from this radiation equals the diameter of the DNA double helix. The reason for the decrease in RBE with more densely ionising radiation is the 'waste' of energy, which occurs for very close ionisation events. Once the double strand of the DNA is broken, subsequent ionising events (e.g. break in the base of the DNA from intermediate ionisation) are wasteful. The toxicity of the radiation per absorbed dose therefore decreases and so does the RBE because of this 'overkill effect'.

As demonstrated by research RBE is a complex, multifactorial-dependent quantity, determined by the following factors: radiation quality (LET), dose, dose rate and tissue type (biologic system).

2.8 THE OXYGEN EFFECT: OXYGEN ENHANCEMENT RATIO (OER)

It is a proven fact that well oxygenated tumours respond better to radiotherapy than poorly oxygenated ones. For tumours with high proportions of hypoxic cells (i.e. cells lacking oxygen), tumour hypoxia is one of the main reasons for treatment failure. The present section will describe the rationale behind the radioresistance of hypoxic tumours.

2.8.1 The oxygen 'fixation' hypothesis

Indirect interactions (Chapter 1) constitute approximately 70% of the total interactions between ionising radiation and DNA. Indirect action of radiation occurs when ionising radiation interacts with other atoms or molecules in the cell, especially water, to produce free radicals, with unpaired valence electrons that are able to damage the DNA in the cell.

The interaction of a photon (or charged particle) with the water molecule removes an outer shell electron to form the electron depleted (HOH+) or electron enhanced (HOH-) ions. These ions, being unstable, form the uncharged radicals OH* and H*. These radicals have an unpaired electron in the valence shell, designated by *. Unpaired electrons are very active, and achieve a lower state of energy by stripping an

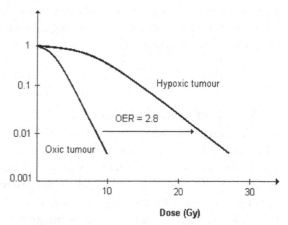

Figure 2.12. Plot of survival curves of oxic and hypoxic cells. Note that OER = 2.8, meaning that hypoxic cells need 2.8 times higher doses of radiation than oxic cells for the same endpoint (i.e. 1% survival) on cell survival.

electron from the neighbouring atom to form a stable pair of electrons with opposing spin.

$$H_2O \xrightarrow{\text{radiation}} H_2O^+ + e^-$$

$$H_2O^+ + H_2O \longrightarrow H_3O^+ + OH\,*$$

The hydroxyl radical can further interact with the cellular DNA, break chemical bonds, and initiate chemical changes that would result in biological damage. As long as the damage consists of a single strand break, this can be easily repaired. However, in the presence of molecular oxygen, the free radical interacts quickly with oxygen producing a more damaging molecule, hydrogen peroxide (H_2O_2), which leads to a non-restorable change in the chemical composition of the DNA exposed to ionising radiation.

Therefore, in the presence of oxygen, the DNA break is 'set', making it unrepairable in response to radiation. This process is called 'the oxygen fixation hypothesis' (here 'to fix' = 'to set', 'to make it permanent').

On the other hand, as the H_2O_2 cannot be formed in the absence of oxygen, hypoxic cells would easily repair the damage to their DNA. Therefore, hypoxic cells are more radioresistant than oxic cells due to their ability to repair radiation-induced damage.

2.8.2 Oxygen enhancement ratio (OER)

To illustrate the extent of radioresistance of hypoxic cells as compared to oxygenated cells, the quantity 'oxygen enhancement ratio' (OER) is defined as the ratio of doses without oxygen (hypoxic conditions) and with oxygen in order to produce the same biological effect (see Figure 2.12). Mathematically, OER is expressed as:

$$OER = \frac{D \ without \ O_2}{D \ with \ O_2}\bigg|_{ISOEFFECT} \quad (2.15)$$

2.8.3   OER as a function of LET

Experimental studies have shown that for most of the cells irradiated with X-rays the OER is around 3. This observation is generally valid for sparsely ionising radiation. With an increase in LET, or more densely ionising radiation, OER decreases (see Figure 2.13). For some high-LET particles (i.e. high energy neutrons, α-particles) OER decreases to unity. This means that the effect of the high-LET radiation is the same whether the tumour is well oxygenated or hypoxic, due to the clustered damage produced to the cell, causing poor repair in either well oxygenated or hypoxic condition.

Considering RBE and OER, one can conclude that for hypoxic and slowly proliferating tumours high-LET radiation might be more advantageous than low-LET radiation. The differences in radiosensitivity between hypoxic and oxic cells is reduced with high-LET radiation and head & neck cancers which have high proportions of hypoxic cells might benefit from high LET radiation such as neutrons. Slowly growing tumours are X-ray resistant, because a large

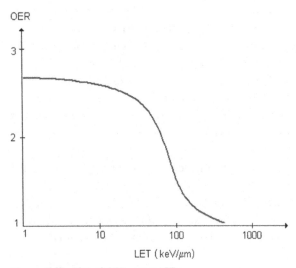

Figure 2.13. Plot of OER versus LET.

population of the cells are in the quiescent phase (G_0 which is resistant). However, the differences in resistance between cycling and non-cycling cells are reduced by high-LET radiation.

2.9   REFERENCES

Brenner D, Hlatky L, Hahnfeldt P, Hall E *et al.* (1995) A convenient extension of the linear-quadratic model to include redistribution and reoxygenation. *IJROBP* **32**: 379–390.

Douglas BG and Fowler JF (1976) The effect of multiple small doses of x rays on skin reactions in the mouse and a basic interpretation. *Radiation Research* **66**: 401–426.

Elkind MM, Sutton-Gilbert H, Moses W, Alescio T and Swain W (1965) Radiation response of mammalian cells grown in culture. V. Temperature dependence of the repair of X-ray damage in surviving cells (aerobic and hypoxic). *Radiation Research* **25**: 359–376.

Hall EJ (2000) *Radiobiology for the Radiologist.* 5th edn. Lippincott Williams & Wilkins, Philadelphia.

Hartwell L and Weinert T (1989) Checkpoints: controls that ensure the order of cell cycle events. *Science* **246**, 629–634.

Hewitt H and Wilson C (1959) A survival curve for mammalian cells irradiated in vivo. *Nature* **183**: 1060–1061.

Hill R and Bush R (1969) A lung-colony assay to determine the radiosensitivity of the cells of a solid tumour. *International Journal of Radiation Biology* **15**: 435–444.

King CR and Fowler JF (2001) A simple analytic derivation suggests that prostate cancer alpha/beta ratio is low. *International Journal of Radiation Oncology Biology Physics* **51**: 213–214.

Nias AHW (2000) *An Introduction to Radiobiology.* Wiley, UK.

Nurse P (2000) A long twentieth century of the cell cycle and beyond. *Cell* **100**: 71–78.

Overgaard M (1985) The clinical implication of non-standard fractionation. *IJROBP* **11**: 1225–1229.

Peters LJ, Ang KK and Thames HD (1988) Accelerated fractionation in the radiation treatment of head & neck cancer. *Acta Oncologica* **27**: 185–194.

Puck TT and Markus PI (1956) Action of x-rays on mammalian cells. *Journal of Experimental Medicine* **103**: 653–666.

Sinclair WK (1969) Dependence of radiosensitivity upon cell age. In *Proceedings of the Carmel Conference on Time and Dose relationships in Radiation Biology as Applied to Radiotherapy*. BNL Report 50203. pp. 97–107. Upton, New York.

Steel GG (Ed.) (2002) *Basic Clinical Radiobiology*. 3rd edn. Hodder Arnold, London.

Till J and McCulloch E (1961) A direct measurement of the radiation sensitivity of normal mouse bone marrow. *Radiation Research* **14**: 213–222.

Travis EL and Tucker SL (1987) Iso-effect models and fractionated radiotherapy. *IJROBP* **13**: 283–287.

Withers HR and Elkind MM (1970) Microcolony survival assay for cells of mouse intestinal mucosa exposed to radiation. *International Journal of Radiation Biology* **17**: 261–267.

3 Elements of radiotherapy physics

3.1 X-RAY AND PARTICLE GENERATORS

As mentioned in Chapter 1, the radiation sources can either be natural or anthropogenic (man-made). The man-made radiation sources are generally produced in nuclear reactors, X-ray tubes and accelerators.

3.1.1 Production of radioisotopes

The radioisotopes that decay via β^- decay mode can be obtained from natural radioactive series that contain a number of β^- emitters amongst the heavy elements of the radioactive chains. Fission reaction products are also rich in β^- emitting radioisotopes, e.g. ^{90}Sr, ^{137}Cs. Radio-carbon ^{14}C is made in nature when nitrogen in the atmosphere is hit by a cosmic ray:

$$^{14}N + n \rightarrow {^{14}C} + p \xrightarrow{\quad 5568y \quad} {^{14}N} + \beta^- + \tilde{\nu} \quad (3.1)$$

However, for most practical purposes, they are produced artificially in nuclear reactors in a neutron rich environment. β^- isotopes have an excess of neutrons, so in order to produce them, a nuclear reaction is used in which a stable isotope will absorb one or more neutrons to form an unstable β^- emitter, e.g.:

$$n + {^{59}_{27}Co} \rightarrow {^{60}_{27}Co} + \gamma \text{ or}$$

$$n + {^{107}Ag} \rightarrow {^{108}Ag} + \gamma \xrightarrow{\quad 2.4 \text{ min} \quad} {^{108}Cd} + \beta^- \quad (3.2)$$

If N is the number of radioactive nuclei in the radioisotope sample being produced in the nuclear reactor, then the rate at which N increases is a balance between isotope production and its depletion by radioactive decay:

$$\frac{dN}{dt} = \sigma N_{\text{Target}}\, n_{\text{flux}} - \lambda N \quad (3.3)$$

Where N_{Target} is the number of target atoms, n_{Flux} is the neutron flux, i.e. the number of neutrons per square meter per second passing through target and σ is the reaction cross-section in m^2 (probability that the reaction will occur). Therefore at time t, the number of radioactive nuclei in the sample will be:

$$N(t) = \frac{\sigma N_{\text{Target}}\, n_{\text{flux}}}{\lambda}(1 - e^{-\lambda t}) \quad (3.4)$$

The maximum obtainable radioisotope concentration (so-called saturation) occurs when the rate of formation equals the rate of decay and the corresponding saturation activity, A, is:

$$A = \sigma N_{\text{Target}}\, n_{\text{flux}} \quad (3.5)$$

When this condition is reached, the sample should be removed from the reactor and the radioisotope leached.

The first artificially created β^+ radioisotope was made by Pierre and Irene Joliot-Curie in Paris, 1932:

L. Marcu et al., *Biomedical Physics in Radiotherapy for Cancer*,
DOI 10.1007/978-0-85729-733-4_3, © CSIRO 2012

$^{10}B + \alpha \rightarrow {}^{13}N + n$, where ^{13}N decays as:

$$^{13}N \rightarrow {}^{13}C + \beta^+ + \nu \qquad (3.6)$$

There are no natural β^+ emitters (apart from negligible 0.001% in ^{40}K) and, as a result, they have to be man-made for any applications. β^+ emitters have an excess of protons compared to the stable isotopes. Consequently, to make a β^+ emitter, a proton needs to be 'inserted' into the stable nucleus and/or some neutrons have to be ejected. This process happens during high energy nuclear reactions using accelerators. Most β^+ isotopes are now produced in cyclotrons using proton and deuteron accelerated beams. β^+ emitters are used in nuclear medicine in Positron Emission Tomography (PET) imaging. Isotopes required are all short-lived, which can create problems with the timely delivery of sufficient amount of the required radioisotope. As a result, hospitals may need small medical cyclotrons on site to have an adequate supply of the emitters required. Some of the isotopes commonly used are:

$$\begin{aligned} {}^{16}O\,(p,\alpha){}^{13}N &\rightarrow T_{1/2} = 10\ \text{min} \\ {}^{18}O\,(p,n){}^{18}F &\rightarrow T_{1/2} = 90\ \text{min} \\ {}^{14}N\,(p,\alpha){}^{11}C &\rightarrow T_{1/2} = 20\ \text{min} \\ {}^{14}N\,(d,n){}^{15}O &\rightarrow T_{1/2} = 2\ \text{min} \end{aligned} \qquad (3.7)$$

3.1.2 Production of X-rays

X-rays are the most common radiation form used in radiation therapy. X-ray sources used in industry and medicine are almost exclusively man-made and their production is a two stage process: 1) electron acceleration; 2) X-ray generation during energetic electron interactions with the target material. The basic apparatus for X-ray generation includes: X-ray tube and accelerators.

3.1.3 X-ray tube

An X-ray tube is a highly evacuated glass bulb that contains essentially two electrodes: an anode made of platinum, tungsten, or another heavy metal of high melting point, and a cathode (see Figure 3.1).

The cathode is a metal filament coated with an electron emitting material (e.g. barium oxide) and it serves as the source of the electrons. These are released from the cathode through thermionic emission; i.e. the filament is heated up by a current passing through it (known as filament current), emitting electrons as the material heats up. The emitted electrons are then accelerated towards the anode in the electrostatic potential, U_a, set between the cathode and the anode. The energy, E, that the electrons will be accelerated to is:

$$E = qU_a\ [\text{eV}] \qquad (3.8)$$

where q is the electron charge and the unit of electron-Volt corresponds to kinetic energy of an electron when moving through potential difference of 1 Volt; i.e. $1\,\text{eV} = 1.6 \times 10^{-19}$ Joules. The stream of electrons between the cathode and the anode is known as the tube current and is usually measured in milliamps. Once the electrons hit the anode, they start interacting with the atomic electrons and the nuclei of the anode material. Much of the energy applied to the tube is transformed into heat at the focal spot of the anode (up to 99% depending on the electrons' energy). The remaining energy is spent in bremsstrahlung X-ray generation. The anode target is commonly made from tungsten, which has a high melting point in addition to a high atomic number. High atomic number maximises the X-ray yield, while high melting point preserves the anode. However, cooling of the anode is still required. Water or oil recirculating systems are often used to cool X-ray tubes.

The voltage/potential applied in the X-ray tube defines the maximum X-ray energy and influences the shape of the X-ray spectrum. Low energy X-rays from a thin anode have a dipole radiation pattern; i.e. the intensity (number) of photons as a function of angle from the original electron trajectory is:

$$I(\theta) \sim \sin^2(\theta) \qquad (3.9)$$

This means that the X-rays will be emitted in a ring around the electron trajectory, with the highest intensity at a 90° angle. No X-rays will be radiated along the initial electron trajectory (0 degrees). For high energy X-rays (electron velocity close to speed of light), relativistic effects cause forward peaking of the angular distribution.

3.1.4 Accelerators

Radioactive sources can yield particle projectiles of up to 15 MeV kinetic energy for some isotopes (however much lower energies of about 4 MeV on average can

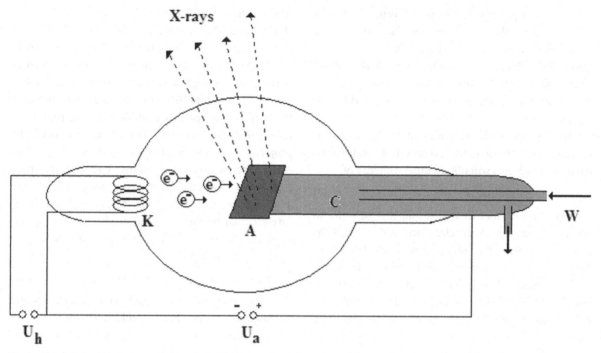

Figure 3.1 Schematic diagram of the principle of operation of an X-ray tube.

generally be obtained). Radioactive sources are to these days used in a specialised area of radiation therapy, known as brachytherapy.

Cosmic rays contain particles and γ rays of energies up to 10^{13} MeV. But intensities are very low (and not really controllable or useful for practical purposes). Consequently, there is a need for another source of high-energy particles and X-rays, where we can control energies, obtain sufficiently high intensities of particles in the beam and/or have a choice of projectiles. That means there is a need for a particle accelerator. Only the very basic accelerator principles will be covered here as there is numerous literature available detailing the operational principles of these devices. For additional reading, for example (Greene and Williams 1997) is recommended.

All particle accelerators use the effect of electric potential on charged particles, i.e. use some sort of accelerating electrodes. Only charged particles or ions (not neutral atoms, neutrons, etc.) can be accelerated. In general the basic components of an accelerator are: 1) particle or ion source, 2) accelerating electrodes, 3) electromagnetic fields to deflect particles (i.e. control their trajectory), 4) beam line with target and detecting system.

The first accelerators were intended to study fundamental interactions and the structure of nuclei. Later accelerators were developed for radiotherapy of cancer patients, implantation of materials for industry and solid state and material sciences (e.g. semiconductor doping). According to the trajectory along which particles are accelerated, accelerators can be divided into two main categories:

1. *Linear*; i.e. the particle beam is accelerated on a linear path. These include electrostatic accelerators (Van de Graaff generator, tandems) and resonant accelerators.
2. *Circular or Cyclic*; i.e. the particle beam is accelerated on a circular path. These include cyclotron, betatron, synchrotron, $e^- e^+$.

Linear accelerators

Static linear accelerators

A typical example of a static linear accelerator is the *Van de Graaff accelerator*. Basically, it is a high voltage generator with an evacuated electrostatic tube (see Figure 3.2). It contains a motor driven pulley, an insulating rubber belt, metal combs and a charge terminal. The first metal comb draws electrons from the belt, thus building positive charge in the belt. The belt is conveyed through to the terminal where the second comb collects the charge and spreads it over the terminal (while the other electrode is grounded). Voltage potentials of up to 1–2 million Volts can be generated in this manner, compared to several hundred kV for an X-ray tube.

Once again, if the terminal of the generator is charged to create a voltage, V, across the tube, then the particle of charge q will obtain kinetic energy of:

$$E = qV \qquad (3.10)$$

It is obvious from this equation, that in order to obtain higher particle acceleration energies, one has to keep increasing the voltage or use particles/ions of larger charge (i.e. atoms stripped of more electrons). Both of these methods have practical and physical limitations, as once a maximum voltage potential is reached for a given design, further voltage increase will result in discharge/sparking. Also for protons, charge larger than 1 cannot be obtained.

In a *tandem accelerator*, an electron is firstly attached to a projectile to create a negatively charged particle (for example a negative carbon ion). The terminal is in the middle section of accelerator (see Figure 3.3) and is charged positively, so the particle is accelerated speeding towards it. At the terminal, the projectile passes through a thin carbon stripper foil, which rids the projectile of some or all of its electrons (for example changing the $12C^{-1}$ ion to $12C^{+6}$ ion). The particle will be now positively charged and therefore repelled by the terminal, yielding further acceleration. The total kinetic energy obtained, if n electrons are stripped, is:

$$E = (1 + nq)V \qquad (3.11)$$

As mentioned above, high voltage electrostatic accelerators may have problems with sparks

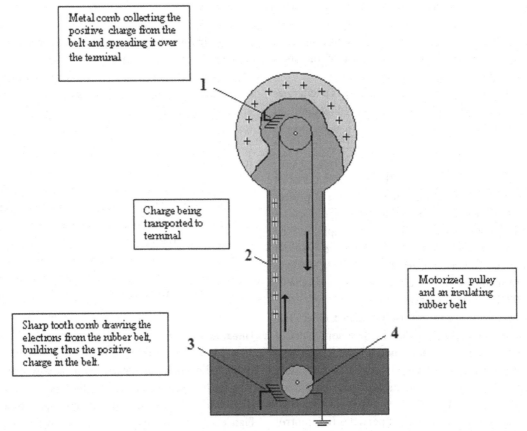

Figure 3.2. Schematic diagram of a Van de Graaff accelerator.

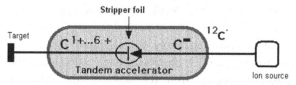

Figure 3.3. Schematic diagram of a tandem accelerator. The example showing the acceleration of carbon ions.

(discharge) and voltage stability. SF_6 gas is used to fill the space between the electrodes in order to prevent discharge between electrodes.

Resonant linear accelerators

In these accelerators, the particles are moving in a high-frequency alternating electromagnetic (EM) field along the accelerating tube. As a result, synchronisation must be achieved between the movement of the particle and the frequency of EM field. The particle trajectory is enveloped by a series of drift tubes of increasing length (see Figure 3.4). The particle is only being accelerated in the space between the tubes. There is no electric field inside the tubes themselves. As the particle moves towards the drift tube it is accelerated, this means that the tube entrance must have an opposite charge to the particle. Once the particle is inside the tube, the EM field reverses its polarity, and the exit of the drift tube will now have the same charge as the particle and will be repelling it. At the same time, the entrance of the subsequent tube will be of opposite polarity, further accelerating the particle.

The length of the tube, L, is related to the particle velocity, v, (on entrance) as:

$$L = vt \qquad (3.12)$$

where $t = \frac{1}{2}T$ is half of the period of the EM field alteration and the time that the particle spends inside the tube. The length is therefore related to the frequency of EM field, f, as:

$$L = \frac{v}{2f} \qquad (3.13)$$

The kinetic energy of a particle going through the kth gap in a potential, V, between the drift tubes will then be:

$$E = \frac{1}{2}mv^2 = kqV \qquad (3.14)$$

To ensure synchronisation (i.e. particle movement between the drift tubes must be in resonance with the phase of the electromagnetic field); the length of the tubes has to increase with the increasing particle velocity. The length of the kth tube then is:

$$L_k = \frac{1}{f}\sqrt{k\frac{q}{m}V} \qquad (3.15)$$

It is clear that unlike electrostatic accelerators or X-ray tubes where the beam of accelerated particles can be continuous, for resonant accelerators, the synchronisation is achieved only for a bunch/group of particles injected into the accelerator at the right time to be captured by the required phase of the EM field. Particles entering the accelerating tube ahead or behind of this moment will not be accelerated. As a result, resonant accelerators operate with pulsed sources of particles.

The relations above are more complicated for relativistic particles. Obviously, the larger the length of

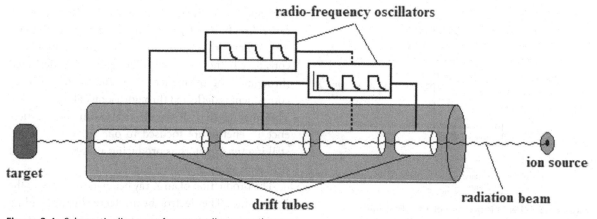

Figure 3.4. Schematic diagram of resonant linear accelerator.

the accelerating structure, the larger the energy of the accelerated particles. However, construction of large length accelerators is not practical; as a result cyclic accelerators have been developed.

Medical Resonant Linear Accelerators for X-ray production

In radiotherapy, X-ray energies in the MV region are required, so that the depth penetration is better and larger doses can be delivered to deep seated tumours. However, megavoltage X-rays of high intensities covering larger areas cannot be easily produced using an X-ray-tube. To increase efficiency of high-energy X-ray production, particle (electron) accelerators are used. Accelerators most commonly used for X-ray production are: linear accelerators (Linac), betatrons, and synchrotrons.

For medical purposes, linear accelerators are used almost exclusively.

A schematic flow chart of the components of a medical linac is shown in Figure 3.5. In linear accelerators, bunches of electrons (b) from the electron gun (a) are accelerated in the copper structure, called the waveguide (c), by means of an energy transfer from the high power oscillating electromagnetic fields of radio frequencies (microwaves).

Microwave generators (d) are used to provide microwave power to the waveguides to accelerate the pulse of electrons from the electron gun. There are two types of microwave generator tubes commonly used in the medical linear accelerators, i.e. the klystron and magnetron. The frequency of the microwaves produced by the klystron is about 3 GHz, and the corresponding wavelength is about 10 cm. The microwaves from the klystrons are fed into the accelerator structure via the waveguide. The linac is under high vacuum at all times.

The electron beam has to be actively steered through the accelerator system by the use of two orthogonal dipoles formed by pairs of beam steering coils (e). Moreover, as the electrons are accelerated through the guide they are subject to forces that will tend to make the beam diverge. Focusing fields required are provided by an additional series of solenoids, known as focusing foils (e). The electron beam leaving the accelerating structure continues through an evacuated bending magnet system (f). It is deflected magnetically either so as to strike a target (g) for X-ray therapy or to exit through the treatment head for electron therapy (h). There are two configurations generally used in medical linear accelerators, i.e. 90° and 270° bending. The radius of curvature of the electron beam is dependent on the electron energy and therefore the 90° bending system acts as an energy spectrometer. The purpose of the 270° angle bending system is to accomplish achromatic bending so that the electrons will strike the X-ray target or pass through the exit window at the same point and in the same direction independently of their energy (Figure 3.6). When the angular and energy distributions are considered, the low energy component is deflected through a loop of smaller radius and the high energy component is deflected through a loop of larger radius. This ensures that all the electrons with slight difference in energy are focused to one small spot when striking the target, thus producing an X-ray treatment field with sharper defined edges.

The production of an X-ray beam itself begins at the X-ray target. The electron beam steered by the bending magnet hits the surface of the X-ray target at 90°. As

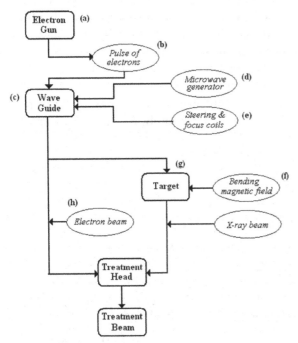

Figure 3.5 Schematic diagram of a medical linear accelerator components.

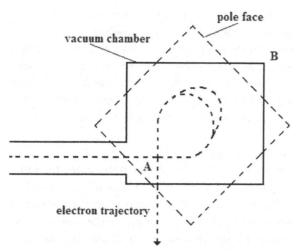

Figure 3.6. Schematic diagram of electron trajectory bending in a 270˚ angle bending system. (Reprinted from Greene and Williams 1997. Copyright (1997), with permission from Taylor & Francis Group LLC – Books)

the electron beam penetrates the target material, Coulomb interactions between the electron beam and the atomic electrons and the protons in the nuclei of the target material occur. Coulomb interactions of accelerated electrons with protons result in bremsstrahlung X-ray generation. This is the main process through which the X-rays in the linac head are produced. A picture of a Varian medical linear accelerator is shown in Figure 3.7. Some components of the linac system will be now discussed.

Waveguide

Waveguides are devices designed to carry electromagnetic waves from one place to another without significant loss in intensity. There are two waveguides employed in linear accelerators. The first waveguide conducts microwaves from the microwave generator and feeds them into the second accelerating waveguide which is used to accelerate electrons to nominal energies. Inside this copper structure microwaves produce currents flowing in the copper that in turn generate oscillating electric fields pointing along the length of the structure as well as oscillating magnetic fields pointing in a circle around the interior of the accelerator pipe. A pattern of alternating electro-magnetic

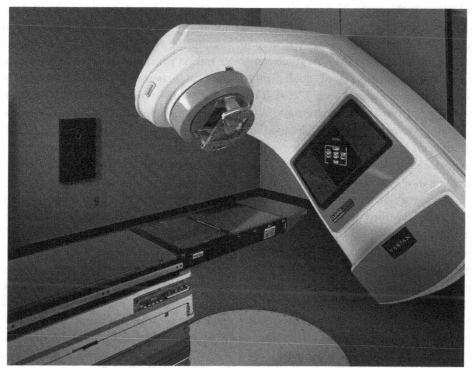

Figure 3.7. A picture of a high energy 2100C Varian medical linear accelerator. (Courtesy and Copyright ©2009, Varian Medical Systems, Inc. All rights reserved.)

waves develops that forces electrons to travel and accelerate down the pipe. The electrons are accelerated along the length of the waveguide. The longer the waveguide the higher the velocity gained. However, at higher energies, the energy gained by acceleration is almost all due to the mass gained, as electrons will be moving close to the speed of light.

The length of the waveguide must be a multiple of the wavelength, so waveguides are only practical for electromagnetic waves in the microwave range, with wavelengths, λ, on the scale of a few centimetres. As mentioned before, if a microwave oscillation is set up at one end of a waveguide, its electric field causes electric currents to flow in the copper walls. These currents in turn induce new electric and magnetic fields in the waveguide, oscillating with the same frequency as the original microwave. The net effect is that the microwave travels along the copper pipe of radius, a, in the transverse magnetic field with the phase velocity, v_p:

$$v_p = \frac{c}{\sqrt{1 - (\lambda/2.16a)^2}} \qquad (3.16)$$

This velocity represents the movement of the electric field pattern along the guide. This velocity must be known and controlled in order to keep electrons in the accelerating phase of the wave.

From the design point of view, the waveguide consists of a series of circular cavities placed equidistantly along the copper tube (see Figure 3.8 on p. 209). It is evacuated to allow free movement of electrons. Two types of accelerating waveguide are generally used in modern linacs that are based on: a) travelling wave; b) standing wave principles.

In the travelling wave system the microwaves propagate through the waveguide towards the final cavity, where they are either absorbed or exit the waveguide and dissipate in a resistive load (there is no wave reflected back into the waveguide). This means that at any one time only one in four cavities has the right phase of the EM field, e.g. maximum positive amplitude, to accelerate the electrons (see Figure 3.9 top).

In the standing wave system both waveguide ends are terminated, using a conducting disc. The microwave power is reflected from both ends, generating standing waves in the waveguide. This means that at all times, there is zero electric field in every second

cavity and therefore it cannot contribute towards electron acceleration. These cavities only transfer electrons between the neighbouring cavities on each side where acceleration does occur. As a result, the current designs have these coupling cavities shifted to the sides of the waveguide structure, shortening the lengths of the waveguide by 50% (see Figure 3.9 bottom).

Treatment head

Once the X-rays are produced in the target, their distribution is strongly peaked forward and requires shaping and absorption of undesired radiation. As a result, following the X-ray target is the primary collimator. It is designed to absorb all unwanted sections of the X-ray field. Tungsten is often used in their design because of its high atomic number providing effective attenuation. The produced X-ray beam has an angular distribution that is strongly peaked forward, which is not desired for current clinical radiotherapy practice. A more uniform angular distribution of the photon beam is achieved by passing it through a flattening filter. The material of the flattening filter is generally lead or copper depending on the beam energy or manufacturer. Following the flattening filter are the monitoring system and the mirror. The monitoring system consists of four quadrants of ion chambers which are fixed in the beam direction. The ion chambers measure the radiation beam dose output in terms of Monitor Units (MU) and symmetry of the radiation beam. They are essential to ensure that the right amount/quantity of radiation has exited the linac treatment head. The mirror underneath the monitor chamber system is used to project light from the optical source to replicate the shape of the radiation field. The angle and position of the mirror and the light source are carefully aligned so that the light field is coincident with the radiation field. These components are designed in such a way so that they have minimal effect on the radiation beam. Below the mirror are two sets of jaws which constitute a secondary collimator (see Figure 3.10). These are movable tungsten blocks with sufficient thicknesses to absorb unwanted radiation and to define the radiation field size. The jaws move in an arc shape to account for the divergence of the X-ray beam. Other components such as the multi-leaf collimators and wedges can also be

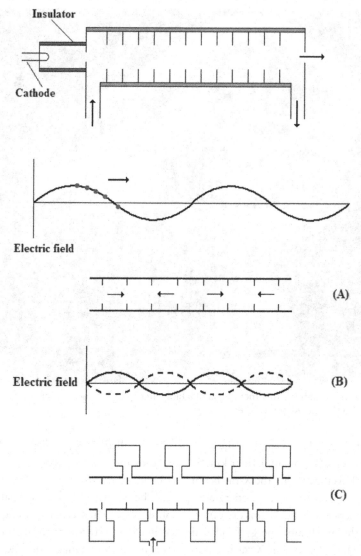

Insulator

Cathode

Electric field

(A)

Electric field (B)

(C)

Figure 3.9. Schematic diagram of a travelling wave (top) and standing wave waveguides (bottom). (Reprinted from Greene and Williams 1997. Copyright (1997), with permission from Taylor & Francis Group LLC – Books)

mounted to the head. These components are generally made of tungsten and steel alloys. They enable customisation and conformation of the intensity and shape of the radiation beam, entering a patient, for complex treatment targets, providing good tumour/target coverage and shielding of healthy tissues. Modern linacs are also capable of producing both X-ray and electron beams. In the electron mode, the X-ray target and the flattening filter are replaced by a pair of electron scattering foils which are mounted on a carousel. The foils cause the narrow accelerated electron

beam to scatter resulting in a broad, uniform dose distribution at a reference plane (see Figure 3.11).

Characterisation of megavoltage X-rays
X-ray beams produced in linear accelerators (and X-ray tubes) are always heterogeneous, polyenergetic; i.e. the beams contain photons with the whole range of energies. The maximum energy possible is given by the energy of the initial accelerated electron beam (and therefore accelerating potential); as the electrons cannot produce X-rays of energies higher than their own

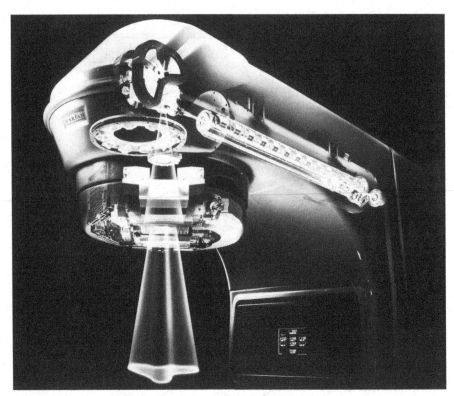

Figure 3.10. A cross-section through the treatment head of a high energy Varian linear accelerator. (Courtesy and Copyright ©2009, Varian Medical Systems, Inc. All rights reserved.)

due to conservation of energy. For example if the electrons are accelerated in a 4 MV potential, their kinetic energy will be 4 MeV. This means that the X-ray beam produced will contain a spectrum of X-ray energies of up to 4 MeV (E_{max}). As a result, X-ray beams are generally characterised by the maximum energy produced (peak voltage) in MV. The polyenergetic X-ray beam in this example would therefore be called a 4 MV X-ray beam. As a rule of thumb, the mean energy of X-rays in the beam is about 1/3 of $E_{max.}$

Cyclic accelerators

Cyclotron
Cyclic accelerators have enabled to increase the acceleration length considerably using a circular trajectory. Particles are maintained on circular paths by means of magnetic fields perpendicular to the plane of their trajectory.

The cyclotron, the most typical example of a cyclic accelerator, consists of two evacuated magnetic semi-

circles called Dees (see Figure 3.12). In each Dee there is a magnetic field perpendicular to its plane. A high frequency electromagnetic field acts on charged particles between the Dees. The particles are only being accelerated when crossing the gap between the Dees. While the particles are inside the Dees, they are under the influence of a magnetic field only, which will cause their trajectory to curve and return back into the space between the Dees. As the particles will be each time entering the accelerating gap in the opposite direction, the phase of the EM field must be modulated (polarity reversed), so that at the very instance of the particle entering the gap, it must find itself in the accelerating field; i.e. must be attracted and accelerated towards the opposing Dee. The diameter, r, of particle trajectory increases with increasing energy. When a diameter close to the dimension of the Dees is reached, the particle will leave the accelerator and hit the target.

The total force acting on a particle of charge, q, and velocity, $\vec{v}$, is the sum of electric ($\vec{E}$) and magnetic forces ($\vec{B}$):

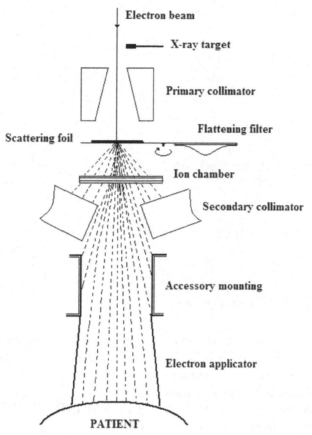

Electron beam

X-ray target

Primary collimator

Flattening filter

Scattering foil

Ion chamber

Secondary collimator

Accessory mounting

Electron applicator

PATIENT

Figure 3.11. A cross-section through the treatment head of a high energy linear accelerator in electron mode.

$$\vec{F}=q\vec{E} + q(\vec{v}\,x\vec{B}) \qquad (3.17)$$

The particle velocity is related to the radius, r, of the trajectory and orbiting frequency, f, as:

$$v = 2\pi r f \qquad (3.18)$$

The diameter of the trajectory is then given by:

$$r = \frac{mv_{x,y}}{qB} \qquad (3.19)$$

The frequency of the electromagnetic field, f_e, must match the orbiting frequency in order to achieve synchronisation and is equal to:

$$f_e = \frac{qB}{2\pi m} \qquad (3.20)$$

For a particle of constant mass, this frequency does not depend on the radius of the particle's orbit, as the time the particles spend inside the Dee is the same for all radii and all particle energies. While the particles continue to accelerate and gain speed, the radius of their trajectory increases and therefore they travel more distance in the same time, so as the particle beam spirals out, the frequency does not need to change.

Synchrotron

A synchrocyclotron is an accelerator in which the frequency of the driving alternating electric field is varied to compensate for the mass gain of the accelerated particles as their velocity approaches the speed of light. This is in contrast to the classical cyclotron, where the frequency is kept constant.

A synchrotron represents the current generation of cyclic accelerators. It consists of an accelerating ring of a given circumference, therefore the radius of rotation is constant (see Figure 3.13). It maintains a constant driving frequency of the electromagnetic field in the accelerating gap and it compensates for the relativistic mass gain of the accelerated particles by increasing the magnetic field, $\vec{B}$, to keep the radius constant as the

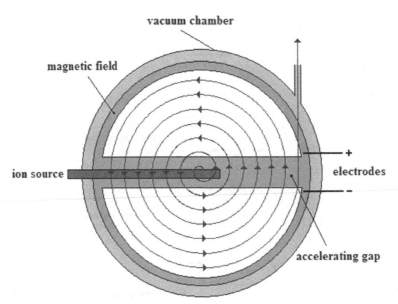

Figure 3.12. Schematic diagram of a cyclotron accelerator.

particle energy increases (equation 3.19); i.e. while magnetic field is constant for cyclotrons, it increases for synchrotrons. Similar to resonant accelerators, in order to achieve synchronisation between the increasing particle energy and changes of the magnetic field, the synchrotron uses pulses/bunches of particles, while in cyclotrons the particle beam can be continuous. Synchrotrons provide variable energy of the accel-

erated particles. They are also capable of producing much greater beam currents than cyclotrons.

3.2   RADIATION QUANTITIES AND UNITS

In general, a radiation beam consists of a large number of particles moving through space/medium in

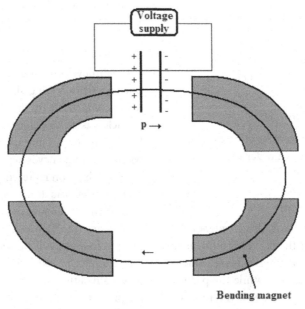

Figure 3.13. Schematic diagram of a synchrotron accelerator.

which it undergoes interactions. Thus there are two general quantities associated with a radiation beam: number of particles and the energy carried by these particles. In addition, basic radiation quantities reflect the ability of ionising radiation to produce free charge and to deposit energy.

3.2.1 Particle fluence

If dN is the number of particles (for example photons) in a radiation beam, incident on a sphere of cross-sectional area, dA, then the particle fluence, Φ, is given by:

$$\Phi = \frac{dN}{dA} \; [\text{m}^{-2}] \qquad (3.21)$$

3.2.2 Energy fluence

If dE is the energy transported by the particles incident on a sphere of cross-sectional dA, then the energy fluence Ψ is defined as:

$$\Psi = \frac{dE}{dA} \; [\text{J/m}^2] \qquad (3.22)$$

If E is the energy of a particle and dN represents the number of particles with energy E then the energy fluence can be calculated from particle fluence by using the following equation:

$$\Psi = \frac{dN}{dA} E = \Phi E \qquad (3.23)$$

However, almost all practical X-ray and particle beams are polyenergetic; i.e. they contain particles with a spectrum of energies. As a result, the particle fluence is replaced by the differential particle fluence, $\Phi_E(E)$, corresponding to a single energy bin E, also known as the particle fluence spectrum:

$$\Phi_E(E) = \frac{d^2 N(E)}{dA dE} = \frac{d\Phi(E)}{dE} \qquad (3.24)$$

The same concept is also used for energy fluence. The differential energy fluence is defined as:

$$\Psi_E(E) = \frac{d\Psi(E)}{dE} = \frac{d\Phi(E)}{dE} E \qquad (3.25$$

The differential energy fluence is also called the energy fluence spectrum.

3.2.3 Exposure

The exposure is a quantity that reflects the ability of radiation to ionise air. It is the absolute value of the charge, dQ, of the ions of one sign produced in air when all of the electrons liberated in a volume element of air (of mass dm) are completely stopped in air:

$$X = \frac{dQ}{dm} \; [\text{C/kg}] \qquad (3.26)$$

The old unit of exposure was 1 R (Roentgen), where $1\text{R} = 2.58 \times 10^{-4}$ C/kg. Since 1 cm^3 of air weighs 1.239×10^{-6} kg (at standard pressure and temperature conditions) in order to produce 1 free ion pair in air, approximately 33.85 eV (i.e. 33.85 Joules/Coulomb) of energy is needed. Consequently exposure of 1 R will result in 0.00873 J/kg dose in the air.

3.2.4 Exposure rate

This is a useful quantity that provides a simple way of calculating the exposure near a radioactive γ source. If Γ is the exposure rate constant in $\text{Jkg}^{-1}\text{m}^2\text{s}^{-1}\text{Bq}^{-1}$, then the exposure rate X/t of the source at a distance, d, is:

$$\frac{X}{t} \propto \frac{\text{Activity}}{(\text{dist})^2} = \frac{\Gamma A}{d^2} \; [\text{Ckg}^{-1}\text{s}^{-1}] \qquad (3.27)$$

Values of Γ are measured and tabulated for various radioactive sources. The formula assumes that the source is a point source. This is a simplification; however, the formula can be used to estimate exposure around an object containing a radioactive source (e.g. person injected with radioisotope). Only γ radiation is taken into consideration in the formula. For example the Γ value for ^{131}I is 7.647×10^{-5} mJkg^{-1} m^2/h/MBq.

3.2.5 Kerma

Kinetic Energy Released in Matter represents the amount of energy transferred, E_{TR}, from the X-ray beam to charged particles in the form of kinetic energy per unit mass in the medium of interest, and so has the unit J/kg, which is given the special name Gray (Gy):

$$K = \frac{dE_{TR}}{dm} \; [\text{J/kg} = \text{Gy}] \qquad (3.28)$$

3.2.6 Absorbed dose

This quantity is a measure of the energy absorbed in a medium by ionising radiation. It is the energy absorbed, E_{AB}, deposited per unit mass of medium, and also so has the unit Gray (Gy):

$$D = \frac{dE_{AB}}{dm} \; [\text{J/kg} = \text{Gy}] \qquad (3.29)$$

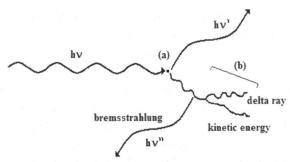

Figure 3.14. Schematic of energy transfer and energy deposition by X-rays. The X-ray of energy, $h\nu$, interacts at point (a), transferring its energy to an electron (kerma) and to a scattered X-ray of energy, $h\nu'$. Energy absorption (dose) occurs along the electron trajectory (b) as it comes to a stop in a medium. Dose is also deposited by secondary electrons if they have sufficient energy to cause ionisation tracks of their own.

3.2.7 Relationship between exposure, kerma and absorbed dose

X-rays do not deposit their energy in a medium directly. In fact, the energy transfer from X-rays to the medium is a two-stage process: Firstly energy is transferred (kerma) to electrons of the medium and then it is absorbed in the medium (dose) through stopping and interactions of electrons. Kinetic energy of electrons is lost by ionisation, excitation, bremsstrahlung, lattice and/or molecular vibrations, heat and therefore absorbed in the medium. This means that the process of energy transfer does not happen at the same place as the energy absorption. The energy is absorbed further down the stream (i.e. at a greater depth into the medium) from the point of initial X-ray interaction. The process is explained in Figure 3.14.

3.2.8 Electronic equilibrium

The quantity kerma is related to energy fluence of an X-ray beam. Absorbed dose can only be related to energy fluence if there is an equilibrium between kerma and dose. This situation happens in a medium, when so-called electronic equilibrium is reached; i.e. in this region of medium as many electrons come to complete rest as are set into motion by impinging photons. The dose can be then related to kerma as:

$$D = K(1 - g) \tag{3.30}$$

where g is the fraction of energy lost in radiative processes (bremsstrahlung).

Electronic equilibrium is established at a certain depth beyond the surface depending on the X-ray energy. The region at the surface of the medium, before the equilibrium is reached is called the **build-up region.** The electrons set in motion may travel up to several centimetres through the medium and may even escape if the medium is thin. The concept is illustrated in Figure 3.15. Note that for the realistic case of photon attenuation, the true (exact) equilibrium is never reached. The absorbed dose will be slightly higher then kerma at a given depth in the absorber, as the dose is related to kerma (energy transferred) further up-stream, where the number of interacting photons was higher.

In the build-up region, the energy deposition increases with depth, until the depth, D, is reached, when the dose will reach its maximum. This depth is called depth of maximum dose, D_{max}. The depth of maximum dose is roughly equal to the range of secondary electrons in the medium, i.e. it will depend on the electron (and therefore on the incident photon) energy. D_{max} for a 6 MV X-ray beam from a linear accelerator is at about 1.5 cm depth in water. D_{max} for an 18 MV X-ray beam is at ~3.5 cm in water (for the radiation field size of about 10×10 cm^2). After reaching D_{max}, the dose will attenuate exponentially, as more and more photons are exponentially removed from the beam. The function describing the dependence of the absorbed dose on the depth into the absorber is known as a depth dose curve. The percentage depth dose curve expresses the dose deposition at depth relative to dose at D_{max} (100%). Percentage depth dose curves of 6 and 18 MV X-ray beams from Siemens KD-2 linear accelerator attenuating in water are shown in Figure 3.16.

The build-up effect, due to the subsequent deposition of secondary particle energies is more marked for higher energy photon beams, where the range of liberated electrons can be up to several cm (this is valid for low Z materials like water). The range of electrons in water is about 0.5 cm per MeV. The build-up effect has a significant consequence in radiotherapy, as the maximum dose is not at the skin surface but deeper inside tissue. This enables sparing of the skin during the treatment and to deposit the dose more effectively at the position of the disease. At low photon energies (200 kV), the secondary electron range is short so the

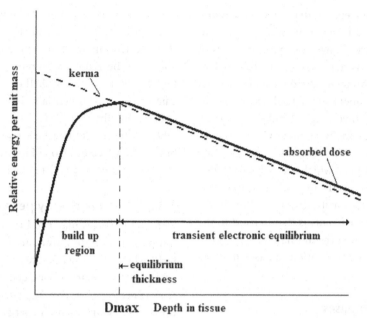

Figure 3.15. The relationship between kerma and dose as a function of depth into the medium, displaying the attenuation of the X-ray beam.

deposited dose as a function of depth has very similar shape to the exponential distribution discussed in Chapter 1.

3.3 RADIATION DOSE MEASUREMENTS

Determination of the absorbed dose is one of the main objectives for the majority of studies or applications of ionising radiation. Even more so, if radiation is used to treat cancer where precise amounts of dose are deposited during the course of treatment. There are three basic methods currently used for determination of absorbed dose to water: calorimetry, chemical dosimetry and ionisation dosimetry. The only direct method of measuring absorbed dose is by calorimetry; i.e. measurement of temperature change of the

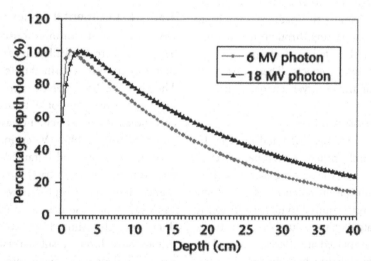

Figure 3.16. Relative percentage depth dose curves of 6 and 18 MV X-ray beams from Siemens KD-2 linear accelerator attenuating in water. The curves are normalised to the maximum dose. (Courtesy Royal Adelaide Hospital)

medium, as a result of energy deposited by passing radiation. This method is not straightforward due to very small temperature changes for typical ranges of radiation doses and has not become widely adopted. At present dose measurements are done using devices called ionisation chambers submerged in water, followed by calculations involving a number of correction factors derived from Bragg-Gray Cavity theory (Gray 1936; Rogers 1995). Determination of dose using ionisation chambers, which are small gas filled instruments, is indirect, as the ionisation produced by radiation within the gas cavity inserted in an irradiated medium is measured. This is then related to the energy absorbed in that surrounding medium. So in order to determine dose, ionisation in gases must be understood first.

3.3.1   Ionisation in gases

An atom is ionised when one or more orbital electrons are removed, leaving a positively charged ion and one or more free electrons. As discussed in Chapter 1, ionisation may be produced through inelastic collisions between a high velocity charged particle such as an electron, a proton, or even a nuclear fission fragment with the atomic electrons of a material. Ionisation may also be produced by collision of energetic particles with a molecule, breaking a bond and leaving the two separate parts with a positive and a negative charge. The bombarding particle, such as heavy ions, may even gain or lose charge as it proceeds through a material, resulting in ionisation of the medium. Ionisation is also caused by X-rays passing through the material and interacting with the atomic electrons through photo-electric or Compton effects. These processes generate free electrons and positively charged ions.

3.3.2   Ionisation potential

Electrons are bound in atomic shells and in order to remove an electron and produce an ion pair, energy must be spent to overcome the binding energy. This is also known as the ionisation potential of the atom. For example, the energy required to ionise a nitrogen atom is 14.5 eV. As atoms have a number of electrons (apart from hydrogen) placed at different energy levels, it is necessary to specify which energy shell the electron has been removed from, since the ionisation

potential is different for different shells; only a few electron volts may be required to remove an outer-shell electron in an atom, while tens of kilo-electron volts may be required to remove a K-shell electron (e.g. it is 88 keV for a K-shell electron of a lead atom). The ionisation potentials have been determined experimentally and can be found in atomic data tables. After ionisation, the ion will eventually recombine with a free electron. The energy of binding the electron is generally emitted as a single photon.

3.3.3   Average energy per ion pair, W

Charged particles may produce tens of thousands of ion pairs before they come to a complete stop. Similarly, when an X-ray liberates a secondary electron, a cascade of ion pairs will be generated along the electron trajectory. The average energy required to produce an ion pair by a high energy particle is known as the W value of the atom or molecule. This average energy loss is of particular relevance in radiation dosimetry. If a charged particle of energy E is stopping in gas (e.g. air), the number of ion pairs, N, produced when all of the energy of the charged particle is absorbed is:

$$E = WN \tag{3.31}$$

The value of W in a gas is always larger than the ionisation potential itself, since some energy is also lost in other processes such as excitation.

3.3.4   Experimental values of W for gases

One of the most common ion-chamber gases is air, because of its ready availability and because of the fact that the exposure is defined in terms of air ionisation. Therefore, air has received more attention in experimental measurements of W than any other gas. Probably the earliest measurement was made by Rutherford and McClung in 1900 (Valentine and Curran 1958). They used X-rays and obtained a value of 88 eV/ip (electron volts per ion pair), a value about 2.6 times higher than that accepted now. Much experimental work on W of various gases, including air, has been done since that time. Improved experimental techniques have brought substantial agreement among careful, independent measurements on many of the more common gases (Valentine and Curran 1958;

Table 3.1. Average W values for some gases.

air	33.85
oxygen	31.8
hydrogen	36.6
ethane	24.6
CO_2	32.9
H_2O (vap)	30.1

Whyte 1963). A sample of average W values for some gases are shown in Table 3.1 (for X-ray and γ-ray interactions only).

3.3.5 Ionisation in solids

In addition to ionisation chambers, semiconductor detectors (e.g. diodes and mosfets) are used for dosimetry purposes. These also work on the principle of ionisation and generation of charge as a result of passing radiation. However, instead of ion pairs, as in gases, electron-hole pairs are generated in a semiconductor. Whenever a charged particle loses energy in a solid, electrons make a transition from the valence band to the conduction band. The hole left in the valence band behaves like a positively charged particle. Recombination happens when an electron makes a transition back to the valence band.

In addition to energy loss in electron-hole pair production, radiation energy is also lost to lattice excitations and vibrations, or into sub-ionisation electron energy. The energy required to produce an electron-hole pair, W, in this case is (Shockley and Queisser 1961):

$$W = E_g + rE_r + 2E_f \qquad (3.32)$$

where, E_g is the energy of the band gap in a semiconductor, r is the number of phonons (generated per ionisation event), E_r is the phonon energy, and E_f is the residual electron (or hole) energy after an electron-hole pair is formed.

3.3.6 Bragg-Gray cavity theory

As mentioned in Section 3.2, it is the electrons liberated in X-ray interactions that deposit dose in a medium. Consequently, the absorbed dose to a

medium, D_{med}, at point P is related to the electron fluence in the medium Φ_{med}, as follows:

$$D_{med} = \Phi \left(\frac{S_{col}}{\rho} \right)_{med} \qquad (3.33)$$

where $(S_{col}/\rho)_{med}$ is the unrestricted mass collision stopping power of the medium at the energy of the electron (introduced in Chapter 1). This relation is valid under the condition that there exists charged particle equilibrium (CPE) within an irradiated medium; i.e. the number of secondary electrons leaving the medium volume around point P is equal to the charged particles entering the volume.

In order to measure the absorbed dose at point P in the medium, it is necessary to introduce a radiation detector (dosimeter) into the medium; i.e. part of the medium volume is replaced by a detector. The sensitive (measuring) volume of the dosimeter is also known as a cavity. If the material of the cavity has a different atomic number, Z, and density, ρ, than that of the irradiated medium (which is usually the case), then the measured absorbed dose inside the cavity will also be different from the absorbed dose to the medium at point P. As a result, a theory, a relation is needed that will relate the absorbed dose in a dosimeter to the absorbed dose in the medium containing the dosimeter. Several cavity theories have been developed over the years, which depend on the size of the cavity under consideration; for example, the Bragg–Gray (Gray 1936) and Spencer–Attix theories (Spencer and Attix 1955) for small cavities and the Burlin theory for cavities of intermediate sizes (Attix and Roesch 1968).

In general the cavities are considered to be small, intermediate or large relative to the ranges of secondary electrons produced by photons in the medium. In the case where the range of electrons is much larger than the cavity dimensions, the cavity is regarded as small. This forms the basis of the Bragg-Gray cavity theory that assumes that the detector is a cavity so small that, when inserted into a medium, it does not disturb the fluence of charged particles in the medium. It also assumes that the absorbed dose in the cavity is deposited solely by charged particles passing through it. This implies that any contribution to the dose due to X-ray interactions themselves in the cavity must be negligible; this volume only detects the electrons generated in the surrounding medium. The consequence of this is that the electron fluence in the cavity is the same and equal to the equilibrium fluence established in the surrounding medium. This condition is only valid in regions of CPE or transient CPE. In reality, the presence of a cavity always causes some degree of fluence perturbation, requiring the introduction of a fluence perturbation correction factor when determining the absorbed dose.

In ideal conditions, all electrons entering the cavity are produced outside the cavity and completely cross the cavity and they do not stop within the cavity (see Figure 3.17). This means that the ideal Bragg-Gray cavity (detector) is one of infinitesimal dimensions, a 'point' detector. In practice, such detectors do not exist but many real detectors may, in a first approximation, be treated as Bragg-Gray detectors to a high degree of accuracy.

If the conditions of the charged particle equilibrium are fulfilled, then the dose to the medium D_{med} is related to the dose in the cavity D_{cav} as follows:

$$\frac{D_{med}}{D_{cav}} = \frac{\left(\frac{S}{\rho}\right)_{med}}{\left(\frac{S}{\rho}\right)_{cav}} \qquad (3.34)$$

This is the ratio of the average mass collision stopping powers (sometimes referred to as unrestricted stopping powers, Podgorsak 2005) of the medium and

the cavity. The use of unrestricted stopping powers rules out the production of energetic secondary charged particles in the cavity and the medium, as they may travel some distance before they deposit dose in the medium. Equation 3.34 reflects the fact that as electrons slow down, the dose they deposit is proportional to the mass collision stopping power of the medium (energy lost per g/cm^2). As a result the ratio of the doses in the cavity and medium is found by averaging these stopping powers over the energy spectrum of all electrons present. Stopping powers are complex functions of electron energies and in a situation where a spectrum of electron energies is present in the medium; they have to be either measured or calculated using special calculation techniques (e.g. Monte Carlo simulations).

As mentioned earlier, the validity of the Bragg–Gray theory depends on the cavity size relative to the range of electrons in the medium. This means that the size of the Bragg-Gray cavity depends on the energy of the X-ray beam; i.e. it will have to have smaller dimensions for low energy X-rays compared to high energy X-rays.

3.3.7 Spencer–Attix cavity theory
The Bragg–Gray cavity theory does not take into account the creation of secondary electrons (also known as delta electrons) generated as a result of hard collisions in the slowing down of the primary

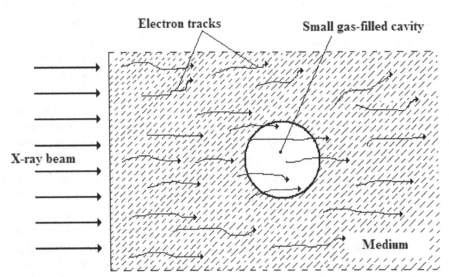

Figure 3.17. Schematic principle of a Bragg-Gray cavity inserted in a medium irradiated by X-rays. Secondary electrons traverse the cavity and deposit dose within its volume.

electrons in the sensitive volume of the dosimeter. The delta electrons have enough energy to generate ionisation tracks of their own. Some of these electrons produced inside may even escape from the cavity, transporting some of their energy with them. This will result in the reduction of the absorbed dose in the cavity. This phenomenon is accounted for by a more general Spencer–Attix cavity theory that uses modified mass stopping powers of the cavity material. The Spencer–Attix theory still operates under the two Bragg–Gray conditions; however, these conditions now apply also to the secondary particle fluence as well as to the primary particle fluence.

3.4 RADIATION DETECTORS AND DOSIMETERS

3.4.1 Ionisation chamber

Ionisation chambers are the most common devices used in radiotherapy and in diagnostic radiology for measurement of radiation dose. A typical ionisation chamber consists of a central electrode and a cylindrical chamber wall with a spherical or conical end mounted on a cylindrical stem (see Figure 3.18), connected to a high voltage supply of several hundreds volts. The cavity between the opposing walls is filled with accurately known air volume, designed to fulfill as close as possible the conditions of a Bragg–Gray detector. In this gas volume ionising radiation creates electron-ion pairs. These are attracted by the electrodes of opposing charge creating thus a current which can be measured by an electrometer. The

conductive outer wall of an ionisation chamber is generally made of graphite or PMMA (thermoplastic material). The wall and the collecting electrode are separated with a high quality insulator to reduce the leakage current when a polarising voltage is applied to the chamber. A guard electrode is also used inside the chamber to further reduce chamber leakage. The guard electrode draws the leakage current and makes it to flow to ground, bypassing the collecting electrode.

For dose measurements, the ionisation chamber is placed in a water or water equivalent phantom. The absorbed dose to water at the reference point can be derived using equation 3.34 and the formalism discussed in the following sections.

Metal Oxide Semiconductor Field Effect Transistors (MOSFET)

A MOSFET is a semiconductor based solid state electronic device which can be either p-type or n-type. A p-type MOSFET has a silicon substrate, p-type source and drain terminals, with a silicon dioxide (SiO_2) insulating layer separating the substrate from an aluminum gate (see Figure 3.19).

An electric field is set up across the SiO_2 when a negative voltage is applied to the gate terminal with respect to the substrate. This electric field attracts any holes present in the substrate to the interface between the SiO_2 and n-type materials. The holes form an *inversion layer* of n-type material that has the properties of p-type, and which connects the source and drain terminals (Figure 3.20).

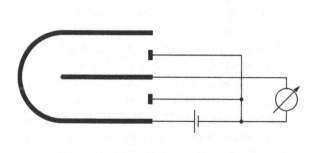
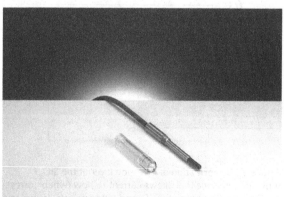

Figure 3.18. Schematic diagram and a photo of a cylindrical Farmer type ionisation chamber. (Courtesy PTW 2010)

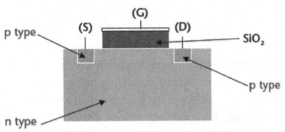

Figure 3.19. Configuration of semiconductor material in a p-MOSFET. Biasing may be applied to the terminals: (S): source, (G): gate, (D): drain. (Courtesy Royal Adelaide Hospital)

This inversion layer allows current to flow from the source to drain terminals. The threshold voltage, V_{th}, is defined as the minimum negative gate voltage which allows a current to flow. The inversion layer is formed only if the gate voltage is more negative than the threshold voltage. From a dosimetric point of view V_{th} is defined as the voltage required to maintain a certain set drain current.

When a MOSFET is exposed to radiation of sufficient energy (>18 eV) electron-hole pairs are created in the SiO_2 layer. The number of pairs produced, N, is proportional to the energy deposited, E_{dep}, and therefore to dose:

$$N\alpha\frac{E_{dep}}{W} \qquad (3.35)$$

Where W is the work required to produce one electron-hole pair in silicon dioxide (~18 eV).

If ***during irradiation*** a positive gate voltage is applied to a p-type MOSFET, the free electrons are

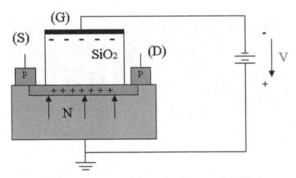

Figure 3.20. Formation of inversion layer at the SiO_2/ substrate interface that allows current to flow (when correct biasing is applied) between (S) and (D) terminals. (Courtesy Royal Adelaide Hospital)

attracted to the gate whilst the holes migrate to the SiO_2 and n-type material interface. The holes may become spatially located in charge traps formed in the oxide near the interface. As a result, the main processes involved as a result of the interaction of ionising radiation and correct biasing of a MOSFET are: a) creation of electron-hole pairs in SiO_2, b) separation of electrons from holes by application of electric field across the oxide (positive gate bias) and subsequent movement of electrons to the gate, c) hole transport through the oxide towards the SiO_2/substrate interface, d) trapping of holes and electrons in the oxide, e) build up of interface and border traps in the Si band gap and e) electron-hole recombination.

After irradiation is complete, if a negative gate bias is applied, the trapped holes (near the SiO_2/substrate interface) repel some of the positively charged carriers that form the inversion layer. Hence, a larger negative gate bias than that applied pre-irradiation is required to form the inversion layer. So to produce the same pre-irradiation current a shift of threshold voltage, ΔV_{th}, will have occurred. This ΔV_{th} is proportional to dose and is the basis for MOSFET dosimetry. ΔV_{th} is measured by taking readings of gate threshold voltage, V_{th}, prior to and after irradiation:

$$\Delta V_{th} = V_{th}^{post} - V_{th}^{pre} \qquad (3.36)$$

Importantly the same (constant) drain current is used to measure pre and post irradiated MOSFETs. ΔV_{th} after radiation exposure is proportional to dose (Savic *et al.* 1995). Repeated exposure to radiation leads to build up of hole traps and eventually to the saturation of a MOSFET. Saturation occurs when the inversion layer cannot be formed sufficiently by any applied voltage to allow current to flow from the source to drain terminals, therefore, the MOSFET can no longer be used as a dosimeter.

MOSFETs are limited not only in lifetime but they are only capable of measuring the dose at a specific point. However, an array of MOSFETs could be used to obtain 2D or 3D dosimetric information.

Advantages of MOSFETs include energy independence for megavoltage X-rays, dose rate independence, only small axial anisotropy (±2% for 360°), and linear dose-response relationship within the voltage ranges specified by manufacturers (Izewska and Rajan 2005).

MOSFETs can exhibit dependence on temperature and changes in the bias voltage during irradiation. The reading must be taken in a specified time after exposure, as it will drift with time.

Diodes

A diode dosimeter is another solid state detector and it is basically a p–n junction diode. The diodes are produced by taking n type or p type silicon and counter-doping the surface to produce the opposite type material. Only the p–Si diodes are used in radiotherapy dosimetry, since they are less affected by radiation damage. Similar to MOSFETS, radiation produces electron–hole pairs within the diode, including the depletion layer. The charges produced diffuse into the depleted region and generate currents in the reverse direction in the diode. Ionising radiation induces an electric current in the diode proportional to the dose rate (~10 pA/cGy/min). Diodes have active detection areas of 2–3 mm^2 (therefore they are useful for measurements of small radiation fields) and are usually assembled at the end of a coaxial cable. The use of semiconductor diodes has also been investigated for dosimetry (Wright and Gager 1977).

The advantages of diodes include high sensitivity to radiation, small size, good mechanical stability, absence of external voltage and real-time dose readout. However, diodes exhibit temperature, dose-rate, and incident radiation angle dependency. As a result they have to be carefully calibrated for given clinical conditions. The deviation of dose determination is reported to be about 1.5% (Essers and Mijnheer 1999). Several devices use diodes arranged in linear and 2D arrays to investigate line dose profiles and 2D dose maps.

Thermoluminescent dosimeters

A Thermo-Luminescent Dosimeter (TLD) is a non-conducting crystal with no electrons in the conduction band. At room temperature, all electrons are positioned in the valence band. When a crystal is exposed to ionising radiation, electrons receive energy and will make a transition from the valence band into the conduction band. This leaves positively charged holes in the valence band. The electrons and holes may move through the crystal until they recombine or until they are trapped in metastable energy states, between the valence and conduction bands. These metastable states are associated with defects in the crystal (e.g. as a result of impurities). If the crystal is heated, the electron can gain sufficient energy to make a transition from its trap to the conduction band. The electron may then move around in the crystal until it recombines with a trapped hole and a thermoluminescence photon is emitted. Alternatively, when the crystal is heated, the hole receives sufficient energy to move until it recombines with a trapped electron and a thermoluminescence photon is emitted (see Figure 3.21).

The width of the energy gap between the trap and conduction band determines the temperature required for releasing the electron and for producing thermoluminescence. This is characteristic of the particular material (its crystalline structure) employed. As the temperature of the crystal is increased, the probability of an electron escaping from a trap increases as well. Hence, the emitted light will be of low intensity at low temperatures, passing through one or more maxima at high temperature corresponding to thermal energies, and then decrease again to zero as no more filled traps remain.

The return of trapped electrons and holes (stimulated by heating) to the stable state, is associated with release of energy. This energy may be released as visible or UV light; a phenomenon known as thermoluminescence. If several traps of different depths are involved in this process, the recording of the light emission as a function of heating time (or temperature) results in a glow curve consisting of several glow peaks. The term 'glow curve' refers to the graph of TL light as a function of either temperature or time. The glow curve of a fluorescent crystal (also known as phosphor) characterises its dosimetric properties. For example, low temperature glow peaks suggest that the phosphor will lose its stored TL with time due to spontaneous transitions at room temperatures. A glow curve with peaks at very high temperatures means that the crystal will produce infrared radiation at the temperature required to release the traps. Ideally, a glow curve should reveal only a single thermoluminescent peak that occurs at a temperature high enough to ensure room temperature stability, but not so high so as to present instrumental problems. An

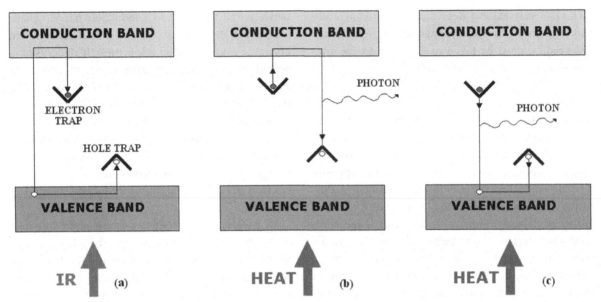

Figure 3.21. Schematic energy level diagram of a material exhibiting thermoluminescence. (a) Exposure to ionising radiation. (b) Electron trap is less stable during heating, and hole trap is the emitting centre. (c) Hole trap is less stable during heating, and electron trap is the emitting centre (Courtesy Mahesh *et al.* 1989).

example of a glow curve for a LiF phosphor is shown in Figure 3.22.

Thermoluminescent sensitivity is defined as the amount of light released by the phosphor per unit of radiation exposure. The lower limit of useful sensitivity depends on the characteristics of the phosphor and the TLD reader (the device that measures the light output from TL during the heating cycle). Most of the commercially available TLD readers can measure

radiation doses of less than 1 mGy. The upper limit of the useful range is generally limited by the phosphor itself. The energy response is the variation of the TL output, for a fixed radiation dose, as a function of the energy of the absorbed radiation. This variation arises from the dependence of the material's absorption coefficient (μ) on beam energy. The effect of the photon energy response is usually defined relative to 1.25 MeV photons from a ^{60}Co source (McKeever *et*

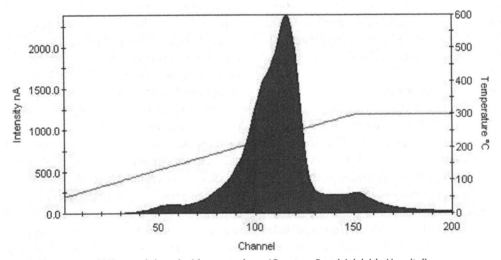

Figure 3.22. A Glow curve of LiF crystal doped with magnesium. (Courtesy Royal Adelaide Hospital)

al. 1995). Lithium Fluoride (LiF), one of the most commonly used TL dosimeters (in part due to its tissue equivalency), has relatively small energy dependence in the MV region but a strong energy response variation for X-rays below 1 MV.

The dose response is defined as the functional dependence of the intensity of measured TL signal on the absorbed dose. The ideal dosimeter should have a linear dose response over a wide dose range, however, most TL phosphors used in practical dosimetry display a variety of non-linear effects. In particular, the response of a TL phosphor is linear, then *supralinear* and then *sublinear* as the dose increases. As a result, the dose calibration curve needs to be measured for a given TLD phosphor and the radiation beam quality of interest.

The rate at which the thermoluminescence energy is released depends on the phosphor temperature and increases sharply at higher temperatures. The phenomenon where the TL signal from a TLD sample decreases with time after irradiation is known as fading. The most prevalent is thermal fading, i.e. the loss of TL signal induced by temperature. The thermal fading rate is influenced by two parameters: trap depth and a temperature-dependent frequency factor. Extensive fading may influence the reading results and corrections have to be applied (e.g. discard the contribution to the TL readout below a certain temperature threshold).

After reading, TLDs can be re-used. The reliable re-use of TL phosphors requires the use of strict thermal annealing procedures to empty the traps and re-establish the thermodynamic defect equilibrium that existed in the material before irradiation and readout. Re-processing of TLDs can be time-consuming.

Most frequently used TLD materials include: LiF:Mg, Ti, MgB_4O_7:Dy, $Li_2B_4O_7$:Mn, $CaSO_4$, CaF_2, Mg_2SiO_4, BeO, Al_2O_3. TLDs can come as powder, rods, discs or chips of very thin thickness suitable for measurements in the steep dose gradient.

Films

Radiographic film is frequently employed in the study of high-energy radiation therapy. It has several advantages over other conventional methods in that it has a low cost, speed of data collection, increased spatial resolution, ease of handling, and the ability to produce two dimensional dose maps in the film plane which is very attractive with regard to the study of dynamic radiation field delivery.

Photographic film typically consists of a transparent material base of cellulose acetate, thinly coated with an emulsion consisting of gelatine. The emulsion consists of silver halide crystals (typically 95% silver bromide and 5% silver iodide) embedded in gelatine. Gelatin is an ideal substrate as it keeps the non-uniform grains of silver halide finely dispersed (see Figure 3.23), preventing clumping and sedimentation. It also protects unexposed grains from reduction by the developer agent and chemically neutral to the crystals in terms of fogging and loss of sensitivity (Das *et al.* 2002).

Upon exposure to ionising radiation the silver bromide directly or indirectly ionises, releasing energetic electrons that produce electron and hole pairs, which subsequently disperse through the silver bromide crystals trapping electrons in the impurity atoms leading to the production of free silver ions and to the formation of a latent image. Film development is a chemical process, which amplifies the latent image by a factor of millions. During the film developing process the free silver ions are reduced to silver atoms, which are unaffected by the fixing solution and therefore remain behind. The emulsion that has not undergone a chemical reaction is removed by the fixing solution. The metallic silver produces a darkened area on the transparent base material.

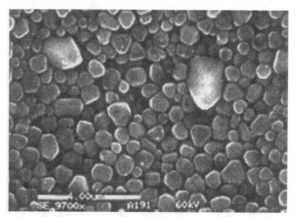

Figure 3.23. Electron micrograph showing silver halide grains evenly dispersed in gelatin substrate of the Kodak XV film. (Reproduced from Cheng and Das 1996. Copyright (1996), with permission from the American Association of Physicists in Medicine)

The degree of film darkening can be measured from the optical density (OD) of the film. This is achieved by using a film densitometer, which measures the amount of light transmitted through an exposed film. The OD is defined as:

$$OD = \log \frac{I_0}{I_t} \qquad (3.37)$$

where I_t and I_o are the amount of light collected by the densitometer with and without the film respectively. Unexposed base material will have a certain OD value, which is termed background or fog. This fog OD value is subtracted from the OD values obtained from the exposed film to provide a corrected response. Ideally, the relationship between the dose and OD should be linear. This varies from emulsion to emulsion as some are linear over a limited dose range and others can be non-linear. The dose versus OD curve is known as the sensitometric or characteristic curve and should be measured for each emulsion (see Figure 3.24).

Apart from the gradient of the slope (also known as gamma), speed of the film, i.e. the amount of exposure required to yield optical density of 1 above the fog, and film contrast, i.e. range of log exposures to provide density range within linear region, are other parameters that characterise film emulsions. When using films as dosimeters, the exposure should be chosen to make all parts of the radiograph lie on the linear portion of the sensitometric curve.

Energy independence and tissue equivalence are ideal qualities in detector materials. In the case of radiographic film, the silver content of the film emulsion has an atomic number of 47, which is much greater than the atomic number of tissue 7.64. The high atomic number of the silver results in a higher cross-section for low energy photon interactions. This results in a very high-energy dependence of film below approximately 400 keV, especially below 200 keV due to photoelectric interactions. This is a serious disadvantage of radiographic film as a radiotherapy dosimeter. In addition, the optical density depends on the film plane orientation with respect to the beam direction; on emulsion differences amongst films of different batches, films of the same batch or even in the same film; as well as densitometer/digitiser artefacts.

Basically, two types of radiographic films have been typically used for dosimetric purposes: firstly, X-OMAT V films (XV2 Film, Eastman Kodak Co., Rochester, NY), Agfa (Agfa Structurix D2, Structurix Film Systems, Ridgefield Park, NJ) and secondly, Kodak Extended Dose Range (EDR2, Eastman Kodak Co., Rochester, NY).

Sensitometric curves for these two films are shown in Figure 3.25.

Although the use of Kodak XV2 films has been reported in the literature for verification of the dose

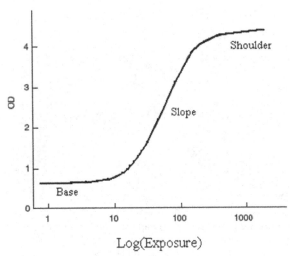

Figure 3.24. Typical sensitometric curve for a radiographic film.

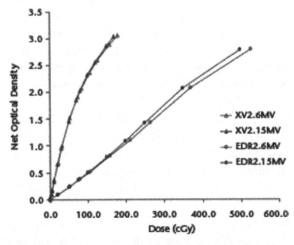

Figure 3.25. Sensitometric curves for Kodak EDR and XV films for 6 and 15 MV photons. (Reproduced from Chetty and Charland 2002. Copyright (2002), with permission from IOP Publishing Ltd.)

distribution in radiotherapy its use is limited due to the response depending on the radiation beam energy. Kodak extended dose range (EDR2) type radiographic film replaced the Kodak XV film as it provides the ease of use as a film dosimeter without some of the disadvantages seen with the XV type film. Dose saturation with the XV film has been quoted by the manufacturer at 200cGy (Kodak, Rochester NY) and in the literature between 100cGy (Dogan *et al*. 2002) and 200cGy (Zhu *et al*. 2002). Literature states for EDR2 film a saturation point at 700cGy (Kodak, Rochester NY, Zhu *et al*. 2002) and 500cGy (Dogan *et al*. 2002).

The two types of film differ in that EDR2 film is composed of uniform cubic crystals of silver halide finely dispersed in a double emulsion layer, coated on a 0.18 mm ester base. The silver halide crystals are approximately 10 times smaller than those found in the XV emulsion rendering the film much less sensitive than the XV film, resulting in a low noise level and higher contrast. Zhu *et al*. (2002) state that the EDR2 film is rendered developable as a result of the double hit process, dominant for mega-voltage X-ray beams.

Radio-chromic films

Radiochromic films (Gafchromic TM) have also been used to verify dose delivery. The film contains a special dye that is polymerised when irradiated. The polymer absorbs light, and the transmission of light through the film can be measured. This means that it does not need to be processed using chemicals. It also has excellent reproducibility, very low energy dependency and is nearly tissue equivalent (Klassen 1997; Niroomand-Rad *et al*. 1998). Radiochromic films are, however, quite expensive and the measured data has to be analyzed by a dedicated spectrophotometer. A good agreement (within 2%) between radiochromic films and ionisation chambers has been reported (Tangboonduangjit *et al*. 2004).

Gel dosimeters

Gel dosimeters are 3-dimensional integrated dosimeter-and-phantom systems suitable for relative dose determination. The gel dosimeter is a radiation-sensitive, self-developing and tissue-equivalent solid gel material that verifies integrated three-dimensional (3D) dose distributions produced in the gel by radiation treatment. There are two basic types of gel dosimeters:

1) Fricke gels (solutions of ferrous ammonium sulphate, xylenol orange and sulphuric acid) in Agarose or gelatin gel.
2) Polymer gels (solutions of ferrous ammonium sulphate, xylenol orange and sulphuric acid) in Agarose or gelatin gel.

When exposed to radiation, a chain of chemical reactions starts in ferrous sulphate solution that results in the conversion of ferrous ions Fe^{2+} into ferric ions Fe^{3+}, resulting in the change of optical density (Appleby and Leghrouz 1991). The conversion yield is proportional to the absorbed dose (until saturation is reached) and therefore the absorbed dose can be indirectly determined. Similarly, when polymer gel dosimeters are irradiated, polymerisation occurs as a result of free radicals production that is proportional to the radiation dose. Once again this causes changes of optical properties of the gel. The change induced by radiation is measurable and can be quantified using different techniques. The most common techniques used to measure this change are: magnetic resonance imaging, X-ray computed tomography and optical computed tomography (CT).

In conventional Fricke dosimetry, the light absorption at about 300 nm is utilised, because a) this absorption was negligible before ferrous ion oxidation and b) it is proportional to the ferric ion concentration and therefore to the absorbed dose. Spectrophotometric analysis (as in optical CT) is used widely and is considered reliable. In addition, the different paramagnetic properties of ferrous and ferric ions mean that nuclear magnetic resonance (NMR) analysis can be used to determine spatial distribution of different paramagnetic species, as they have a different effect on the spin relaxation times of the hydrogen nuclei of the solution (Schulz *et al*. 1990; Gum *et al*. 2002).

The advantage of gel dosimeters is that they are the only real 3D dosimetry system available for providing good spatial and dose accuracy. This is of particular importance for modern treatment techniques including stereotactic radiosurgery and intensity modulated radiotherapy.

The main disadvantages of gel dosimeters are the sensitivity to time, method of preparation and temperature, resulting in readout differences from batch to batch for the same delivered dose; cylindrical containers are required for optical readers and the results are less accurate readout at the gel/container interface. If MRI is used to read gels, MR time is often limited and expensive with long scan times required for accurate readout, e.g. 5% accuracy is achieved for over 10 hr scan time (Gum *et al.* 2002). They are relative dosimeters and as such require a reliable cross-calibration technique. A major limitation of Fricke gel systems is the continual post-irradiation diffusion of ions, resulting in a blurred dose distribution. Polymer gels can be toxic and special precautions are required for their handling. Cost may also prove to be a prohibitive factor.

3.5   DETERMINATION OF ABSORBED DOSE

Determination of absorbed dose using calibrated ionisation chambers will be briefly discussed in this section. This topic has been covered extensively and rigorously in numerous publications and textbooks (Khan 2003; Johns and Cunningham 1983; Metcalfe *et al.* 1997; Podgorsak 2005) so only a basic summary will be provided here. For detailed derivation of the mathematical formalism it is recommended that the reader studies the relevant sections of the references provided.

3.5.1   Absorbed dose in free space

As mentioned earlier, calorimetry is the true direct method of measuring absorbed dose in a medium. However, in practice the dose is measured using calibrated ionisation chambers and measuring the charge produced by X-rays in the medium. If the medium is air, then the measurement of dose can be related to exposure in air.

If one has an ionisation chamber that has a known exposure calibration factor, N_x, then exposure, X, at some point in air can be measured and determined:

$$X = MN_X \qquad (3.38)$$

where M is the corrected ionisation chamber reading corrected for the effect of ambient temperature and pressure and ion recombination.

The air kerma, K_{air}, at low X-ray energies (below 1 MeV) is directly related to exposure/ionisation at the point of interest as (this kerma is also known as collision kerma):

$$K_{air} = X\frac{W_{air}}{q} \qquad (3.39)$$

where the energy required to produce one ion pair (W_{air}/q) is 33.85 J/C for air.

If a small mass of medium of radius r_{med} (e.g. the detector) is inserted inside the air volume at the measurement point, the kerma in the medium is given by:

$$K_{med} = K_{air}\left(\frac{\mu_{ab}}{\rho}\right)_{air}^{med} k(r_{med}) \qquad (3.40)$$

Where

$$\left(\frac{\mu_{ab}}{\rho}\right)_{air}^{med}$$

is the ratio of averaged mass energy absorption coefficients for medium and air defined in Chapter 1. Finally, assuming that the ratio of absorbed dose to kerma at the measurement point is equal to 1, the dose in free space (air) can be calculated as:

$$D_{FS} = X\left(\frac{W_{air}}{q}\right)\left(\frac{\bar{\mu}_{ab}}{\rho}\right)_{air}^{med} k(r_{med}) \qquad (3.41)$$

Where $k(r_{med})$ is the correction factor for the perturbing effect of the medium.

3.5.2   Absorbed dose in a phantom

In most practical situations, including calibration of radiation output from linear accelerators, one wishes to determine in a medium other than air. Consequently, the formalism introduced in the previous section needs to be extended to an absorbing medium. (In radiation therapy, one is interested in dose absorbed to tissues and therefore water, due to similarity in density and Z, is used as the surrogate medium for measurements). If an ionisation chamber is used that is calibrated to measure exposure (see equation 3.38), then the dose in the medium can be determined as follows:

$$D_{med} = MN_X\left(\frac{W_{air}}{q}\right)\left(\frac{\bar{\mu}_{ab}}{\rho}\right)_{air}^{med} k(c_{med})b \qquad (3.42)$$

where $k(c_{med})$ accounts for the perturbing effect of the chamber of outer radius diameter c_{med} and b is the ratio of kerma and dose at the point of measurement (often considered to be equal to 1).

3.5.3 Determination of absorbed dose for megavoltage X-rays

From a radiation therapy point of view, accurate determination of radiation dose from megavoltage X-rays, such as those coming from high energy accelerators (typical range of energy spectra from 4 MV to 25 MV) is of utmost importance. This could be achieved, for example, using the equation 3.42 above, providing that the exposure calibration factor, N_x, of a chamber is known and that this calibration factor is valid for megavoltage X-rays. The exposure calibration factor enables to convert the charge collected (i.e. meter reading) by the ionisation chamber to exposure at a given photon energy, which generally is the energy of ^{60}Co gamma rays (1.17 and 1.33 MeV). It is however important to know what corrections to apply for the change in the beam energy, if the chamber calibrated with ^{60}Co source is used to calibrate e.g. an 18 MV X-ray beam. In addition, the $k(c_{med})$ correction factor needs to be elaborated. Experimentally, charge, Q, produced by an X-ray beam needs to be accurately measured. A short discussion of this issue is provided below.

The cavity-gas calibration factor, N_{gas}

Johns and Cunningham (1983) have derived two expressions relating dose absorbed in a homogeneous medium to measurements of either charge per unit mass of gas (air) in a chamber or to the response of a chamber calibrated for exposure against a standard chamber, namely

$$D_{med} = (33.85 \ JC^{-1}) \frac{Q}{m} \overline{S^{wall}_{air}} \left(\frac{\overline{\mu_{ab}}}{\rho} \right)^{med}_{wall} k_c \quad (3.43)$$

where

$$\overline{S^{wall}_{air}}$$

is the ratio of the mean stopping powers of the electrons in the wall of the ionisation chamber and air (averaged over photon and electron spectrum) to account for the effect of chamber wall material. The correction factor k_c, for the finite size of the ionisation chamber of outer radius, c, containing the air cavity of radius, a, is:

$$k_c = \frac{k(a_{wall}) \, k(c_{med})}{k(c_{wall})} \quad (3.44)$$

And:

$$D_{med} = MN_x (0.00873 \ Jkg^{-1}R^{-1}) \left(\frac{\overline{\mu_{ab}}}{\rho} \right)^{med}_{air} k(c_{med}) \, b \quad (3.45)$$

which is essentially equation 3.42. Both these expressions involve the medium in which the chamber is placed. In order to derive a factor independent of the medium, these two expressions can be equated to solve for what is known as the cavity-gas calibration factor (QW/mM) or N_{gas} (where Q/mM is the charge Q per unit mass of air, m, per meter reading, M):

$$N_{gas} = N_x 0.00873 \frac{1}{\overline{S^{wall}_{gas}}} \left(\frac{\overline{\mu_{ab}}}{\rho} \right)^{wall}_{air} \frac{k(c_{wall})}{k(a_{wall})} \quad (3.46)$$

which is the absorbed dose to the gas in the chamber per unit reading on the chamber meter. Note that this expression does not depend on the medium one wants to measure the dose in. N_{gas} can be determined for any **energy for which N_x is available** and is independent of energy, so can be applied at energies above 3 MeV. To calculate dose in a medium in terms of N_{gas}, substitution is made in (3.45) yielding:

$$D_{med} = MN_{gas} \overline{S^{wall}_{gas}} \left(\frac{\overline{\mu_{ab}}}{\rho} \right)^{med}_{wall} k_c \quad (3.47)$$

For any other energy E, this equation is:

$$D_{med} = MN_{gas} \left[\overline{S^{wall}_{gas}} \right]_E \left[\left(\frac{\overline{\mu_{ab}}}{\rho} \right)^{med}_{wall} \right]_E [k_c]_E \quad (3.48)$$

There has been an assumption made in deriving equation (3.43) that all secondary electrons were generated in the chamber wall. However, at higher energies a very significant proportion of the electrons are liberated in the medium beyond the chamber walls so that:

$$D_{med} = MN_{gas} \overline{S^{med}_{gas}} k(a_{med}) \quad (3.49)$$

If the ionisation chamber is calibrated in terms of dose (rather then exposure), then $D_{med} = M \, N_D$, and the dose to the gas cavity for a reference calibration energy is given by:

$$N_{gas} = N_D \frac{1}{\left[\overline{S^{wall}_{gas}}\right]_{ref}} \left[\left(\frac{\overline{\mu_{ab}}}{\rho}\right)^{med}_{wall}\right]_{ref} [k_c]_{ref} \quad (3.50)$$

3.5.4 Absorbed dose in the neighbourhood of an interface between different materials

It needs to be mentioned that electronic equilibrium is not present a at an air-phantom interface. Neither it is present at an interface between two different materials (e.g. bone and soft tissue). The analysis of this is quite complex and requires either carefully set-up measurements or Monte Carlo simulations. The effects at the interface depend on the density of the interfacing materials as well as on the energy of the X-ray radiation.

3.5.5 Dosimetry for electron beams

Dosimetry of electrons is different to that of high energy photons. Firstly, while the electron bean is narrow and nearly monoenergetic when exiting the accelerating structure, electrons after passing through scattering foils and other structures in the linac treatment head will lose some of their energy, resulting also in broadening of the spectrum. When the beam enters the medium, the energy of the electrons within the beam will continue to decrease with depth until they come to a complete stop. As the electrons' energy changes, their corresponding mass stopping powers change accordingly.

The dose deposited in water due to electrons at certain depth in a phantom is given by:

$$D_W = \frac{Q}{m}\left(33.85\,\frac{J}{C}\right)\overline{S}^{water}_{air} \quad (3.51)$$

Where $\overline{S}^{water}_{air}$ is the ratio of the mass stopping powers averaged over the energy spectrum of electrons when exiting the chamber. As the spectrum of electrons changes with depth, so does the $\overline{S}^{water}_{air}$ factor, so good knowledge of electron energy spectrum at depth (or the mean energy of the beam) and of the stopping power ratios is important. It is also important that a specially designed chamber, especially with respect to the height of the collecting volume, is used to minimise the averaging in the dose gradient. Plane parallel chambers are to be used for electron dosimetry, that have the air cavity in a shape of a disc with one flat surface facing the radiation source and serving as the entrance window as well as one of the electrodes. The distance between the entrance window and the second electrode should be 2 mm or less. The disc design also ensures that the electron fluence is sampled through the front window and the contribution from electrons entering through the side walls is minimal.

The value of Q/m in the equation 3.51 is difficult to determine accurately as it depends on accurate knowledge of the air volume inside the chamber. Therefore, if the N_{gas} factor of the chamber is known (for example from equation 3.50), then the dose can be determined from:

$$D_{med} = MN_{gas}\,\overline{S}^{med}_{air}\,k_e \quad (3.52)$$

where k_e is the correction factor for chamber perturbation effect.

3.6 RADIOTHERAPY DOSIMETRY PROTOCOLS

Determination of absorbed dose from X-ray or electron radiation sources is one of the major and most important tasks of a medical physicist. In previous sections, mathematical equations have been provided that enable the calculation of radiation dose to water based on the exposure produced by ionising radiation in the gas volume of the ionisation chamber inserted into the medium. Even though the equations are relatively simple, many parameters have to be known to calculate the dose correctly, e.g. stopping powers of a given radiation beam for air and water, various chamber related correction factors, and factors that convert the data from reference calibration conditions to particular measurement set-up. As a result, several dosimetry protocols have been developed from the nineteen-sixties to this date, depending on how the data, knowledge and technology evolved.

Early dosimetry protocols have tended to be based on the C_λ concept, where C_λ is an overall conversion factor from the reference radiation calibration conditions. C_λ simply converts from ionisation current in the chamber (exposure in Roentgen), to absorbed dose at the reference point in water:

$$D = RNC_\lambda \quad (3.53)$$

where D is dose in rads (this is an old unit of dose; 1 rad = 0.01 Gy) at the centre of the ion chamber, R is the pressure and temperature corrected ion chamber reading, and N is the calibration factor from the National Standards Laboratory. C_λ depends on the X-ray energy and the absorption medium (water was though generally used as the standard medium).

The IAEA TRS 277 protocol published in 1987 (IAEA 1987) was designed to be a unified, simple and easily executable protocol for use across the world for a variety of dosimeters. It also promoted a consistent policy towards the sources of data for stopping powers and other parameters used in dosimetry measurements. In this protocol the absorbed dose determination was based on standards calibrated in air and the so-called *absorbed-dose-to-air ionisation chamber factor*, $N_{D,air}$ is used:

$$N_{D,air} = \frac{D_{air,c}}{M_c} = N_k(1-g)\,k_{att}\,k_m \qquad (3.54)$$

Subsequently, the following expression gives dose to water at the reference depth d_o:

$$D_w(d_0) = M_u N_{D,air}(S_{w,air})_u P_u P_{cell} h_m \qquad (3.55)$$

where M_u is the meter/ion chamber reading corrected for temperature and pressure, ion recombination, polarity and humidity effects; p_{cell} allows for the non-air equivalence of the central electrode material; h_m is defined for electron beams only and is related to the change in spectrum from a plastic phantom material to water; P_u is a perturbation term to allow for the lack of water-equivalence of the chamber wall leading to a change in the electron spectrum.

In 2000 IAEA released a new document TRS 398: *Absorbed Dose Determination in External Beam Radiotherapy: An International Code of Practice for dosimetry based on Standards of Absorbed Dose to Water.*

The major characteristic of this protocol is (as the title suggests) that **the dose determination is based on standards calibrated in water.** Having the secondary standards calibrated in water means that no conversion from stopping powers in air to stopping powers in water is required, making the calibration more accurate since the uncertainty in stopping powers is no longer included.

National laboratories now calibrate ionisation chambers in water using a Co^{60} beam for high energy photon dosimetry. A chamber's $N_{D,w}$ (dose-to-water

calibration factor) is provided, replacing $N_{k,air}$ (exposure factor) or $N_{D,air}$ (dose-to-air factor) used previously. However, since the calibration is performed at Co^{60} energies a new correction factor is introduced, $k_{q/qo}$, to account for different radiation quality/energy of the calibrated beams (e.g. 6 MV X-rays) compared to Co^{60} radiation (1.17 and 1.33 MeV). Reference measurement depth of 10 cm is recommended for all photon energies above Co^{60}. The absorbed dose to water at depth of maximum dose is then calculated as:

$$D_{w,q}(d_{max}) = \overline{M}_{ave}\, C_{TP}\, p_s\, C_{EC}\, N_{D,w,qo}\, K_{q,qo}\, \frac{1}{PDD}$$
$$(3.56)$$

Where $\overline{M}_{ave}$ is the average meter/ion chamber reading, C_{EC} is the electrometer calibration factor, C_{TP} is the standard correction for temperature and pressure, p_s is the recombination factor and $k_{q,qo}$ is the mentioned radiation quality correction factor. The list of correction factors is provided in TRS 398 for a variety of ion chambers. $N_{D,w,qo}$ is the chamber calibration factor (i.e. Gy/nC) determined in water for a beam quality q_o (i.e. Co^{60}). Since the measurement is performed at 10 cm depth in water, a percentage depth dose (PDD) correction must also be applied do determine the dose at d_{max}. The measurement set-up for an NE2611 ionisation chamber is shown in Figure 3.26. Note that it is the chamber centre that is positioned at 10 cm depth. A radiation field size of 10×10 cm^2 is used.

Similar changes are applied to absolute dose determination of electron beams. The reference conditions for these beams have beam changed as well and are related to R_{50} (half value of the depth dose distribution) rather than the practical electron range R_p. This protocol is now adopted internationally.

3.6.1 Calibration of low energy X-rays

Low energy X-rays of up to 0.3 MeV energies are generally divided into two groups: low energy (up to 100 kV) and medium energy X-rays (up to 300 kV) reflecting two distinct treatment modalities in radiation therapy: superficial and deep (orthovoltage). Special/different calibration conditions apply due to the much lower energy of these X-rays (having different absorption and interaction properties) compared

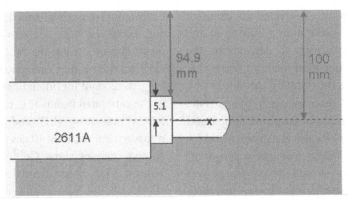

Figure 3.26. Schematic of absolute dose calibration set-up of NE2611 ionisation chamber using IAEA TRS 398 protocol. (Courtesy Royal Adelaide Hospital)

to megavoltage X-rays. There are two major protocols used internationally. The first one has been published by IPEMB in 1996 and is based on standards calibrated in air (IPEMB 1996 and 2005). The second one is the IAEA TRS 398 protocol based on standards calibrated in water (IAEA 2000).

3.7   QUALITY ASSURANCE

'In order to obtain best possible results from radiotherapy, a programme of quality assurance is essential. Such a programme aims to ensure consistency of the medical prescription and the safe fulfilment of that prescription, as regards dose to the target volume, together with minimal dose to normal tissue and minimal exposure of personnel.' (From Quality Assurance in Radiotherapy, World Health Organization, Geneva, 1988.)

Quality Assurance (QA) is a system of all planned and systematic actions necessary to provide adequate confidence that a product or service will satisfy the given requirements for quality. QA is one part of quality management systems (ISO 9000:2005). In radiation therapy, for example, quality assurance means all those procedures that ensure consistency of the medical prescription and delivery of that prescription, in regards to dose to the target volume, while minimising the dose to normal tissue and exposure of personnel. It also assumes that adequate patient monitoring is implemented to determine the treatment outcome.

Written instructions, for the most common procedures in radiotherapy, must cover all stages of the radiotherapy process, as the planning and implementation of treatment requires many kinds of technically demanding apparatus and procedures, and effective collaboration by several vocational groups. The written instructions must also include practical directions for responding to and preventing accidents.

Various national or international organisations, such as the World Health Organization (WHO) in 1988, AAPM in 1994 and 2009, European Society for Therapeutic Radiation Oncology (ESTRO) in 1995 and Clinical Oncology Information Network (COIN) in 1999, have issued recommendations for quality standards in radiotherapy. Other organisations, such as the International Electrotechnical Commission (IEC) in 1989 and the Institute of Physics and Engineering in Medicine (IPEM) in 1999, have issued recommendations for certain parts of the radiotherapy process. Numerous technical reports and technical documents regarding quality assurance, establishment of facilities, audits of facilities, acceptance testing and commission of radiotherapy apparatus and associated software have been published by the International Atomic Energy Agency. Where recommended standards are not available, local standards need to be developed, based on a local assessment of requirements.

Regulatory measures and recommendations are generally not legislative but have been mostly prepared by various intergovernmental and non-governmental bodies, e.g. the (IEC), the International Commission on Radiological Protection (ICRP), the

International Commission on Radiation Units and Measurements (ICRU), the World Health Organization (WHO), and by professional organisation like the American Association of Physicists in Medicine or the Australasian College of Physical Scientists and Engineers in Medicine (ACPSEM).

3.7.1 Secondary standard equipment and calibration

An international code of practice, developed by IAEA should guarantee a degree of uniformity of dose delivery throughout the world. The procedures described in the IAEA publication TRS 398 should be included in any radiotherapy quality assurance programme.

The absorbed dose to water from radiation therapy devices is determined through the use of a chamber/electrometer combination at the reference point under reference conditions, as specified in the appropriate dosimetry protocols (e.g. AAPM TG-51, AAPM TG-61, or TRS 398). Local or secondary standards are chamber/electrometer combinations that have a calibration coefficient in terms of air-kerma or absorbed dose to water directly traceable to a primary standards dosimetry laboratory (PSDL) or an accredited secondary standards dosimetry laboratory (SSDL). As it is the charge produced that is being measured when a chamber is irradiated, the calibration of an ionisation chamber basically relates the absorbed dose to measured charge under reference calibration conditions. The ionisation chamber may be calibrated together with the electrometer or separately. The calibration factor is given in units of the radiation dose (Gy) per unit charge.

These standards, which comprise a unique chamber/electrometer combination, are the basis of accurate dose delivery and are generally removed from routine clinical use. Routine calibration of radiation therapy devices in the clinical setting is typically performed with field grade chambers and electrometers (also known as tertiary instruments) which have a combined calibration coefficient transferred from the secondary standard equipment.

The national primary standards laboratories in turn implement international recommendations and guidelines, for example that of the International Bureau of Weights and Measures (Bureau International des Poids et Mesures, BIMP) that ensures

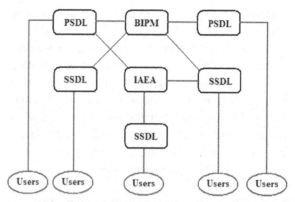

Figure 3.27. Schematic of traceability chain of calibration of dosimetric instruments (BIPM = Bureau International des Poids et Mesures).

world-wide uniformity of measurements and their traceability to the International System of Units (SI), as shown in Figure 3.27.

National primary standards laboratories maintain primary standards for ionising radiation and perform calibrations of therapy dosimetry equipment that are traceable to these standards. Calibrations at ^{60}Co energy are generally used as the basis for megavoltage dosimetry, and are suitable for use with protocols TRS-277, TRS-381, and TRS-398.

The secondary standard or reference dosimeter usually consists of three basic units: the ionisation chamber, the measuring assembly (electrometer and cables), and may also include a portable stability check source.

3.7.2 Ionisation chamber

The ionisation chamber used as secondary standard dosimeter must have excellent long term stability and low energy dependence. Any variation in the response should not be greater than 0.5% per year. It also needs to be unsealed and able to promptly equilibrate with outside ambient pressure and temperature.

For cylindrical Farmer type chambers (frequently used as secondary standards), the change in response with energy should be less than ±2% in the range of half-value layers from 2 mm Al to 3 mm Cu, i.e. from approximately 70 kV to 250 kV X-ray tube potentials. For chambers used for absolute calibration of high-energy X-ray beams, the total wall thickness (including build-up cap if available) must be sufficient to generate electron equilibrium for at least Co^{60} gamma rays.

Ionisation chambers for measuring low-energy radiation should have an entrance window consisting of a thin membrane through which the radiation enters the measuring volume (thin-window chambers). The response variation of these chambers should be within ±2% in a range of half-value layers from 0.05 mm to 2 mm Al, i.e. from approximately 12 kV to 70 kV X-ray tube potentials.

3.7.3 Measuring assembly (electrometer)

The electrometer measures the charge or current from the ionisation chamber. It generally also provides polarising potential for the ionisation chamber. The long-term stability of the measuring assembly must be better than ±0.5% per year. The performance of the electrometer should be checked regularly with a current source in the ranges of values obtained during routine irradiation conditions (e.g. in a nano-Coulomb range).

3.7.4 Portable stability check source

The stability check source is used to perform constancy checks of the ionisation chamber and electrometer assembly and to verify that no significant change/drift has occurred since the calibration of the secondary standard at the national laboratory (PSDL).

Typically, a $^{90}Sr + ^{90}Y$ radioactive source encapsulated in silver foil is used as a check source. This source is a pure beta-particle emitter (i.e. emits electrons only), with ^{90}Sr half-life of about 28 years. As a result the required decay correction is of only a few tenths of a percent per month and the check source does not have to be replaced frequently. During a measurement, the source is assembled, using special holders, with a chamber. The maximum energy of the ^{90}Y β particles of 2.2 MeV is adequate to penetrate the silver foil and the chamber wall. The geometrical relationship between the radioactive source and the chamber must be reproducible in order to minimise the effect of small changes in chamber position. The electrons from the $^{90}Sr + ^{90}Y$ source irradiate the chamber for a given time and charge is collected by the electrometer. The readings are corrected for ambient atmospheric conditions at the chamber position. The relative standard deviation of a check source reading, determined from repeated measurements, should not exceed 0.5% from the baseline value established for the source/chamber/electrometer assembly. Higher deviations should be investigated.

3.7.5 Transfer of secondary standard calibration to field instruments; measuring the output of an X-ray machine with cross-calibrated field ionisation chambers

Secondary standard, as explained in the previous section, is not used for routine QA measurements of an output from an X-ray machine (e.g. linear accelerator). Routine measurements are performed with so-called field instruments, which most commonly an ion chamber/electrometer assembly. Before the field instrument can be used for dosimetric measurements, it needs to be cross-calibrated against the secondary standard equipment.

A field chamber may be cross-calibrated against a calibrated reference chamber at the reference beam quality Q_o. The chambers are compared by alternately placing the chambers in a water phantom with their reference points at z_{ref} (a side-by-side chamber intercomparison is a possible alternate configuration). The calibration factor in terms of absorbed dose to water for the field ionisation chamber is given by:

$$N_{D,w,Qo}^{field} = \frac{M_{ref}}{M_{field}} N_{D,w,Qo}^{ref} \qquad (3.57)$$

where M_{ref} and M_{field} are the meter readings per monitor unit (MU) for the reference and field chambers, respectively, corrected for the influence of temperature and pressure, electrometer calibration, polarity effect and ion recombination as described in Chapter 6, TRS 398 (IAEA 2000).

$N_{D,w,Qo}^{ref}$, is the calibration factor in terms of absorbed dose to water for the reference chamber. Preferably, the readings M_{ref} and M_{field} should actually be the averages

$$\overline{M_{ref}/M_{em}} \text{ and } \overline{M_{field}/M_{em}}$$

where $(M_{ref}/M_{em})_i$ and $(M_{field}/M_{em})_i$ are, respectively, the ratios of the reading of the reference detector and the field instrument to the reading of an external monitor. The external monitor should preferably be positioned inside the phantom approximately at the depth z_{ref} but at a distance of 3 to 4 cm away from the chamber centre along the major axis in the transverse plane of the beam. Note that in the case of a side-by-side measurement an external monitor is not needed provided that the beam profile is adequately uniform.

The field chamber with the calibration factor $N_{D,w,Qo}^{field}$ may be used subsequently for the determination of absorbed dose to water in the user beam.

3.7.6 Quality assurance tests on radiotherapy treatment machines

While the calibration of the X-ray output from a linear accelerator is one of the most important tasks that a medical physicists is responsible for, there are many other physics and technical aspects of the radiotherapy equipment performance that must be checked at regular intervals. For example: energy/HVL of the treatment beams, flatness and symmetry of the X-ray profiles, light and radiation coincidence, wedge stability and transmission, mechanical and radiation isocentres, safety interlocks as well as calibration and QA of ancillary devices like electronic portal imaging detectors or multileaf collimators. Many of these tests are performed also as part of the linac commissioning and acceptance testing. As mentioned earlier, many international and professional groups have developed guidelines for regular quality assurance that state the frequency and details of the tests to be performed. Students should refer to the literature list recommended below (AAPM 40 (Kutcher 1994), 142 (Klein 2009)).

3.8 REFERENCES

Appleby A and Leghrouz A (1991) Imaging of radiation dose by visible color development in ferrous-agarose-xylenol orange gels. *Medical Physics* **18**: 309–312.

Attix FH and Roesch WC (1968) *Radiation Dosimetry.* Academic Press, New York.

Cheng CW and Das IJ (1996) Dosimetry of high energy photon and electron beams with CEA films. *Medical Physics* **23**: 1225–1232.

Chetty IJ and Charland PM (2002) Investigation of Kodak extended dose range (EDR) film for megavoltage photon beam dosimetry. *Physics in Medicine and Biology* **47**: 3629–3641.

Cunningham JR and Johns HE (1970) The calculation of absorbed dose from exposure measurements: practical problems in dosimetry. *Physics in Medicine and Biology* **15**: 71–77.

Das I, Cheng CW and Pai S (2002) Basic film dosimetry. AAPM meeting 2002, http://www.aapm.org/meetings/02am/pdf/8321-71068.pdf

Dogan N, Leybovich LB and Sethi A (2002) Comparative evaluation of Kodak EDR2 and XV2 films for verification of intensity modulated radiation therapy. *Physics in Medicine and Biology* **47**(22): 4121–4130.

Essers M and Mijnheer BJ (1999) In vivo dosimetry during extenal photon beam radiotherapy. *International Journal of Radiation Oncology Biology Physics* **43**(2): 245–259.

Gray LH (1936) An ionization method for the absolute measurement of γ-ray energy. *Proceedings of the Royal Society A*, 156: 578–596.

Greene D and Williams PC (1997) *Section, Linear Accelerators for Radiation Therapy.* 2nd edn. Institute of Physics Publ.

Gum F, Scherer J, Bogner L, Solleder M, Rhein B and Bock M (2002) Preliminary study on the use of an inhomogeneous anthropomorphic Fricke gel phantom and 3D magnetic resonance dosimetry for verification of IMRT plans. *Physics in Medicine and Biology* **47**: N67–77.

International Atomic Energy Agency (1987) 'Absorbed dose determination in photon and electron beams: an international code of practice'. Technical Reports Series 277, STI/DOC/010/277. IAEA, Vienna, Austria.

International Atomic Energy Agency (2000) 'Absorbed dose determination in external beam radiotherapy: an international code of practice for dosimetry based on standards of absorbed dose to water'. Technical Report Series 398, STI/DOC/010/398. IAEA, Vienna, Austria.

International Commission on Radiation Units and Measurements (1984) 'Radiation dosimetry: electron beams with energies between 1 and 50 MeV'. ICRU Rep 35. ICRU, Washington, DC.

International Electrotechnical Commission (1989) 'Medical electron accelerators on the range 1 MeV to 50 MeV – Guidelines for functional performance characteristics'. International Electrotechnical Commission (IEC) Technical Report no 977. Geneva.

International Organization of Legal Metrology (1990) 'Secondary standard dosimetry laboratories for the calibration of dosimeters used in radiotherapy'. OIML D 21 Edition. Paris, France.

International Organization for Standardization (2005) 'Quality management systems – fundamentals and vocabulary'. ISO 9000:2005, http://www.iso.org/iso. Geneva, Switzerland.

IPEMB (1996) The IPEMB code of practice for determination of absorbed dose for X-rays below 300 kV generating potential (0.035 mm Al – 4 mm Cu HVL; 10–300 kV generating potential). Physics in Medicine and Biology 41: 2605–2625, 1996.

IPEMB: Aukett RJ, Burns JE, Greener AG, Harrison RM, Moretti C, Nahum AE and Rosser KE (2005) Addendum to the IPEMB code of practice for the determination of absorbed dose for x-rays below 300 kV generating potential (0.035 mm Al–4 mm Cu HVL), Physics in Medicine and Biology 50: 2739–2748.

Izewska J and Rajan G (2005) Chapter 3: Radiation dosimeters, quality assurance of external beam radiotherapy. In: Radiation Oncology Physics: A Handbook for Teachers and Students. (Ed. EB Podgorsak) STI/PUB/1196. pp. 71–99. International Atomic Energy Agency Vienna, Austria.

Johns HE and Cunningham JR (1983) The Physics of Radiology. 4th edn. Thomas, Springfield, Illinois.

Khan FM (2003) The Physics of Radiation Therapy. 3rd edn. Lippincott, Williams and Wilkins, Philadelphia.

Klassen N, van der Zwan L and Cygler J (1997) Gaf-Chromic MD-55: investigated as a precision dosimeter. Medical Physics 24(12): 1924–1934.

Klein EE, Hanley J, Bayouth J, Yin FF, Simon W, Dresser S, Serago C, Aguirre F, Ma L, Arjomandy B and Liu C (2009) Task Group 142 report: quality assurance of medical accelerators. Medical Physics 36: 4197–4212.

Kutcher GJ, Coia L, Gillin M, Hanson WF, Leibel S, Morton RJ, Palta JR, Purdy JA, Reinstein LE, Svensson GK, Weller M and Wingfield L (1994) Comprehensive QA for radiation oncology, Report of AAPM Radiation Therapy Committee Task Group 40. Medical Physics 21: 581–587.

Ma C-M and Nahum AE (1991) Bragg-Gray theory and ion chamber dosimetry for photon beams. Physics in Medicine and Biology 36: 413–428.

McKeever SWS, Moscovitch M and Townsend PD (1995) Thermoluminescence Dosimetry Materials: Properties and Uses. Nuclear Technology Publishing, England.

Mahesh K, Weng PS and Furetta C (1989) Thermoluminescence in Solids and Its Applications. Nuclear Technology Publishing, Ashford, Kent, UK.

Metcalfe P, Kron T and Hoban P (1997) The Physics of Radiotherapy X-rays from Linear Accelerators. Medical Physics Publishing, Madison, Wisconsin.

Nahum AE (1978) Water/air mass stopping power ratios for megavoltage photon and electron beams. Physics in Medicine and Biology 23: 24–38.

Niroomand-Rad A, Blackwell C, Coursey B et al. (1998) Radiochromic film dosimetry: recommendations of AAPM Radiation Therapy Committee Task Group 55. American Association of Physicists in Medicine. Medical Physics 25(11): 2093–2115.

Podgorsak EB (Ed.) (2005) Chapter 12: Quality assurance of external beam radiotherapy. In: Radiation Oncology Physics: A Handbook for Teachers and Students. STI/PUB/1196. International Atomic Energy Agency Vienna, Austria.

PTW-Freiburg (Physikalisch-Technische Werkstätten) (2008) Ionizing radiation detectors catalogue, 2009–2010, D165.229.00/03 2008-12. PTW, Germany.

Rogers D (1995) Ionizing radiation dosimetry and medical physics. Physics in Canada 51(4): 178–181.

Savic Z, Radjenovic B, Pejovic M and Stojadinovic N (1995) The contribution of border traps to the threshold voltage shifts in PMOS dosimetric transistors. IEEE Transactions Nuclear Science 42: 1445–1454.

Schulz RJ, deGuzman AF, Nguyen DB and Gore JC (1990) Dose-response curves for Fricke-infused gels as obtained by nuclear magnetic resonance. *Physics in Medicine and Biology* **35**: 1611–1622.

Shockley W and Queisser HJ (1961) Detailed balance limit of efficiency of p-n junction solar cells. *Journal of Applied Physics* **32**: 510–519.

Spencer LV and Attix FH (1955) A theory of cavity ionization. *Radiation Research* **3**: 239–254.

Tangboonduangjit P, Metcalfe P and Butson M (2004) Matchline dosimetry in step and shoot IMRT fields: a film study. *Physics in Medicine and Biology* **49**(17): N287–92.

Valentine JM and Curran SC (1958) Average energy expenditure per ion pair in gases and gas mixtures. *Reports on Progress in Physics* **21**: 1–29.

Whyte GN (1963) Energy per ion pair for charged particles in gases. *Radiation Research* **18**: 265–271.

World Health Organization (1988) *Quality Assurance in Radiotherapy*. WHO, Geneva.

Wright AE and Gager LD (1977) Silicon diode detectors used in radiological physics measurements. Part II: measurement of dosimetry data for high-energy photons. *Medical Physics* **4**(6): 499–502.

Zhu X, Jursinic P, Grimm D *et al.* (2002) Evaluation of Kodak EDR2 film for dose verification of intensity modulated radiation therapy delivered by a static multileaf collimator. *Medical Physics* **29**(8): 1687–1692.

4   Tumour characteristics, development and response to radiation

4.1 THE INDUCTION OF CANCER

Cancer arises as a result of sequential accumulation of genetic changes. These changes include a combination of inherited and acquired alterations in the DNA sequence, ranging from point mutations to deletions, amplifications, and translocations.

The first recurrent chromosome aberration found in a human tumour (chronic myeloid leukaemia) was the 'Philadelphia chromosome' (Nowell and Hungerford 1960). This chromosome is an abnormally small chromosome 22, which is one of the two chromosomes involved in a translocation with chromosome 9. This translocation occurs in a single bone marrow cell which, through clonal expansion, causes leukaemia. The revolutionary chromosome banding technique introduced in the 1970s allowed the discovery of several other consistent chromosome aberrations in various tumour types.

A general characteristic of many cancers is the presence of aneuploidy (abnormal number of chromosomes). Genes which are affected by chromosome aberrations are grouped in two categories:

- oncogenes, and
- tumour suppressor genes.

Oncogenes were initially described as any genes capable of causing cancer (Knowles 2005). Later on, when tumour suppressor genes were identified as genes which encode proteins whose absence, inactivation or mutation promotes carcinogenesis (therefore loss of function), the oncogenes were redefined as genes promoting carcinogenesis via gain of function (Figure 4.1).

Tumour-specific chromosome aberrations act as tumour markers therefore the identification of genes affected by these aberrations provide novel targets in cancer treatment.

4.2 NORMAL CELLS VERSUS MALIGNANT CELLS

The challenge in treating cancer consists in the fact that the characteristics of malignant cells differ from their normal cell counterparts, which makes the behaviour of cancer more unpredictable. Differences between normal and malignant (tumour) cells can be found in relation to cell cycle, population kinetics and their architectural organisation (Nias 2000). Tumour cells in cultures are considered 'immortal' since they can be passaged indefinitely. Lower concentrations of serum or growth factors than normal cells are required for tumour cells to grow *in vitro*. Cell communication and movement is governed, partly, by plasma cell surface membrane properties. The structure and functions of

L. Marcu et al., *Biomedical Physics in Radiotherapy for Cancer*,
DOI 10.1007/978-0-85729-733-4_4, © CSIRO 2012

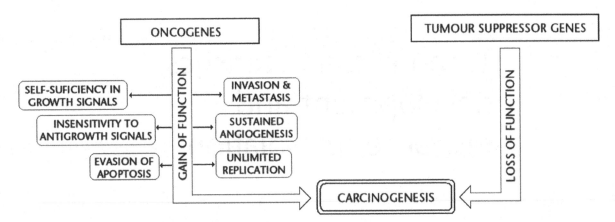

Figure 4.1. Basic illustration of molecular cytogenetics of cancer.

cell membrane in tumour cells is also altered, leading to abnormal cellular behaviour. Malignant cell invasiveness through the normal tissue barrier is one consequence. Loss of contact inhibition by tumour cells compared to normal cells which stop growing once they make contact results in growth to high densities. The control on the mitotic cycle is also lost by tumours. Malignant cells fail to stop at cell cycle checkpoints, so their growth cannot be restricted anymore. In this way, any damaged DNA in cancer cells is replicated and further mutations are accumulated.

Thus cancer cells have defects in regulatory mechanisms governing normal cell proliferation and homeostasis. Hanahan and Weinberg (2000) suggested six fundamental alterations in cell physiology which collectively dictate malignant cell growth and which are shared by the majority of human tumours:

1. *Self-sufficiency in growth signals*
    While normal cells require mitogenic growth signals before transiting from the quiescent phase into the cell cycle, tumour cells generate their own growth signals, disturbing the homeostatic mechanism.
2. *Insensitivity to antigrowth signals*
    The role of growth-inhibitory signals is to maintain tissue homeostasis and cellular quiescence. Normal tissues are sensitive to antigrowth signals, however, malignant cells have disruptions in the antigrowth signalling pathways, leading to unrestrained growth.

3. *Evasion of apoptosis*
    Apoptosis, also called programmed cell death, is a genetically driven 'cell suicide' mechanism, which allows regulation of cell number within a tissue or organ. In normal tissues, the balance between cell production and cell death is dictated by pro-apoptotic regulators. Many tumours, however, acquire resistance towards apoptosis through gene mutations that alter the ability of the cell to undergo programmed cell death. As a consequence, instead of dying, the malignant cell continues to proliferate by evading the apoptotic pathway.
4. *Unlimited replicative potential*
    All the above presented acquired characteristics such as growth signal autonomy, insensitivity to inhibitory signals and resistance to apoptosis, lead to another property of malignant cells which is the infinite replicative potential. Observations made in the 60's on the replicative potential of normal human fibroblasts grown as monolayers in tissue cultures showed that they hold a limit ('Hayflick' limit) for proliferation. It contrast, cell culture experiments demonstrated that tumour cells are often immortal, suggesting that the limitless replicative potential was acquired *in vivo* during tumour progression.
5. *Sustained angiogenesis*
    Angiogenesis is the process of new blood vessel formation (neovascularisation), critical during organogenesis to ensure a continuous supply of oxygen and nutrients. Once the organ is formed,

the process of angiogenesis stops and the nutrients are supplied by the already formed vasculature. Tumours manage to grow to lethal sizes due to angiogenesis. In order to develop, tumours recruit and sustain their own private blood supply, usually from already existing healthy vessels. Tumours activate the angiogenic 'switch' by changing the balance of angiogenic inducers and inhibitors through altered gene transcription.

6. *Tissue invasion and metastasis*
    Malignant cells from the primary site of origin of the tumour have the ability to traverse the normal cell barrier and to migrate to distant sites. Through capillary beds, cells are transported to various sites where they invade the normal cell population and develop as metastases. Invasion and metastasis are highly complex processes, the underlying molecular mechanisms of which are still not fully understood. Both of these processes are potential threats to the survival of the host.

4.3 TUMOUR GROWTH CHARACTERISTICS

4.3.1 Tumour kinetic parameters

Tumours are complex, diverse and heterogeneous entities, yet all share the characteristic of proliferation beyond the constraints which limit growth in normal tissue. The growth of tumours is best represented by exponential increase of cell numbers with time. The exponential pattern of growth assumes no cell loss or infertility and represents the simplest mode of tumour growth. By growing exponentially, the tumour volume increases by a constant fraction at equal time intervals. Volume doubling time is a kinetic parameter representing the time for the tumour volume to double. The volume doubling time is generally longer than the cell cycle time because of cell loss and migration of cells out of the cell cycle into a non-proliferating phase (G_0).

Many human tumours during their development show exponential growth. However, tumours also undergo irregular or decelerating growth (Steel 1977). A more accurate representation of irregular tumour growth is given by the Gompertzian growth curve (Figure 4.2). In Gompertzian growth doubling time

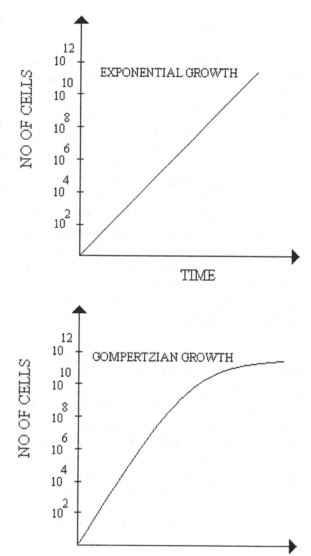

Figure 4.2. Tumour growth curves.

initially increases steadily until the tumour reaches a critical size when there is progressive slowing of growth. The slowing of growth has been attributed to decreased cell production rather than increased cell loss (Steel 1977).

Potential doubling time, T_{pot}, is a cell kinetic parameter representing the time for the tumour to double its size when there is no cell loss. T_{pot} can be expressed as a function of the length of the S phase, T_S, and the thymidine labelling index, LI, which is the percentage of cells in the S phase:

$$T_{\mathrm{pot}} = \lambda \frac{T_S}{LI}$$

where λ is a correction factor for the irregular age distribution of growing cell population and is usually within the range of (0.7–1).

Tumour cell loss is estimated from the cell loss factor (Steel 1977), which is defined as a function of T_{pot} and the volume doubling time, T_d:

$$\text{Cell loss factor} = 1 - \frac{T_{\mathrm{pot}}}{T_d}$$

The main mechanisms of cell loss are necrosis (cell death produced by the progressive degradative action of enzymes) and differentiation (cells attaining adult structural and functional capacity). Additionally, tumour cells can go through apoptotic death ('programmed', potentially controllable death), similarly to normal cells in the tissue of origin.

4.3.2 Tumour composition and characteristics of tumour cells

Tumour cells can be classified into two main categories: proliferating cells and nonproliferating cells. Non-proliferating cells can be either quiescent (resting) but retain the capacity to divide by re-entering into cell cycle, or sterile cells that are no longer able to divide. There are also stromal cells that would not contribute towards tumour growth and, finally, dying cells which in time are eliminated from the tumour through the circulatory and lymphatic systems.

Figure 4.3 shows a classification of tumour cells as a function of their proliferative ability (Begg 1997).

Cells with indefinite proliferative potential are mentioned in the literature as either clonogenic or stem cells. Stem cells are defined as the cells that have the ability to perpetuate themselves through self-renewal. Clonogenic cells are described as the cells that can divide indefinitely. The terminology is still debated since the existence of stem cells within the tumour is still hotly disputed (Kummermehr 2001).

However, there are some aspects to support the 'cancer stem cell' concept (Reya et al. 2001):

- The mechanisms that regulate self-renewal of normal cells and cancer cells are similar.
- There is a possibility that tumour cells arise from normal stem cells.
- There are cancer cells within the tumour with indefinite proliferative ability that drive the formation and growth of tumours.

The main contributors to tumour growth and development are indisputably the stem (clonogenic) cells, due to their self-renewal property. Although finitely proliferating cells contribute to the total population of malignant cells, they are not capable of regrowing the tumour due to their division-limited life. Therefore, the main target for radiotherapy is the tumour stem population.

Initially, nonproliferating cells appear harmless since, by definition, they are not proliferating. How-

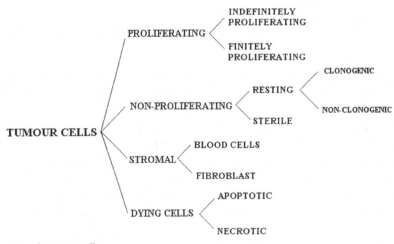

Figure 4.3. Classification of tumour cells.

ever, quiescent cells have higher radioresistance than cycling cells, because of conservation of cells in the G_0 phase until an internal stimulus triggers them back into the cycle. The genetic signalling received by resting cells from the shrinking tumour in response to radiation is one such stimulus. Resting cells react to the signal by re-entering the cycle and contribute towards tumour repopulation. Since resting cells can originate from either stem cells or finitely proliferating cells, recruitment of these cells is a significant contributor towards tumour recurrence and treatment failure.

4.4 TUMOUR KINETIC PARAMETERS

Tumour cell kinetic parameters for various tumour types have been determined by several research groups using methods such as percentage labelled mitoses, thymidine analogues, flow cytometry. Although average values for cell kinetic parameters have been determined for a typical human tumour (see Table 4.1), there is a range of variations among tumours due to the differences in their proliferative ability. Therefore, some tumours are slowly proliferating with a low cell turnover (such as prostate cancer) and others are rapidly proliferating with short mitotic cycles (such as head & neck carcinomas). The characteristic of rapid proliferation is often retained even during therapy, and successful management of these types of cancer depends on appropriate choice of

treatment regimens to overcome any potential for accelerated tumour repopulation.

The knowledge of tumour kinetics in general, and most importantly, the knowledge of tumour kinetics on an individual basis is a step towards individualisation of treatment planning, one of the goals of improving radiotherapy in the future.

4.5 TUMOUR BEHAVIOUR DURING RADIOTHERAPY

The target in radiotherapy is obviously the tumour, and the aim of radiotherapy is to achieve a high therapeutic ratio by either increasing the probability of tumour control, or decreasing the probability of normal tissue complications. The increase in tumour control is achieved by high tumour cell kill (reflected by low surviving fraction), thus maximising the chances of successful treatment. Cell killing would therefore appear to be the simplest observable evidence of response of the tumour to radiotherapy. However, in order to die, cells go through complex processes, which are dependent not only on the characteristics of cells but also their surrounding environment.

As previously discussed, division delay is a common response of cells damaged by radiation. In this process, cells are arrested at various points of the cell cycle (usually before entering mitosis or during the S phase) to allow time for possible cellular repair. Depending on the functionality of the checkpoints,

Table 4.1. Cell kinetic parameters for various tumours (Tannock and Hill 1998; Hall 2000; Begg and Steel 2002).

Kinetic parameter/ Tumour type	Volume doubling time (days)	Potential doubling time (T_{pot})(days)	Labelling index (%)	Cell loss factor (%)	T_S (length of the S phase)(h)
Typical tumour	60	5	–	90	–
Breast	82	10.4 (8.2–12.5)	3.7 (3.2–4.2)	89	10.4 (8.7–12)
Prostate	1100	28	1.4	97	11.7
Head & neck	45 (33–150)	4.5 (1.8–5.9)	7 (5–17)	91	11.9 (8.8–16.1)
Melanoma	52	7.2	4.2	84	10.7
Colorectal	90	4 (3.3–4.5)	13.1 (9–21)	96	15.3 (13.1–20)
Lymphoma	28	15.6	3	29	12

cells can repair the damage successfully, trigger apoptotic death, or progress through the cycle with unrepaired (or misrepaired) DNA.

Cell recruitment is another recognised process by which tumours respond to radiation. The pictures below define the process of recruitment and illustrate its effect on distribution of cells in the cycle.

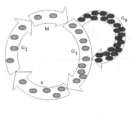

Clonogenic (stem) cells and finitely proliferating cells are distributed along the cell cycle, while the quiescent cells (dark circles) are resting in the G_0 phase, out of the mitotic cycle. Cytotoxic treatment such as radiotherapy and chemotherapy are the usual triggers that bring the quiescent cells back into the cycle.

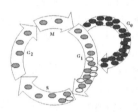

During radiotherapy quiescent cells are re-cycled (white circles) as a response to tumour shrinkage in order to repopulate the tumour. This process is called cell recruitment. Recruitment can occur either in 'batches', when groups of cells are re-cycled at the same time, or through a continuous cell flow into the cycle.

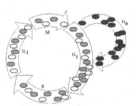

As radiation treatment progresses, more quiescent cells re-cycle and regain their proliferative capacity. Therefore a redistribution of the previously resting cells along the mitotic cycle can be observed (note the distribution of the white circles).

Loco-regional failure in the treatment of the rapidly proliferating tumours has been attributed to accelerated repopulation (Withers 1993). Accelerated repopulation is a marked increase in the growth rate (15 to 20 times faster) after the commencement of radiotherapy. Accelerated repopulation is not *clinically* evident at the beginning of the treatment because the vast majority of tumour cells are sterilised and the tumour is regressing before the small number of sur-

viving stem cells begin to repopulate. Repopulation is a cumulative process in response to the progressive radiation damage during fractionated radiotherapy. However, there is no indication that repopulation cannot be triggered from the beginning of the treatment, and rapid, inherent growth is a characteristic of a small proportion of tumours.

The first study confirming the ability of surviving clonogenic cells to repopulate the tumour after irradiation was conducted in 1969 (Hermens and Barendsen) on rat R1 rhabdomyosarcoma transplants. After a single dose of 20 Gy X-rays, they measured the clonogen surviving fraction (SF) over the following weeks observing that the post-irradiation SF = 0.01 increased in 12 days to SF = 1. Another notable experiment was undertaken on Lewis lung tumours (Stephens *et al.* 1978) when, besides surviving fraction, the number of viable cells in the tumour was also determined, estimating therefore the contribution of clonogenic cells to repopulation.

Repopulation becomes measurable usually 3–4 weeks after the start of the treatment. Nevertheless, compensatory proliferation in tumours may also be due to a decrease in the level of hypoxia and malnutrition, which have previously been the factors inhibiting growth.

Figure 4.4 represents a theoretical curve of tumour growth, regression and regrowth during treatment. If

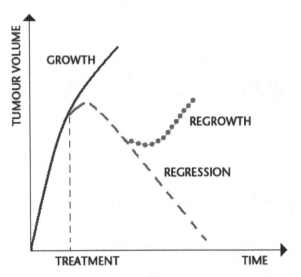

Figure 4.4. Theoretical curve illustrating tumour growth, regression and regrowth.

tumour growth is disturbed by treatment (*blue curve*), the majority of tumours would respond by regression (*green curve*). The optimal scenario is the one with full regression (complete tumour response), when all the clonogenic cells are killed, so that none remains to be able to regrow the tumour. Unfortunately this situation is not applicable for most tumours except for small ones ($\leq$ 3 cm). Many cancers respond to the killing effect of radiation by stimulating the surviving stem cells in order to regrow the tumour (*red curve*). Tumour regrowth (or repopulation) after radiotherapy is common for some rapidly proliferating cancers, and is one of the main reasons for treatment failure. One typical example of rapidly proliferating tumour with the above described properties is head & neck cancer.

Experimental data on squamous epithelia have shown that the accelerated repopulation response is analogous to the acute response of normal tissue after injury (Dörr 1997). It is suggested that squamous cell carcinomas retain some of the homeostatic control mechanisms attributed to their tissue of origin (Trott and Kummermehr 1991). Similarly, several other papers support the evidence that normal and cancerous squamous epithelia share the same behaviour in response to injury (Trott and Kummermehr 1991; Trott 1999; Denham *et al.* 1996). Therefore, the mechanisms responsible for normal tissue repopulation may be considered pertinent to tumour repopulation. Dörr (1997) categorise the main regrowth mechanisms as the three A's of repopulation: asymmetry loss, acceleration of stem cell division and abortive division (limited number of cell divisions by stem cells destined to die). Hansen (Hansen *et al.* 1996) considers recruitment and accelerated stem cell division as the responsible mechanisms for repopulation. The results obtained by Withers and Elkind (1969) from crypt cell experiments indicate that division cycle synchrony is a source for repopulation. Trott's work (Trott 1999) also underlines that the most plausible explanation for accelerated regrowth is loss of asymmetric stem cell division (Table 4.2).

The paragraphs below briefly describe the repopulation mechanisms listed in Table 4.2.

- Cell recruitment is the re-entry of the quiescent cells (cells in the G_0 phase) into the mitotic cycle.

Table 4.2. Possible mechanisms responsible for the accelerated tumour growth.

Mechanism	Source
Cell recruitment	Hansen *et al.* 1996
Accelerated stem cell division	Withers, Elkind 1969 Dörr 1997 Hansen *et al.* 1996
Asymmetry loss in stem cell division	Withers, Elkind 1969 Trott, Kummermehr 1991 Dörr 1997
Abortive division	Dörr 1997

- Accelerated stem cell division refers to the shortening of the cell cycle after the start of radiotherapy.
- Loss in asymmetrical division expresses the change in division pattern of the stem cell, from an asymmetrical division (one stem and another finitely proliferating/nonproliferating cell) to a symmetrical division (two stem cells).

The difficulty in assessing accelerated regrowth is that the process starts when the tumour population has decreased to a few thousand of cells in number, which is not clinically detectable (Withers 1993). Therefore, theories on the qualitative appraisal of repopulation need more substantiation.

Bladder carcinoma was also shown to repopulate during radiotherapy following a lag period of about 5–6 weeks after the start of treatment (Maciejewski and Majewski 1991). The study reported a clonogen doubling time of 5–8 days, suggesting that time protraction might have a significant impact on tumour control. Similarly to head & neck cancer, in the radiotherapy for bladder carcinoma an accelerated regimen (with more than 5 days/week fractions) is recommended.

To assess the extent and mechanisms of repopulation in **cervical cancers**, experiments in human cervical squamous cell carcinoma (SiHa) xenografts were conducted in SCID mice (Sham and Durand 1999). Tumours were treated with 25 Gy in 10 fractions over 5 days and regrowth and cell kinetics parameters were followed during treatment, and for 10 days after completion. It was noticed that while cell cycle time remained constant, a rapid repopulation began during irradiation, which was largely attributable to an increased growth fraction and decreased potential doubling time, triggered by increased cell loss. It was concluded that tumour regrowth occurred more rapidly than predicted by pre-treatment kinetic parameters (such as T_{pot}).

As therefore expected, prolongation of treatment time in **cervical cancers** treated with either external beam radiotherapy or brachytherapy have been reported to lead to adverse effects (Chen *et al.* 2003). While there were several debates regarding the radiobiological superiority of low dose rate (LDR) brachytherapy over high dose rate (HDR), the normal-tissue toxicity data resulting from continuous hyperfractionated accelerated radiotherapy (CHART) regimen has elucidated some of the questions. The analysis of morbidity for patients treated with CHART regimen demonstrates that repair half-times for late-reacting normal tissue cells are of the order of 4–5 h, significantly larger then initially thought. It was demonstrated that, for a repair half-time of 1.5 h for tumour cells, if the half-time for repair of late-reacting normal tissue cells surpasses 2.5 h, LDR becomes radiobiologically inferior to HDR, which might explain the success of HDR in clinical practice (Orton 2001).

As mentioned above, accelerated repopulation in rapidly proliferating tumours is one of the reasons for treatment failure. However, there are ways to overcome repopulation. A successful method is to alter the conventionally fractionated schedule, and to deliver it either in an accelerated regimen (larger doses/day, and shorter overall time) or as a hyperfractionated schedule (two or more fractions a day). These treatment modalities will be discussed in more detail in Chapter 5.

4.6   TUMOUR CELL DEATH

Tumour cell death can occur either as a response to irradiation (mitotic death, apoptosis) or through lack of oxygen and nutrients (necrosis).

Tumour cell death following irradiation has been shown experimentally to be tumour-type dependent. After irradiation, cells with damaged chromosomes may die attempting the next (or a subsequent) mitosis. This mode of cell death is called *mitotic death*, and is the most common form of cell death. Cell survival in this case is dose-rate dependent and is also a linear-quadratic function of dose. The cell survival curve therefore has a shoulder. When irradiated cells die before reaching mitosis, *interphase death* is said to have occurred.

Apoptosis, or programmed cell death, is a genetically regulated pathway which leads to cell lethality, and is the dominant mode of cell death for some cell types such as lymphoid cells. Apoptosis is a natural process to eliminate an excess of normal cells and abnormal or maldeveloped cells.

Once apoptosis is initiated, the cell's nuclear chromatin is condensed, the cytoplasmic organelles are compacted and the cell shrinks. Apoptotic cells maintain their cell membrane integrity following nuclear fragmentation.

During their development tumours encounter many stresses which can trigger the genetic signalling leading towards eradication of potentially damaged cells by programmed cell death. One of the most important regulators of apoptotic death in tumours is the tumour suppressor gene, p53. When DNA damage is detected by the cell, concomitant signals cause an increase in the levels of p53. Elevated levels of p53 suppress growth of tumour cells by either arresting their progression in the cell cycle until the damage is repaired (see division delay) or by inducing apoptosis. While programmed cell death is a critical component of normal tissue homeostasis, tumour cells often develop mutations in the key genes that regulate apoptosis thus providing the potential for further mutations.

Many cell lines are affected by both apoptotic and mitotic death. However, an indirect relationship between the extent of apoptosis and cellular radioresistance has been observed. While apoptotic death is virtually absent in radioresistant cell lines, this mode of death predominates in radiosensitive cell lines.

In contrast to apoptosis which involves the activation of a genetic program, *necrosis* is a passive response to injury. This type of cell death occurs commonly in solid tumours, when the levels of oxygen and nutrients reaching the cells have fallen to critically low values. Tumours, therefore, often present with a necrotic core surrounded by hypoxic cells in locations at a critical distance from blood vessels whilst well oxygenated tumour cells located close to blood vessels are more responsive to treatment.

During necrosis cells swell and lyse, releasing their cellular content into the intercellular space where they stimulate an inflammatory response.

4.7 TUMOUR HYPOXIA AND ANGIOGENESIS

It has been well established both in pre-clinical and clinical studies that most tumours have a considerable proportion of hypoxic cells that show resistance to both radiation and chemotherapy. Moreover, hypoxia is a marker of an aggressive tumour phenotype also associated with a poor outcome following surgery. Tumour hypoxia, therefore, is a strong negative prognostic factor for treatment outcome. Also, when oxygen delivery within the tumour is suppressed, the tumour responds by angiogenesis – the formation of new blood vessels. Once the angiogenic switch is turned on, the tumour develops its own vascular network which allows for further growth and invasiveness.

Measurement of oxygen tension (pO_2) was the first way to characterise tumour hypoxia clinically. Based on polarographic electrode measurements Gatenby *et al.* (1988) was the first to show that hypoxia was associated with a poor prognosis after radiotherapy in advanced head & neck tumours. Since then, pO_2 measurements by the Eppendorf probe are extensively used, and the relationship between oxygen tension, hypoxia and treatment outcome is being quantified. A recent comprehensive study (Nordsmark *et al.* 2005) has analysed the relationship between pre-treatment measurements of tumour oxygen tension and survival in advanced head & neck cancer. pO_2 measurements have been undertaken and analysed in 397 patients using the fraction of pO_2 values ≤ 2.5 mmHg ($HP_{2.5}$), ≤ 5 mmHg (HP_5) and median tumour pO_2 (mmHg) as descriptors. The study has shown that tumour hypoxia is associated with a poor prognosis in patients with advanced head & neck cancer, and the factor with the greatest prognostic significance was found to be $HP_{2.5}$. It is, therefore, of crucial importance to develop therapeutic strategies for overcoming or targeting hypoxia.

4.7.1 Tumour hypoxia

Hypoxic cells are more resistant to radiation than well oxygenated cells. The difference in radiosensitivity between hypoxic and oxic cells is attributable to the greater capacity of hypoxic cells for repair the DNA damage caused by OH radicals resulting from radiation treatment (in the presence of oxygen the DNA damage is set and oxic cells therefore cannot undergo successful cell repair).

Hypoxia occurs in tumours due to lack of oxygen and nutrients. Tumours are characterised by the presence of two types of hypoxia:

- chronic hypoxia (diffusion-limited)
- acute hypoxia (perfusion-limited).

Limited diffusion of oxygen into tumour leads to *chronic hypoxia*. The main reason for limitation in oxygen diffusion is the distance from the cancerous cells to the closest blood vessel. As the tumour grows, cells are pushed away from blood vessels so oxygen and nutrients are not able to reach the tumour by simple diffusion. Tumour hypoxia was initially thought to arise in cells situated at distances of at least 100–150 μm from functional blood vessels. However, more recent quantitative studies done on hypoxic tumours showed that hypoxic cells are already present within a 25–50 μm rim from blood vessels (Ljungkvist *et al.* 2002). It was also observed that the hypoxic cell fraction increases with the distance from blood vessels. Hypoxia can be also detected close to non-functional vessels. Permanent occlusions of blood vessels create areas with low oxyhemoglobin levels, leading to chronically hypoxic cells.

Acute hypoxia is considered a more dynamic form of hypoxia because of its transient nature. Transient hypoxia occurs in tumour cells which are dependent on blood vessels that are subject to partial decrease in functionality. This partial (or temporal) decrease in functionality limits oxygen perfusion to the tumour, making it transiently hypoxic. Consequently it is hard to quantify acute hypoxia within a tumour. However, experimental studies designed to monitor oxygen tension were able to quantify transient hypoxia in human cell lines transplanted in mice (xenografts) (Bennewith and Durand 2004). The studies concluded that the changes in tumour blood flow and oxygen tension within the monitored tumours are highly heterogenous, occurring with different magnitudes and periodicities in different regions of the same tumour. These results show that acute hypoxia is highly unpredictable, both spatially and temporally, making it hard to control.

Although it was thought that the two types of hypoxia have the same radioresistance, chronically hypoxic cells were found more sensitive to radiation damage than the acute ones. Therefore it would be useful if the measuring techniques used to detect hypoxia could differentiate between diffusion-limited and perfusion-limited hypoxia.

Methods to detect (measure) tumour hypoxia

To accurately plan a treatment for a hypoxic tumour it is crucial to localise the hypoxic population and to measure the extent of hypoxia. There are several techniques to determine the degree of tumour hypoxia, although none of them are used routinely in clinics:

- *Polarographic electrode (Eppendorf)*
  The polarographic electrode (the oxygen microelectrode based on a polarographic method) is one of the most widely used devices for tumour oxygenation measurements. Polarography, in general, is an electrochemical technique for identifying chemical elements in which the electric potential is varied in a regular manner between two electrodes while the current is monitored (Daşu 2004). The oxygen electrode used in practice nowadays was manufactured by Eppendorf in Germany and is also known as the pO2 histograph. The reason the Eppendorf electrode has become a gold standard in determining the oxygen tension is because of its good correlation with the clinical outcome. Also, the polarographic electrode allows quantitative assessment of oxygen distribution levels within the tumour. Some of the disadvantages consist of its limited applicability to superficial tumours and the inability to distinguish between necrotic and viable cancerous tissues.

- *Endogenous markers*
  Endogenous markers are gene products that are up-regulated in the presence of hypoxia. Hypoxia is involved in the transcriptional regulation of several genes. Hypoxia-inducible factor-1α (HIF-1α) is a transcription factor which mediates cell response to hypoxia. Cells express HIF-1α regularly, however, the protein degrades in a normally oxygenated environment (Isa *et al.* 2006). In hypoxic conditions the protein is stabilised, inducing the transcription of several genes (related to angiogenesis, hypoxia, pH control). The expression of HIF and the proteins it regulates can be measured using immunohistochemistry. Therefore a single biopsy, which, however, might not be representative of the whole tumour, is all that is required. Since HIF-1α plays an essential role in oxygen homeostasis *in vitro*, its importance for predicting treatment outcome in head & neck cancers has been also investigated (Aebersold *et al.* 2001). The study concluded that HIF-1α is overexpressed in the majority of patients with squamous cell cancer, particularly of the oropharynx, and that the level of expression has prognostic significance for treatment outcomes in patients undergoing curative radiotherapy.

- *Exogenous (bioreductive) markers (nitroimidazole)*
  Nitroimidazoles (misonidazole, pimonidazole, etanidazole) are nitro aromatic compounds that bind to hypoxic cells. These markers diffuse easily into hypoxic cells due to their high solubility and low metabolism (Stone *et al.* 1993). Nitroimidazole is administered, prior to biopsy or resection of a tumour, and hypoxic cells in histological sections can be identified using immunohistochemistry, flow cytometry and immunofluorescence (Isa *et al.* 2006). Though biopsies are not always reliable representatives of the tumour as a whole, head & neck studies have shown a good correlation between the extent of pimonidazole binding and treatment outcome. Kaanders *et al.* (2002) have shown that biopsies from patients with high levels of pimonidazole binding had only 48% locoregional tumour control over 2 years, compared to the 87% locoregional control presented by those with low levels of pimonidazole binding.

- *Hypoxia-selective imaging (PET, SPECT)*
  PET has the ability to image tumor metabolism quantitatively in any part of the body. Hypoxic cells can be imaged with PET using radiolabelled nitroimidazole compounds, of which ^{18}F-labelled

fluoromisonidazole ([^{18}F]FMISO) has been successfully used in clinical settings for head & neck cancers (Lehtio *et al.* 2001).

Also, bioreductive markers, like nitroimidazoles, are radiolabelled to be imaged by single-photon emission computed tomography (SPECT). Through their non-invasiveness, imaging methods like PET and SPECT are soon becoming the methods of choice for assessing the oxygenation status of tumours.

All of the above methods for measuring the extent of hypoxia in human tumours were trialled and implemented in several centres. Unfortunately, currently, there is no clinically usable way of estimating the proportion of acute hypoxia *in vivo* (Brown and Le 2002). The existing methods for quantifying hypoxia present with numerous advantages, but also drawbacks, which underscores the head for further research.

Methods to overcome tumour hypoxia

As tumour hypoxia is one of the main reasons for treatment failure, an enormous effort has been expended to develop strategies to overcome the resistance of hypoxic cells to treatment. Some of the approaches to control hypoxia were:

- *Carbogen breathing*
  Carbogen is a gas mixture of 5% carbon dioxide and 95% oxygen which has been demonstrated to improve the oxygenation of both experimental and human tumours mostly by increasing the oxygenation of the blood. The rationale for the use of a high oxygen-content gas to improve tumour oxygenation is that the increase in arterial oxygen pressure will enhance the diffusion of oxygen into the tissue. The addition of 5% CO_2 was originally proposed to counteract any vasoconstriction induced by pure oxygen breathing.
- *Hypoxic cell sensitisers (misonidazole, etanidazole)*
  The role of hypoxic cell sensitisers is, obviously, to sensitise the tumour to radiotherapy, therefore these drugs have been developed as adjuncts to radiotherapy. In order to sensitise the tumour to radiation they should be administered prior to treatment. The number of hypoxic cell sensitisers tested so far in clinical trials is high, the reason being the conflicting results given by some of the

drugs. For example, although misonidazole has been shown to be in general insufficiently powerful to sensitise hypoxic cells, a Danish trial has proven the effectiveness of the drug for pharyngeal and laryngeal cancers (Overgaard *et al.* 1989). Similarly, other clinical trials concluded that neither etanidazole nor pimonidazole have definite efficacy when combined with conventional radiotherapy while nimorazole has been proven to be effective in carcinomas of the supraglottic larynx and pharynx (Overgaard *et al.* 1998). Therefore, more studies are needed to clearly define the clinical role of hypoxic cell sensitisers.

- *Vasoactive agents (nitric oxide, endothelin-1)*
  Nitric oxide (NO•) is known to be a key molecule controlling vascular tone in normal tissues. Its role in the control of tumour blood flow is under investigation.
  Endothelin-1 is a vasoactive agent predominately secreted by endothelial cells *in vivo*. Several human cancers and animal tumour cell lines have been shown to secrete high levels of endothelin-1. The regulation of endothelin production by endothelial cells has been shown to be modified under hypoxia. Additionally, endothelin receptors have been demonstrated to be down regulated in tumour vasculature. Therefore, abnormalities in the local concentration of endothelin-1 and the density of the receptors in tumour vasculature will modify the response of the tumour vasculature to exogenously administered endothelin.

The success using these methods has been limited by either normal tissue toxicity or limited tumour radiosensitisation. In the mid 1980s, through the discovery of a hypoxic cytotoxin, **tirapazamine** (TPZ), Brown and Le (2002) have 'turned hypoxia from problem to advantage'. They showed that specifically killing the hypoxic cells has greater therapeutic potential than radio- or chemo-sensitising them. The rationale behind this statement is that hypoxic cytotoxins target and kill cells which normally are resistant to radio/chemotherapy, therefore complementing the cytotoxic effect of the treatment. In addition, hypoxic cytotoxins also target acutely hypoxic cells which otherwise are more resistant to radiation and harder to control than chronically hypoxic cells (Denekamp and Dasu 1999).

While testing the drug which they initially called SR 4233, Brown and Le observed that the killing potential of tirapazamine is much higher than that of any existing radiosensitising agent (the same concentration of tirapazamine killed a much larger number of hypoxic cells than any radiosensitising drug tested before). Furthermore, the differential toxicity to hypoxic cells presented by tirapazamine was much larger than that of any other known drug. Further studies showed that the cytotoxicity of tirapazamine resides in its ability to produce DNA double-strand and chromosome breaks under hypoxic conditions (Wang *et al.* 1992). While under hypoxic conditions tirapazamine is reduced to a highly reactive radical that produces strand breaks in the DNA, under aerobic conditions, the radical is back-oxidised to the non-toxic parent compound with the concomitant production of the superoxide radical, which is much less toxic than the tirapazamine radical (Brown 1999).

Developed as an adjunct to radiotherapy, tirapazamine has proven its role in overcoming tumour hypoxia (Marcu and Olver 2006). One of the pioneering experiments testing the efficacy of tirapazamine has compared, in a fractionated regimen, two radiation response modifiers: the bioreductive cytotoxin tirapazamine, and nicotinamide with carbogen, a tumour oxygenation enhancer (Dorie *et al.* 1994). Tirapazamine and nicotinamide were each administered before radiation treatment while carbogen was administered immediately before as well as during irradiation. The study showed that both treatment strategies improved tumour control as compared to the effect of radiation alone. However, out of the three tumour types examined, two of them showed significantly greater enhancement of tumour response after exposure to tirapazamine, while the remaining tumour type responded equally to both treatment modalities. The authors noted that the least responsive tumour had the lowest hypoxic fraction, consequently the bioreduction of tirapazamine was not that efficient as in the other, more hypoxic tumours. This experiment was a demonstration of the way hypoxia can be turned from a problem to an advantage: it showed that killing hypoxic cells leads to a greater (or at least similar) enhancement of the effect of fractionated radiotherapy on tumour control than radiosensitising (or oxygenating) the cells.

4.7.2 Tumour angiogenesis

Introduction

Angiogenesis is the term which describes the growth of new capillary blood vessels, a process that is essential for tumour growth and development. Cancer cells progress through a series of mutations by activating certain oncogenes and losing specific suppressor genes. However, in order to grow to a detectable size, tumours need to recruit and sustain their own blood supply. Tumours unable to induce angiogenesis remain *in situ* and dormant at a microscopic size.

Most certainly the inhibitors of blood-vessel growth found naturally in our bodies defend normal individuals against progression of cancer to a lethal stage. Autopsies of women aged 40 to 50 who died of causes other than cancer showed that more than one third of them had *in situ* breast tumours. However, breast cancer is diagnosed in only 1% of women in this age range. Moreover, practically all autopsies of individuals aged 50 to 70 have *in situ* carcinomas of the thyroid, whereas only 0.1% of those in this age group are actually diagnosed with thyroid cancer during their life. The fact that many people carry *in situ* tumours which do not develop to invasive disease suggests that these minuscule tumours are dormant and need additional signals to grow to a

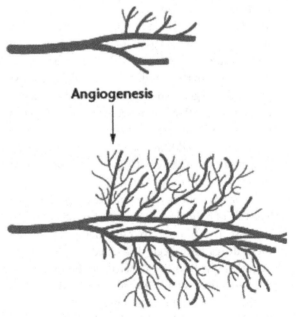

Figure 4.5. The development of new blood vessels from the previously existing normal vasculature.

lethal size. Therefore one can define cancer as having two critical phases:

- the first phase of mutation acquisition which generally results in microscopic tumours, and
- the second phase which involves the switch to the angiogenic phenotype.

The progression of cancer depends on the balance between angiogenic activators and inhibitors within the body. The angiogenesis balance is controlled by the genetic make-up of any individual cancer cell and its microenvironment within the tumour. This could explain the various growth rates observed for tumours with the same histopathologic type.

Early research

It is now widely accepted that an increasing vascular supply is critical for the progressive growth of solid tumours. Just as in normal tissue, cells in solid tumours must receive oxygen and nutrients to survive and grow. The first connection between oxygen supply and tumour growth was made by Thomlinson and Gray in 1955. They postulated that necrotic cells, found at 90–150 μm from blood vessels, are a result of tumour starved of oxygen. They showed that the oxygen diffusion distance was one of the crucial factors determining the viability of the cell. It was concluded that at the boundary of oxic and necrotic cells there is a rim of hypoxic cells which have limited oxygenation, but in contrast to necrotic cells, the hypoxic ones are still viable.

Later in the 1970s, Judah Folkman investigated the connection between hypoxia and tumour growth in a more quantitative manner, stating that a tumour without an adequate blood supply would grow only around 1–2 mm^3 (this is the approximate distance that nutrients could enter tumour cells by passive diffusion).

Any further increase in size would require the tumour to provide its own blood supply via angiogenesis.

For a tumour to become vascularised there is need for some of the constituent cells to switch to an angiogenic phenotype and to stimulate endothelial cells in order to form new blood vessels. This 'angiogenic switch' involves a change in the local equilibrium between proangiogenic factors (such as vascular endothelial growth factor (VEGF)) and negative regulators of angiogenesis (such as angiostatin, endostatin and thrombospondin). VEGF is regarded as one of the most potent growth factors for endothelial cell activation and is secreted by almost all solid tumours. Angiostatin, endostatin and thrombospondin are all naturally occurring proteins which inhibit endothelial proliferation therefore they are potent angiogenesis inhibitors.

Characteristics of tumour vasculature

Figure 4.6 shows the architectural differences between normal vasculature and tumour-stimulated blood vessels.

Tumour vasculature has several abnormal features such as occlusions, blind ends, breaks in the vessel walls, and arteriovenous shunts. Vessel strangulation (occlusion) leads to acute hypoxia. The occlusion within a blood vessel can last from minutes to hours, and once it resolves, another occlusion can occur in a different part of the tumour. As previously discussed, acute hypoxia is hard to control because of its unpredictable nature temporally as well as spatially.

4.8 TUMOUR METASTASIS

Metastasis is the transfer of malignant cells from the affected organ to other organs, via circulatory or lymphatic systems. It was shown that tumour spread leads

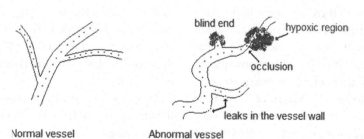

Figure 4.6. Comparison between a normal blood vessel and an abnormal vessel produced through tumour angiogenesis.

Table 4.3. Organ selectivity of metastatic spread (Tannock and Hill 1998; Hart 2006).

Primary tumour	Preferential organ for metastasis
breast	bone, brain, lung, liver
neuroblastoma	liver
osteosarcoma	lung
bowel	liver
prostate	bone
melanoma (skin)	liver, brain, bowel
lung	brain, liver, bone marrow
thyroid	lung, bone

to secondary cancer development through a metastatic cascade (Hart 2006):

1. invasion of cancer cells into surrounding healthy tissue with infiltration of capillaries or lymphatic channels
2. release of cancer cells into the lumen of the penetrated vessels
3. survival of cancer cells in the circulation
4. arrest of the surviving cancer cells in the capillary beds of distant organs
5. invasion and growth of the disseminating cells at the distant site.

In about 80% of tumours the probability to metastasise is directly proportional to the size of the primary tumour population. However, modern techniques like microarray analysis of gene expression have shown that even small tumours have the capacity to metastasise if the primary tumour expresses the gene for metastatic spread.

Clinical observations indicated that certain tumours have preferential metastatic spread to particular target organs (Plesnicar 1989) (see Table 4.3).

Although the reasons for this organ selectivity of metastasis are unknown, there are some hypotheses proposed to expound the phenomenon (Hart 2006). The first hypothesis is the mechanistic theory which states that the site of metastatic spread is a consequence of the anatomical location of the primary tumour, being therefore dictated by the pattern of blood flow (hemodynamic model). This theory, however, is insufficient, as does not explain the metastatic pattern of all tumours (there are well vascularised organs and tissues, such as kidney and muscle tissue, which are very seldom involved in metastatic invasion). The second theory is based upon the observation that vascular endothelial cells express specific receptors which bind to particular ligands. Therefore, organ endothelia could, potentially, exhibit differences in their ability to bind vascular agents. The third hypothesis, also called the 'seed and soil' hypothesis is backdated to 1889 and is based on the consideration that for a tumour to metastasise there is need for a favourable environment. It means that the characteristics of the invading tumour cells have to be compatible with the ones of the invaded organs (organ preference model).

Although metastatic spread is the most common cause of death in cancer patients, there are very limited ways to specifically target this process. While radiotherapy is the first-choice treatment for the unresectable primary tumours, metastatic disease cannot be controlled with radiation. There is, therefore, need for antimetastatic drugs, able to inhibit the process of tumour dissemination. Since successful metastasis is dependent on the balance and interplay of the promoter and suppressor genes in each step during the metastatic process, the basic anti-metastatic strategy is aimed at either blocking the promoters or potentiating the suppressors.

One drug category to play a role in the reduction in metastases is the anticoagulant and antiplatelet drugs, by inhibiting the arrest of circulating tumour cells (Dickson *et al.* 1996).

Experiments on melanoma cell lines have shown that the expression of specific genes is reduced in tumour cells which have acquired the ability to metastasise, meaning that the reintroduction of such genes can suppress the metastatic phenotype (Steeg *et al.* 2003). Such metastasis suppressor gene is Nm23, which is one out of 20 genes discovered until today. The in vitro metastasis suppression ability of the Nm23 gene was evidenced in melanoma, breast, oral squamous carcinoma and also colon cancer, through decreased motility, colonisation and invasion (Berger *et al.* 2005).

While some metastasis suppressor genes trigger dormancy in metastatic tumour cells by causing growth arrest of solitary cells at the secondary site, others promote dormancy of micrometastatic colonies, after disseminated tumour cells have undergone proliferation. One way or the other, the molecular advances in anti-metastatic studies indicate that metastasis suppressor genes may serve as a substrate for targeted therapy.

4.9   REFERENCES

Aebersold DM, Burri P, Beer KT, Laissue J, Djonov V, Greiner RH *et al.* (2001) Expression of hypoxia-inducible factor-1alpha: a novel predictive and prognostic parameter in the radiotherapy of oropharyngeal cancer. *Cancer Research* **61**: 2911–2916.

Begg AC (1997) Cell proliferation in tumours. In: *Basic Clinical Radiobiology.* 2nd edn. (Ed. GG Steel) pp. 14–23. Oxford University Press, New York.

Begg AC and Steel GG (2002) Cell proliferation and growth rate of tumours. In: *Basic Clinical Radiobiology.* 3rd edn. (Ed. GG Steel) pp. 8–22. Hodder Arnold, London.

Bennewith KL and Durand RE (2004) Quantifying transient hypoxia in human tumour xenografts by flow cytometry. *Cancer Research* **64**: 6183–6189.

Berger J, Vander Griend D, Robinson V, Hickson J *et al.* (2005) Metastasis suppressor genes: from gene identification to protein function and regulation. *Cancer Biology and Therapy* **4**: 805–812.

Brown JM (1999) The hypoxic cell: a target for selective cancer therapy. *Cancer Research* **59**: 5863–5870.

Brown JM and Le QT (2002) Tumour hypoxia is important in radiotherapy, but how should we measure it? *International Journal of Radiation Oncology Biology Physics* **54**: 1299–1301.

Chen SW, KoLiang JA, Yang SN HL and Lin FJ (2003) The adverse effect of treatment prolongation in cervical cancer by high-dose-rate intracavitary brachytherapy. *Radiotherapy and Oncology* **67**(1): 69–76.

Daşu I (2004) Theoretical modelling of tumour oxygenation and influences on treatment outcome. PhD thesis, Umea University, Sweden.

Denekamp J and Daşu A (1999) Inducible repair and the two forms of tumour hypoxia-time for a paradigm shift. *Acta Oncologica* **38**: 903–918.

Denham J, Walker Q, Lamb D, Hamilton C *et al.* (1996) Mucosal regeneration during radiotherapy. *Radiotherapy and Oncology* **41**: 109–118.

Dickson RB, Johnson MD, Maemura M and Low J (1996) Anti-invasion drugs. *Breast Cancer Research and Treatment* **38**: 121–132.

Dorie MJ, Menke D and Brown JM (1994) Comparison of the enhancement of tumor responses to fractionated irradiation by SR 4233 (tirapazamine) and by nicotinamide with carbogen. *International Journal of Radiation Oncology Biology Physics* **28**: 145–150.

Dörr W (1997) Three A's of repopulation during fractionated irradiation of squamous epithelia: Asymmetry loss, Acceleration of stem-cell divisions and Abortive divisions. *International Journal of Radiation Biology* **72**: 635–643.

Gatenby RA, Kessler HB, Rosenblum JS, Coia LR *et al.* (1988) Oxygen distribution in squamous cell carcinoma metastases and its relationship to outcome of radiation therapy. *International Journal of Radiation Oncology Biology Physics* **14**: 831–838.

Hall EJ (2000) *Radiobiology for the Radiologist.* 5th edn. Lippincott, Williams and Wilkins, Philadelphia.

Hanahan D and Weinberg RA (2000) The hallmarks of cancer. *Cell* **100**: 57–70.

Hansen O, Grau C, Bentzen S and Overgaard J (1996) Repopulation in the SCCVII squamous cell carcinoma assessed by an in vivo-in vitro excision assay. *Radiotherapy and Oncology* **39**: 137–144.

Hart I (2006) The spread of tumours. In: *Introduction to the Cellular and Molecular Biology of Cancer.* (Eds M Knowles and P Selby) pp. 278–288. Oxford University Press.

Hermens A and Barendsen G (1969) Changes of cell proliferation characteristics in a rat rhabdomyosarcoma before and after X-irradiation. *European Journal of Cancer* **5**: 173–189.

Isa AY, Ward T, West C, Slevin N and Homer J (2006) Hypoxia in head & neck cancer. *British Journal of Radiology* **79**: 791–798.

Kaanders JH, Wijffels KI, Marres HA, Ljungkvist AS, Pop LA, van den Hoogen FJ *et al.* (2002) Pimonidazole binding and tumor vascularity predict for treatment outcome in head & neck cancer. *Cancer Research* **62**: 7066–7074.

Knowles M (2005) Molecular cytogenetics of cancer. In *Cellular and Molecular Biology of Cancer*. 4th edn. (Eds M Knowles and P Selby) pp. 95–116. Oxford University Press.

Kummermehr JC (2001) Tumour stem cells – the evidence and the ambiguity. *Acta Oncologica* **40**(8): 981–988.

Lehtio K, Oikonen V, Gronroos T, Eskola O, Kalliokoski K *et al.* (2001) Imaging of blood flow and hypoxia in head & neck cancer: initial evaluation with [15O]H2O and [18F]Fluoroerythronitroimidazole PET. *Journal of Nuclear Medicine* **42**(11): 1643–1652.

Ljungkvist AS, Bussink J, Rijken PF *et al.* (2002) Vascular architecture, hypoxia, and proliferation in first-generation xenografts of human head-and-neck squamous cell carcinomas. *International Journal of Radiation Oncology Biology Physics* **54**: 215–228.

Maciejewski B and Majewski S (1991) Dose fractionation and tumour repopulation in radiotherapy for bladder cancer. *Radiotherapy and Oncology* **21**(3): 163–170.

Marcu L and Olver I (2006) Tirapazamine: from bench to clinical trials. *Current Clinical Pharmacology* **1**: 71–79.

Nias AHW (2000) *An Introduction to Radiobiology*. John Wiley & Sons Ltd., West Sussex.

Nordsmark M, Bentzen S, Rudat V, Brizel D, Lartigau E *et al.* (2005) Prognostic value of tumor oxygenation in 397 head & neck tumors after primary radiation therapy. An international multi-center study. *Radiation and Oncology* **77**: 18–24.

Nowell PC and Hungerford DA (1960) A minute chromosome in human chronic granulocytic leukemia. *Science* **142**: 1497.

Orton CG (2001) High-dose-rate brachytherapy may be radiobiologically superior to low-dose rate due to slow repair of late-responding normal tissue cells. *International Journal of Radiation Oncology Biology Physics* **49**(1): 183–189.

Overgaard J, Sand Hansen H and Overgaard M (1989) Misonidazole combined with split-course radiotherapy in the treatment of invasive carcinoma of larynx and pharynx: report from the DAHANCA 2 study. *International Journal of Radiation Oncology Biology Physics* **16**: 1065–1068.

Overgaard J, Sand Hansen H, Overgaard M *et al.* (1998) A randomized double-blind phase III study of nimorazole as a hypoxic radiosensitizer of primary radiotherapy in supraglottic larynx and pharynx carcinoma. Results of the Danish Head & Neck Cancer Study (DAHANCA) Protocol 5-85. *Radiotherapy and Oncology* **46**: 135–146.

Plesnicar S (1989) Mechanisms of development of metastases. *Critical Reviews in Oncology* **1**: 175–194.

Reya T, Morrison SJ, Clarke MF and Weissman IL (2001) Stem cells, cancer, and cancer stem cells. *Nature* **414**: 105–111.

Sham E and Durand R (1999) Repopulation characteristics and cell kinetic parameters resulting from multi-fraction irradiation of xenograft tumors in SCID mice. *International Journal of Radiation Oncology Biology Physics* **43**: 617–622.

Steeg PS, Ouatas T, Halverson D, Palmieri D and Salerno M (2003) Metastasis suppressor genes: basic biology and potential clinical use. *Clinical Breast Cancer* **4**: 51–62.

Steel GG (1977) *The Growth Kinetic of Tumours*. Oxford University Press, Oxford.

Steel GG (2002) *Basic Clinical Radiobiology*. Arnold, London.

Stephens T, Currie G and Peacock J (1978) Repopulation of gamma irradiated Lewis lung carcinoma by malignant cells and host macrophage 1 precursors. *British Journal of Cancer* **38**: 573–582.

Stone HB, Brown JM, Phillips TL and Sutherland RM (1993) Oxygen in human tumours: correlations between methods of measurement and response to therapy. *Radiation Research* **136**: 422–434.

Tannock I and Hill R (1998) *The Basic Science of Oncology*. 3rd edn. McGraw-Hill International.

Tomlinson RH and Gray LH (1955) The histological structure of some human lung cancers and the possible implications for radiotherapy. *British Journal of Cancer* **9**: 539–549.

Trott K (1999) The mechanisms of acceleration of repopulation in squamous epithelia during daily irradiation. *Acta Oncologica* **38**: 153–157.

Trott K and Kummermehr J (1991) Accelerated repopulation in tumours and normal tissues. *Radiotherapy and Oncology* **22**: 159–160.

Wang J, Biedermann KA and Brown JM (1992) Repair of DNA and chromosome breaks in cells exposed to SR 4233 under hypoxia or to ionizing radiation. *Cancer Research* **52**: 4473–4477.

Withers HR (1993) Treatment-induced accelerated human tumour growth. *Seminars in Radiation Oncology* **3**: 135–143.

Withers HR and Elkind MM (1969) Radiosensitivity and fractionation response of crypt cells of mouse jejunum. *Radiation Research* **38**: 598–613.

5 Fractionation and altered fractionation in radiotherapy

5.1 INTRODUCTION

'The object of treating a tumour by radiotherapy is to damage every single potentially malignant cell to such an extent that it cannot continue to proliferate' (Munro and Gilbert 1961). In order to achieve complete eradication of a tumour, all clonogenic cells within it must be rendered incapable of continued proliferation. As previously discussed in Chapter 4, each tumour originates from a single cell which underwent multiple mutations. It therefore follows that the survival of even one single clonogenic (stem) cell leads to regrowth of the tumour.

Consequently, the highest tumour control probability (TCP) and the lowest normal tissue complication probability (NTCP) is the major goal of radiotherapy. This represents the optimal approach to radiotherapy of any site including the head & neck. The therapeutic ratio, defined as the ratio between TCP (tumour control probability) and NTCP (normal tissue complication probability), can be used to indicate the extent to which the optimal is achieved. High therapeutic ratios can be achieved either by increasing radiation dose for better tumour control whilst keeping the normal tissue complication probability constant, or by reducing NTCP whilst keeping TCP constant. For optimal results, one would aim for increase in TCP whilst decreasing NTCP.

Several treatment-related parameters need to be considered in order to improve the effectiveness of radiotherapy. These include accurate staging of the cancer, radiobiological characteristics of the tumour, radiation modality (whether external beam or brachytherapy), energy of radiation, treatment technique, overall prescribed dose, fractionation regimen (dose per fraction, number of fractions, time interval between fractions), treatment modalities other than radiation (chemotherapy, hyperthermia, gene therapy, immunotherapy, etc), tumour hypoxic cell sensitisers and radiosensitisers, tissue radioprotection. Radiobiological models are useful tools in understanding the influence of the various parameters on the same and different tumour sites. The effect of various treatment modalities is simulated and used to calculate biologically equivalent fractionation schedules as well as to predict treatment outcomes based on experimentally derived input parameters.

5.2 THE 5 R'S OF RADIOBIOLOGY

The concept of fractionation is a consequence of radiobiological experiments conducted on rams in the 1920s. The aim of these French experiments was to sterilise rams using a single dose of kilovoltage radiation, a process that could not occur without

L. Marcu et al., *Biomedical Physics in Radiotherapy for Cancer*,
DOI 10.1007/978-0-85729-733-4_5, © CSIRO 2012

considerable skin damage. It was observed that the goal could be achieved by dividing the single dose into multiple fractions, thus sparing the skin. Fractionation in radiotherapy started to be used in order to spare normal tissue (by repair and repopulation) and also to increase the damage to the tumour (by reoxygenation and redistribution).

The 5 R's of radiobiology are considered to be the following:

- Repair of sublethal damage.
- Repopulation by surviving cells.
- Redistribution of cells along the cell cycle.
- Reoxygenation of hypoxic cells.
- Radiosensitivity.

Repair and repopulation tend to confer resistance to the tissue between two radiation doses, while redistribution and reoxygenation are likely to make the tissue more sensitive to a subsequent dose. These four factors modify the response of a tissue to repeated doses of radiation. Different tissues (both normal and cancerous) behave differently during radiotherapy. The main factor responsible for the difference is considered to be the fifth R, radiosensitivity, as the response to radiotherapy is influenced by the sensitivity of the individual.

5.2.1 Repair

The damage produced in a mammalian cell nucleus by 1 Gy of low LET radiation consists of approximately 1000 DNA single-strand breaks and 40 double-strand breaks (1 DSB per chromosome per Gy) (Olive 1998). It was shown by track structure analysis that 50% of DSB will have other types of DNA damage in close proximity (clustered damage) (Hill 1999). **Repair** refers to the process by which the function of the cell is restored. Repair of DNA strand breaks illustrates the ability of cells to repair the radiation damage. Although ionising radiation can produce a broad spectrum of DNA lesions including damage to nucleotide bases, unrepaired or misrepaired DNA double-strand breaks (DSB) are thought to be the principal lesions responsible for the induction of genetic changes in mammalian cells, including chromosomal abnormalities and gene mutations.

Cells possess a complex set of signalling pathways for recognising DNA damage and initiating its repair.

The ATM gene is one of the main sensors of DNA damage, which activates by phosphorylation a variety of proteins involved in cell cycle control and DNA repair. Unrepaired or misrepaired DSB lead primarily to large-scale genetic changes that are frequently manifested by chromosomal aberrations. The pathway used to repair DNA damage depends on the stage of the cell cycle.

The double-helical structure of DNA is ideally suited for repair because it carries two separate copies of all the genetic information – one in each of its two strands. Thus, when one strand is damaged, the complementary strand retains an intact copy of the same information, and this copy is generally used to restore the correct nucleotide sequences to the damaged strand. Single strand breaks do not disrupt the integrity of the double helix and therefore they repair with ease. However, if there are more than one single strand breaks affecting the DNA, depending on their location (directly opposite breaks or distantly opposite breaks) they can lead to double strand breaks which undergo a more complex repair process as the double helix is cleaved into two segments (Figure 5.1). It is to be noted that the probability for two separate track events to hit opposite strands of the DNA at a dose of a few Gy (thus causing a double strand break) is very low due to the small diameter of the DNA molecule (about 2.5 nm) (Joiner 2002).

The major categories of DNA repair systems involved in the cellular response to ionising radiation are the following: excision repair (excises damaged nucleotide segments followed by re-synthesis), mismatch repair (corrects error of replication) and recombination repair (restores double strand breaks) (Figure 5.2). The fourth category, which is a direct repair system, converts the damaged nucleotides into their original structure in a direct way, which is, however, very uncommon after radiation-induced DNA damage (Lindahl and Wood 1999).

Nevertheless, rejoining of DNA strand breaks does not necessarily mean that gene function is restored. A significant additional factor is repair fidelity. If the repair is not complete, a subsequent radiation dose can easily cause a lethal damage to the cell. If repair of the damage is correct, the cell recovers. For a sublethally damaged cell, *in vitro*, it takes at least 1 hour to repair the damage. *In vivo* the repair time is supposed

I. Double strand break

II. Single strand break

A. distantly opposite breaks

B. directly opposite breaks

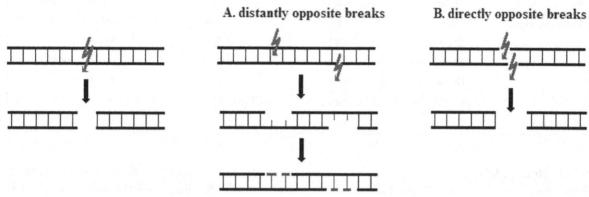

Figure 5.1. DNA single and double strand breaks.

to be longer, therefore in the case of hyperfractionation (radiation twice a day) a 6 hour time gap is kept between the two fractions. The aim here is to allow the normal tissue time to repair damage, but unavoidably, repair can take place in cancerous tissue as well.

As described in § 2.1 the linear-quadratic model presented in equations (2.5) to (2.6) assumes that there is full repair of sublethal damage between subsequent radiation fractions. This means that there is a time gap of at least 6 hours between two consecutive fractions to allow for normal tissue repair, although some organs/tissues need longer times to complete sublethal damage repair (for instance, the spinal cord may need up to 24 hours repair time) (Joiner 2002). If the interfraction interval is reduced below the time necessary for sublethal damage repair (usually when multiple fractions per day are delivered) the damage created by one fraction might not be fully repaired before the delivery of a subsequent radiation dose. Therefore the residual damage interacts with the newly created lesion leading to *incomplete repair*. An important parameter which characterises the ability of normal tissues to repair radiation-induced damage is *repair half-time* ($T_{1/2}$) and is defined as the inter-fraction time required for half of the repair processes to take place.

Based on animal studies it has been proposed that for certain normal tissues, sublethal damage repair may involve a bi-phasic process (two repair rates) consisting of a fast process (short repair half-time) followed by a slow repair (long repair half-time) (Table 5.1).

EXCISION REPAIR

MISMATCH REPAIR

RECOMBINATION REPAIR

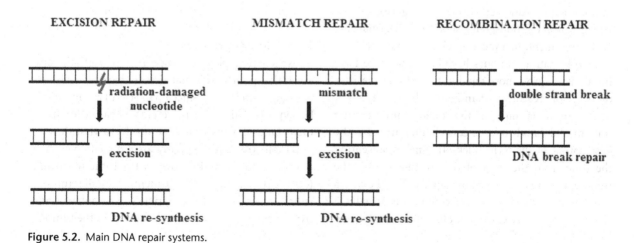

Figure 5.2. Main DNA repair systems.

Table 5.1. Bi-phasic sublethal damage repair times for normal tissue.

Tissue/organ	Short $T_{1/2}$	Long $T_{1/2}$	α/β ratio	Reference
Mouse lung	24 min	4 h	3.8 Gy	Van Rongen 1993
Mouse kidney	9 min	5 h	2.1 Gy	Millar 1994
Rat spinal cord	42 min	3.8 h	2 Gy	Ang 1992
	22 min	6.5 h	2 Gy	Landuyt 1997
	12 min	4.3 h	1.3 Gy	Kim 1997
	12 min	2.2 h	2.47 Gy	Pop 2000
Pig epidermis	10.2 min	5.4 h	5.19 Gy	Millar 1994

5.2.2 Repopulation

Repopulation occurs when cells that survive irradiation proliferate. In normal tissue repopulation is an essential effect as healthy cells can repopulate the affected tissue or organ between fractions. This occurs especially in normal tissues with high cell turnover (gastrointestinal tract, bone marrow) so the side effects of the treatment (nausea, vomiting, hematologic symptoms) can be diminished. For the late responding tissues the fractionation of radiotherapy can be vital, as slowly proliferating cells hardly regrow the damaged tissue, if they ever do.

Repopulation, however, can occur in malignant tissue as well. Thus the number of cells that must be killed increases. Stem cells or clonogenic cells are those able to regrow the whole tumour if they are not destroyed. Although the percentage of stem cells in a tumour is usually 2% (or even less), due to their infinite proliferative capacity, they can restore the tumour. The aim of radiotherapy is to target the clonogenic cells, in order to successfully eradicate the tumour. Repopulation can occur between two successive radiation fractions, but also towards the final part of the treatment, in a more accelerated manner. Rapidly proliferating tumours have been shown to have the ability to grow more rapidly at a certain time after the start of treatment, than before therapy. Head & neck cancer is one of the rapidly proliferating tumours. The study of head & neck tumours led to the designation of the term 'kick-off time', representing the time from the start of the treatment until the tumour begins to grow more rapidly than before, a time period which for these tumours is usually 3 weeks. This accelerated proliferation influences

strongly the local control of the tumour, so the treatment should be adjusted for the final part of radiotherapy in accordance with tumour properties.

5.2.3 Redistribution

Redistribution (or reassortment) of cells along the cell cycle occurs regularly. Normal cells as well as tumour cells propagate according to an internal clock, proceeding through a sequence of phases constituting the cell cycle. The cell cycle time varies as a function of tumour type (and also normal tissue), lasting between several hours and a couple of days. The four phases have different sensitivities to radiation. Thus the M phase is the most sensitive, and the S phase is the most resistant. Cells that survive a first dose of radiation will tend to be in a resistant phase but within a few hours they may progress into a more sensitive phase when they can be killed. For rapidly proliferating cells (with shorter cell cycle times) the fractionation schedule seems to be important again, as between two fractions cells are travelling from one phase to another, thus every fraction will hit some cells in the sensitive phase.

5.2.4 Reoxygenation

Reoxygenation plays a major role in radiotherapy, given that poorly oxygenated cells (hypoxic cells) are resistant to radiation. Since up to 30% of a tumour can be hypoxic, this often represents a reason for treatment failure. Thus cells that survive a first dose of radiation are mainly poorly oxygenated, but their oxygen supply may improve as the tumour shrinks (during the fractionated treatment). A smaller tumour is better perfused by capillaries, so the nutrient and oxygen supply can easily reach the core of the tumour,

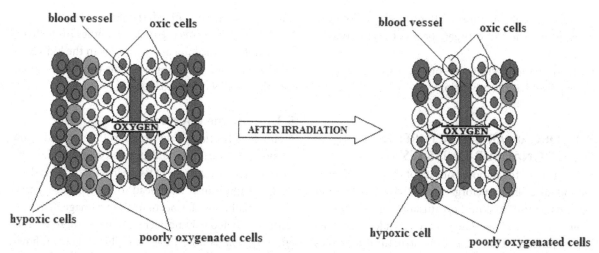

Figure 5.3. Schematic illustration of reoxygenation within a tumour cell population. The radiation-induced cell kill of oxic cells situated close to the blood vessels will enable the oxygen to reach poorly oxygenated and hypoxic cells (thus reoxygenating them), making them more radiosensitive to the subsequent dose.

making it more radiosensitive. The speed of reoxygenation varies widely, occurring within a few hours in some tumours and taking several days in others. If reoxygenation occurs rapidly then it may be due to recirculation of blood through vessels that were temporarily closed. Reoxygenation during longer periods of time is usually the result of cell death leading to the above mentioned tumour shrinkage. For more effective radiotherapy hypoxic cell sensitisers should be given to the patient, immediately before radiotherapy.

Hypoxia is considered to be one of the treatment challenges for several tumours. Chronic hypoxia or diffusion-limited hypoxia is easier to control through reoxygenation as its location within the tumour is known, therefore fractionated radiotherapy leads to tumour shrinkage and, eventually, the hypoxic core becomes close to the oxygen-carrying blood vessels allowing for reoxygenation (Figure 5.3). Acute hypoxia is more of a problem than chronic hypoxia, since the length of time during which a particular blood vessel is occluded is hard to predict. Fractionated radiotherapy could, partially, overcome acute hypoxia if the occluded vessel becomes functional before the subsequent radiation dose. However, there is no certainty about the appearance and location of another temporally hypoxic region within the tumour, increasing the likelihood of it being 'missed' by the radiation treatment.

5.2.5 Radiosensitivity

Radiosensitivity of human tumours is dependent on multiple factors including:

- tumour-related factors: hypoxia, tumour kinetics, number of clonogenic cells
- host-related factors: defence, volume effect, genetic predisposition.

The degree of radiosensitivity is best studied by predictive assays, individualising the cancer treatment as required for each particular tumour, even with the same histopathological type.

Radiosensitivity of normal tissues is influenced by genetic factors. The main parameters influencing the appearance of early and/or late effects after irradiation relate to the characteristics of the treatment and of the patient. The most common treatment-related characteristics include the following:

- dose of radiation (high dose versus low dose)
- type of radiation (low LET versus high LET)
- fractionation schedule (late effects are more sensitive to changes in fractionation than early effects).

Host-related characteristics determining normal tissue reaction are mediated through:

- intra-patient variability (differences in tolerance of tissues or organs of the same patient)

- inter-patient variability (differences in radiosensitivity of the same organ or tissue type among patients)
- fractionation sensitivity of the tissue or organ expressed as the α/β ratio.

5.3 ORGAN ARCHITECTURE: FUNCTIONAL SUB-UNITS (FSU)

In addition to the radiosensitivity of their constituent individual cells, tissue/organ sensitivity to radiation depends on the structural organisation of the cells (or group of cells). Tissues/organs are considered to consist of functional sub-units, the structural architecture of which contributes significantly to the radiosensitivity of that specific organ/tissue.

The effects of radiation on an organ operate at the following levels:

- cellular, causing individual cell death
- functional sub-unit (FSU), leading to damage of one or more functional sub-units
- organ, resulting in organ malfunction.

A functional sub-unit of a tissue or organ each containing a certain number of cells, is that component which is integral to tissue/organ function. The following characteristics of FSUs determine the effects of radiation on tissue/organ function:

- All cells within an FSU need to be killed for it to be inactivated;
- The number of FSUs inactivated for malfunction depends on the architecture of the tissue/organ (organisation of FSUs);
- Any surviving cell within an FSU is able to repopulate.

A simple way of representing the organisation of functional sub-units within tissues/organs is to classify them into serial or parallel structures. This organisation of the FSUs is called *organ architecture* (Figure 5.4). Although purely serial or parallel arrangements of FSUs are ideal considerations, such modelling allows for convenient assessment and prediction of the effect of radiation on such structures. With the possible exception of the spinal cord as a typical example of a serial organ, the majority of ana-

tomical organs are mixed structures. Nevertheless, because of the arrangement of the lobules in the liver, bronchioles in the lung and nephrons in the kidney in parallel manner, these three organs can be classified into the parallel organ category.

5.3.1 Volume effects

A simple definition of the volume effects of radiation on normal tissues is the dependence of any damage sustained on the volume of tissue irradiated. This definition would immediately lead to the conclusion that the threshold dose for normal tissue damage increases as the irradiated volume decreases in size (*dose-volume effect hypothesis*) (see Table 5.2). This statement, however, is debatable, since the response of various organs to ionising radiation depends more on their structural architecture. As previously discussed, parallel organs are less radiosensitive than serial organs, because of the organisation of their FSUs. To impair the function of a parallel organ, there is need for several FSUs to be lethally damaged. Therefore, there is a threshold number of FSUs damaged beyond which the overall function of the organ would be impaired. Consequently, the volume effect is much more pronounced in parallel organs. On the other hand, the volume effect is virtually absent in serial organs, since even one lethally damaged FSU can lead to the impairment of the whole organ, there being no threshold limit for the number of FSUs damaged (see also Table 5.3).

There is a large number of publications in the literature presenting various **models for NTCP** based on FSUs of different organ architecture. Radiobiological models such as the Lyman-Kutcher-Burman (LKB) model (Lyman 1985; Kutcher and Burman 1989), the relative seriality NTCP model (Källman *et al.* 1992) or the critical volume NTCP (Niemierko and Goitein 1993), all have been extensively analysed however, their acceptance in clinical practice is still pending due to clinicians preference towards dosimetric models (Miller *et al.* 2009).

5.4 FRACTIONATION IN RADIOTHERAPY

Dose fractionation in radiotherapy originated in the first decade of the 20th century. One of the rationales for changing single-dose radiation treatments into

SERIAL ORGAN ARCHITECTURE

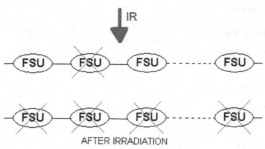

FSUs are dependent on each other. If any one FSU is inactivated, the function of the whole organ is impaired.

PARALLEL ORGAN ARCHITECTURE

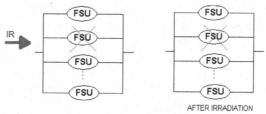

FSUs are independent of each other. If some FSUs are inactivated the organ can still perform its task. There is a threshold for the number of FSUs for parallel organs that can be destroyed beyond which the organ will not be able to function.

MIXED ORGAN ARCHITECTURE

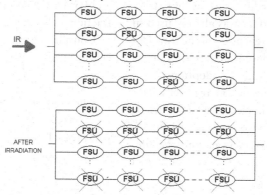

Mixed organ architectures are the most commonly found, since it is difficult to categorise an organ as purely serial or parallel.

Figure 5.4. Diagrammatic representation of organ architecture.

fractionated ones was based on the observation of the association between the proliferative activity of cells and susceptibility to radiation-induced injury. Robert Kienböck first reported the higher radiosensitivity of cells with high mitotic activity in 1901 (Thames 1987). Several fractionation studies have been undertaken by Schwartz who consistently expressed his preference for dose fractionation: 'in the same tumour there will be cells more radiosensitive than others, depending on the phase of the division cycle. Therefore it is not recommended to use one, or a few large doses separated by long intervals, since the most advantageous time for irradiation may be missed entirely or occur during one of the intervals. Instead we recommend a method of small daily doses' (Thames and Hendry 1987).

One of the milestones in the history of the treatment of rapidly proliferating cancers occurred in the 1920s when Coutard developed a technique using external beam radiation (Röntgen) therapy using one or two low-dose-rate fractions per day over two weeks, or over a longer period of time for larger tumours. His method was rapidly adopted by several cancer

Table 5.2.   Tolerance doses for various organs (Emami *et al.* 1991).

Organ	TD$_{5/5}$ (Gy) Volume irradiated			TD$_{50/5}$ (Gy) Volume irradiated			End point
	1/3	2/3	3/3	1/3	2/3	3/3	
Brain	60	50	45	75	65	60	Necrosis/infarction
Esophagus	60	58	55	72	70	68	Clinical stricture/ perforation
Heart	60	45	40	70	55	50	Pericarditis
Larynx	79	70	70	90	80	80	Cartilage necrosis
Lung	45	30	17.5	65	40	24.5	Pneumonitis
Skin	10 cm^2 70	30 cm^2 60	100 cm^2 55	10 cm^2 –	30 cm^2 –	100 cm^2 70	Necrosis/ulceration
Spinal cord	5 cm 55	10 cm 50	20 cm 47	5 cm 70	10 cm 70	20 cm –	Myelitis/necrosis

institutions across the world and used as a gold standard for dose fractionation for about a decade.

Altered fractionation schedules such as hyperfractionation as is understood today was already used in the 1930s. With better comprehension of the time factor (the time over which a dose is delivered in determining a biological effect) and the adoption of cell survival models, other fractionation regimens have since been developed and implemented for various tumour sites. For tumours undergoing rapid proliferation during treatment, altered fractionation schedules have become widespread clinically as they counteract the time factor.

Table 5.3.   Volume effects in normal tissues as a function of organ architecture.

Parallel organs	Serial organs
There is a threshold limit for the number of FSU's damaged to impair the function of the organ.	*There is no threshold limit* for the number of FSU's damaged to impair the function of the organ (even a single lethally damaged FSU can lead to organ impairment).
The *volume effect is very pronounced.*	The *volume effect* is almost *non-existent.*
The risk of complications depends on *dose distribution* throughout the *whole organ.*	The risk of complications depends strongly on *high-dose regions* (hot spots).

The most commonly used cell survival model is the linear-quadratic one, originally developed by Douglas and Fowler (1976) to interpret skin isoeffect doses for fractionated radiotherapy.

Considering the linear quadratic formulation for cell survival after the exposure to a total dose D:

$$S = \exp(-\alpha D - \beta D^2)$$

when radiotherapy is fractionated in 'n' number of fractions each delivering a dose 'd', the above equation is expressed as:

$$S = \exp[-n(\alpha d + \beta d^2)] = \exp[-nd(\alpha + \beta d)] \tag{5.1}$$

For fractionated treatment, the greater the number of fractions the larger the shoulder of the survival curve because of repair of cell damage between each consecutive fraction. Therefore, when fractionating radiotherapy, the survival curve becomes less steep than for a single dose treatment (Figure 5.5).

The vertical pulses of the survival curves are due to cell regrowth in between consecutive fractions. Thus, increasing the number of fractions (and reducing the dose size) reduces the level of cell kill through the repair of sublethal damage. The historical basis for dose fractionation – to spare the normal tissue adjacent to tumours – is supported by experimental data that tumour cells are less able to repair sublethal damage (Pekkola-Heino *et al.* 1998), thus validating the linear quadratic formula.

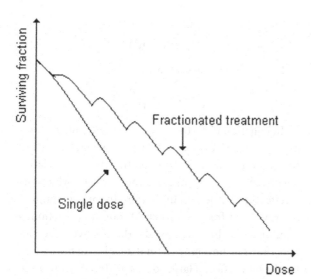

Figure 5.5 Cell survival curves: single dose versus dose fractionation.

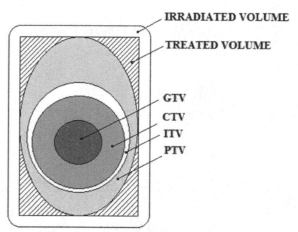

Figure 5.6. Definition of target volumes.

One of the most important aspects of radiotherapy planning and treatment in order to avoid systematic errors especially when it comes to fractionation is to correctly define the target volumes involved and implicitly the organs at risk (OAR). In the ICRU Report 50 (1993) the International Commission on Radiation Units and Measurements has defined three distinct target volumes suitable for today's widely employed conformal radiotherapy techniques (Figure 5.6):

- the *gross tumour volume* (GTV) which is the clinically detectable/visible tumour and is determined through direct visualisation or indirectly, via imaging techniques;
- the *clinical target volume* (CTV) defined as the volume that accounts for the subclinical microscopic tumour spread (such as lymph nodes); ICRU 62 recommends the addition of an internal margin to the CTV accounting for internal movement and changes in size and position of the CTV during treatment. The volume incorporating the CTV and the internal margins is termed the **internal target volume** (ITV);
- the *planning target volume* (PTV) defined as the volume which accounts for various uncertainties.

While the gross tumour volume and the clinical target volume are anatomical-clinical concepts which are defined before establishing the treatment modality, the planning target volume is a geometric concept defined for the purpose of treatment planning and evaluation and accounts for various uncertainties that might occur during treatment, such as organ or tumour motion, patient set-up, and inaccuracies in beam delivery. The PTV is a useful instrument to shape dose distributions, ensuring that the prescribed dose will be delivered to the CTV. All the above target volumes are incorporated in the treated volume which is *'the tissue volume that [...] is planned to receive at least a dose selected and specified by radiation oncology team as being appropriate to achieve the purpose of the treatment, e.g., tumour eradication or palliation, within the bounds of acceptable complications'* (ICRU Report 62).

The 1999 ICRU Report 62, which came to supplement some of the target definitions, has taken into consideration the radiobiological impact of organ architecture on normal tissue complications, therefore making a classification of organs into serial, parallel and serial-parallel (mixed). The OAR has been defined by the aforementioned report as *'normal tissues whose radiation sensitivity may significantly influence treatment planning and/or prescribed dose'* (Figure 5.7). Furthermore, ICRU 62 suggests the consideration of margins around organs at risk, similarly to tumour movement uncertainty. Thus, the **planning organ at risk volume** (PRV) is formulated to account for movements of organs at risk. Therefore, PRV for OAR is equivalent to PTV for CTV.

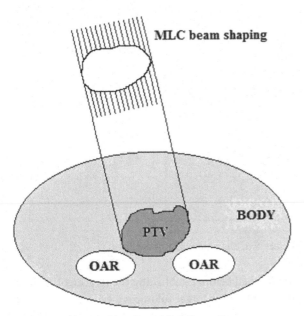

Figure 5.7. PTV conformality with OAR sparing.

A major challenge in radiotherapy planning occurs when the PTV overlaps with an organ at risk. In this case, highly conformal techniques such as IMRT or proton therapy have the ability to improve the dose achievable across the PTV while restricting the dose to the adjacent organs.

5.5 BIOLOGICALLY EFFECTIVE DOSES IN RADIOTHERAPY

The effect of fractionated radiotherapy on various normal tissues can be characterised by the total dose delivered in equal increments (fractions). When the appropriate values for the α and β parameters are known, the linear-quadratic model can be a valuable means of showing the difference between early and late responding tissues.

Each successive fraction in fractionated radiotherapy has been shown to be equally effective. The equation representing the dependence of cell survival on radiation dose can be written as: E = -lnS, where E is the biologic effect of radiation on a tissue and S is the surviving fraction of cells in the tissue. Taking equation (5.1) into consideration, the biologic effect (E) can be expressed as:

$$E = nd(\alpha + \beta d) \qquad (5.2)$$

or,

$$E = \alpha D + \beta D d \qquad (5.3)$$

Rearranging equation (5.3):

$$\frac{E}{\alpha} = D\left[1 + \frac{d}{(\alpha/\beta)}\right] \qquad (5.4)$$

In equation (5.4), the E/α ratio represents the biologically effective dose or BED. D is the total dose, and the term $1 + d/(\alpha/\beta)$ in parentheses is the relative effectiveness. The term gives the factor by which the isoeffect dose is less than that for an infinite number of very small fractions when 'd' dose per fraction is administered. In other words, the relative effectiveness shows by how much a total dose has to be reduced for the same effect if larger doses per fraction are used. Therefore, the Biologically Effective Dose (BED) is the parameter by which different fractionation regimens can be compared.

A sensible way of determining biologically effective doses is to convert the treatment parameters into the isoeffective dose in 2 Gy fractions (EQD$_2$). This has the advantage that the 2 Gy fractional doses are often applied in clinical practice, and dose-response data are available. Considering equation (5.4) for isoeffect calculations:

$$D\left(1 + \frac{d}{\alpha/\beta}\right) = D_2\left(1 + \frac{d_2}{\alpha/\beta}\right) \qquad (5.5)$$

where d_2 = 2 Gy, D_2 is the isoeffective dose given in 2 Gy fractions and is expressed as:

$$D_2 = D\frac{1 + \dfrac{d}{\alpha/\beta}}{1 + \dfrac{d_2}{\alpha/\beta}} = D\frac{(\alpha/\beta) + d}{(\alpha/\beta) + d_2} \qquad (5.6)$$

The α/β ratio is the only parameter which has to be found as a function of the end-point (whether relating to tumour or normal tissue effects) of concern.

5.6 INCOMPLETE REPAIR MODEL

The incomplete repair model, based on the linear quadratic formalism was introduced by Thames (1985) and modified later to account for overnight repair (overnight interfraction interval) (Thames 1989). When considering mono-exponential repair kinetics of sublethal damage, the correction (h) to the β component of the linear quadratic model will append the equation for biological effect with a function of repair half-time ($T_{1/2}$) and interfraction interval Δt:

$$E = nd\{\alpha + \beta d[1 + h(T_{1/2}, \Delta t)]\} \qquad (5.7)$$

The function h accounts for incomplete repair between both daily fractions (θ_1) and overnight fractions (θ_2) and is expressed as:

$$h(T_{1/2}, \Delta t) = (1 + \theta_1^2)\left[\frac{\theta_1}{1 - \theta_1\theta_2}\right]\left(1 - \frac{2}{n} \cdot \frac{1 - (\theta_1\theta_2)^{n/2}}{1 - \theta_1\theta_2}\right) + \theta_1 \qquad (5.8)$$

In the above relation θ_1 and θ_2 are functions of $T_{1/2}$ and Δt:

$$\begin{cases} \theta_1 = \exp\left(-\Delta t \dfrac{\ln 2}{T_{1/2}}\right) \\ \theta_2 = \exp\left(-(24 - \Delta t)\dfrac{\ln 2}{T_{1/2}}\right) \end{cases} \qquad (5.9)$$

For tissues with bi-phasic repair times (also see § 5.2.1) equation (5.7) becomes more complex as both slow and fast repair half-times have to be taken into consideration. Therefore:

$$E = nd\{\alpha + \beta' d[1 + h'(T'_{1/2}, \Delta t)] + \beta'' d[1 + h''(T''_{1/2}, \Delta t)]\} \qquad (5.10)$$

where β' quantifies the extent of slow repair half-time ($T'_{1/2}$), β'' of fast repair half-time ($T''_{1/2}$) and the quadratic component β is the sum of the two repair components $\beta = \beta' + \beta''$.

5.7 THE LQ MODEL AT HIGH DOSE PER FRACTION REGIONS

The large single-doses used in radiosurgery raised the question whether the linear quadratic model applies to this treatment or whether adaptation is needed. There are various papers published which have debated this matter and there is no common consensus upon the validity of the LQ model in the high dose region. In their paper on hypofractionated radiotherapy Gay et al. (2009) have assumed that the linear-quadratic model is valid up to a dose per fraction of

28 Gy. However, as underlined by Brenner (2008) the LQ model is well validated up to 10 Gy per fraction and it has acceptable outcome when used up to 18 Gy per fraction for the design of clinical trials. The challenge at high doses stays in the fact that the data behind the LQ model are obtained in vitro at much smaller doses than those used in radiosurgery. Therefore, in clinical settings, the LQ model often underestimates tumour control after SRS excluding also the vascular and stromal damage produced at radiosurgical doses (Kirkpatrick et al. 2008).

In their effort to modify the LQ model to better describe tissue response to large doses of radiation per fraction Guerrero and Li (2004) have included a new parameter based on both in vitro cell survival data of human tumour cell lines and in vivo animal iso-effect curves. They showed that the predictions of the modified LQ model are consistent with the lethal-potentially lethal (LPL) model which was initially proposed to describe radiation response at radiosurgical doses (Curtis 1986). The basis of the extended model is the LQ model for constant dose rate exposure which includes the dose protraction factor G to account for dose-rate effects:

$$S = \exp[-\alpha D - \beta G(\lambda T)D^2] \qquad (5.11)$$

where

$$G(\lambda T) = \frac{2(\lambda T + e^{-\lambda T} - 1)}{(\lambda T)^2} \qquad (5.12)$$

where λ is the repair rate, T represents the delivery time and D is the dose (Sachs et al. 1997).

The extended LQ model retains the α and β dependence at low fraction doses and includes a new parameter by inducing a shift in the dose protraction factor G: $G(\lambda T) \rightarrow G(\lambda T + \delta D)$, with δ being the new parameter. This new parameter was determined by adjusting both low-dose and high-dose regions of the modified LQ model with the LPL survival curves, reproducing the LPL behaviour for infinite dose rates. A possible interpretation given by the authors to the δ parameter is by means of an effective repair rate defined as $\lambda_{eff} = \lambda + \delta \dot{D}$. The equivalence between the modified LQ model and the LQ model is obtained if the repair rate increases linearly with the dose rate $\dot{D}$.

Based on the above extended model, Carlone *et al.* (2005) demonstrated that when derived from a mechanistic basis, the model presents a linear-quadratic-linear (LQL) behaviour, due to the linear pattern of sublethal lesion interaction.

5.8   ALTERED FRACTIONATION SCHEDULES

The continuous search to increase the therapeutic ratio between tumour control and late normal tissue injury led to the development and subsequent adoption of altered (modified) fractionation schedules. Variations in fractionation schedules are among a number of similar approaches to improve tumour control including radiation sensitisers, bio-reductive drugs and molecular targeting methods which have not been validated by clinical trials.

The main factors influencing the design of an altered fractionation schedule include the following:

- dose per fraction
- number of fractions
- time interval between consecutive fractions
- overall time and dose.

Improvement in tumour control should not be the only consideration when employing a new fractionation schedule; normal tissue toxicity should be limited if not reduced. When dealing with normal tissue complication, one has to consider both early and late responding tissues, as well as their particular characteristics in response to radiation damage.

As discussed in Chapter 4, early treatment reactions result from cell depletion in rapidly proliferating tissues (skin, mucosa). This property, of rapid proliferation allows *early responding tissues* to regenerate during treatment, if the necessary conditions are met. While the latent period before expression of the functional damage is independent of dose and depends on the turnover of the functional cells, the rate of recovery is dose-dependent and is dictated by the number of surviving stem cells (Steel 2002). Therefore, the clinical impact of early reactions can be reduced by:

- prolonging treatment (to enhance repopulation)
- keeping the interfraction interval at least 6 hours apart (to encourage repair of sublethal damage)

- decreasing total dose (to increase rate of recovery).

As tumours are also early responding tissues, all of the above considerations apply to radiation tumour response as well. Therefore, the focus should be on limiting normal tissue toxicity whilst limiting treatment duration. Also, overall radiation dose shall be established with a high therapeutic ratio in mind, without compromising tumour control.

Late reactions occur in slowly proliferating tissues. The damage caused by ionising radiation to cell populations in tissues with long cell cycle times will show up only months or years after treatment, depending on the extent of the damage and also the tissue type. *Late responding tissues* therefore, have a latent period before the functional damage caused by radiation is expressed and its extent is dose dependent. Late reactions, therefore, can be reduced by:

- keeping dose/fraction <2 Gy
- decreasing total dose
- keeping the interfraction interval at least 6 hours apart (to encourage repair of sublethal damage).

In summary, early and late reactions show different patterns of response to fractionated radiotherapy, which is reflected in differences in the α/β ratio of the linear quadratic model. As evident in Figure 5.8 the dose-response relationship for late responding tissues is more curved than for early responding tissues, since the α/β ratio for late reaction is smaller (the β parameter has greater influence at lower doses) than the α/β for early reacting tissues.

After a significant increase in loco-regional control in head & neck cancers, altered fractionation schedules including hyperfractionated radiotherapy, accelerated fractionation, accelerated-hyperfractionated or hypofractionated radiotherapy are being explored for other tumour sites. The subchapters below present the most common cancers where the employment of altered fractionation schedules offered improved therapeutic results (Marcu 2010).

5.8.1   Altered fractionation schedules for head & neck cancers

One of the main reasons for treatment failure in the radiotherapy of head & neck cancers is their inherent aggressive behaviour manifested through accelerated

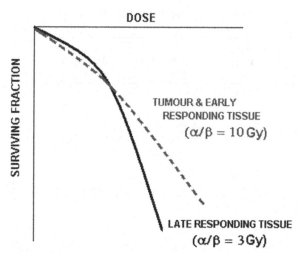

Figure 5.8 Fractionation sensitivity in early versus late responding normal tissue.

repopulation and radioresistance by having a high hypoxic fraction of cells. Altering conventionally fractionated radiotherapy to shorten the duration of treatment (accelerated radiotherapy) has been shown to limit tumour repopulation (Peters *et al.* 1988). The increase in acute toxicity of these more aggressive radiation schedules was accepted as a reasonable trade-off for improved tumour control especially as it was managed with appropriate medical support and did not lead to irreversible damage to late responding tissues.

The most commonly used altered fractionation schedules for the radiotherapy of advanced head & neck cancers are:

- *hyperfractionated radiotherapy* to exploit the differences in radiosensitivity of cancer and normal cells in order to increase the therapeutic ratio
- *accelerated radiotherapy* to overcome tumour repopulation
- *accelerated hyperfractionated radiotherapy.*

Conventionally fractionated radiotherapy is defined as radiotherapy given in week-daily incremental doses (fractions) of one fraction/week-day, over a duration of several weeks (usually 6-7). *Hyperfractionated radiotherapy* involves the delivery of multiple (2 or 3) daily fractions of small doses. The total dose given is usually the same or moderately increased compared to conventional treatment, while overall treatment duration is the same. *Accelerated radiotherapy* is defined as a radiotherapy regimen in which the duration of treatment is reduced by the delivery of 2 or more week-daily treatments on some or all of the treatment days. One way of accelerating treatment is to treat 6 days/week instead of week-daily (5 days/week). Sometimes the total dose in accelerated radiotherapy is reduced. Table 5.4 presents the main characteristics of the altered treatment regimens in comparison with conventional radiotherapy.

CHART (Continuous Hyperfractionated Accelerated Radiation Therapy) combining the two most common approaches of altered fractionation with greater emphasis on accelerated fractionation, underwent phase III trial in the late 1990s (Dische *et al.* 1997). The CHART protocol applied 36 fractions of 1.5 Gy/fraction over 12 consecutive days, for a total overall dose of 54 Gy. Compared to conventional treatment schedules, the total dose in CHART is significantly less in order for the effects on acutely responding tissues to be able to be tolerated. While the accelerated hyperfractionated regimen was expected to increase loco-regional tumour control, the success of CHART in achieving this was limited because of the low total dose delivered. In fact, local tumour control in patients treated with CHART was identical to that of patients receiving conventionally fractionated radiotherapy, of 2 Gy/fraction each

Table 5.4. Main characteristics of the conventional and altered fractionation schedules for head & neck cancers.

Fractionation regimen	Dose/fraction	Number of fractions/day	Days of treatment/week	Overall dose	Overall treatment time
Conventional	2 Gy	1	5	70 Gy	7 weeks
Hyperfractionated	<2 Gy (1.2 Gy commonly)	2–3	5	≥70 Gy	7 weeks
Accelerated	<2 Gy	1	6	<70 Gy	5 weeks
Accelerated hyperfractionation	<2 Gy	2	5–6	<70 Gy	<5 weeks

Table 5.5. Trials of accelerated radiotherapy regimens for head & neck cancer: great versus modest acceleration and associated therapeutic gain.

Trial/reference	Regimens compared	Overall dose (Gy)	Treatment duration (weeks)	Local tumour control	Therapeutic gain
DAHANCA	Accelerated	66	6	70%	Yes
(Overgaard 2003)	Conventional	66	7	60%	
RTOG	Accelerated-with	72	6	54.5%	Yes
(Fu 2000)	concomitant boost				Yes
	Hyperfractionated	81.6	7	54.4%	
	Conventional	70	7	46%	
Skladowski et al.	Accelerated	70	5	82%	Yes
(2000)	Conventional	70	7	37%	
TROG	Accelerated-	59.4	3.5	no difference	No
(Poulsen 2001)	hyperfractionated				
	Conventional	70	7		
EORTC	Accelerated-	72	5	59%	No (late toxicity
(Horiot 1997)	hyperfractionated				nullified gain in
	Conventional	70	7	46%	tumour control)
CHART	Accelerated-	54	1.7	no difference	No
(Dische 1997)	hyperfractionated				
	Conventional	66	6.5		

week-day over 7 weeks (Dische et al. 1997). However, increasing the overall dose in CHART, even if its tolerability by acute responding tissues could be overcome, would have increased the probability of late normal tissue complication. The increase in late normal tissue injury is a general problem encountered in trials that incorporated a greatly accelerated treatment schedule. The Trans-Tasman Oncology Group (TROG) (Poulsen et al. 2001) delivered 1.8 Gy twice a day to a total dose of 59.4 Gy in 33 fractions over 24 days, also reported no differences in loco-regional control between the hyperfractionated, accelerated and conventionally fractionated regimens.

The general conclusion from results of clinical trials of altered fractionation with highly accelerated treatment schedules without a reduction in total dose is that the expected increase in loco-regional tumour control will be offset by increased late tissue injury. On the other hand, regimens employing significant total dose reduction, though well tolerated, do not result in better tumour control.

This is supported by the results of several clinical trials of accelerated radiotherapy (RTOG, Skladowski, DAHANCA) (see Table 5.5) involving accelerated

fractionation schedules and total doses equivalent to conventional regimens of 70 Gy which have reported improvement in local tumour control. Therefore, the best results in accelerated radiotherapy are obtained with regimens that deliver the conventional total dose with a modest reduction in the duration of treatment with fractions delivered 6 days/week (Corry and Rischin 2004).

Table 5.5 underscores the general conclusion from clinical trials that moderately accelerated radiotherapy offers an improved therapeutic ratio over conventional treatment schedules. The latter should no longer be a standard of care for head & neck cancers. Clinical investigations have shown that to further increase the therapeutic gain for advanced head & neck cancers concurrent radio-chemotherapy should be employed, altered fractionation as a stand alone treatment being the treatment choice for intermediate-stage tumours (Nguyen and Ang 2002; Budach et al. 2006).

5.8.2 Altered fractionation schedules for prostate cancers

The last decade of prostate cancer treatment was a remarkable learning experience for both the scientific

Table 5.6. Trials of hypofractionated radiotherapy regimens for prostate cancer and associated therapeutic gain as compared to conventionally fractionated radiotherapy.

Trial/reference	Regimens compared	Treatment schedule	Treatment outcome	Therapeutic gain
Prospective phase III randomised trial 168 patients (*Arcangeli* **2010**)	Hypo-fractionated *versus* Conventional	62 Gy in 20 fractions over 5 weeks, 4 fractions per week (**3.1 Gy/ fraction**) *versus* 80 Gy in 40 fractions over 8 weeks	**TCP:** 3-year freedom from biochemical failure (FFBR) 87% – hypo-fractionation 79% – conventional **NTCP:** no differences in late toxicity	*Yes*
Randomised trial 91 patients (*Norkus* **2009**)	Hypo-fractionated 3D-CRT *versus* Conventional 3D-CRT	57 Gy in 17 fractions over 3.5 weeks: 13 fractions of **3 Gy** + 4 fractions of **4.5 Gy** *versus* 74 Gy in 37 fractions at 2 Gy/ fraction over 7.5 weeks	**NTCP:** min. 3 months follow-up (acute toxicity) grade 2 GU: 19.1% (hypo) versus 47.7% (conventional) duration of acute GI toxicity shorter with hypofract. (3 weeks versus 6 weeks)	*Yes* (but longer follow-up is needed for decisive results)
Randomised hypo-fractionated dose escalation trial 100 patients (*Pollack* **2006**)	Hypo-fractionated IMRT *versus* Conventional IMRT	70.2 Gy in 26 fractions at **2.7 Gy/ fraction** *versus* 76 Gy in 38 fractions at 2.0 Gy/ fraction	**NTCP:** small increase in GI toxicity in the hypo-fractionated arm	*Not conclusive* (the target endpoint was acute toxicity; longer follow-up is needed for decisive results).
Randomised trial 217 patients (*Yeoh* **2006**)	Hypo-fractionated *versus* Conventional	55 Gy in 20 fractions over 4 weeks (**2.75 Gy/fraction**) *versus* 64 Gy in 32 fractions over 6.5 weeks	**TCP:** similar in the two groups **NTCP:** GI toxicity worse in the hypo-fractionated group	*No* (the two schedules were equivalent in efficacy)
Randomised trial 936 patients (*Lukka* **2005**)	Hypo-fractionated *versus* Conventional	52.5 Gy in 20 fractions over 28 days (**2.63 Gy/ fraction**) *versus* 66 Gy in 33 fractions over 45 days	**TCP:** clinical/ biochemical failure (5 years) 59.95% (hypo) versus 52.95% (conventional); no difference in overall survival **NTCP:** similar late toxicity	*Not conclusive* (hypo-fractionation may be inferior to conventional regimen)

GU = genitourinary (toxicity); GI = gastrointestinal (toxicity)

and medical communities thanks to new developments in radiobiology and technology. Concepts such as bystander effect and adaptive response to treatment and also the questioned value of the α/β ratio established by several research groups to a very low figure have greatly changed the image of prostate treatment (Brenner and Hall 1999; Fowler *et al.* 2001). Direct measurements of cellular proliferation in prostate tumours suggest a slow growth rate, with a T_{pot} ranging from 16 to 61 days, the largest T_{pot} measured in

Table 5.7. Estimated α/β ratios for prostate carcinoma and late rectal toxicity, respectively.

α/β (Gy) Prostate carcinoma	α/β (Gy) Late rectal toxicity	References
1.5 (assumed)	2.3	Marzi 2009
–	5.4	Brenner 2004
3.1 (1.7–4.5)	–	Wang 2003
1.2	–	Brenner 2002
1.49 (1.25–1.76)	–	Fowler 2001
1.5 (1.4–1.7)	–	Brenner and Hall 1999
–	3.87	Deore 1993

human tumours (Haustermans *et al.* 1997). It was hypothesised that the α/β ratio of a cell population is determined by its age distribution, therefore, tissues with slow proliferation and large population of quiescent cells have a low α/β ratio (Duchesne and Peters 1999). The low α/β ratio of prostate cancer implies a higher radiosensitivity to fraction size than the adjacent late responding organs at risk such as rectum and bladder. It was, therefore, suggested to change the conventionally fractionated treatment into smaller number of fractions delivering larger doses of radiation thus *hypo-fractionating* the overall dose.

The range of dose per fractions used in trials varies from clinic to clinic (from 2.7 Gy/fraction to 4.5 Gy/fraction) and so does the outcome (see Table 5.6). Livsey and colleagues (2003) have analysed the 5-year outcome of hypofractionated conformal radiotherapy delivered to a large cohort (705 patients) using 3.13 Gy per fraction (50 Gy in 13 fractions over 22 days). While their results have indicated that a similar tumour control and normal tissue complications are achieved as with 65–70 Gy delivered in 1.8–2 Gy fractions, Arcangeli *et al.* (2010), with the same 3 Gy /fraction has achieved therapeutic gain. This result might be due to the overall treatment dose delivered within the hypofractionated regimen, which in Arcangeli's trial was 12 Gy larger.

While some clinical trials show no benefit from hypofractionated radiotherapy, others suggest that delivering larger doses in smaller number of fractions can increase tumour control without detrimental effects to normal tissue, results which support the low α/β ratio of prostate cancer.

Still a major concern for the use of hypofractionation is the late rectal toxicity. Hypofractionation does not lead to increased therapeutic ratio in prostate cancer treatment unless the α/β ratio of prostate cancer is lower that the α/β ratio of the surrounding normal tissue (see Table 5.7 for estimates). Since the α/β ratio for late rectal effects is subject to numerous debates it is difficult to accurately assess the risk of toxicity for non-conventional fractionation schedules (Marzi *et al.* 2009). Therefore, to validate the efficiency of hypofractionation in prostate cancer management there is need for well-designed trials delivering a wide range of doses per fraction to a sufficiently large number of patients as well as adequate follow up for clinical and statistical analysis (Ritter *et al.* 2009).

5.8.3 Altered fractionation schedules for breast cancer

Breast cancers are among those tumours which are shortlisted for altered fractionation schedules. Both accelerated partial breast irradiation (an advanced form of hypofractionation) and hypofractionated radiotherapy are currently undergoing extensive investigation in clinics (Table 5.8).

Cell kinetic parameter studies of human breast cancer suggest a larger-than-average potential doubling time (10.4 days) (Rew and Wilson 2000) which can be an indication towards hypofractionation. Volume doubling time measurements indicate large variations (44–295 days) (Peer *et al.* 1993) suggesting very different pretreatment patterns of tumour kinetics. These are the situations when predictive assays would come as a real help in assessing the proliferation ability of

Table 5.8. Trials of hypofractionated radiotherapy regimens for breast cancer and associated outcome as compared to conventionally fractionated radiotherapy.

Trial/reference	Regimens compared	Treatment schedule	Treatment outcome
Randomised trial RTOG – 0413 (initiated in **2005**)	Hypo-fractionated PBI *versus* Conventional WBI	34 Gy in **3.4 Gy fractions** using multi-catheter brachytherapy *or* 34 Gy in **3.4 Gy fractions** using MammoSite® balloon catheter *or* 38.5 Gy in **3.85 Gy fractions** using 3D conformal external beam radiation *versus* 50 Gy (2.0 Gy/ fraction) or 50.4 Gy (1.8 Gy/fraction) to whole breast	trial in progress
Randomised trial 1234 patients (*Whelan 2010*)	Hypo-fractionated *versus* **Conventional**	**42.5 Gy in 16 fractions over 22 days** (2.66 Gy/ fraction) *versus* **50.0 Gy in 25 fractions over 35 days**	At 10 years: *risk of local recurrence* 6.7% in the conventional group and 6.2% in the hypofractionated group; **comparable** *cosmetic* **outcome**
International Standard Randomised Controlled Trial *Trial A* 2236 patients (*START Trialists' Group 2008*)	Hypo-fractionated *versus* Conventional	**41.6 Gy in 13 fractions of 3.2 Gy/ fraction over 5 weeks** *or* **39 Gy in 13 fractions of 3.0 Gy/ fraction over 5 weeks** *versus* **50 Gy in 25 fractions of 2.0 Gy in 5 weeks**	*local-regional tumour relapse at 5 years:* 3.6% in conventional 3.5% in hypo-fractionated 41.6 Gy 5.2% in hypo-fractionated 39 Gy; **lower total dose (41.6Gy) in larger fraction sizes leads to similar outcome as the standard dose**
International Standard Randomised Controlled Trial *Trial B* 2215 patients (*START Trialists' Group 2008*)	Hypo-fractionated *versus* **Conventional**	**40 Gy in 15 fractions of 2.67 Gy/fraction over 3 weeks** *versus* **50 Gy in 25 fractions of 2.0 Gy over 5 weeks**	**possible therapeutic gain:** rate of local-regional tumour relapse at 5 years was 2.2% in the hypofractionated group and 3.3% in the conventional group
Randomised trial 258 patients (*Polgar 2007*)	Hypo-fractionated PBI *versus* **Conventional WBI**	**36.4 Gy in 5.2 Gy fractions (7 fractions) high dose rate multi-catheter brachytherapy** *versus* **50 Gy in 25 fractions over 5 weeks**	PBI produces **similar** outcome at 5-years as WBI **however with much better** cosmetic results
Randomised trial 1410 patients (*Yarnold 2005*)	Hypo-fractionated *versus* Conventional	39 Gy in 13 fractions over 5 weeks (**3 Gy/ fraction**) *or* 42.9 Gy in 13 fractions over 5 weeks (**3.3 Gy/fraction**) *versus* 50 Gy in 25 fractions over 5 weeks	42.9 Gy in 13 fractions is **equivalent** with 50 Gy in 25 fractions regarding tumour control and tissue toxicity

PBI - partial breast irradiation; WBI - whole breast irradiation

tumours prior to radiotherapy and also in deciding upon the most appropriate fractionation schedules for the individual. By determining the growth rates of primary breast cancer, Peer and colleagues have come to the conclusion that volume doubling times are age-dependent, a result which would dictate a different radiobiological approach to a young patient (<50 years old, with volume doubling times ranging from 44 to 147 days) and an old one (>70 years old, with volume doubling times ranging from 120 to 295 days). Accelerated partial breast irradiation was shown to be a feasible treatment due to the small volume irradiated (Budrukkar 2008). Hypofractionated radiotherapy delivered over a short time (usually over 5 to 10 days) can be employed through various modalities such as: multi-catheter brachytherapy, MammoSite balloon catheter (see also Chapter 9) or 3D-CRT. The RTOG group is currently conducting a randomised trial of conventional whole breast irradiation versus partial breast irradiation for women with early stage breast cancer (NSABP B-39, RTOG 0413) having as primary endpoint the time from randomisation to the diagnosis of in-breast tumour recurrence and as secondary endpoints: distant disease-free interval, recurrence-free survival, overall survival, quality of life and treatment toxicities (both acute and late).

In the randomised trial reported by Yarnold and colleagues the group has tested various radiation fraction sizes (50 Gy in 25 fractions, 39 Gy in 13 fractions and 42.9 Gy in 13 fractions all delivered over 5 weeks) and their effect on tumour control in patients with early stage breast carcinoma after local tumour excision (Yarnold *et al.* 2005; Owen *et al.* 2006). Their long-term results indicate that breast cancer tissue is probably similarly sensitive to fraction size (estimating the α/β ratio to 4 Gy) as dose-limiting healthy tissue, meaning that larger fractions could be safely delivered for a better therapeutic ratio. A similar outcome was achieved by the International Standard Randomised Controlled Trialists' group after the implementation of various hypofractionated radiotherapy schedules, with different fraction sizes. Therefore, decreasing total dose and increasing fraction size can lead to similar tumour control as with standard fractionation (50 Gy delivered in 2 Gy/fraction) however with possibly better cosmetic outcome

(Polgar *et al.* 2007). Given the fact that breast carcinoma is the leading cancer in women (Kamangar *et al.* 2006) and radiotherapy plays a critical role in the long-term management of breast cancer, it is important to take into consideration treatment schedules which are (at least) similarly as effective as standard (conventional) schedules. This increases patients' comfort by reducing overall treatment time while possibly leading to better cosmetic outcome.

5.9   SUMMARY

The implementation of altered fractionation schedules in clinics occurred as a need to increase the therapeutic ratio of those tumours for which radiobiological rationales have indicated a potentially better outcome after modified radiation schedules. While for some cancers altering conventional fractionation resulted in therapeutic gain (head & neck, prostate) or cosmetic advantage (breast cancer) for other cancers modification of fractionation regimen showed no improvement in survival. Despite the fact that the five R's of radiobiology support the choice of hyperfractionated radiotherapy also in the management of brain tumours, shorter overall treatment times and larger fraction sizes did not result in better response of the tumour (Lang *et al.* 1998; Nieder *et al.* 2004). Nonetheless, a positive endpoint observed with hypofractionation was a better quality of life of glioma patients, which is a valuable result (Lang *et al.* 1998). Also, due to shorter treatment course, hyperfractionation for malignant gliomas can be advantageous for those patients who are not suitable for aggressive therapies (Nieder *et al.* 2004).

For further implementation of altered fractionation schedules and evaluation of the efficacy of non-standard radiotherapy parameters there is need for valid radiobiological foundations and more conclusive trials, especially for the new candidates (such as breast cancer).

5.10   REFERENCES

Ang K, Jiang G, Guttenberger R *et al.* (1992) Impact of spinal cord repair kinetics on the practice of altered fraction schedules. *Radiotherapy and Oncology* **25**: 287–294.

Arcangeli G, Saracino B, Gomellini S, Petrongari MG et al. (2010) A prospective phase III randomized trial of hypofractionation versus conventional fractionation in patients with high-risk prostate cancer. *International Journal of Radiation Oncology Biology Physics* Jan 2 [online]

Bourhis J, Overgaard J, Audry H, Ang K et al. (2006) Hyperfractionated or accelerated radiotherapy for head & neck cancer: a meta-analysis. *Lancet* **368** (9538): 843–854.

Brenner DJ (2004) Fractionation and late rectal toxicity. *International Journal of Radiation Oncology Biology Physics* **60**(4): 1013–1015.

Brenner DJ (2008) The linear-quadratic model is an appropriate methodology for determining isoeffective doses at large doses per fraction. *Seminars in Radiation Oncology* **18**: 234–239.

Brenner DJ and Hall EJ (1999) Fractionation and protraction for radiotherapy of prostate carcinoma. *International Journal of Radiation Oncology Biology Physics* **43**(5): 1095–1101.

Brenner DJ, Martinez AA, Edmundson GK, Mitchell C et al. (2002) Direct evidence that prostate tumors show high sensitivity to fractionation (low alpha/beta ratio), similar to late-responding normal tissue. *International Journal of Radiation Oncology Biology Physics* **52**(1): 6–13.

Budach W, Hehr T, Budach V, Belka C et al. (2006) A meta-analysis of hyperfractionated and accelerated radiotherapy and combined chemotherapy and radiotherapy regimens in unresected locally advanced squamous cell carcinoma of the head & neck. BMC Cancer **6**: 28.

Budrukkar A (2008) Accelerated partial breast irradiation: an advanced form of hypofractionation. *Journal of Cancer Research Therapy* **4**: 46–47.

Carlone M, Wilkins D and Raaphorst P (2005) The modified linear-quadratic model of Guerrero and Li can be derived from a mechanistic basis and exhibits linear-quadratic-linear behaviour. *Physics in Medicine and Biology* **50**(10): L9–13.

Corry J and Rischin D (2004) Strategies to overcome accelerated repopulation and hypoxia – what have we learnt from clinical trials? *Seminars in Oncology* **9**: 802–808.

Curtis SB (1986) Lethal and potentially lethal lesions induced by radiation – a unified repair model. *Radiation Research* **106**: 252–270.

Deore SM, Shrivastava SK, Supe SJ, Viswanathan PS et al. (1993) Alpha/beta value and importance of dose per fraction for the late rectal and recto-sigmoid complications. *Strahlentherapie und Onkologie* **169**(9): 521–526.

Dische S, Saunders M, Harvey A et al. (1997) A randomised multicentre trial of CHART versus conventional radiotherapy in head & neck cancer. *Radiotherapy and Oncology* **44**: 123–136.

Douglas BG and Fowler JF (1976) The effect of multiple small doses of X-rays on skin reactions in the mouse and a basic interpretation. *Radiation Research* **66**: 401–426.

Duchesne GM and Peters LJ (1999) What is the alpha/beta ratio for prostate cancer? Rationale for hypofractionated high-dose-rate brachytherapy [editorial]. *International Journal of Radiation Oncology Biology Physics* **44**(4): 747–748.

Emami B, Lyman J, Brown A, Coia L, Goiten M et al. (1991) Tolerance of normal tissue to therapeutic radiation. *International Journal of Radiation Oncology Biology Physics* **21**: 109–122.

Fowler J, Chappell R and Ritter M (2001) Is α/β for prostate tumors really low? *International Journal of Radiation Oncology Biology Physics* **50**: 1021–1031.

Fu K, Pajak T, Marcial V, Ortiz H et al. (1995) Late effects of hyperfractionated radiotherapy for advanced head & neck cancer: long-term follow-up results of RTOG 83-13. *International Journal of Radiation Oncology Biology Physics* **32**: 577–588.

Fu KK, Pajak T, Trotti A et al. (2000) Radiation Therapy Oncology Group (RTOG) phase III randomized study to compare hyperfractionation and two variants of accelerated fractionation to standard fractionation radiotherapy for head & neck squamous cell carcinomas: first report of RTOG 9003. *International Journal of Radiation Oncology Biology Physics* **48**: 7–16.

Gay HA, Sibata CH, Allison RR and Jeremic B (2009) Isodose-based methodology for minimizing the morbidity and mortality of thoracic hypofractionated radiotherapy. *Radiotherapy and Oncology* **91**: 369–378.

Guerrero M and Li XA (2004) Extending the linear-quadratic model for large fraction doses pertinent to stereotactic radiotherapy. *Physics in Medicine and Biology* **49**(20): 4825–4835.

Haustermans KM, Hofland I, Van Poppel H *et al.* (1997) Cell kinetic measurements in prostate cancer. *International Journal of Radiation Oncology Biology Physics* **37**: 1067–1070.

Hill MA (1999) Radiation damage to DNA: the importance of track structure. *Radiation Measurements* **31**: 15–23.

Horiot JC, Bontemps P, van der Bogaert W *et al.* (1997) Accelerated fractionation compared to conventional fractionation improves loco-regional control in the radiotherapy of advanced head & neck cancers: Results of the EORTC 22851 randomized trial. *Radiotherapy and Oncology* **44**: 111–121.

ICRU Report 50 (1993) 'Prescribing, recording and reporting photon beam therapy (Report 50)'.

ICRU Report 62 (1999) 'Prescribing, recording and reporting photon beam therapy (Report 62)'.

Joiner M (2002) Models of radiation cell killing. In: *Basic Clinical Radiobiology*. 3rd edn. (Ed. GG Steel) pp. 64–70. Arnold Publ., London.

Joiner M and Bentzen S (2002) Time-dose relationships: the linear-quadratic approach. In: *Basic Clinical Radiobiology*. 3rd edn. (Ed. GG Steel) pp. 120–133. Arnold Publ., London.

Källman P, Ågren A and Brahme A (1992) Tumour and normal tissue responses to fractionated non-uniform dose delivery. *International Journal of Radiation Biology* **62**: 249–262.

Kamangar F, Dores GM and Anderson WE (2006) Patterns of cancer incidence, mortality, and prevalance across five continents: defining priorities to reduce cancer disparities in different geographic regions of the world. *Journal of Clinical Oncology* **24**: 2137–2150.

Kirkpatrick JP, Meyer JJ and Marks LB (2008) The linear-quadratic model is inappropriate to model high dose per fraction effects in radiosurgery. *Seminars in Radiation Oncology* **18**: 240–243.

Kim J, Hao Y, Jang D and Wong C (1997) Lack of influence of sequence of top-up doses on repair kinetics in rat spinal cord. *Radiotherapy and Oncology* **43**: 211–217.

Kutcher GJ and Burman C (1989) Calculation of complication probability factors for non-uniform normal tissue irradiation (The effective volume method). *International Journal of Radiation Oncology Biology Physics* **16**: 1623–1630.

Landuyt W, Fowler J, Ruifrok A, Stüben G *et al.* (1997) Kinetics of repair in the spinal cord of the rat. *Radiotherapy and Oncology* **45**(1): 55–62.

Lang O, Liebermeister E, Liesegang J and Sautter-Bihl M (1998) Radiotherapy of glioblastoma multiforme. Feasibility of increased fraction size and shortened overall treatment. *Strahlentherapie und Onkologie* **174**(12): 629–632.

Lindahl T and Wood RD (1999) Quality control by DNA repair. *Science* **286**: 1897–1905.

Livsey J, Cowan R, Wylie J, Swindell R *et al.* (2003) Hypofractionated conformal radiotherapy in carcinoma of the prostate: five-year outcome analysis. *International Journal of Radiation Oncology Biology Physics* **57**: 1254–1259.

Lukka H, Hayter C, Julian JA, Warde P *et al.* (2005) Randomized trial comparing two fractionation schedules for patients with localized prostate cancer. Journal of Clinical Oncology **23**: 6132–6138.

Lyman JT (1985) Complication probability as assessed from dose-volume histograms. *Radiation Research* **104**: S13–S19.

Marcu L (2010) Altered fractionation in radiotherapy: from radiobiological rationale to therapeutic gain. *Cancer Treatment Reviews* (in press), doi: 10.1016/j.ctrv.2010.04.004.

Marzi S, Saracino B, Petrongari MG, Arcangeli S *et al.* (2009) Modeling of alpha/beta for late rectal toxicity from a randomized phase II study: conventional versus hypofractionated scheme for localized prostate cancer. *Journal of Experimental and Clinical Cancer Research* **28**: 117.

Millar W, Jen YM, Hendry J and Canney P (1994) Two components of repair in irradiated kidney colony forming cells. *International Journal of Radiation Oncology Biology Physics* **66**: 189–196.

Millar W, Hopewell J, Van den Aardweg G and Canney P (1996) A two component analysis for the repair of radiation induced sublethal damage in pig epidermis. *International Journal of Radiation Biology* **69**: 123–140.

Miller J, Fuller M, Vinod S, Suchowerska N *et al.* (2009) The significance of the choice of Radiobiological (NTCP) models in treatment plan objective functions. *Australasian Physical and Engineering Sciences in Medicine* **32**: 81–87.

Munro TR and Gilbert CW (1961) The relation between tumor lethal dose and the radiosensitivity of tumor cells. *British Journal of Radiology* **34**: 246–251.

Nguyen L and Ang K (2002) Radiotherapy for cancer of the head & neck: altered fractionation regimens. Lancet Oncology **3**: 693–701.

Nieder C, Andratschke N, Wiedenmann N, Busch R *et al.* (2004) Radiotherapy for high-grade gliomas. Does altered fractionation improve the outcome? *Strahlentherapie und Onkologie* **180**(7): 401–407.

Niemierko A and Goitein M (1993) Modeling of normal tissue response to radiation (the critical volume model). *International Journal of Radiation Oncology Biology Physics* **25**: 135–145.

Norkus D, Miller A, Kurtinaitis J, Haverkamp U *et al.* (2009) A randomized trial comparing hypofractionated and conventionally fractionated three-dimensional external-beam radiotherapy for localized prostate adenocarcinoma: a report on acute toxicity. *Strahlentherapie und Onkologie* **185**(11): 715–721.

NSABP B-39, RTOG 0413 (2006) A randomized phase III study of conventional whole breast irradiation versus partial breast irradiation for women with stage 0, I or II breast cancer. *Clinical Advances in Hematology and Oncology* **4**: 719–721.

Olive P (1998) The role of DNA single- and double-strand breaks in cell killing by ionizing radiation. *Radiation Research* **150**(5 Suppl): S42–51.

Overgaard M (1985) The clinical implication of non-standard fractionation. *International Journal of Radiation Oncology Biology Physics* **11**: 1225–1229.

Overgaard J, Hansen HS, Specht L *et al.* (2003) Five compared with six fractions per week of conventional radiotherapy of squamous cell carcinoma of head & neck: DAHANCA 6 and 7 randomised controlled trial. *Lancet* **362**: 933–940.

Owen JR, Ashton A, Bliss JM, Homewood J *et al.* (2006) Effect of radiotherapy fraction size on tumour control in patients with early-stage breast cancer after local tumour excision: long-term results of a randomised trial. *Lancet Oncology* **7**(6): 467–471.

Peer PG, van Dijck JA, Hendriks JH, Holland R *et al.* (1993) Age-dependent growth rate of primary breast cancer. *Cancer* **71**(11): 3547–3551.

Pekkola-Heino K, Servomaa K, Kiuru A and Grenman R (1998) Sublethal damage repair capacity in carcinoma cell lines with p53 mutations. *Head Neck* **20**: 298–303.

Peters LJ, Ang KK and Thames HD (1988) Accelerated fractionation in the radiation treatment of head & neck cancer. *Acta Oncologica* **27**: 185–194.

Polgar C, Fodor J, Major T, Nemeth G *et al.* (2007) Breast-conserving treatment with partial or whole breast irradiation for low-risk invasive breast carcinoma-5-year results of a randomized trial. *International Journal of Radiation Oncology Biology Physics* **69**: 694–702.

Pollak A, Hanlon A, Horwitz E, Feigenberg S *et al.* (2006) Dosimetry and preliminary acute toxicity in the first 100 men treated for prostate cancer on a randomized hypofractionation dose escalation trial. *International Journal of Radiation Oncology Biology Physics* **64**(2): 518–526.

Pop LA, Millar WT, van der Plas M and van der Kogel AJ (2000) Radiation tolerance of rat spinal cord to pulsed dose rate (PDR-) brachytherapy: the impact of differences in temporal dose distribution. *Radiotherapy and Oncology* **55**(3): 301–315.

Poulsen MG, Denham JW, Peters LJ, Lamb DS *et al.* (2001) A randomized trial of accelerated and conventional radiotherapy for stage III and IV squamous carcinoma of the head & neck: a Trans-Tasman Radiation Oncology Group Study. *Radiotherapy and Oncology* **60**: 113–122.

Rew DA and Wilson GD (2000) Cell production rates in human tissues and tumours and their significance. Part II: clinical data. *European Journal of Surgical Oncology* **26**: 405–417.

Ritter M, Forman J, Kupelian P, Lawton C *et al.* (2009) Hypofractionation for prostate cancer. *The Cancer Journal* **15**: 1–6.

Sachs RK, Hahnfeld P and Brenner DJ (1997) The link between low-LET dose-response relations and the underlying kinetics of damage production/repair/misrepair. *International Journal of Radiation Biology* **72**: 351–374.

Skladowski K, Maciejewski B, Golen M *et al.* (2000) Randomized clinical trial on 7-day-continuous accelerated irradiation (CAIR) of head & neck cancer – report on 3-year tumour control and normal tissue toxicity. *Radiotherapy Oncology* **55**: 101–110.

START Trialists' Group, Bentzen SM, Agrawal RK, Aird EG *et al.* (2008) The UK Standardisation of Breast Radiotherapy (START) Trial A of radiotherapy hypofractionation for treatment of early breast cancer: a randomised trial. *Lancet Oncology* **371**(9618): 1098–1107.

Steel GG (Ed.) (2002) *Basic Clinical Radiobiology.* 3rd edn. Arnold Publ., London.

Thames HD (1985) An 'incomplete-repair' model for survival after fractionated and continuous irradiations. *International Journal of Radiation Biology* **47**: 319–339.

Thames HD (1989) Repair kinetics in tissues: alternative models. *Radiotherapy and Oncology* **14**: 321–327.

Thames HD and Hendry JH (1987) *Fractionation in Radiotherapy.* Taylor & Francis.

Travis EL and Tucker SL (1987) Iso-effect models and fractionated radiotherapy. *International Journal of Radiation Oncology Biology Physics* **13**: 283–287.

Van Rongen E, Thames H and Travis E (1993) Recovery from radiation-damage in mouse lung-interpretation in terms of 2 rates of repair. *Radiation Research* **133**: 225–233.

Wang JZ, Li XA, Yu CX and DiBiase SJ (2003) The low alpha/beta ratio for prostate cancer: what does the clinical outcome of HDR brachytherapy tell us? *International Journal of Radiation Oncology Biology Physics* **57**(4): 1101–1108.

Whelan TJ, Pignol JP, Levine MN, Julian JA *et al.* (2010) Long-term results of hypofractionated radiation therapy for breast cancer. *New England Journal of Medicine* **362**(6): 513–520.

Yarnold J, Ashton A, Bliss J *et al.* (2005) Fractionation sensitivity and dose response of late adverse effects in the breast after radiotherapy for early breast cancer: long-term results of a randomised trial. *Radiotherapy and Oncology* **75**: 9–17.

Yeoh E, Holloway R, Fraser R, Botten R *et al.* (2006) Hypofractionated versus conventionally fractionated radiation therapy for prostate carcinoma: updated results of a phase III randomized trial. *International Journal of Radiation Oncology Biology Physics* **66**: 1072–1083.

6 Three-dimensional conformal radiotherapy: technical and physics aspects of treatment

6.1 INTRODUCTION

Radiotherapy is a medical specialty that uses radiation to treat cancer and other diseases. The treatment approaches, based on the radiation source used, can be divided into two main categories: external beam radiotherapy and brachytherapy. In the external beam radiotherapy (EBRT) the radiation source is located at a distance from the patient and the radiation beam penetrates the patient from the outside (externally) in order to deliver radiation dose to the treated volume inside a patient. In brachytherapy (see Chapter 10) radiation sources are placed inside a patient directly into the treated volume. External beam radiotherapy is sometimes also called *teletherapy* and it represents the most frequently used form of radiation therapy. External beam radiotherapy uses primarily high energy (megavoltage) photon beams and for specific purposes also electron beams of MeV energies. There is also an increasing trend towards use of other charged particles such as protons, heavier ions (e.g. ^{12}C) or neutrons.

Radiation therapy is typically delivered in a series of short treatment sessions (10–15 minutes) five days a week over a period of five-to-eight weeks (depending on the tumour site), as discussed in Chapter 5. In general, multiple radiation beams are used that are directed at the tumour volume from several different angles, converging on the area to be treated. Multiple angles are used because of the exponential attenuation of X-rays, as tissues closer to the radiation source will receive larger doses than those lying at larger depths within the body. This would mean that healthy tissue might receive more dose than the deeper seated tumour itself if a single X-ray beam is used. Multiple beams spread the dose around larger volumes of healthy tissues while converging (delivering the maximum dose) within the tumour. Radiation therapy always aims to deliver a high dose of ionising radiation to the tumour while minimising the radiation dose delivered to normal surrounding tissues.

In the early days, rectangular or square shaped radiation beams (also called fields) were used. The dose delivered was of uniform intensity across each radiation field so the side effects from damage to healthy tissue surrounding a tumour could be harmful – this was limiting the amount of dose that could be delivered to tumours themselves. In the seventies, with the onset of two-dimensional (2D) radiotherapy techniques, lead blocks and wedges were used to shape beams to fit roughly a two-dimensional profile of the tumour. This resulted in reduced healthy tissue toxicities. The blocks, however, had to be individually

L. Marcu et al., *Biomedical Physics in Radiotherapy for Cancer*,
DOI 10.1007/978-0-85729-733-4_6, © CSIRO 2012

manufactured for every single beam angle used. The process was labour-intensive and time-consuming. It also required the therapists to re-enter the treatment room for each new beam in order to make the needed adjustments. In this era, the doctors prescribed tumour doses based on the clinical experience (in regards to dose, fractionation, field size) and judgement without full knowledge of three-dimensional volumes and doses (Marks and Ma 2007).

The planning process of a course of radiotherapy involves selection of radiation beams of certain energy distribution, collimated to a desired field size, and arranged around the patient to deliver a desired radiation dose to the tumour volume whilst minimising the dose to the surrounding healthy tissue. Initially, radiotherapy treatment planning consisted of manually combining data on superimposed measured isodose charts (Tsien 1955). Such manual methods provided limited accuracy, due to the limited degree of complexity, and also the lack of dose distribution optimisation (Metcalfe et al. 1997). Later, major improvements were possible due to developments of computer technology. Basic corrections for heterogeneities where first introduced that took account of the primary radiation. The effective depth method was introduced that corrected for heterogeneities by applying a correction factor to the geometrical depth to a point within the patient (Milan and Bentley 1974).

The introduction of the computed tomography (CT) technology in the late seventies was a major breakthrough in treatment planning, enabling to visualise and delineate the extent of disease relative to normal tissue (Goiten et al. 1979). The CT also provided the means of obtaining the electron densities of tissues within the patient. As Compton scattering is the primary photon interaction for mega-voltage X-rays, the absorbed dose to tissue depends on the electron densities of irradiated tissues of different composition (Sontag et al. 1977). Hounsfield (1973) defined the so-called CT number scale that related the gray scale of the CT image to the X-ray attenuation coefficients (Chapter 1), and thus to electron densities. As a result, CT technology aided greater accuracy in dose calculations in treatment planning by providing quantitative data that could be utilised in heterogeneity corrections.

In the late seventies the first interactive colour graphics 3D treatment planning computer was introduced that also enabled input of transverse contours that could be viewed 3-dimensionally with varying colours corresponding to different anatomical structures (McShan et al. 1979). Changes in the dose distributions could be viewed on screen as a result of changes in accelerator parameters/settings.

Other advances in radiotherapy included dynamic wedge implementation and the introduction of a computer controlled multileaf collimator (MLC). Dynamic wedge model was developed in late seventies (Kijewski et al. 1978) providing an alternative to the manual placement of physical wedges. However, as computers were not at that time commercially integrated with the linear accelerator the benefit of the technique was not available clinically. In the late eighties, the computers had become fully integrated with the linear accelerator and the technique was implemented for clinical treatments (Leavitt et al. 1989).

Several other rapid developments have affected the further development of radiation therapy, and the evolution from the 2D therapy to 3D conformal planning and dose delivery, to intensity modulated radiotherapy and image guided radiation therapy have aided in minimising healthy tissue injury, while allowing to increase tumour dose and thus improving the treatment outcome for the cancer patients.

6.2 THREE-DIMENSIONAL RADIATION THERAPY

Three-dimensional conformal radiation therapy (3D-CRT), has revolutionised radiation treatments in the late eighties, and is still the most widely used treatment technique to this date. In this technique, high-resolution images, using for example a computed tomography scanner, of a tumour are acquired, that are reconstructed in such a way that a 3D view (volume) of the tumour as well as of the adjacent anatomy is obtained. These images are then exported into a so-called radiation treatment planning system where dose calculations are performed as well as shaping of the individual X-ray beams to conform to the contours of the 3D image (Purdy 1996; Webb 1997; Purdy 2008).

The delivery of highly conformed radiation beams was enabled through the development of a sophisticated and ingenious device known as the multi-leaf collimator (MLC). It consists of a computer-controlled and motor-driven array of up to ~60–150 parallel tungsten leaves arranged in two opposing banks (Helyer and Heisig 1995; AAPM report no 72, 2001). The tungsten leaves can be moved into a desired position and block the path of an X-ray beam. The individually moving leaves can be programmed to generate unique, patient specific apertures through which radiation beams are directed at a tumour volume from a given direction (gantry angle). This means that the shape of the MLC aperture matches the 2D projection of the tumour volume as seen from the direction from which radiation is being delivered (see Figure 8.1). For each

beam angle, the MLC aperture is changed to align as precisely as possible to the outline of the planning target volume (PTV, see Chapter 5), resulting in a highly conformal 3D radiation dose matching the 3D shape of the PTV. Consequently this treatment technique enables to achieve significant reduction of doses delivered to healthy tissues. Generally, the MLCs are incorporated into the linear accelerator treatment heads.

Similar to 2D therapy, 3D CRT is also delivered using a series of fixed-shape fields (typically between four to eight static fields are applied). From the treatment planning point of view, optimisation of 3D CRT plans is performed iteratively, by manually varying the weights, wedges used, numbers and directions of beams until a satisfactorily uniform dose to the target is achieved without exceeding the dose tolerance of

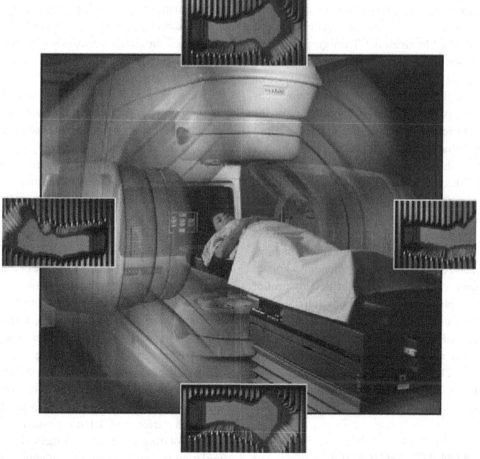

Figure 6.1. Illustration of the 3D-CRT principle using conformal radiation beams generated with multileaf collimators. (Courtesy and Copyright ©2009, Varian Medical Systems, Inc. All rights reserved.)

neighbouring sensitive tissues. This is also known as *forward treatment planning*. This technique in general requires more beams and smaller radiation field sizes compared to those used in conventional radiation therapy, requiring more accurate patient positioning.

The aim of 3D-CRT, to deliver a prescribed dose as high and as uniform as possible to the target volume while minimising dose to healthy tissue, does not represent a new concept; this has always been the goal of radiotherapy within the limitations of technology of treatment machines and within the ability to calculate and display dose. In earlier practice dose was matched as closely as possible to the target volume through selection of field sizes, beam directions and weights, wedge filters, shielding blocks and compensator filters. Further improvements were due to developments in technology, namely: new generation of linear accelerators with improved mechanical precision and stability, computing on mainframe and minicomputer systems, treatment simulators, CT imaging of target volume and organs at risk (healthy tissues), CT imaging and dose calculation based on CT number to density conversion, computer workstations with elementary 3D display of target etc, so-called beam's eye view of anatomy from radiation source with divergent beam outline superimposed, digitally reconstructed sagittal and coronal dose planes and others. Computer control of equipment has enabled an emphasis on three-dimensional conformal radiotherapy through advances in imaging technology and the associated diagnostic skills, including multimodality imaging (computed tomography, magnetic resonance imaging, single photon emission computed tomography, ultrasound, positron emission tomography and others) and their co-registration (also known as fusion) for use in combination. The development of 3D treatment planning systems (both software and hardware) in advancing of conformal radiation therapy was crucial and it included faster processors and increased RAM, advanced 3D graphics and multi-window displays. The new calculation algorithms also included new accelerators capabilities, including the use of dynamic wedges and MLCs.

6.3   TREATMENT SIMULATION

Simulation is the first step in the planning for radiation therapy treatment. In the 1960s, a dedicated X-ray simulator, utilising the X-ray imaging technology, was introduced into the clinics, changing the approaches to treatment planning and soon becoming an essential equipment and step in the radiotherapy process. A simulator, as the name suggests, simulates the process of transmitting X-rays through a patient during therapy. The acquired X-ray images are called projections. Using these, a clinician was able to localise and define a patient's tumour and surrounding anatomy and to determine the position of treatment beams, radiation field sizes and position of shielding blocks. In addition, during simulation all custom treatment positioning aids such as masks and immobilisation devices are measured and custom made. These aids are then used during every treatment fraction, ensuring that the patient lies in the correct position each time.

This conventional simulator was essential during the era of 2D dose planning systems and was superseded in the late nineties by a so-called CT Simulator, enabling 3D visualisation (Stephenson and Wiley 1995).

CT based simulation requires a different approach from an oncologist, as target volumes and organs at risk are delineated on each individual slice of acquired CT images, as opposed to drawing a portal (treatment field outline) on a simulator radiograph. CT scanner is used to obtain patient anatomical data, preferably in a intended treatment position. During image acquisition, CT contrast agents may be used to assist with visualisation and contouring of tumour volume and normal tissue contours. After that the treatment simulation itself happens as a 'virtual process' as it is fully performed with a dedicated computer workstation and software developed specifically for simulation (Sherouse *et al.* 1990) and the presence of the patient is not required to complete the treatment planning process. The modern software packages enable very efficient contouring of key structures, e.g. using so-called segmentation-based algorithms that might detect edges/structures in the image using edge detection operators; the isocentre can be positioned manually or can be determined by a computer. Other tools include viewing of the contours on planar images from both anterior-posterior and lateral projections, moving, scaling, rotating images and others. Since the CT simulation is a virtual process, patients should spend less time in the clinic compared to conventional simulator sessions for most treatment sites. This is because beam angles and treatment field shapes can be determined after the patient has left the simulation room.

6.3.1 CT scanner

In general, the CT simulation system consists of a CT scanner (the imaging device), a flat table top (identical to that used for treatments on a linac), virtual simulation software interfaced to a precision marking system using computer controlled moveable lasers as well as interface and export functions via network to a radiation therapy treatment planning software. Most CT simulator systems contain simulator workstations interfaced to a CT scanner.

During simulation, it is essential that the patient is positioned on the flat-top couch in the treatment position, so that the information acquired can be used to reproduce this position on a daily basis in a linac suite and also to ensure that the relative positions of individual anatomical structures are the same during simulation and planning as during treatment. This has lead to a development of large bore CT scanners with apertures larger than 80 cm so that radiotherapy positioning can be achieved (e.g. for breast and mantle techniques). At present, all major manufacturers offer large bore

options. Initially, the larger aperture size has lead to a decrease in image quality; however the latest generation of CT scanners, using improved reconstruction algorithms, provides the same image quality as for many diagnostic CT scanners. Multislice scanning as well as breath gating options, useful to determine the extent of tumour motion during a breathing cycle, with prospective and/or retrospective scanning/reconstruction options are also available (see Figure 6.2). The CT therapy couch top should also allow for use of the standard accessories needed to position the patient, for example breast boards and head rests. These accessories significantly enhance positioning accuracy throughout the treatment course (Aird and Conway 2002).

Alignment of the patient, during simulation, is achieved using a set of orthogonal lasers mounted on the walls and ceiling of the CT room, or on a special rigid gantry. The ceiling laser (so-called sagittal line) moves laterally under computer control so that the isocentre for a particular plan can be accurately marked. The position of the isocentre can be then exported into the planning system.

Prior to scanning, a scout view scan is made to determine the region over which axial or helical slices

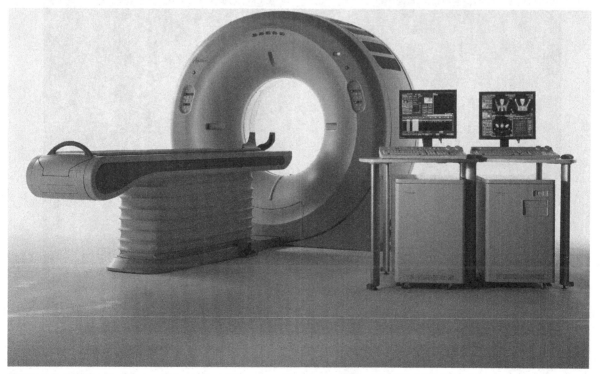

Figure 6.2. Toshiba Aquilion multislice helical CT scanner. (Courtesy and Copyright Toshiba. All rights reserved)

will be scanned. The CT operator will select a protocol particular for the site to be treated, e.g. breast, in order to use standard scanning parameters including slice thickness. Modern CT scanners allow the slice thickness to be as low as 1 mm. The oncologist will identify the target volume and the isocentre from the scan data and the patient will be marked/tattooed where the lasers intersect the skin.

Once the oncologists contoured the gross target volume (GTV) on the CT images, GTV must be expanded to generate a planning target volume to account for contouring uncertainties, patient set-up errors, movements of the target during the treatment. Then the beam orientation, dimensions and shapes of treatment fields can be then determined and dose can be calculated using the radiotherapy planning system.

6.3.2 Virtual simulator software

The virtual simulator should be capable of fast reconstruction of any section, should provide options for automatic outlining of skin, lungs, bones, semi-automatic outlining of critical organs and tumour volumes, as well as automated volumetric margins expansion. Current virtual simulator softwares allow for different margins to be added in different directions. The system must be capable to reconstruct rendered 3D views with appropriate CT slices superimposed and allow rotating the 3D view for visualisation from any angle (Figure 6.3). Display of all the required structures can be turned on or removed as required with viewing possible in multiple windows on the same screen page.

CT simulator system must be connected to the radiotherapy treatment planning system. Most manufacturers of radiation therapy products produce so-called *open systems*, meaning that regardless of the manufacturer all equipment units linked together should connect and communicate seamlessly, including image and data transfer. While this was not always the case, development of standards such as Digital

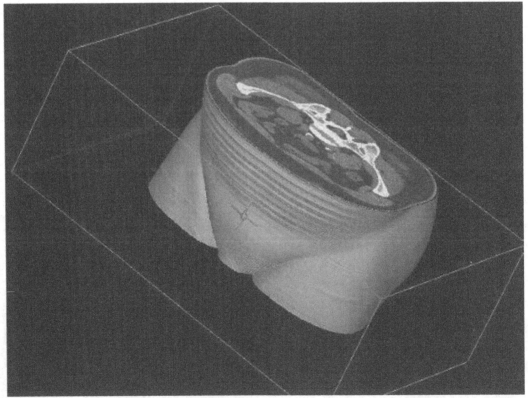

Figure 6.3. An example of a 3D display reconstructed and rendered from a CT scan data. (Courtesy the Royal Adelaide Hospital)

Imaging and Communications in Medicine (DICOM v3), and the standard for data transfer in radiotherapy (DICOM-RT) assisted to establish communication of digital image information, regardless of device manufacturer. DICOM, as the communications standard for transferring images and information between equipment, provides rules regarding the formats of specific data sets and also rules on how systems communicate and exchange data sets. In addition, DICOM-RT also allows export of radiotherapy images, treatment plans and structure contours.

6.4 DIGITALLY RECONSTRUCTED RADIOGRAPHS (DRR)

With the onset of 3D CRT, computed tomography imaging has become essential for radiotherapy treatment planning because of its ability to localise, define, and reconstruct a patient's tumour and co-located anatomy more accurately and in three dimensions as compared to a conventional radiotherapy simulator. The role of the simulator was to produce images of the proposed treatment fields for verification prior to the treatment and to use them for comparison with images from a linear accelerator. However, the individual CT images represent narrow anatomical cross-sections only and are not beams eye view. Therefore they do not directly show projections of the radiotherapy beams and cannot be compared with 2D megavoltage images acquired during the course of treatment in order to verify patient set-up. As a result, special algorithms had to be developed for computing/reconstructing 2D images from CT data that would correspond to a conventional simulation film. Such re-computed images, known as digitally reconstructed radiographs (DRRs) represent an approximation of an X-ray image from CT data (Stanley 1999).

In other words, a digitally reconstructed radiograph is a recreation of a conventional 2D X-ray image (i.e. a radiograph) from CT data (Figure 6.4). These images then serve as reference images for verification of treatments designed in a planning system. Current softwares also contain utilities that enable to superimpose graphic overlays of anatomic structures, field edges, beam crosshairs, and linear scales onto DRRs (Figure 6.5 on p. 210).

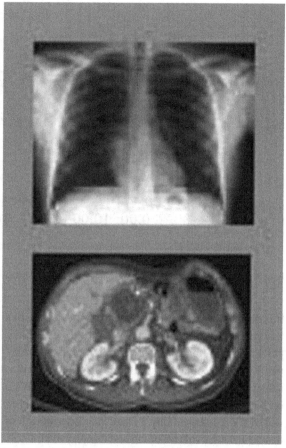

Figure 6.4. Sectional CT slices (bottom) are used, using special computational algorithms, to reconstruct 2D X-ray images of the anatomy (top), known as digitally reconstructed radiograph. (Courtesy the Royal Adelaide Hospital)

Between 50 and 100 slices are generally required to achieve accurate organ volume delineation and good quality DRRs. Whilst the main use of DRRs is for treatment verification, it is important to understand that DRR is only a snapshot of the patients' anatomy and position at the time of the scan and can never be matched exactly with images acquired during treatment with linear accelerator.

6.5 DOSE-VOLUME HISTOGRAMS

The outcome of radiation treatment (including normal tissue complications) does not depend on the delivered dose only, as there is a definite relationship between the dose and the volume of tissue exposed to

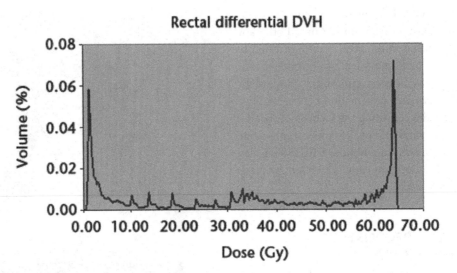

Figure 6.6. An example of a differential dose-volume histogram for a critical structure (rectum).

this dose. As a result, when evaluating the quality of a treatment plan, it is the distribution of dose within a particular volume of interest that is a measure of plan's clinical suitability. In clinical practice this is achieved by analyzing *dose-volume histograms* (DVH) of the target volume as well as critical structures, where DVH is essentially a frequency distribution of dose within the volume of interest (Shipley *et al.* 1979). In other words, a dose-volume histogram summarises a 3D dose distribution, calculated by the planning system, in a 2D graphical format

DVHs can be presented in two ways: differential DVHs or cumulative DVHs. A dose-volume histogram consists of equidistant dose bins (e.g. 0–0.1 Gy, 0.1–0.2 Gy,...) ranging from zero dose to the maximum delivered dose. In a differential histogram, the column/bin height (vertical axis) corresponds to the volume of a given structure receiving a dose assigned to the bin (horizontal axis) (Figure 6.6).

For cumulative DVHs, the column height of any dose bin (e.g. 1–1.1 Gy) represents the volume of a given structure receiving a dose greater than or equal to that dose. For fine small bin sizes, the cumulative DVH looks like a smooth line plot. In 3D-CRT, it is desired that the whole target volume (100%) is exposed uniformly to the prescribed dose (100% dose). Therefore the cumulative DVH will look like a horizontal line at the top of the graph, at 100%, with a

sharp vertical drop at around maximum dose (see Figure 6.7 and the DVH for prostate). For critical structures, it is desired that very little volume receives maximum dose, and most of the volume receives small doses only, as a result, an optimum DVH should drop sharply from the first (0 Gy) dose bin to the last (maximum dose) (see Figure 6.7 and the DVH for rectum).

Since their introduction, dose–volume histograms (DVHs) have been used extensively as a tool for treatment planning evaluation and plan comparison.

6.6 DOSE CALCULATION

Nowadays radiotherapy departments routinely use commercial dose calculation (also known as treatment planning) systems to calculate radiation dose inside a patient.

In 3D-CRT the dose calculations are performed using computer models. In order to calculate a dose distribution inside a patient, two components are essentially required: a) a model of a radiation source, i.e. linear accelerator and radiation spectrum produced and b) a model/representation/image of a patient, generally obtained using computed tomography. In addition, sound understanding of high energy photon interactions and electron transport in human body as well as in other materials is necessary. In the

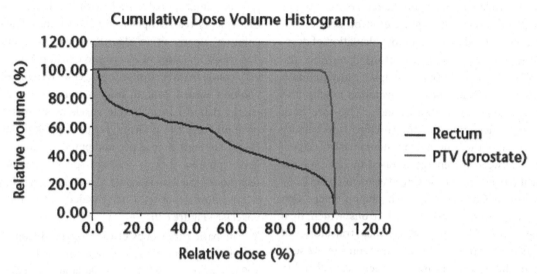

Figure 6.7. An example of a cumulative dose-volume histogram for a target volume (prostate) and a critical structure (rectum).

pre-3D-CRT days, patient dose distributions were generally estimated from extensive measurements in water and corrected for patient body contours, beam modifiers (e.g. use of wedges and shielding blocks) and for different densities of body tissues (e.g. bone, muscle and lung). In 3D-CRT, rather than applying corrections to measured data, the dose distributions are calculated from first principles and measurements are used to determine individual parameters in the dose calculation algorithms and also to verify the accuracy of calculated dose profiles.

In the current clinical practice, the trend is to use an increased number of fields and more complex shielding using multileaf collimation. It is now accepted that computed tomography has an essential role in radiotherapy treatment planning, not only for its role in the detection of malignant disease but for its relevance in therapy dose calculation; as the determination of anatomical cross-sections of a patient in the form of an electron density maps enables an accurate calculation of the dose distribution in three dimensions.

The image is usually presented on a computer screen using a gray scale, with air displayed in black, muscles in gray and bones in white. The grey scale (or the shades of gray from black to white) is calibrated in terms of CT numbers also known as Hounsfield units (Hounsfield 1973). Typically, the highest number is

assigned to white and the lowest number to black with all numbers in-between corresponding shades of gray on a linear scale. The most important property of these units is that they correlate electron densities within an object to X-ray linear attenuation coefficients.

If density of water is taken as a reference, then a Hounsfield or a CT number of a point within an image is defined as:

$$H = 1000 \frac{\mu_m - \mu_{water}}{\mu_{water}} \qquad (6.1)$$

where μ_m and μ_{water} are the X-ray linear attenuation coefficients for a material (i.e. tissue) and for water, respectively. Often, the CT number of water is chosen as zero. The relationship between CT numbers and electron densities is determined individually for each CT scanner using specially designed CT phantoms.

Once the 3D image (reconstructed from individual CT slices) of a patient has been acquired, information has been obtained both about the geometrical representation of a patient as well as about the distribution of electron densities of individual tissues inside a patient. This information is then used for calculation of dose. In general, in order to calculate the attenuation of a primary photon beam in media other than water, the photon dose calculation algorithms apply so-called path-length scaling (known also as the effective path length) based on the ratio of densities of the media to water. The relative electron density at a given point is used as an input for calculation of dose.

Current model based algorithms determine the dose distribution from first principles. Most common models are the pencil beam convolution models and collapsed cone convolution models. They are both based on convolution (i.e. the combined probability distribution of the sum of two random variables) performed between the energy released in each volume element (voxel) and a dose spread element (kernel). As discussed in Chapter 3, at each photon interaction site, energy is transferred to electrons which then deposit/spread this energy along their trajectories at some distance away from the interaction site. As such the convolution is performed between the probability of energy release/transfer and the probability distribution of energy absorption in a medium. In other words, the convolution/superposition method separates primary photon interactions from the interaction of secondary particles (charged particles and scattered photons) liberated and generated at the interaction point of a primary photon.

Primary interactions are relatively easy to calculate and are based on basic physics discussed in Chapter 1. The secondary effects are accounted for by convolving

pre-computed spread kernels with the distribution of total energy released per unit mass (terma). The convolution superposition algorithms can compute the dose even for cases of electronic disequilibrium and very complex three dimensional geometries. The convolution kernels contain information on the relative energy deposited in discrete voxels as a function of position from the point of primary photon interactions. The kernels are pre-computed for monoenergetic photon beams using special calculation techniques known as Monte Carlo. The kernels yield relative dose deposited when divided by the mass of a voxel (see Figure 6.9).

The basic three steps of the Collapsed Cone Convolution Superposition dose algorithm (Mackie *et al.* 1998; Mackie *et al.* 2001; Papanikolaou *et al.* 1993) will be discussed briefly.

1) **Modelling the incident energy fluence**

The X-ray spectrum and the energy it carries (i.e. energy fluence) must be determined as it exits the head of the linear accelerator. This is estimated from the inputted information on the design of a given linear accelerator and from the measured photon beam data. As mentioned above, the photon spectrum is represented by a set of beams

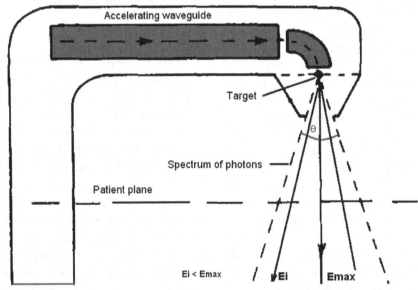

Figure 6.8. Schematic drawing of a photon spectrum exiting the treatment head of a linear accelerator. Photons emitted at an angle, θ, relative to the central axis of the beam have lower energies compared to photons emitted closer to the central axis.

of discrete energies (usually 15–20) that are assigned relative photon fluence values. These relative fluence weights can be adjusted to fit model calculations to the measured beam data (specifically depth dose curves). The photon spectrum is assumed to soften (i.e. photon energy decreases) with the transverse distance from the beam's central axis (see Figure 6.8). In order to account for this, each spectral (fluence) weight, W_p, is reduced by an off-axis factor, $F(\theta)$, of:

$$F(\theta) = \left[\frac{1}{1 + (E_i/E_{MAX})}\right]^{S\theta} \qquad (6.2)$$

where E_i is the energy of the ith energy bin, E_{MAX} is the highest energy in the beam, θ is the angle that a ray line makes with the central axis, and S is an off-axis softening parameter, which can be modified by the user in fitting the measured dose profiles (Starkschall et al. 2000).

The off-axis dependence of the photon fluence travelling through air and incident on the patient is modelled as a cone that is increasing linearly with distance from the central axis to a maximum cone radius. Both the cone angle and the cone diameter are adjustable model parameters. The treatment field itself is defined by the position of the collimators in the linac treatment head. The attenuation of the fluence by the collimators is modelled using a user defined transmission factor through the collimator blocks.

2) **Projection of incident fluence through the density representation of a patient and computation of Total Energy Released per unit MAss (TERMA) volume**

Considering the vector representation shown in Figure 6.9, the absorbed dose, $D(\vec{r})$, to a volume element at a point, $\vec{r}$, resulting from an interaction of a monoenergetic photon of energy, E, at an interaction point, $\vec{r}'$, is expressed as the convolution of the total energy released per unit mass (known as terma) with a dose spread kernel. The terma is defined as the *total* energy liberated by a photon during an interaction with a material of unit mass, (i.e. it represents the kinetic energy of resultant secondary electrons as well as energy lost in other process like excitations). Quantitatively,

terma depends on the primary photon energy fluence. The dose spread or convolution kernel, on the other hand, represents the probability per unit volume that this energy will be deposited in the vicinity of the site of the primary photon interaction. The dose, $D(\vec{r})$, is expressed as follows:

$$D(\vec{r}) = \iint\limits_{V,E} \vec{r}' \frac{\mu}{\rho}(\vec{r}',E)\frac{d\Psi(\vec{r}',E)}{dE} A(\vec{r}-\vec{r}',E)\, dE\, d^3\vec{r}'$$

$$(6.3)$$

where μ/ρ is the mass attenuation coefficient of the interaction medium, and

$$\frac{d\Psi(\vec{r}',E)}{dE}$$

is the energy fluence spectrum at point $\mathbf{r}'$, and $A(\vec{r}-\vec{r}',E)$ represents the dose spread or convolution kernel. This is a complex integral, so it is useful to separate the energy integration from the spatial integration and the dose can be calculated as:

$$D(\vec{r}) = \int\limits_{V} T(\vec{r}')\overline{A}(\vec{r},\vec{r}-\vec{r}')\, d^3\vec{r} \qquad (6.4)$$

where $T(\vec{r}')$ is the terma distribution, expressed as:

$$T(\vec{r}') = \int\limits_{E} \frac{\mu}{\rho}(\vec{r}',E)\frac{d\Psi(\vec{r}',E)}{dE}\, dE \qquad (6.5)$$

and $\overline{A}(\vec{r},\vec{r}-\vec{r}')$ is the polyenergetic dose-spread kernel, averaged over the local spectrum of the beam. Because the energy spectrum is position dependent (as shown in Figure 6.8), the spectrally averaged kernel is also position dependent.

Other beam parameters such as scatter from the flattening filter, scatter from the beam modifiers (e.g. wedges) as well as electron contamination are also modelled as separate functions.

3) **A three-dimensional superposition of the TERMA with an energy deposition kernel using a ray-tracing technique to incorporate the effects of heterogeneities on lateral scatter**

The photon beam penetrating a patient body will interact with organs and structures of varying densities which can cause large variations to the beam attenuation and lateral scattering effects. As

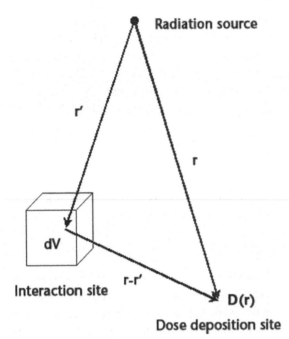

Figure 6.9. Vector representation of the convolution/superposition dose calculation technique.

a result, the equation 6.4 requires adjustment to account for the presence of structures of varying density. This is achieved through a so-called ray tracing technique between the TERMA primary interaction site and the dose deposition site. In this technique, three-dimensional rays are projected from the dose deposition site, which is tilted on its axis to align with the divergent primary beam to account for the changing direction of the incident particle. The dose spread function is then obtained from the expression:

$$\overline{A}(\vec{r} - \vec{r}') = \overline{A}(\rho_{ave}, \vec{r} - \vec{r}')\frac{\rho_e^W(\vec{r})}{\rho_{ave}} \qquad (6.6)$$

where $\overline{A}(\rho_{ave}, \vec{r} - \vec{r}')$ is the polyenergetic dose-spread kernel, averaged over the local spectrum of the beam and $\rho_e^W(\vec{r})$ is the ratio of the local electron density to water for the unit volume element with average density ρ_{ave}. The use of electron density in equation 6.6 is due to the fact the energy is deposited predominantly through electron-electron interactions, and thus, is incorrect to assume the mass density can be used to quantify electron energy loss. As

the average density ρ_{ave} is determined between two points with a displacement of $\vec{r} - \vec{r}'$, it can be calculated from the following expression:

$$\rho_{ave} = \frac{1}{\vec{r} - \vec{r}'}\int_{r'}^{r}\rho(\vec{r}'')d\vec{r}'' \qquad (6.7)$$

where $\rho(\vec{r}'')$ is the density of the volume element located at point $\vec{r}''$ along the projected line.

Finally, the equation for dose within a medium containing heterogeneities is given by the following expression:

$$D(\vec{r}) = \frac{1}{\rho(\vec{r})}\int_V T(\vec{r}')\rho_e^W(\vec{r}')\overline{A}(\rho_{ave}, \vec{r} - \vec{r}')\frac{\rho_e^W(\vec{r})}{\rho_{ave}}d^3\vec{r}$$

$$(6.8)$$

In this expression, the terma is multiplied by the electron density relative to water for the volume element at point $\vec{r}'$. This is because the terma is the energy imparted per *unit mass*. So in order to determine the terma for a material of *unit volume*, other than water, the terma must multiplied by the number of electrons per volume relative to that of water (and as discussed above CT numbers from a patient image are used to determine the electron density of a given volume element).

6.7   DYNAMIC WEDGE

Wedge filters are designed to produce a gradient of dose distribution across the treatment field (Figure 6.10). The wedge angle is used to quantify the effect of a particular wedge filter on the dose distribution. It is defined (IEC report 976, 1989) as the angle through which an isodose curve is tilted at the central axis of the beam at a specified depth (generally 10 cm).

Initially physical removable wedges have been used. These were made of lead, brass or steel alloys. The insertion of the wedge into the treatment head of a linac will result in a reduced beam transmission and also in the hardening of the radiation beam as the photons of lower energies will be absorbed within the wedge. A standard set of wedges generally provides profile angles of 15, 30, 45, and 60 degrees.

Nowadays dynamic wedges are commonly used that produce a wedged beam by dynamic motion of

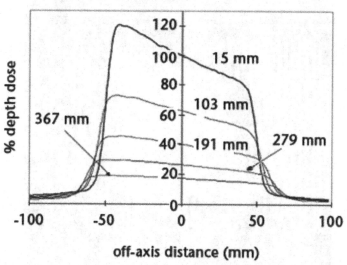

Figure 6.10. Dose profiles measured at different depths for a 45 degree wedge using 6 MV photon beam. (Courtesy the Royal Adelaide Hospital)

the collimators during irradiation, meaning that there no longer is an object attached to the treatment head requiring manual manipulation by staff. Dynamic wedge production can be very flexible as the collimator movement is programmed to produce any required beam shape. Furthermore, as the wedge is not produced by differential attenuation through an absorber, the energy of the beam does not change.

6.8　MULTI LEAF COLLIMATOR

The multileaf collimator (MLC) is a computer-controlled device capable of providing photon beam shielding on linear accelerators using high density leaves (typically tungsten alloy) projected into the radiation field (see Figures 6.11 and 6.12). While MLCs may have a number of uses in radiation therapy, the primary is to replace conventional mounted blocks for critical organ shielding. They eliminate the need for mounted block manufacturing, manipulation and storage. The computer control of the device means that changes in the blocking pattern can be easily produced. Secondary use of MLCs is in the production of intensity modulated beams (Chapter 7), where as a result of adjustment of the position of the MLC within the radiation field during the beam-on time, complex

dose distribution patterns can be achieved. In general, the required MLC field shape is first generated on a treatment planning computer, and then sent to a record and verify system (see section 6.10) interfaced with the linac control system. The linac will then upload the information about the location of individual leaves and will deploy them to planned positions.

Over the years manufacturers have developed different approaches to multileaf collimator design and functionality. When evaluating performance of a particular MLC system, the following should be considered: MLC design, leaf radiation transmission, leaf sizes, number of leaves, extent leaf travel, leaf abutment, source-to-leaf distance/isocentre clearance, leaf positioning mechanism and its accuracy, leaf positioning limitations and leaf speed.

When it comes to design, a variety of commercial MLC configurations is available. Some designs may involve the replacement of the upper or lower pair of conventional accelerator jaws (Siemens, Elekta) while others have added an MLC to the conventional jaws (Varian). Some configurations even use no conventional jaws at all and use multileaf collimation as a single source of field shaping (e.g. tomotherapy). MLC designs involving upper or lower jaw replacement influence　the　monitor　unit　calculation　as

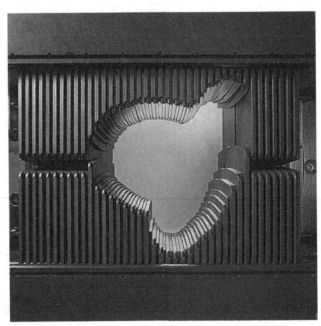

Figure 6.11. A picture of Varian multileaf collimator, consisting of two banks of opposing tungsten leaves. Movement of the leaves in different positions generates an aperture for radiation beam; i.e. defines the shape of the radiation field. (Courtesy and Copyright ©2009, Varian Medical Systems, Inc. All rights reserved.)

the proximity of the MLC to the flattening filter is sufficient to obscure part of the extra-focal radiation. In addition, the MLC design affects isocentre clearance as, when they are used as tertiary collimators (see Figure 6.13), they will reduce the space between the bottom of the treatment head and the isocentre.

The radiation beam diverges from the focal spot in the accelerator treatment head towards the patient. As a result, the MLC shape needs to conform to the beam direction. MLCs can be made divergent in one or two direction: as a distance from the source and as a distance from the central axis. This is achieved by making leaf sides match the field divergence along the leaf height and by the manner of individual leaf travel; i.e. leaves are flat ended but need to move in an arc motion so that the edge of the leaf end is parallel to the beam direction). When arc motion is not available in a design, manufacturers mimic divergence by rounding the leaf edges (see Figure 6.14). For rounded leaf ends the MLC motion is restricted to a single plane. Consequently, the MLC penumbra (the width of the radiation field edge defined as the distance between 80 and 20% isodose line) is slightly bigger than that of custom made focused blocks and there is

also larger radiation leakage when the opposing leaves are touching each other (abutting leaves). Also, the field penumbra is larger for rounded than for flat-end designs.

The term double focused MLC is used to describe systems with leaves moving along an arc centred on the X-ray target, while the term single focus MLC is used for systems with leaves moving perpendicularly

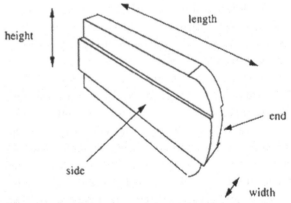

Figure 6.12. Schematic of a typical leaf from a multileaf collimator. (Reproduced from Boyer *et al.* 2001. Copyright (2001), with permission from the American Association of Physicists in Medicine)

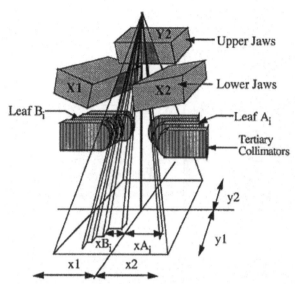

Figure 6.13. Schematic of a multileaf collimator system used as a tertiary collimator in addition to upper and lower jaws. (Reproduced from Boyer *et al.* 2001. Copyright (2001), with permission from the American Association of Physicists in Medicine)

to the beam central axis; i.e. single focus MLCs have leaves that move in a plane and have rounded ends.

Computer control is an essential component of the MLC design and performance. There must be feedback on the leaf position, and beam interlocks initiated when leaf misplacement is detected. There also must be interlock system installed to detect leaf carriage positions that could lead to unintentional irradiation outside the shielded area. Other safety interlocks must recognise the unintentional use of the MLC in electron mode. Leaf position can be verified by the MLC system in a variety of ways. Some vendors use optical encoders which are useful for monitoring individual leaf position. Other designs monitor leaf position by means of a CCD camera.

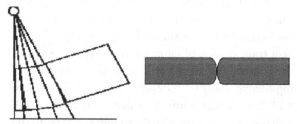

Figure 6.14. Divergent movement of a multileaf collimator (left) and rounded leaf edges of opposing MLC leaves mimicking the radiation beam divergence (right).

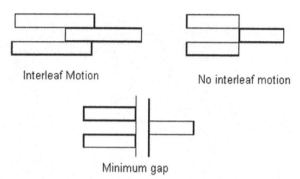

Figure 6.15. Schematic of possible leaf motion for opposing bank of leaves.

6.8.1 Leaf travel

The performance of the MLC as well as its ability to generate complex field shapes for small as well as large radiation fields depends on design limitation on the motion of individual leaves as well as on the motion of the leaf carriages. The maximum field size will depend on the permissible distance between the most extended leaf and the most retracted leaf, how far the leaves can extend across the centre line of the treatment field as well as on the total travel distance for the carriages. Other motion features include possibility of leaf interdigitisation (or interleaf motion) or whether the leaves from the opposing banks can abut (touch) as illustrated in Figure 6.15.

Another major characteristic is related to a radiation delivery method: a) if the irradiation (beam on) and the MLC leaf motions are executed simultaneously, this is known as *dynamic* delivery b) if the radiation and leaf motions are executed sequentially, this is known as *static* delivery. In dynamic delivery, the accuracy of the leaf positions and the correlation between the leaf positions and the accumulated dose, must be monitored by the linac control system.

6.8.2 MLC radiation transmission

As discussed before, MLCs remove the need for production and manual positioning of cerrobend blocks, thus saving machine time, and providing a healthier environment for radiation therapy staff. However, the use of MLCs increases the penumbra region of the treatment fields as well as radiation leakage between (inter) and through (intra) individual leaves. Interleaf transmission is a result of the diverging leaf design of

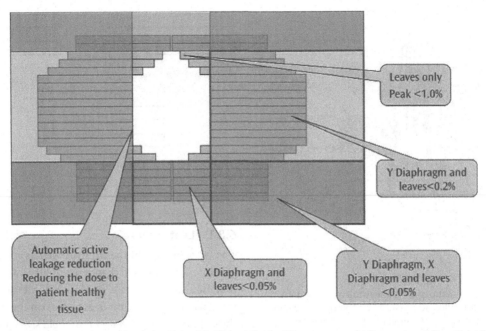

Figure 6.16. Radiation transmission levels for Elekta MLCi2 multileaf collimator system. (Courtesy and Copyright ©2008 Elekta AB (publ). All rights reserved.)

the MLC leaves. As the radiation beam is diverging, leakage occurs between each leaf. As a result, in any design it must be assured that the leaves provide an acceptable degree of attenuation that is comparable to that of conventional blocks.

In MLCs with a double focus and flat leaf-end design, there is full radiation transmission on the open side of the leaf. This is reduced immediately to the 'shielded' transmission underneath the leaf. Single focus MLCs have leaves with rounded ends. In this case, the radiation transmission through the leaf end changes gradually from full in the open field to the fully shielded value over a certain distance.

In MLCs designed to replace a set of conventional collimators, the back-up jaws are generally designed as part of the MLC system that can be controlled by the MLC controller. The jaws must be coordinated with the leaves to minimise the leaf transmission and interleaf leakage.

According to AAPM report no 72; the following limits are recommended:

- the intraleaf transmission should be: the same as for conventional collimators, if MLC replaces the jaws and less than 5% for tertiary MLC;

- the intraleaf transmission should be the same as for conventional collimators, if MLC replaces the jaws and less than 5% for tertiary MLC;
- abutting leaves transmission can be up to 25%.

An example of radiation transmission levels for Elekta MLCi2 multileaf collimator system are shown in Figure 6.16.

6.8.3   Tongue-and-groove effects

In addition to the rounded leaf design the construction of the individual leaves results in another important design feature, the leaf side edge. As the construction of the MLC is of a divergent design any gap between adjacent leaves could result in an unhindered path of radiation to a patient. This is the reasoning as to why the leaves are generally not constructed with flat sides and edge-to-edge. To prevent transmission of radiation in between the leaves, the construction of the MLC edge is of an interlocking *tongue-and-groove* design as displayed in Figure 6.17. This design limits, to a degree, the amount of radiation that is transported through the MLC to the patient by providing a physical barrier that attenuates the beam.

X-rays

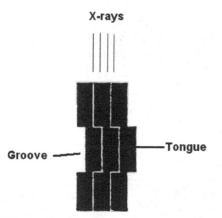

Figure 6.17. A schematic diagram of a tongue and groove design of an MLC system.

6.8.4 Multileaf collimator dose undulation

As a result of finite width of individual leaves, an undulated (scalloped) dose pattern occurs at the edge of a radiation treatment field defined by the MLC. This is the consequence of using stepping leaves of finite width to shape the radiation field. This is an MLC disadvantage compared to blocks that can be moulded smoothly and exactly to the required field shape (see Figure 6.18).

This jagged field edge of an MLC produces larger penumbra and is visible on radiographs at any depth. The dose undulation can be quantified by undulation index (UI) that is defined as the ratio of the width of the 50% undulation to the 20 to 80% penumbra width. Techniques have been developed to reduce the undulation (using software and mechanical solutions, e.g. couch movement). Also smaller leaf size reduces the dose undulation as shown in Figure 6.19.

While the dose undulation might seem as a major disadvantage, it has been shown that variations in daily set-up will blur the block edges and MLC edges

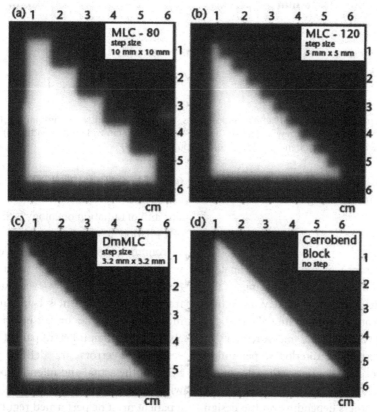

Figure 6.18. Radiographic films irradiated with 6 MV X-rays showing radiation field edge and corresponding undulation of the dose pattern (a) Multileaf collimator (MLC) with 80 1 cm wide leaves. (b) MLC with 120 0.5 cm wide leaves width. (c) Dual-layer micro-MLC with 0.32 cm leaf width. (d) Cerrobend blocks. (Courtesy Liu *et al.* 2008)

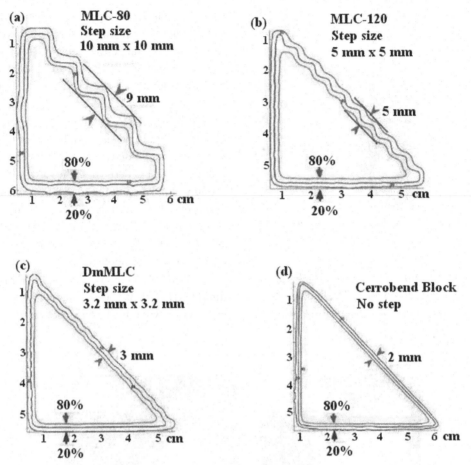

Figure 6.19. Penumbra measurements of 20% 80% isodose lines, and the dose undulation amplitude of 50% isodose line; a) Multileaf collimator (MLC) with 80 1 cm wide leaves. (b) MLC with 120 0.5 cm wide leaves width. (c) Dual-layer micro-MLC with 0.32 cm leaf width. (d) Cerrobend blocks. (Courtesy Liu *et al.* 2008)

(there will be no difference in treated field edge) to the extent that they are indistinguishable (Galvin *et al.* 1998).

6.8.5 MLC QA

Regular quality assurance of multileaf collimators must be implemented in any department using MLCs. Tests should include: position accuracy including readout, and investigation of gravitational sag, light and radiation field coincidence, measurement of radiation leakage, testing of interlocks, penumbra measurements and dose distribution at the edge of the field, leaf speed, generation of leaf shapes and the file transfer process and others depending on the design and intended use within department.

6.9 ELECTRONIC PORTAL IMAGING DEVICES

The aim of radiation oncology is to deliver a high dose of radiation to the tumor while preserving normal surrounding tissues. Accurate patient positioning and field placement is crucial in order to achieve desired treatment outcomes. However, during the course of fractionated treatment, set-up variations as well as motion of organs occur. Set-up errors, while undesirable, represent an inherent part of the treatment process. These errors are defined as the difference between the actual and intended position of a patient with respect to radiation fields. As a result imaging of a patient must be performed regularly to confirm the treatment set-up. Verification of the correct patient

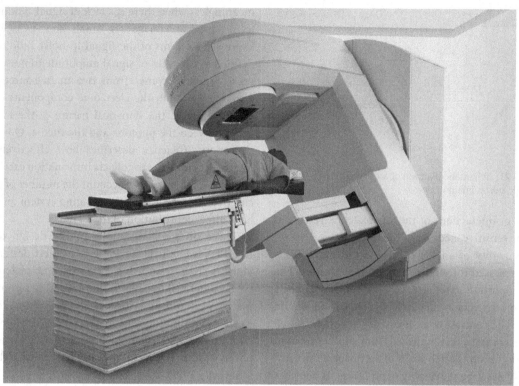

Figure 6.20. Siemens accelerator with an electronic portal imaging device extended underneath the treatment couch. (Courtesy and Copyright © Siemens AG, 2002–2008. All rights reserved.)

positioning relative to the radiation beam has traditionally been performed by placing an X-ray film beyond the patient to produce an image with the exit radiation, called a port film.

The film cassette system was labour and time consuming involving film loading, positioning of a patient, exposure, film development (at some distance away from the treatment room), evaluation of the processed film, mostly using manual (ruler) analysis. This process could take several minutes overall, during which a patient, while immobilised could have still moved. This can lead to increased probability of positioning error and set-up accuracy limitations of up to 5 mm.

Electronic portal imaging devices (EPIDs) were introduced into clinical practice more than 20 years ago. They were first used only as a replacement for port films, but as these devices produce digital images and require no chemical processing, the possibility of performing *on-line* treatment verification and *automatic analysis* became a possibility. In addition, vari-

ous image enhancement software tools have been developed that enable improving the image quality and contrast after exposure. Digital images can also be readily deployed, viewed and shared via computer network.

Electronic portal imaging device is essentially 2D radiation detector array mounted on a motorised robotic arm, which allows it to be positioned with precise movements in the vertical and/or longitudinal and lateral directions. The arm is attached to the linac gantry and extracts underneath the patient (see Figure 6.20). Image taken by the EPID is the result of a high energy X-ray beam (mega voltage range) passing through a patient and interacting with the EPID sensitive layer containing the detector array. The differences in the attenuation of the photons due to varying densities and thicknesses in the object (i.e. patient) give rise to different grey scale or EPID pixel values which form the image. The pixel value is proportional to the amount of free charge formed in the detector as

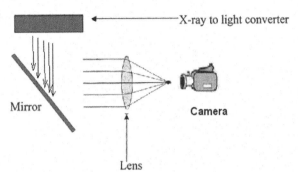

Figure 6.21. Schematic diagram of a camera-based electronic portal imaging device.

a result of interactions of the attenuated X-ray beam with the sensitive medium of the EPID.

The quality of an Electronic Portal Image (EPI) can be assessed through a number of quantities. The most important ones are contrast, signal-to-noise ratio, detective quantum efficiency (DQE) and photon scatter. The contrast of an image represents how well one object can be distinguished from another or from the background. The contrast of an image alone cannot fully describe the quality of an image. It becomes meaningless when there is a lack of signal. The ability to produce an image for small signals is better expressed in terms of the signal-to-noise ratio that is defined as the ratio of signal amplitude to noise. The noise generally comes from two main sources; the dark current from the electronic components of the EPID and from the statistical nature of the interactions between the photons and the media. Quantum Detection Efficiency describes how effectively the image receptor detects/collects information carried by photons. QDE takes into account the number of particles that are detected by the imaging system and that have direct contribution to the signal.

Three different variations in the design of the EPID evolved since the 1980s. The first design is a video based system using a fluoroscopic plate and a CCD camera (Baily 1980). The second design uses a matrix of liquid ionisation chambers and is known as the Scanning Liquid Ion Chamber (SLIC) system (van Herk 1988). The third design uses an amorphous silicon (a-Si) solid state flat panel detector (Taborsky 1981).

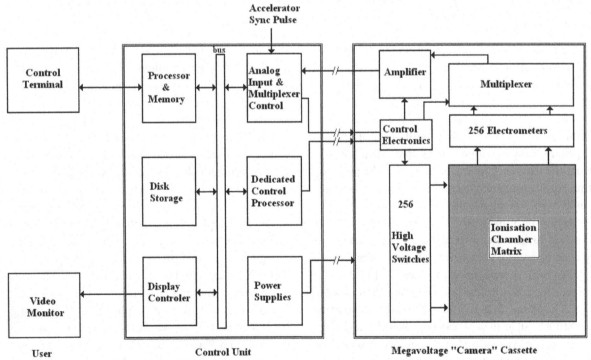

Figure 6.22. Schematic diagram of the internal structure of the scanning liquid ionisation chamber EPID consisting of a control unit and the ion chamber matrix. (Reproduced from Boyer *et al.* 1992. Copyright (1992), with permission from the American Association of Physicists in Medicine)

1) *The video-based EPID* consists of a fluoroscopic plate serving as an X-ray-to-light converter, a mirror and a CCD camera (see Figure 6.21). The fluoroscopic plate is a metal plate with a phosphor material attached to it. X-rays reaching the EPID are converted to visible light which is then reflected into the CCD camera, generating the image. The biggest problem for this EPID type is very low quantum efficiency and poor resolution. While attempts have been made to increase the efficiency of the light output of these EPIDs by increasing the thickness of the phosphor layer, only about 10–20% of the light generated in the phosphor can escape the phosphor and will reach the camera.

2) *The Scanning Liquid Ion Chamber EPID* consists of control electronics system, a 256-channel electrometer, a 256-channel high voltage switch and an ionisation chamber matrix (Figure 6.22). The ionisation chamber matrix is formed by 256 electrode plates and 256 high voltage plates positioned at right angle to each other. The electrode plate and the voltage plate are connected to the electrometer and high voltage switch, forming a single ionisation chamber at every cross point. This arrangement creates a total number of 256×256 image pixels over a surface area of $32.5 \times 32.5 \text{ cm}^2$. The maximum resolution is thus 1.27 mm. The ion chamber matrix is submerged in 0.08 cm thick iso-octane liquid film acting as the radiation sensitive layer of the EPID. The sensitive layer is sandwiched between two printed circuit boards (PCB) and an additional 0.1 cm thick radiation build-up layer made of plasto-ferrite is positioned on top of the PCB layer.

When radiation is present at the EPID sensitive layer, the iso-octane liquid is ionised producing free ions and electrons. The image is acquired by connecting the high voltage electrodes (positioned in one line) to the 300 V voltage supply and collecting the charge using each of the 256 electrometers for about 20 ms. The high voltage is then switched to the next line and the process repeated until all 256 lines have been used. This requires the EPID to be synchronised with the pulse repetition frequency of the linac. The system makes repeated measurements along every row and the signals are averaged over a number of measurements until an image (of reasonable quality) is obtained.

Electrons created in the liquid can be lost through recombination with ions. The time taken for electrons to recombine defines the electron lifetime. Therefore to achieve high charge collection efficiency, it is important that there is sufficient voltage across the ion chamber array (~300 V) to ensure that the electron's mobility in the liquid is large so that the travel/collection time is shorter compared to the electron lifetime.

The Control Unit has a built-in microcomputer with essential data analysis programs and sufficient memory to store and process signals from the electrometers in the Camera Cassette.

3) *The amorphous silicon EPID* is a flat panel imager consisting of a matrix of hydrogenated amorphous silicon (a-Si:H) photodiodes and thin film transistors (TFTs) (Langmack 2001). The imager generally consists of a front metal sheet (e.g. 1 mm copper or tungsten) and a gadolinium oxysulphide phosphor that converts X-rays to light (see Figure 6.23). The light is then detected using an array of a-Si:H photodiodes controlled by a-Si:H TFT switch (the light will generate free electrons in the a-Si:H material that are collected to form an image). The photodiodes are electronically read and form the pixels of the image. Matrix arrays of up to 1024×1024 pixels are available with a pixel size of less than 0.5 mm^2. The photodiode layer is made of amorphous silicon (but other semiconductors have been used as well), which means that it is non-structured and highly irregular. However, defects in silicon act as holes for electrons and once the electrons are trapped they cannot be detected to form an image. As a result, the Si layer needs to be hydrogenated. aSi:H absorbs visible photons very efficiently and is used in many solar cell applications.

Superior imaging quality (high contrast) is the main advantage of this EPID type. This is the consequence of the limited quantum noise (~1% of total noise), smaller pixel size and high efficiency of light detection (e.g. 70–80% greater compared to camera based systems) of aSi:H flat panel detectors.

Initially, the major disadvantage of EPIDs was poor contrast of produced images. As portal imaging uses linac beams in the megavoltage energy range, the main photon interaction (as discussed in Chapter 1) is Compton scattering. This is almost independent of atomic number, Z, so there is intrinsically less object contrast in portal images compared to images acquired using diagnostic X-rays. Diagnostic X-rays

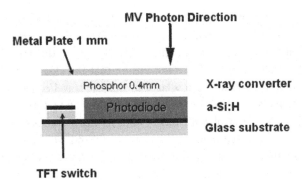

Figure 6.23. A schematic diagram of an amorphous Silicon based EPID.

are of kV energy range and therefore interact primarily via photoelectric effect that is strongly Z dependent, providing good contrast e.g. between soft and bony tissues.

As a result, extensive efforts were made to improve the technology for acquisition of portal images with megavoltage X-rays. Eventually, the development of aSi:H flat panel detectors resulted in generation of high quality images leading to widespread acceptance of EPIDs that have now become an essential linac component. As a latest development, diagnostic X-rays are being used to image the same area as the therapy beam to provide high resolution images. This is generally done by adding an X-ray tube onto the linac gantry. This will be discussed in more details in Chapter 7.

As mentioned earlier, an on-line digital image of the patient anatomy acquired with an EPID can be used for direct position verification against the planned treatment position using digitally reconstructed radiographs. Regular imaging is used to identify and reduce set-up errors. The set-up errors consist of *systematic errors* and *random errors*. Random errors represent statistical fluctuations in all directions in the patient position from one treatment fraction to another. Random deviations are not reproducible. Systematic errors are consistent deviations in the same direction (i.e. are reproducible). Systematic error is a result of a condition which exists throughout the entire course of treatment (this could be, for example an error/tolerance in the CT couch calibration in one direction, translated onto a reference image).

Determination of patient displacement from the intended position is performed using so-called image registration. Firstly, the treatment radiation field edge is identified in the portal image. This is aligned with the radiation field outlines in the reference image (i.e. DRR) in order to identify any differences in the size and shape of the radiation fields being compared. Secondly, anatomical structures in both images are matched in order to quantify shifts and rotations in patient position. This can be done by aligning the anatomical structures (e.g. pelvic rim or ribs) on the two images by translating and/or rotating the portal image onto the reference image; i.e. co-registration of the reference image with the electronic portal image is performed using landmarks. Bony anatomy represents the most common landmark; however this may not accurately represent the true position of the treated organ (e.g. position of the prostate relative to the pelvic rim). As a result, fiducial markers in the form of gold seeds or coils can be implanted into the tumour prior to treatment to serve as landmarks (Figure 6.24). Positioning accuracy of less then 1 mm can be achieved with the use of fiducial markers.

When bony anatomy is used for co-registration, double exposures may be required: firstly with a larger open field to capture the bony anatomy in the image; second exposure is then performed using the treated field aperture only. This gives a darker outline of the treatment field within the imaged anatomical region. In general, treatment staff is required to outline and align the anatomy. The accuracy of this process depends on their experience and on the quality of the portal image. Special software is used (provided by EPID manufacturers) to perform auto-analysis; i.e. it confirms patient position and suggests shifts. Once shifts have been performed another portal image might be acquired to confirm that the shifts were made in the right direction. A typical workflow is shown in Figure 6.25.

The set-up errors are the reason for the need to generate a Planning Target Volume (PTV) from the Clinical Target Volume (CTV); as defined in Chapter 5. The radiation field used must cover the PTV in order to ensure that the tumour is always irradiated regardless of the set-up uncertainties. However, the margins/distances by which a CTV is expanded to form a PTV have to be carefully investigated in order

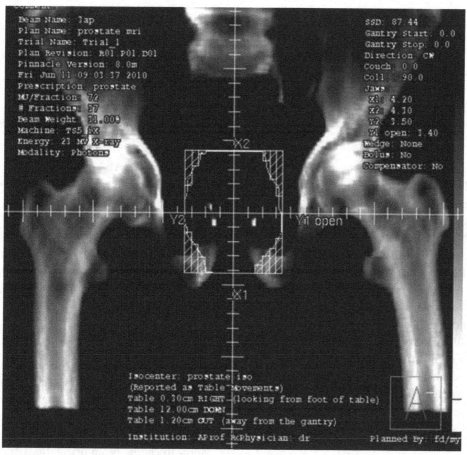

Figure 6.24. An electronic portal image of pelvic area with gold seeds implanted inside a prostate. (Courtesy Royal Adelaide Hospital)

to prevent unintentional irradiation of surrounding healthy tissues.

Several mathematical formulae have been suggested for calculation of CTV-PTV margins. The ICRU 62 (ICRU 1999) states that systematic (Σ) and random (σ) errors should be added in a quadrature and used for margin (M) calculation. This approach assumes that random and systematic errors have an equal effect on dose distribution, which may not be the case, as their impact is different. While random errors blur the edges of dose distribution, the systematic errors cause a directional shift of the dose distribution relative to the tumour. It has been demonstrated that systematic errors have higher dosimetric impact than random errors.

As a result, a formula was proposed by Stroom (Stroom and Heijmen 2002), ensuring that on an average, 99% of the CTV receives more than or equal to 95% of the prescribed dose:

$$M = 2\Sigma + 0.7\sigma \qquad (6.9)$$

The most commonly used formula has been introduced by van Herk (van Herk 2000 and 2004):

$$M = 2.5\Sigma + 0.7\sigma \qquad (6.10)$$

This formula ensures that 90% of patients in the population receive a minimum cumulative CTV dose of at least 95% of the prescribed dose.

6.10 RECORD AND VERIFY SYSTEM

As a result of increased complexity of radiation treatments, including the use of multileaf collimators, a need arose for the use of network systems in radiotherapy that would handle input and transfer of

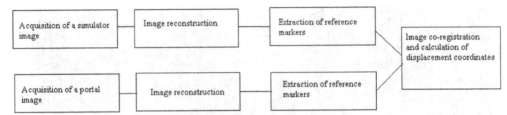

Figure 6.25. Workflow diagram for patient set-up verification using electronic portal imaging and on-line analysis.

patient imaging and demographic data, transfer of and up-load of treatment plans and patient set-up in the treatment room, verification and recording of treatment parameters, including devices for accurate and repeatable patient positioning, as well as verification and recording of delivered dose. These systems, known as Record and Verify systems, have been designed to detect and prevent mistakes in the delivery of external beam radiation therapy and aim to prevent accidental delivery of radiation dose, to improve quality control, and to provide record keeping and report generating capabilities.

Once a treatment plan is completed, the Record and Verify system will be used to generate treatment prescriptions, treatment calendars, will drive machine set-ups, will verify machine parameters, and record actual treatments. The system inhibits a machine from being turned on if the settings do not agree with the prescribed values to within specified maximum permissible deviations.

Record and Verify systems also provide immediate and continuous on-line feedback to a radiation therapist at the treatment console. If any of the treatment parameters during the treatment is outside its tolerance limit (e.g. a position of a particular MLC leaf is not reached), the treatment will be interrupted.

6.11   IMPLEMENTATION OF 3D CRT

Clinical evidence of improved survival benefit, better local tumour control or reduced normal tissue complications from 3DCRT over conventional radiotherapy is increasing for many tumour sites and will be discussed in more details in Chapter 8. As a result, the three dimensional conformal radiation therapy is now considered an essential standard treatment in any clinic.

According to IAEA-TECDOC-1588, *Transition from 2-D Radiotherapy to 3-D Conformal and Intensity Modulated Radiotherapy* (IAEA 2008), the design and delivery of a 3D-CRT treatment requires a whole system of procedures that must be in place so that the treatments can be delivered safely and accurately. The following summary lists essential components that need to be established when implementing 3D-CRT into clinical practice:

- adequate immobilisation of patients throughout the whole process
- the use of high quality 3D medical imaging (CT, MRI, PET) to determine the gross tumour volume, clinical target volume, planning target volume and planning organ at risk volume (see Chapter 5)
- the use of 3D treatment planning systems that allow to choose beam orientations and to display beam's-eye-views of the treatment beams
- the 3D dose calculation using advanced dose calculation algorithms
- the evaluation of the dose plan and/or the biological effect using dose volume histograms, tumour control probability and normal tissue complication probability
- the transfer of these planning data to the delivery machine using DICOM RT standards and Record and Verify system
- the digital linear accelerator with multileaf collimator and electronic portal imaging device
- the established verification process of patient position, beam placement and dosimetry
- the evaluation of treatment outcome
- sufficient resource of adequately trained staff (oncologists, therapists, physicists).

Based on the above, the introduction of 3D CRT does represent a financial as well as workforce pressure that needs to be carefully evaluated by the service providers when planning and designing 3D CRT service.

6.12   REFERENCES

Aird EGA and Conway J (2002) CT simulation for radiotherapy treatment planning. British Journal of Radiology 75: 937–949.

Baily NA and Horn RA (1980) Fluoroscopic visualization of megavoltage therapeutic x ray beams. *International Journal of Radiation Oncology Biology Physics* 6: 935–939.

Boyer AL, Antonuk L, Fenster A, van Herk M, Meertens H, Munro P *et al.* (1992) A review of electronic portal imaging devices (EPIDs). *Medical Physics* 19: 1–16.

Boyer A, Biggs P, Galvin J, Klein E, LoSasso T, Low D, Mah K and Yu C (2001) 'Basic applications of multileaf collimators'. Report of Task Group No. 50 Radiation Therapy Committee, AAPM Report No. 72. American Association of Physicists in Medicine by Medical Physics Publishing.

Galvin JM, Han K and Cohen R (1998) A comparison of multileaf-collimator and alloy-block field shaping. *International Journal of Radiation Oncology Biology Physics* 40: 721–731.

Goitein M and Abrams M (1983) Multi-dimensional treatment planning: 1. Delineation of anatomy. *International Journal of Radiation Oncology Biology Physics* 9: 777–787.

Goitein M, Abrams M, Rowell D, Pollari H and Wiles J (1983) Multi-dimensional treatment planning: II. Beam's eye view, back projection, and projection through CT sections. *International Journal of Radiation Oncology Biology Physics* 9: 789–797.

Goiten M, Wittenberg J, Mendiondo M, Doucette J, Friedberg C, Ferrucci J *et al.* (1979) The value of CT scanning in radiation therapy treatment planning: a prospective study. *International Journal of Radiation Oncology Biology and Physics* 5(10): 1787–1798.

Helyer SJ and Heisig S (1995) Multileaf collimation versus conventional shielding blocks: a time and motion study of beam shaping in radiotherapy. *Radiotherapy and Oncology* 37: 61–64.

Hounsfield GN (1973) Computerized transverse axial scanning (tomography). *British Journal of Radiology* 46: 10–16.

Hounsfield GN (1980) Nobel Award address. Computed medical imaging. *Medical Physics* 7(4): 283–290.

International Atomic Energy Agency (2008) *Transition from 2-D Radiotherapy to 3-D Conformal and Intensity Modulated Radiotherapy.* IAEA-TECDOC-1588, IAEA, Vienna, Austria.

International Commission on Radiation Units and Measurements (1999) 'ICRU Rep 62, Prescribing, recording and reporting photon beam therapy'. ICRU, Washington, DC.

Kijewski PK, Chin LM and Bjarngard BE (1978) Wedge-shaped dose distributions by computer-controlled collimator motion. *Medical Physics* 5(5): 426–429.

Langmack KA (2001) Portal imaging. *British Journal of Radiology* 74: 789–804.

Leavitt DD, Stewart JR, Moeller JH and Earley L (1989) Optimization of electron arc therapy doses by multi-vane collimator control. *International Journal of Radiation Oncology Biology and Physics* 16(2): 489–496.

Liu Y, Shi C, Tynan P and Papanikolaou N (2008) Dosimetric characteristics of dual-layer multileaf collimation for small-field and intensity-modulated radiation therapy applications. *Journal of Applied Clinical Medical Physics* 9(2): 15–29.

Mackie TR, Liu HH and McCullough EC (1998) Treatment planning algorithms: model-based photon dose calculation algorithms. In: *Treatment Planning in Radiation Oncology.* (Eds FM Khan and RA Potish) pp. 90–112. Williams & Wilkins, Baltimore.

Mackie TR, Olivera GH, Reckwerdt PJ and Shepard D (2001) Understanding radiation therapy optimization/inverse treatment planning. In: *3-D Conformal and Intensity Modulated Radiation Therapy.* (Eds J Purdy, W Grant III, J Palta, B Butler and C Perez) pp. 247–262. Advanced Medical Publishing Inc., Madison.

Marks LB and Ma J (2007) Challenges in the clinical application of advanced technologies to reduce radiation-associated normal tissue injury. *International Journal of Radiation Oncology Biology and Physics* 69(1): 4–12.

McShan DL, Silverman A, Lanza DM, Reinstein LE and Glicksman AS (1979) A computerized three-dimensional treatment planning system utilizing interactive colour graphics. *British Journal of Radiology* **52**: 478–481.

Metcalfe P, Kron T and Hoban P (1997) *The Physics of Radiotherapy X-Rays from Linear Accelators*. Medical Physics Publishing.

Milan J and Bentley RE (1974) The storage and manipulation of radiation dose data in a small digital computer. *British Journal of Radiology* **47**: 115–121.

Papanikolaou N, Mackie TR, Meger-Wells C, Gehring M and Reckwerdt P (1993) Investigation of the convolution method for polyenergetic spectra. *Medical Physics* **20**: 1327–1336.

Purdy JA (1996) Defining our goals: volume and dose specification for 3-D conformal radiation therapy. *Frontiers of Radiation Therapy and Oncology* **29**: 24–30.

Purdy JA (2008) Dose to normal tissues outside the radiation therapy patient's treated volume: a review of different radiation therapy techniques. *Health Physics* **95**(5): 666–676.

Sherouse GW, Novins K and Chaney EL (1990) Computation of digitally reconstructed radiographs for use in radiotherapy treatment design. *International Journal of Radiation Oncology Biology Physics* **18**(3): 651–658.

Shipley WU, Tepper J E, Prout GR, Verhey LJ, Mendiondo OA, Goitein M, Koehler AM and Suit HD (1979) Proton radiation as boost therapy for localized prostatic carcinoma. *Journal of the American Medical Association* **241**: 1912–1915.

Sontag MR, Battista JJ, Bronskill MJ and Cunningham JR (1977) Implications of computer tomography for inhomogeneity corrections in photon beam dose calculations. *Radiology* **124**(1): 143–149.

Stanley NS (1999) The role of Digitally Reconstructed Radiographs in the verification process. *Journal of Radiotherapy in Practice* **1**: 103–108.

Starkschall G, Steadham RE, Popple RA, Ahmad S and Rosen II (2000) Beam-commissioning methodology for a three dimensional convolution/superposition photon dose algorithm. *Journal of Applied Clinical Medical Physics* **1**: 8–27.

Stephenson JA and Wiley LA (1995) Current techniques in three-dimensional CT simulation and radiation treatment planning. *Oncology* **9**(11): 1225–1240.

Stroom JC and Heijmen BJM (2002) Geometrical uncertainties, radiotherapy planning margins, and the ICRU-62 report. *Radiotherapy and Oncology* **64**: 75–83.

Taborsky SC (1981) Digital imaging for radiation therapy verification. *Proceedings of SPIE* **314**: 164–171.

Tsien KC (1955) The application of automatic computing machines to radiation treatment planning. *British Journal of Radiology* **28**: 432–439.

van Herk M and Meertens H (1988) A matrix ionisation chamber imaging device for on-line patient setup verification during radiotherapy. *Radiotherapy and Oncology* **11**(4): 369–378.

van Herk MP, Remeijer P, Rasch C and Lebesque JV (2000) The probability of correct target dose: dose population histograms for deriving treatment margins in radiotherapy. *International Journal of Radiation Oncology Biology Physics* **47**: 1121–1135.

van Herk M (2004) Errors and margins in radiotherapy. Semin Radiat Oncol **14**: 52–64.

Webb S (1997) *The Physics of Conformal Radiotherapy – Advances in Technology*. IOP Publishing, Bristol, UK.

7 Image guided radiotherapy: radiobiology and physics aspects of treatment

7.1 INTRODUCTION

Successful radiation therapy depends on the ability to deliver substantially more dose to a tumour than to surrounding normal tissues. Generally, the greater the tumour dose, the greater chance of killing the tumour. However, increase in tumour dose is only possible if radiation field margins can be reduced (ICRU 62, 1999). In order to be able to reduce field margins, accurate alignment of the treatment field with the target volume is necessary. However, tumours can move throughout a treatment course. In general, the movement includes *interfraction motion* (changes in position from day-to-day) and *intrafraction motion* (changes in position during a treatment fraction itself).

Interfraction variations are due to variations in bladder and rectal filling, weight loss or gain, or skill of therapists to accurately set up a patient. Intrafraction variations are due to respiratory, cardiac and peristaltic motions, swallowing, as well as the patient's voluntary body movement. Tumour motion therefore represents a limit for the minimum radiation field size that can be used in order to cover the tumour and its movement completely. Because of interfractional motion in particular, in order to reduce the field margins further, it has become necessary for some cancers to accurately identify the location of a tumour relative

to healthy tissues on a daily basis. This successive imaging and determination of positional correlation of the target volume relative to normal structures is the main focus of a treatment approach perfected in the past decade known as the Image Guided Radiation Therapy (IGRT) (Jaffray *et al.* 2007; Steinke and Bezak 2008). In other words, image guided radiotherapy is targeting of the tumor using images with the patient in treatment position immediately prior to or during treatment. The goal of IGRT is to manage inter- and intra-fraction motion to reduce margins and optimise treatment designs. It is fair to say that image guidance in radiation treatment is not a completely new concept. It has always been applied in a variety of forms: surface and skin marks, portal imaging, electronic portal imaging, fluroscopy and conventional CT.

Several forms of IGRT are available at present, depending on the imaging technology used; for example X-rays, magnetic resonance or ultrasound can all be used for image guidance in radiotherapy. Systems can also be based on localisation and tracking of special markers; for example seeds, coils, infrared markers, clips or electromagnetic beacons.

In terms of architecture, some systems incorporate imaging technologies that are fully integrated with the simulation and planning systems. Other set-ups utilise

L. Marcu et al., *Biomedical Physics in Radiotherapy for Cancer*, DOI 10.1007/978-0-85729-733-4_7, © CSIRO 2012

combinations of treatment and imaging devices as well as stand-alone planning systems from different manufacturers communicating via DICOM RT compliant interfaces. In addition, so-called 3D or 4D systems are available, where 3D systems enable volumetric geometrical position identification of the target volume, while 4D systems enable position determination in space and time (e.g. can monitor and account for anatomical changes due to breathing).

As a result, there are many approaches available for image guidance, each having its advantages, disadvantages and limitations. Current IGRT approaches include:

- film imaging acquired using conventional port films
- electronic imaging using electronic portal imaging devices
- video and surface guidance (infrared, ultrasound)
- digital projection imaging (Radiographic and fluoroscopic)
- CT guided (Cone beam CT, CT-on rails, MV CT)
- MRI or US Guided
- 4D (gating, tracking, breath hold)
- marker localisation and marker tracking (seeds, coils, infrared, clips, electromagnetic beacons).

When selecting a suitable imaging IGRT tool, the following should be considered:

- compromise of clinical objectives, product availability, existing infrastructure and manpower
- clinical objectives (dose escalation/normal tissue sparing)
- structures of interest (target/surrogates)
- desired level of precision
- safety of use
- method of intervention/correction
- available treatment capacity
- application for all or some patients
- development and implementation of commissioning and QA procedures
- clinical protocols development; i.e. system of responsibility delegation with respect to measurement, analysis, decision, and correction.

The most common approach uses a diagnostic X-ray tube attached to a linear accelerator that images the tumour immediately prior to therapy. The X-ray tube can be used in different modes either to acquire 2D portal images or a 3D (volumetric) CT scan. In cases where the patient position is shifted or the tumour volume has moved, the patient position can be corrected before the radiation is delivered. The shift is identified by comparing the daily portal or CT image with the reference portal or CT image obtained during treatment planning from a simulator.

7.2 USE OF X-RAY IMAGING IN RADIATION THERAPY

When using X-ray radiography, it is possible to differentiate tissues of varying densities for diagnostic purposes. However, depth information is lost since 3D objects are projected on a 2D film, resulting in an image of super-imposed tissue. This problem can be resolved using computed tomography (CT) scanning, a technique yielding cross-sectional images of a patient. In this technique, the object is exposed from many different directions and the image is reconstructed from superposition of measured X-ray transmission images. The term 'tomography' originates from the Greek words tomos (slice) and graphe (drawing). Stacking large numbers of 2D 'tomographic' slides generates volumetric images. Although the mathematical principle of computing these images was discovered early in the 20th century (Radon 1917), it took until 1972 to build the first CT scanner. Both G.N. Hounsfield and Alan McCormack received the Nobel Prize for Physiology or Medicine (1979) for their independent work.

One of the most important applications of CT in radiation oncology (Figure 7.1) is treatment planning (identification of Planning Target Volume, PTV, as well as calculation of dose distribution) and more recently patient positioning (alignment of PTV) during radiation therapy (RT) treatment (van Dyk 1999).

7.2.1 Development of computed tomography

First generation CT scanners are assembled of a pencil beam X-ray source and a single detector. In order to acquire an image of an object, linear translation of the beam (line sweep) for each projection angle as well as

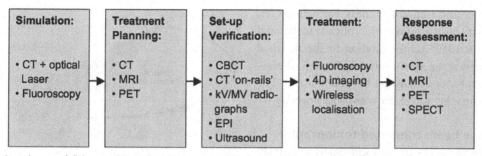

Figure 7.1. Imaging modalities used in radiation therapy. (CT: computed tomography, MRI: magnetic resonance imaging, PET: positron emission tomography, CBCT: cone beam computed tomography, EPI: electronic portal imaging, SPECT: single photon emission tomography). (Courtesy Steinke and Bezak 2008)

rotations in 1° intervals were required. The separation of translational and rotational measurements resulted in scan times of up to 4 minutes. The second generation of CT scanners used a narrow fan beam and multiple detectors. While the translational motion was still necessary (as the fan beam did not cover the whole object), scanning times were reduced significantly. The 3rd generation CT scanners completely eliminated the translational movement of the X-ray source, by increasing the fan-beam angle and introducing arc-shaped detector arrays. Scan times were reduced to ~1 s per slice due to high-speed rotation of the X-ray source and detector array (Kalender 2006). The fourth generation design, was based on a large 360° stationary detector with the X-ray source orbiting around the patient within the detector ring (Figure 7.2).

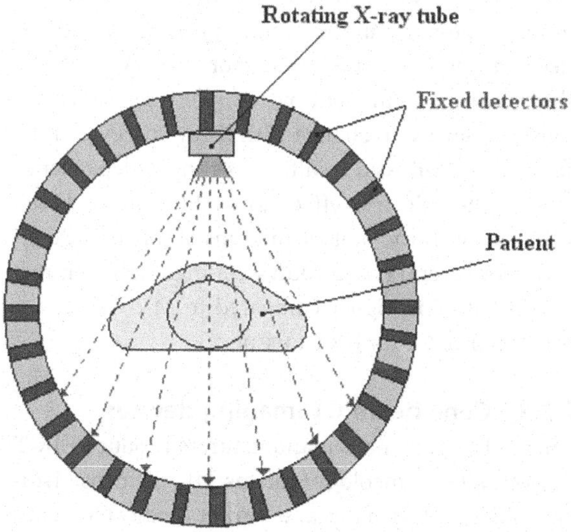

In conventional CT 2D images are simply stacked in order to create a quasi-volumetric image. As a result, in the early 1990s continuous scanning along the patient's longitudinal axis was introduced. The introduction of so-called slipring scanner technology allowed rotations greater than 360° for the first time. Continuous scanning along the patient's longitudinal axis, results in a *helical (spiral)* scanning pattern (Prokop and Galanski 2003) as shown in Figure 7.3. In addition, instead of scanning one slice at a time, the introduction of array detector technology in 1998 opened up the possibility of scanning several slices at one time. Scan times per volume for four-slice helical scanners (0.5 s per rotation) were smaller compared to a single-slice conventional scanner (1 s per rotation) by a factor of 8. Gradually, larger slice numbers became available and 64-slice technology is now state-of-the-art.

With the introduction of spiral techniques, the concept of *pitch* was developed. Its value affects

Figure 7.2. Schematic diagram of a fourth generation CT.

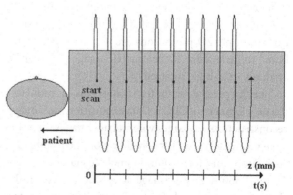

Figure 7.3. Schematic diagram of spiral (helical) CT scanning.

scanning time and section thickness. For helical CTs, the pitch factor is the ratio of the couch translational movement per 360° gantry rotation to the nominal slice thickness at the axis of rotation. In clinical practice the pitch factor usually lies between 1 and 2. The pitch <1 means that successive scans/slices overlap.

7.2.2   Cone beam computed tomography

The possibility of 3D tumour localisation and tracking in the course of RT treatment requires an imaging device to be part of the radiotherapy apparatus, i.e. the linear accelerator (linac). Attaching conventional fan-beam CTs to linacs proved difficult. As a result, a different approach was needed, utilising a simple X-ray tube that could be attached to the linac structure. As the X-ray tube produces a cone of X-rays (rather than a pencil or fan beam), this approach is known as Cone Beam Computed Tomography (CBCT) (Jaffray *et al.* 2002).

A cone beam CT device consists of an X-ray source (X-ray tube) and a digital flat-panel detector (FPD), as shown in Figure 7.4. The detector consists of a large array of amorphous silicon (a-Si) thin-film transistors and optically coupled photodiodes (working on the same principle as a-Si EPIDs discussed in Chapter 6). It contains a sensor that transforms incoming X-rays into electric charge; a capacitor which stores the charge and finally, read-out electronics, which converts charge-information into a digital image. The detector is also mounted on the linac. Both the X-ray tube and the detector rotate with linac gantry rotations. The patient (object) lies between the X-ray tube and the flat panel detector, with the cone of X-rays generating a 2D projection of the patient's anatomy. If the patient is imaged repeatedly during a linac rotation, multiple 2D projections are acquired and combined to generate a 3D volumetric image of patient's anatomy in a single rotation.

The flat panel detector technology was essential for the development of CBCT. Data acquisition and image reconstruction of large volumetric images can be achieved within 1–2 min depending on the number of projections and total rotation angle (usually between 180 and 360 degrees). Image acquisition is generally slower compared to helical CT scans, because rotational speeds are severely limited by the heavy linac

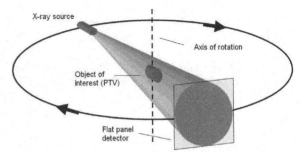

Figure 7.4. Schematic diagram of cone beam computed tomography.

gantry (generally one rotation per minute only). Since the X-ray tube produces kilovoltage X-rays, interacting via photoelectric effect, the low-contrast resolution of this system is superior to electronic portal imaging that uses X-rays of megavoltage energies produced by a linear accelerator. The use of either kilovoltage (30–140 kV) or megavoltage (1–6 MV) imaging modalities also significantly impacts on the signal-to-noise ratio. Similarly, the quantum efficiency of the flat panel detector varies from ~60% for kV energies to only ~1% for MV energies. CBCT also offers 3D spatial information since every point of the volume exposed is reconstructed (Groh *et al.* 2002).

At MV X-ray energies, the Compton effect is the dominant interaction process. Its interaction probability (i.e. the photon attenuation coefficient, $\mu(E)$) is inversely proportional to the photon energy E and, especially for low-Z materials, is nearly independent from the atomic number Z and proportional to the electron density of the attenuator. For kV energies, absorption is dominated by the photoelectric effect, causing contrast to change with X-ray energy and the atomic number. As a result, the strong Z-dependence of the photoelectric effect gives kilovoltage based CBCT a natural advantage in terms of soft-tissue contrast. For several tissue equivalent materials, contrast for kV-CBCT is higher compared to MV-CBCT, e.g. by a factor of 6.5 for breast tissue.

7.2.3   Cone beam CT imaging devices

Currently, three main manufacturers produce CBCT devices: Elekta Oncology Systems, UK, Siemens Medical Solutions, Germany, and Varian Medical Systems, USA (see Figure 7.5). Interestingly, two completely

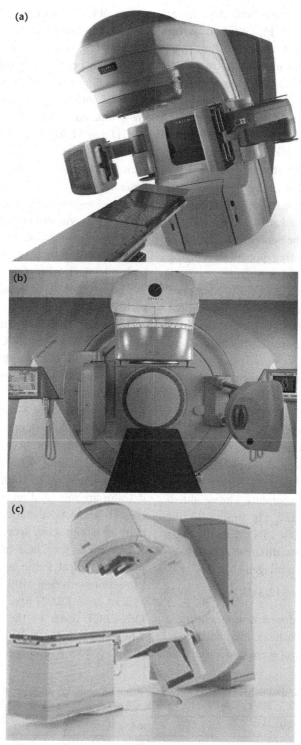

Figure 7.5. a) Figure of Varian On-Board Imaging system (courtesy and Copyright ©2007, Varian Medical Systems, Inc. All rights reserved.); b) Picture of Elekta XVI system (courtesy and Copyright©2008 Elekta AB (publ). All rights reserved.); c) Picture of Siemens MVision system on Siemens Oncor linac (courtesy and Copyright © Siemens AG, 2002–2008. All rights reserved.).

different CBCT technologies have been developed. While Varian and Elekta use kV-CBCT imaging modalities mounted at 90° with respect to the treatment beam, Siemens uses the megavoltage treatment beam to produce MV-CBCT images. However, with their latest product, ARTÍSTE™, Siemens has also incorporated linac-mounted kV-CBCT imaging. The newly emerging Mitsubishi MHI-TM2000 (Mitsubishi Heavy Industries, Japan) IGRT system also features kV-CBCT imaging (Takayama *et al.* 2007).

The Elekta Synergy™ is a radiotherapy linac with an integrated kV-CBCT imager, called X-ray Volume Imaging (XVI). XVI is mounted at 90° with respect to the X-ray treatment beam. The Synergy system uses a kV X-ray tube with accelerating potentials varying from 40 to 130 kVp and 0.1–3.2 mAs (milliampere × seconds) per projection. The X-ray tube is positioned at 100 cm from the linac isocentre. The opposing flat panel detector uses amorphous silicon technology and the active array has the area of 41 cm × 41 cm (1024 × 1024 pixels, 400 μm pitch/pixel) and is located 53.6 cm from the isocentre. The source-to-imager Distance (SID) of 153.6 cm is fixed. The size of exposed area (field-of-view) is set up with collimators on the X-ray tube. A typical CBCT acquisition uses 330 projections per full rotation.

Amer *et al.* (2007) investigated patient doses arising from Elekta's XVI cone beam CT. Measurements were taken using phantoms or patients. The weighted-cone beam dose index, $CBDI_w$, is similar to the weighted-CT dose index, $CTDI_w$. Its definition takes into account dose deposition at different depths (central and peripheral) within the imaged object:

$$CBDI_w = (1/3) D_{central} + (2/3) D_{peripheral} \quad (7.1)$$

Table 7.1 summarises the dose measurements for a 26 cm^2 exposure field size for head, lung and pelvis. CBDI doses for head and lung scans are lower than

comparable electronic portal images using megavoltage X-ray treatment beams, as comparable wide-field EPI images result in average imaging doses of 20–40 mGy per two orthogonal EPIs.

Table 7.2 compares the dose indices from a cone beam CT with those for standard CTs. CBCT doses are low compared to dose resulting from a Single-Slice CT (SSCT) and Multi-Slice CT (MSCT) scanning of head and lung by factors >10 and 2, respectively. For anatomical sites where soft tissue detail is required, CBCT doses proved to be 50% higher due to the need to enhance low-contrast resolution. Typical CBCT imaging for the pelvis could result in a surface dose of up to 30 mGy per scan. If cone beam CT scanning is used on a daily basis (up to 40 fractions), as required in some protocols, the total surface dose approaches the deterministic level of 2 Gy for transient skin erythema (Valentin 2001).

Varian's On-Board Imager™ (OBI) represents another approach to kV-CBCT imaging. OBI produces digital kV radiographic, CBCT and fluoroscopic images. The kV-CBCT apparatus is mounted on a Varian linac at 90° with respect to the treatment beam. A standard kV X-ray tube (60–140 kVp, 2 mAs per projection) and an opposing a-Si flat-panel detector are used. Default settings for the source-imager distance (SID) are 150 cm and 100 cm for the source-axis distance (SAD). Both the X-ray tube and the detector are mounted on moveable robotic arms and the SID and SAD distances are user adjustable. The detector has an active array of 29.8 cm × 39.7 cm (1024 × 1536 pixels for CBCT-mode, 291 × 193 μm pitch/pixel). A typical 1 min acquisition features 650–700 projections covering a full rotation.

Kan *et al.* (2008) have measured effective Varian OBI-CBCT doses to the body and absorbed OBI-CBCT doses to 26 organs, using OBI's standard mode (125 kVp, 80 mA, 25 ms, 150 cm SID) and a low-dose

Table 7.1. Site, beam settings and CBDI$_w$ for Elekta's XVI-CBCT scanning protocols adopted at the Christie Hospital (courtesy Amer *et al.* 2007).

Site	kV	mAs	CBDI$_w$ [mGy]
Head	100	38	1.6
Lung	120	152	6
Pelvis	130	456	25

Table 7.2. Comparison of Elekta XVI-CBDI$_w$ at Christie Hospital (Manchester, UK) and a UK survey of single-slice CT (SSCT) and multi-slice CT (MSCT) CTDI$_{vol}$ for different anatomic sites (courtesy Amer *et al.* 2007).

	SSCT	MSCT	CBCT
	CTDI$_{vol}$ [mGy]	CTDI$_{vol}$ [mGy]	CBDI$_w$ [mGy]
Head	59	80	1.6
Lung	10	13	6
Pelvis	13	14	25

mode (125 kVp, 40 mA, 10 ms, 150 cm SID). The absorbed dose measurements were performed using a female anthropomorphic humanoid phantom (RANDO) with at least two thermoluminescent dosimeters for each organ. Effective doses to the patient for neck, chest and pelvis imaging were estimated. Table 7.3 summarises effective doses to the patient for standard and low-dose CBCT and fan-beam CT (120 kVp, 300 mAs). The larger delivered doses in the standard mode are largely due to a higher number of projections (~700 to ~330) and higher mAs settings in Varian's default settings. Clinicians and medical physicists should be aware of these additional doses delivered to a patient when planning a treatment so that any radiation risks are minimised.

Siemens ARTÍSTE™ is the third major kV-CBCT device that incorporates a unique 'in-line' concept for linac-integrated kV-CBCT imaging (Tücking 2007). The term 'in-line' refers to the geometry of MV treatment beam and kV beam (see Figure 7.6).

The kV X-ray tube is mounted at 180° with respect to the treatment beam. A flat panel imager is installed between Multi-Leaf Collimator (MLC) and isocentre (with its front plane pointing to the kV X-ray tube). The MV and kV beam are thus monitored by a single imaging detector. As the megavoltage treatment beam always traverses the detector, the shape and intensity of the radiation treatment beam are monitored during radiation delivery. Rotating the gantry allows for acquisition of inter and possibly intra-fraction kV-CBCT images. Optionally, a second flat panel detector (with its front plane pointing towards the linac beam) can be installed between kV X-ray source and the isocentre. This detector can perform either MV-CBCT (before treatment) or fluoroscopy (during treatment) imaging. It can also be used to measure MV beam parameters with better spatial resolution than the upper detector. While monitoring beam delivery is a main advantage of the in-line concept, it is also capable of tracking tumour and organ motion perpendicular to the treatment beam. The other 90° solutions (i.e. XVI and OBI) are able to monitor motion along the MV treatment beam axis.

Siemens' MVision™ system has a different approach to cone beam CT. In contrast to 90° solutions, MVision utilises the 6 MV X-ray treatment beam (SAD=100 cm) and an amorphous silicon detector mounted 45 cm from the isocentre and at 180° with respect to the treatment beam to generate volumetric images. It can be used on conventional Siemens linacs, i.e. Primus™ and Oncor™. If used on established linac equipment, MVision represents the least expensive CBCT imaging device as no additional kV source or detector panel are needed. In addition, MVision uses the same coordinate system for imaging and treatment, so the isocentre matching procedures can

Table 7.3. Effective patient doses for Varian's OBI (standard-mode and low-dose) and fan-beam CT. Only one fan-beam measurement has been performed (no error-bars) (courtesy Kan *et al.* 2008).

	Effective dose (mSv)		
Mode	Standard-mode	Low-dose	Fan-beam
Head scan	10.26 ± 0.46	2.10 ± 0.08	3.6
Chest scan	23.56 ± 0.35	5.23 ± 0.122	6.9
Pelvis scan	22.72 ± 0.29	4.89 ± 0.163	10.7

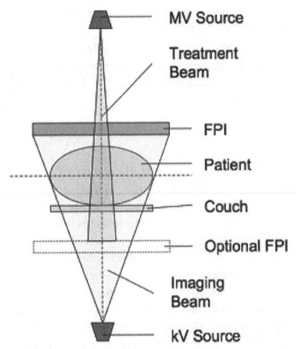

Figure 7.6. Schematic view of in-line kV-CBCT imaging. (Courtesy Steinke and Bezak 2008)

be simplified. The a-Si flat panel detector has an active area of 41 cm × 41 cm (1024 × 1024 pixels, 400 μm pitch/pixel). The MV-CBCT mode features a 200° gantry rotation from 270° to 110° (clockwise) and acquires one projection for each degree. As a result, acquisition and reconstruction time is down to approximately 2 min (Pouliot *et al.* 2005).

Because the Compton effect, which does not depend on the Z of the material, is dominant for MV energies, the quality of the images is worse relative to the kV-CBCT images. This is decreased further because of the presence of scattered X-rays and annihilation radiation caused by pair production. How-

ever, working with MV X-rays reduces the sensitivity to high-Z materials, like in metallic implants or, generally speaking, normally non-compatible CT objects. For kV energies (i.e. photoeffect), implants like hip prosthesis, teeth fillings or orthopaedic hardware cause massive artefacts in CT images.

As mentioned above, using megavoltage photon beams lowers image quality for imaging doses comparable to kV-CBCT. Table 7.4 shows mean daily imaging doses to prostate patients using MVision and conventional electronic portal imaging (Morin *et al.* 2007). Obviously, doses delivered in MV-CBCT protocols are higher than EPI-doses. While EPI acquisition is generally faster, neither soft-tissue nor volumetric information is obtained. Low doses are sufficient to resolve high-contrast areas like bony anatomy, whereas low-contrast regions such as soft-tissue boundaries require increased doses.

Achieving sufficient MV-CBCT image contrast for soft tissue involves using relatively high doses of 60–100 mGy per scan. Prostate patients, who are treated with 77.4 Gy in 43 fractions, would receive an additional dose of up to 4.3 Gy at the isocentre due to MV-CBCT (Miften *et al.* 2007). However, incorporating MV-CBCT dose in the treatment planning as part of therapy itself can reduce additional patient dose. Dosimetric result for plans optimised with and without cone beam CT showed that the average mean dose for cone beam CT is higher for bladder (1.6 ± 1.0 Gy) and femoral heads (1.9 ± 0.8 Gy), but comparable for the rectum (-0.3 ± 1.4 Gy).

In summary, although similar in concept, designs of individual manufacturers yield different imaging doses largely depending on different default beam parameters, number of projections and mAs settings. OBI's moveable gantry arms offer greater flexibility in

Table 7.4. Mean dose to selected anatomical sites received in daily verification imaging for prostate patients (courtesy Morin *et al.* 2007).

Site	MV-CBCT [mGy] 9 MU	EPI [mGy] 2 x 3 MU
Prostate	69	46
Rectum	59	41
Bladder	78	51
Small bowel	83	54

terms of X-ray source and detector position. It is expected that increases in imaging doses are offset by reduced planning target volume margins and more accurate treatment dose delivery. However, this needs to be evaluated carefully for each treatment site and imaging protocol. Increased tumour control and sparing of normal tissue is expected to result in improved patient treatment outcomes. Keeping imaging doses 'As Low As Reasonably Achievable' (ALARA) must be a top priority. Similar to helical CT scanning, cone beam CT image quality can be improved by increasing the number of projections and mAs setting used. In practise, image quality and the risk of inducing fatal cancer from a single radiographic exposure of 5×10^{-5}/mSv (according to ICRP 60) must be balanced. This is an important issue to be considered when implementing CBCT in clinical practise.

7.3 ADAPTIVE RADIATION THERAPY

Cone beam CT scans help to localise the position of a tumour in 3D and to register changes in tumour and patient anatomy during treatment. They can assist to minimise adverse effects on healthy tissues by 'guiding the treatment beam' or by modifying/adapting the treatment plan based on the current patient anatomy as observed on a cone beam CT scan. The modification of treatment as a result of new patient information, obtained for example from cone beam CT scanning, is known as Adaptive Radiotherapy (ART).

Adaptive radiotherapy is a 'closed-loop' feedback mechanism that monitors treatment response (e.g. tumour shrinkage) and/or changes in patient anatomy and implements changes in prescription (i.e. in treatment parameters such as dose distribution, margins, number of fractions) throughout the treatment course (Yan *et al.* 1997) (Figure 7.7). Optimal treatment modification can be determined *off-line* or *on-line*.

If patient imaging is performed daily, sufficient anatomical information can be accumulated to re-optimise treatment parameters for a given patient. After several treatment fractions (~5), the prescription can be modified to conform better to the patient-specific planning target volume (PTV) determined from the images acquired. This approach is known as 'off-line' adaptive radiation therapy (Yan *et al.* 2000). The adapted treat-

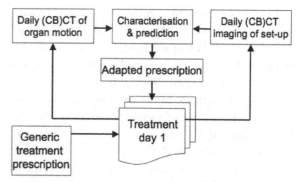

Figure 7.7. Schematic view of the Adaptive Radiation Therapy (ART) workflow. Prescription can be adapted after ~5 treatment days (off-line ART) or daily (on-line ART). (Courtesy Steinke and Bezak 2008)

ment plan accounts for estimated systematic errors in the original plan. Generally, in radiation therapy, large generic margins are used to account for inter-patient set-up variations. Generic margins are based on clinical experience and vary depending on the anatomical site. By accounting for systematic errors in an individual treatment plan, off-line ART allows for a patient-specific margin to be applied to accommodate random set-up variations. As a result PTV margins can be reduced sparing normal tissue.

Ideally, as the tumour position can vary from day to day, the prescription should be adapted and dose distribution recalculated for an individual patient immediately prior to each treatment fraction. This approach is known as 'on-line' adaptive radiation therapy. On-line ART can account for the organ motion, set-up errors as well as for anatomical changes (e.g. tumour growth or shrinkage, changes in patient's weight) during the course of treatment.

Pre-treatment cone beam CT images may be used for both on-line and off-line adjustments to the treatment plan. Once the CBCT image of a patient has been acquired, changes (deformations) in the anatomy that cannot be corrected by simple shifts in position can be identified. This is done by comparing/overlaying the CBCT dataset with the planning CT and differences between planned and on-the-day tissue volumes and their impact on delivered dose distribution are evaluated. If required, the dose delivery can be recalculated using a treatment planning system or recalculation software provided with a given imaging system.

In order to be able to compare individual CT data-sets, special software algorithms known as *image fusion* are used. Fusion software is able to overlay or merge multiple images obtained using the same or different imaging modalities (e.g. CT and MRI). Fusion of different modality images is often used to improve visualisation of various materials or tissues. For example, if CT and MRI images of the same patient are combined, the fused image will display both bones, fat and soft tissue clearly. However, the images that are being fused (*co-registered*) are often not of the same size and shape as patient position and/or image scales (magnification factors) might be different for each imaging modality. In addition, there can be internal changes due to organ move-ment, phase of respiration, bowel/bladder content and others. As a result, in order for the images to be combined, specific feature points must be defined on the two images (for example, a well defined anatomi-cal point). The registration software then distorts one of the images until the points on both data sets match. The underlying algorithm utilises a number of coor-dinate transformations (translation, rotation, scaling, shearing and others) to map feature points on both images (also known as *rigid registration*). The algo-rithm, in effect, correlates the coordinate system of one image to the coordinate system of the second image. Basic fusion algorithms use 2D translation and 2D rotation and are good for combining images of the head/brain and regions close to bones; how-ever, they have limited accuracy in other regions of the body.

In order to fuse two images that might be quite different (as a result of anatomical change, e.g. weight loss or tumour shrinkage during radiation therapy) a more complex algorithm known as *deformable registration* must be used. In deformable registration, points or regions representing the same anatomy in the sequential (day-to-day) image data-sets are identified. These points however will be in various states of change (so-called deformation) from the original reference planning CT dataset. The deformable registration identifies the differences between the datasets and then correlates voxels from one image to voxels on another one using complex mathematical algorithms (Huntzinger *et al.* 2006).

Deformable registration enables even mapping lines onto curves and is suitable for the whole body and can account for organ movement. It can be used for automatic updating of a plan throughout the treat-ment course as it also enables the transfer of target and organ at risk contours between images as well of dose patterns so that a clinician can determine the impact of day-to-day changes on dose delivery.

Finally, while cone beam CT is increasingly used for patient set-up verification, its use in on-line adap-tive replanning is still under development. As a result of the large volume of X-ray exposure (cone beam versus pencil/fan beam), scattered radiation repre-sents a serious problem resulting in deterioration of the CBCT image quality and potentially significant variation of Hounsfield numbers, depending on the amount of scatter. Since the Hounsfield units are related to the electron density at a given pixel, the dose calculation accuracy is affected. Several scatter cor-rection algorithms have been proposed but there is no uniformly accepted solution at present.

7.4 ALTERNATIVE APPROACHES TO IGRT

Alternative approaches to image guidance using con-ventional fan-beam CT scanners have also been inves-tigated. Cone beam CT is indeed not the only possible pathway to obtain an on-line CT before or during radiotherapy fraction.

7.4.1 Tomotherapy

Literally meaning 'slice' therapy, tomotherapy is a treatment technique developed by Mackie *et al.* (1999). TomoTherapy's Hi-ART II™ (TomoTherapy Inc., Madi-son, WI, USA) integrates MV helical fan-beam CT and radiation treatment unit (linac) into a single device. The unit looks fairly similar to a conventional CT scan-ner (Figure 7.8). The ring gantry contains a slip-ring linac producing a 6 MV X-ray narrow fan-beam. As the patient couch is translated through the gantry, the rotating ring-mounted MV source is turned on creat-ing a helical beam pattern (Mackie 2006). This unique helical delivery pattern minimises normal tissue irra-diation. A specially designed 64-leaf binary multi-leaf collimator shapes the treatment beam to yield a desired dose distribution. The unit can deliver highly confor-

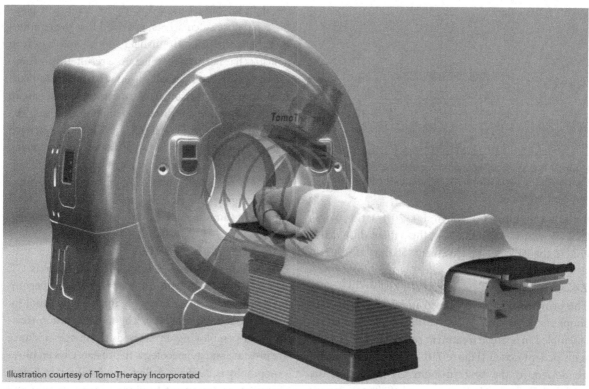

Figure 7.8. TomoTherapy® treatment system. (Courtesy and Copyright ©2008 TomoTherapy Incorporated. All rights reserved.)

mal dose patterns as well as modulated (non-uniform) radiation intensities as used in the intensity modulated radiation therapy (Chapter 8). The slice thickness of the MV beam is defined by a jaw (secondary collimator) in the range of 0.5–5 cm. The MV treatment beam (reduced to 3.5 MV energy) can also be used for daily helical MV-CT imaging, allowing for online treatment adaptation.

The major drawback of Tomotherapy is the beam-on time for treatment delivery that can be up to 15 times larger than that for conventional treatment delivery (Ramsey *et al.* 2006). Typical beam-on times for helical tomotherapy lung treatment (2 Gy per fraction) range from 200 s to 300 s. A similar treatment delivered with a conventional linac takes 20–60 s. The increased beam-on times also increases in-field radiation scatter and the risk of patient movement during treatment. Additionally, the overall treatment time is increased by up to 25 min (using an on-line IGRT approach), limiting the patient throughput. Around 19 patients per treatment day per tomotherapy unit

can be expected (Bijdekerke *et al.* 2008) compared to 35–40 for a conventional linac.

The image noise and low-contrast resolution due to use of megavoltage X-rays for imaging is an issue for tomotherapy. Hi-ART's default pixel setting is 512 × 512 resulting in 0.78 mm in-plane pixel resolution. The signal-to-noise ratio (SNR) is between 2 and 4 depending on the size of the reconstruction matrix and pitch. For settings comparable to standard CT simulators, SNR is worse by a factor of 2.

Typical patient doses for helical tomotherapy are in the range of 10–20 mGy (Shah *et al.* 2007). Higher doses for head & neck were found to be up to 35 mGy (imaged with a fine pitch). The pitch, defined as the ratio of table movement per 360° rotation to slice thickness, is the only free parameter in Hi-ART II's image acquisition mode. There is no flexibility in MV or mAs settings. Doses increase with image quality and are inversely proportional to the pitch. A 'fine' pitch (e.g. 1.0) results in good image quality and higher dose. The total imaging dose to normal tissue

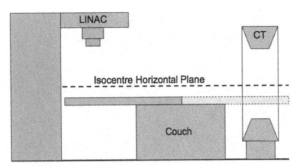

Figure 7.9 Conceptual idea of in-room CT. A sliding couch top moves the patient from the CT unit to the linac.

for a craniospinal CT (pitch 1.0, 20 fractions) was 0.72 Gy, which is about 2 % of the patient dose delivered to the PTV during treatment (Shah *et al.* 2007).

7.4.2   In-room CT

The principal idea of so-called in-room CT is quite simple: a linac and a conventional CT device are assembled in a single treatment room, sharing a common patient couch (Figure 7.9). In 1996, Uematsu *et al.* developed the first in-room CT device at the National Defence Medical College (Saitama, Japan) utilising a Toshiba CT scanner, a motorised couch and a linac (Uematsu *et al.* 1996).

In their procedure, the patient remained on the couch after the CT image was taken. While CT image-guided treatment planning took place, the couch was moved to the linac. Any physical movement of the patient between imaging and irradiation was avoided by using standard treatment immobilisation. The whole concept relied heavily on the mechanical precision of the system.

More modern concepts incorporate the use of 'on-rail' CT devices (e.g. Siemens Somatom™ or GE Smart Gantry™) (Kuriyama *et al.* 2003). Instead of using a sliding couch top to move the patient from the CT unit to the linac, a sliding-gantry helical CT scanner is moved (on-the-rail). The scanning is performed without either couch or patient movement, improving so the spatial accuracy. The patient couch is rotated 90° or 180° (depending on system) immediately after image acquisition to allow for linac treatment. Currently, rotational and other mechanical uncertainties are below 0.5 mm.

The use of kilovoltage X-rays results in good image quality with high soft-tissue contrast. In addition, the

CT data set can be used directly for treatment planning and dose calculations, provided that the relationship between CT Hounsfield units and electron densities has been determined. As a result, the in-room CT can be used for patient set-up verification and correction of interfraction PTV variations due to organ motion, as well as for dose recalculation. Not surprisingly, imaging doses are comparable to moving-couch CT scanners (~3–5 mGy for prostate), thus allowing for daily imaging (Thieke *et al.* 2006). Although, in-room CT can reduce inter-fraction set-up variations, since imaging and treatment are separated, it is not capable of tumour tracking or intra-fraction imaging.

7.4.3   US-guided EBRT

Besides other modern imaging methods such as CT, PET, MRI and fMRI, ultrasonography (US) is becoming greatly accepted and widely implemented tool for image guided radiotherapy. The most common treatment sites employing ultrasounds for image guidance are prostate and gynaecology. In prostate cancer, ultrasonography is used for daily target localisation before radiotherapy treatment to correct organ motion and set-up errors via specialised US-IGRT systems which allow for real-time visualisation of the prostate gland (Peignaux *et al.* 2006). The US probe is localised relative to the treatment isocentre so the 3D position/coordinates are known. After the ultrasound images are obtained, they are superimposed with the 3D CT images acquired for treatment planning, using the isocentre coordinates as reference. Once the anatomical structures on the two image sets are matched, set-up errors are determined and the patient is repositioned according to the initial set-up. The localisation and positioning adjustment are usually done within 10 minutes, making US guided IGRT a safe and feasible method for daily target localisation prior to treatment.

The capability of ultrasound to distinguish soft tissue structures and the high specificity in differentiating solid from fluid-filled structures makes it a good candidate for breast imaging (Yang and Dempsey 2007). Furthermore, despite advancements in CT, PET and MR imaging, ultrasonography remains the most accurate and, undoubtedly, the most cost effective tool for breast cancer imaging, complementing or even replacing the other techniques used for treatment guidance. Berrang *et al.* (2009) reports on 20 early stage breast cancer patients scheduled for partial breast radiotherapy which have been examined post-operatively with 3D ultrasound technology for target definition. They have found that interobserver variability in partial breast radiotherapy target contouring has considerably decreased with US when compared to CT. Besides treatment planning, the US technology is used to image the lumpectomy cavity during daily treatment to eliminate motion-induced errors, knowing the fact that after lumpectomy the cavity changes both shape and location. Therefore, the accuracy of target localisation increases and treatment margins are reduced lowering also the dose to normal tissue.

Colour Doppler imaging can assist in differentiating between benign and malignant breast tumours through the evaluation of angiogenesis in breast tissue. Given that the vasculature presents with different characteristics in malignant compared to benign tissue (see Chapter 9), a high-frequency transducer (7–13 MHz) Doppler ultrasound is required to evaluate flow signals originating from small vessels and those with low flow velocity (Yang and Dempsey 2007).

Ultrasounds are used to guide radiation boost planning (electron therapy) after breast lumpectomy since the early 1990s (Leonard *et al.* 1993). US image-guidance is done by placing the transducer within the electron cone, above the surgical scar which is positioned at the linac isocentre. Once the biopsy site is localised, the central axis is aligned with the axis of the transducer intersecting the scar and the biopsy site. The electron boost field placement is therefore, accurately achieved.

New ultrasound-based systems comprise of abdominal ultrasound probe allowing for IGRT for liver and pancreas treatment. Since the development of the curved linear-array echoendoscope in the 1990s, several centres have reported on successful endoscopic ultrasound-guided (EUS) intratumoural therapy for pancreatic adenocarcinoma, EUS playing a key role in the diagnosis and staging of this cancer (Yan and Van Dam 2008; Ashida and Chang 2009; Al-Haddad and Eloubeidi 2010). The feasibility and safety of endoscopic ultrasound-guided fiducial placement (gold markers) in the delivery of image guided radiotherapy for pancreatic cancers has been assessed by a recent study

(Varadarajulu *et al.* 2010). Fiducial placement was successful, without any complications in all patients and the markers served to identify the movement of the pancreas relative to bony landmarks between fractions, movement which could be accounted for during treatment. EUS-guided gold fiducial insertion for IGRT for pancreatic cancers eliminates the need for fluoroscopic imaging (Park *et al.* 2010), reducing the total dose of radiation received by patients as well as personnel.

3D ultrasound imaging for patient set-up and target motion tracking via internal fiducial marker insertion (using EUS) has been shown to significantly reduce treatment uncertainties during radiotherapy, decreasing therefore, the probability of normal tissue complication.

7.4.4   US-guided brachytherapy

Prostate brachytherapy has adopted ultrasound imaging for several tasks such as: visualising the prostate gland, assessing its dimensions, assisting in treatment planning and also for needle orientation and angulation during treatment. The prostate volume study is part of the interstitial LDR brachytherapy planning and consists of a transrectal ultrasound assessment of the prostate anatomy and its volume which is also an indication of a patient's eligibility to undergo permanent seed implant. Ultrasound images of the prostate are further used for target delineation in support of treatment planning (see Figure 7.10). This ultrasound-defined volume of interest serves as a reference image for subsequent scans. During implant, the orientation and angulation of the needles are ultrasound-guided, allowing for instant adjustments and corrections. Post-implant dosimetry is also based on ultrasound images which are fused with post-treatment CT images for better seed visualisation.

HDR brachytherapy for breast cancer is gaining popularity as an additional treatment to breast-conserving surgery, replacing whole breast external beam irradiation. Usually, interstitial multi-catheter brachytherapy requires a CT scan during treatment planning, meaning that the patient has to be moved with catheters inserted in their breasts. Another alternative is the use of ultrasound imaging for brachytherapy planning and verification purposes. Consequently, 3D ultrasound imaging has been assessed as a primary

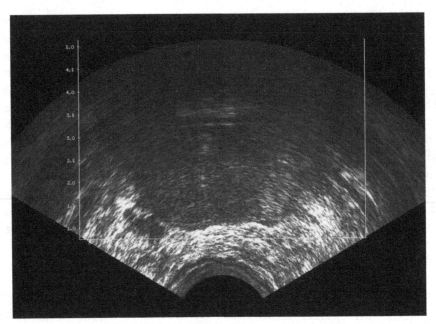

Figure 7.10. Pre-treatment ultrasound image of the prostate gland.

treatment planning imaging technique in breast brachytherapy and found to be clinically feasible (De Jean *et al.* 2009).

While US imaging has its limitations, one of which being the operator-dependent organ assessment, the cost effectiveness, safety, user friendly characteristics and soft tissue specificity are properties which encourage current clinical trends towards broader implementation of US in IGRT.

7.4.5 Beacon guided radiation therapy

One of the latest technological implementations in IGRT is the **Calypso system** (Calypso Medical Technologies, Inc.) which uses a GPS for the Body® technology in order to provide real-time, continuous and accurate information about tumour location during external beam radiotherapy. The localisation system is based on three miniature electromagnetic devices (Beacon transponders) which are implanted into the tumour and allow for non-ionising treatment guidance throughout therapy. The electromagnetic transponders of about 8.5 mm length are able to detect and display organ location and movement with a sub-millimeter localisation accuracy (Balter *et al.* 2005), permitting therefore, both inter and intrafraction patient positioning with high precision. The electromagnetic array of the main device

contains an energy source which is able to excite the transponders and receivers which detect the individual radiofrequency signals of the transponders for location coordinate identification (along lateral, longitudinal and vertical axes) (Figure 7.11). Any movement outside the planned target volume is detected and indicated through visual and audio signals by the tracking station. Adaptive Couch Repositioning hardware allows clinicians to remotely reposition the tumour as indicated by the transponders.

The real-time tumour tracking allows better tumour localisation, more focused dose delivery, increased sparing of the normal tissue and thus higher therapeutic ratio. A clinical study has been undertaken to assess the effect on acute morbidity of reduced planning target volume margins in prostate cancer patients using electromagnetic tracking system and treated with IMRT (Sandler *et al.* 2010). This first outcome-based study showed that patients treated with reduced margins (nominal 3 mm margin) under electromagnetic tracking had less radiation-related morbidities than patients treated with conventional margins. When compared to other daily localisation techniques for PTV margin evaluation for prostate IMRT, such as: skin mark alignment, bony anatomy alignment and implanted fiducial marker positioning,

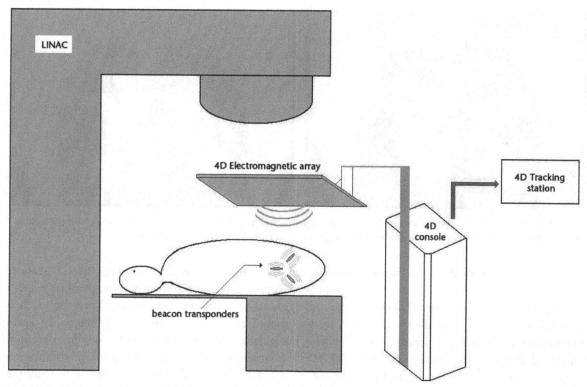

Figure 7.11. Schematic representation of tumour localisation using the Calypso system.

the electromagnetic transponder detection system was found to be the most reliable and rapid, with the smallest margin requirements accounting for intra-fraction motion (Tanyi *et al.* 2010).

The main advantages of the Calypso tracking system are summarised below:

- non-ionising treatment guidance
- real-time, continuous tumour tracking throughout radiotherapy
- possibility to position the patient with high accuracy
- improved tumour targeting
- possibility to deliver higher doses with smaller planning treatment volume margins
- reduced treatment side effects, even with high IMRT doses.

While mainly used for prostate and post-operative prostatic bed tracking during treatment, the system is designed to suit any body site which is treated with radiotherapy. A future step in Calypso's implementation in clinical oncology is towards tumour sites for which organ motion constitutes a treatment challenge (such as lung).

7.5 FOUR-DIMENSIONAL IMAGING AND TUMOUR TRACKING

Respiratory motion in radiation therapy represents a significant challenge for imaging and treatment of tumours, e.g. lung and abdominal tumours, as they can move up to several centimetres as a result of patient breathing. Ideally, the CT planning dataset should accurately indicate the tumour position where it would be during treatment. This is not possible with standard CT scanning. Firstly, the respiratory motion results in artefacts in the CT images (Figure 7.12). Consequently, target volumes based on these images may be distorted and larger than necessary. Secondly, in order to ensure complete coverage of the planning target volume, large radiation field margins have to be used to encompass the tumour for all positions during the breathing cycle. As a result, to be able to account for tumour and organ motion, in addition to 3D

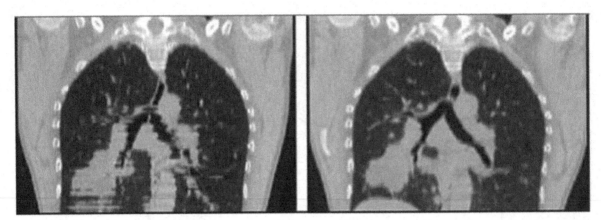

Figure 7.12. The CT scan on the left shows numerous motion artefacts as a result of respiration. The CT scan on the right is corrected for motion and shows a clear image of the target volume. (Courtesy Huntzinger 2003)

spatial data, time information (the fourth dimension) is required as well.

The problem shown in Figure 7.12 can be resolved using CT scanners with so-called respiratory gating functionality also known as 4-dimensional (4D) scanning (Keall 2004). During image acquisition with 4D scanners, information on a patient's breathing pattern/cycle is acquired as well and each image slice is correlated to respiratory information.

In 4D CT technology, the acquisition of CT data is synchronised with a respiratory phase signal, using technologies available on the current market (Huntzinger *et al.* 2006). The associated software sorts the images according to the phase in the respiratory cycle at which they were acquired (for example all images acquired at full expiration will be put together to generate one image dataset). Using these sorted images, the volumetric CT images can be reconstructed with motion artefacts significantly reduced (Figure 7.12).

4D CT image acquisition can be performed prospectively and retrospectively. During prospective scanning, the CT scanner acquires images only at a specific phase of the patient's respiratory cycle. The scanner takes several images at the selected phase and then the couch is moved to the next position. Images are taken when the breathing motion reaches the selected phase; i.e. the acquisition is not continuous. The resultant dataset is a 3D CT image with anatomic geometry (relative positions of individual organs) corresponding to a specific phase of the respiratory cycle.

During retrospective scanning, the CT scanner acquires images continuously through all respiratory phases with the couch stationary. Then the couch is moved to the next position and images are again acquired through all phases and so on until the entire volume of interest is scanned. Each acquired image is correlated to a phase in the breathing cycle. Once the image acquisition is complete, the system can sort the images according to the phase of the respiratory cycle and the position of the imaging couch in which they were obtained. Each phase can then be separately reconstructed. In retrospective scanning mode, multiple volumetric CT images, each representing one phase of the respiratory cycle will be produced (Huntzinger *et al.* 2006).

Using 4D CT scanning information, clinicians are able to define the treatment margins more accurately as they can identify the extent of the tumour motion. However, in order to target accurately the moving tumour during treatment itself (real time tumour tracking), beam gating and/or fluoroscopy imaging mode must be available on the linac (Ford *et al.* 2002).

In fluoroscopy mode, the kV X-ray source of the cone beam CT can be turned on for long periods of time to obtain real-time moving images of the internal structures of a patient. An X-ray image of a patient is captured by the a-Si detector and displayed on a monitor in the control room. To run the kV cone beam CT hardware in a fluoroscopy mode during treatment fraction requires the linac MV radiation beam and the cone beam kV X-ray beam to be turned on simultaneously.

Radiation beam gating is the process of turning the radiation beam on and off based on a *gating signal*. Respiratory gating uses signals from the patient's breathing cycle to switch radiation on and off. The onset and duration of the radiation beam on time are determined by monitoring the patient's respiratory motion. Frequently, optical tracking of infrared markers, positioned on patient's surface (e.g. chest), is used to monitor breathing. The position of the point of reflection on a marker is determined using a camera system. The information from the camera is fed into the gating control system of a linac. Markers on the body are, however, external surrogates only for the internal motion of the organs and the tumour. A relationship between the two needs to be carefully established for each individual case. Other systems use fiducial markers implanted directly into the region of interest and therefore their motion represents the tumour motion more accurately. Monitoring of these internal markers, however, can only be performed with fluoroscopy, thus increasing the radiation dose to a patient.

Usually the radiation is *gated* to turn on at the end of expiration portion of the breathing cycle where the tumour motion is estimated to be less. However the gate can be set at other portions of the breathing cycle if clinically beneficial (e.g. increased sparing of organs at risk). The radiation will be turned on (i.e. the gate will open) for a certain amount of time, until the patient's breathing motion (and the correlated signal) exceeds a preset threshold value, sending a 'radiation off' command to the linac (i.e. the gate closes). Some residual tumour movement will still occur during irradiation (gate open). The width of the gate is a compromise between the amount of acceptable residual tumour motion and the beam on-time (duty cycle). The resultant radiation duty cycle is ~30%–50% and consequently session times will increase compared to standard treatments by up to 10 minutes depending on individual circumstances.

There are two main approaches to gating: a) *Phase-based* gating (automatic gating of treatment delivery based on the same phase of the patient's respiratory cycle) and b) *Amplitude-based* gating (automatic gating based on the absolute position of the marker block on the patient's chest or abdomen, regardless of the phase of respiratory cycle).

Varian Medical Systems, USA have developed the so-called Real-time Position Management (RPM) respiratory gating system. The RPM system uses two infrared light-reflecting markers attached on a plastic box positioned midway between the umbilicus and lower part of the sternum. The reflective markers are illuminated by infrared-emitting diodes surrounding a CCD camera. Vertical motion of these markers is captured by the camera and the RPM software calculates the respiratory phase based on the observed amplitude. Once a reproducible patient breathing pattern is verified, the RPM system will trigger beam on/off signals when the selected gating widows are in range.

Elekta Oncology Systems, UK, have developed the so-called Active Breathing Control (ABC) system that uses relative spirometry. In this technique, the patient inhales or exhales beyond a set threshold, and then a balloon valve inflates actively preventing the patient from further inhaling or exhaling for a specified duration. Beam delivery would only occur during the breath hold.

In summary, 4D-CT imaging can be used to verify tumour motion as a function of the breathing cycle as part of treatment planning, but it cannot verify treatment delivery, since the 4D-CT device and linac are two separate devices. The integration of the CBCT and the linac allows for the assessment of tumour motion immediately before and after treatment. If the cone beam CT device can be used in fluoroscopy mode during irradiation with linac beams, dose delivery to moving tumours can be verified.

7.6 RADIOBIOLOGICAL ASPECTS OF IMAGE-GUIDED RADIOTHERAPY (IGRT)

Multimodality imaging techniques, both anatomic and functional, allow a precise delineation of target volume enabling highly localised irradiation and excellent sparing of the normal tissue. In order to achieve high therapeutic ratio with today's technological potential, the ideal scenario is to combine imaging methods with treatment delivery, obtaining therefore an image-guided therapy. Whether the option is planar IGRT (such as EPID) or volumetric IGRT (such as CT) they both offer the likelihood of a superior treatment outcome. A major advantage of EPID-based IMRT is the use of the treatment beam to align the target. Volumetric IGRT offers the possibility to define the relationship between target volume and organs at risk from a spatial perspective and to assess the potential exposure risk to normal tissue (especially soft tissue) before treatment (Verellen *et al.* 2008).

The reason for employing IGRT in radiotherapy in either of its forms is to increase the therapeutic ratio by both decreasing PTV margins and thus reducing normal tissue toxicity, and by escalating dose to the target, thus increasing tumour control. As with any new technological advances, the implementation of IGRT into clinical settings raises certain issues such as risks from possible additional doses to the patient which are associated with the procedure. Perks and colleagues (2008) have determined the peripheral dose from IGRT using volumetric cone beam CT, as an added contribution to the dose outside the target and compared it with the out-of-field IMRT dose. Based on TLD measurements using an anthropomorphic phantom, a dose of the order of mGy (over 1 cGy/scan) has been found beyond the edge of the IGRT field, which is comparable to the peripheral dose from IMRT, suggesting that this dose contribution has to be taken into account for long term risk assessment.

7.6.1   Clinical trials/studies

To be in line with the current principles of evidence-based medicine the efficacy of IGRT should be assessed through various levels of evidence, starting from expert opinion to the highest levels of evidence which are meta-analysis of randomised clinical trials (Baumann *et al.* 2008).

7.6.2   IMRT-IGRT

The development of image-guided radiotherapy in conjunction with IMRT has further improved treatment outcome in various cancers. The use of on-board CT-imaging IGRT allows for monitoring of tumour behaviour during treatment which provides valuable radiobiological information for adaptive radiotherapy. Cone beam CT provides volumetric imaging during treatment creating the basis for image- and dose-guided radiotherapy.

The clinical experience with cone beam CT is still limited and concerns mainly head & neck, prostate and lung tumours (de Crevoisier *et al.* 2009). However, the results are promising and they justify further research for broader clinical use. A significant dosimetric advantage of four-dimensional adaptive IGRT using cone beam CT over 3D-CRT for lung cancer patients was reported with focus on planning target volume reduction (Harsolia *et al.* 2008). The study showed better normal tissue sparing with adaptive radiotherapy, showing 39% (offline adaptive radiotherapy) and 44% (online adaptive radiotherapy) mean relative decrease in PTV volumes compared to 3D-CRT.

Acute toxicity was assessed in patients undergoing post-prostatectomy radiotherapy with image guidance, showing very good normal tissue sparing given that the majority of patients experienced only grade 1 toxicity (with 7.7% having grade 2) without any grade 3 or higher acute side effects (Sandhu *et al.* 2008). A dose escalation study involving image-guided radiotherapy for prostate carcinoma with a primary endpoint of 5-year biochemical No Evidence of Disease (bNED), concluded that a 79.8 Gy dose delivered in 42 fractions results in low grade acute toxicity (no grade 3 or higher), favourable late toxicity compared with non-IGRT treatments and 79.4% biochemical control at 5 years (Martin *et al.* 2009).

On the other hand, a non-randomised comparative study between image-guided hypofractionated radiotherapy and conventional fractionation without IGRT for prostate cancer showed no significant differences regarding acute toxicity noting, however, that both groups had low rate toxicities (Jereczek-Fossa *et al.* 2010). There is need for further studies to conclusively demonstrate the efficacy of IGRT in reducing the incidence of adverse events.

A proven advantage of IGRT is the improvement of treatment outcome for those tumours which exhibit large geometrical variations. Bladder cancer studies on volume variation and its relation to margins were conducted by Muren *et al.* (2007) showing large margin reduction in bladder radiotherapy under IGRT. Results from other studies investigating target dose increase/normal tissue toxicity decrease and target volume margin decrease with image-guidance are presented in Table 7.5.

Table 7.5.   Target volume margin decrease and outcome improvement with IGRT for various tumour sites using IMRT.

Treatment site (reference)	Margins without IGRT	Margins with IGRT	Target dose increase with IGRT/ normal tissue toxicity decrease
Rectal cancer (Engels 2009)	15 mm(X), 15 mm(Y), 10 mm(Z)	8 mm(X), 11 mm(Yant), 7 mm(Ypost), 10 mm(Z)	NTCP for grade 2 diarrhea reduced from 39.5% to 18%
Bladder cancer (Redpath 2006)	30 mm for full CTV coverage	16 mm for full CTV coverage	only 1% increase in mean average dose but spread in daily mean dose between 96%–106%
Bladder cancer (Burridge 2006)	15 mm (CTV to PTV margin)	10 mm (CTV to PTV margin)	–
Prostate cancer (Ghilezan 2004)	10 mm (CTV to PTV margin)	no CTV to PTV margin	13%

A recent study has compared various online image-guided radiotherapy strategies to illustrate the benefits of online treatment for prostate cancer patients (Schulze et al. 2009). Accordingly, online IGRT has been classified into three precision levels such as bony alignment (with the lowest requirement for online image quality), target alignment (requires higher quality images and fiducial markers) and re-planning (needs online volumetric images). Two 3D-CRT with IGRT and four IMRT-IGRT approaches have been implemented to compare planned and delivered doses to the rectum and bladder. The comparative results of IMRT-IGRT techniques are summarised in Table 7.6.

As shown in Table 7.6, daily IMRT re-optimisation of the treatment plan, closely followed by IMRT with target alignment are the most efficient IGRT approaches which can lead to improved therapeutic ratio in prostate cancer treatment. Similar results have been reported by Thongphiew et al. (2009) after com-

paring adaptive (bony alignment and soft tissue alignment) versus repositioning corrections during prostate cancer treatment. They showed that re-optimisation techniques are highly favourable in hypofractionated radiotherapy when daily corrections are required.

7.6.4   Image guided stereotactic body radiotherapy (IG-SBRT)

Stereotactic body radiotherapy has been implemented among external beam therapies with the aim of managing small lesions outside the brain under stereotactic conditions. The most commonly treated lesions with SBRT are lung, liver, prostate and spine (Timmerman et al. 2007). Similar to IMRT, the goal of SBRT is to achieve a higher tumour control with decreased normal tissue toxicity through steep dose gradients. The accuracy in delivering such treatment necessitates image guidance, reason why the number of studies on image-guided SBRT is on the rise. As with IMRT, either planar or volumetric imaging

Table 7.6.   IMRT-IGRT approaches and their respective doses delivered to the rectum and bladder (Schulze et al. 2009).

IMRT-IGRT approach	CTV – PTV margin (cm)	Organs at risk (OAR)	Mean dose delivered to the bladder (% of target dose)	Mean dose delivered to the rectum (% of target dose)
IMRT with bony alignment	1	Bladder and rectum volumes	65.5	79.6
IMRT with target alignment	0	Bladder and rectum volumes	51.7	71.1
IMRT with re-planning (OAR volumes as constraints)	0	Bladder and rectum volumes	49.9	69.0
IMRT with re-planning (OAR walls as constraints)	0	Bladder and rectum walls	49.2	68.0

modalities are employed for treatment adjustment. Furthermore, ultrasound-based image-guidance is gaining space to avoid the added exposure from ionising radiation which originates from the imaging techniques.

SBRT has replaced conventional radiotherapy for early stage non-small cell lung cancer in several centres due to improved local control and higher survival rates (Hoyer 2008). Breathing-induced motion of lung tumours drives the need for image-guidance during treatment for better outcomes. Image-guided SBRT for unresectable stage I NSCLC with the delivery of a BED greater than 100 Gy showed not only superior local control at 3–5 years and greater overall survival rates than conventional treatments, but also minimal toxicity (Chang and Roth 2007). Image-guided SBRT allows considerable reduction in safety margins for tumour delineation. Consequently, Guckenberger *et al.* (2009) reported a decrease of margins around CTV from a 9–14 mm range without image guidance to a 7–10 mm range with on-line corrections of set-up errors based on bony anatomy. Furthermore, when targeting tumour itself, safety margins have been reduced to below 5 mm, with further reductions with real-time corrections of intra-fractional base-line drifts to 2.6 mm. The authors recommend the 4D image-guided technique used for target verification prior to every fraction and on-line correction of errors to reduce margins as a standard procedure in pulmonary SBRT (Guckenberger *et al.* 2009). The data in Table 7.7 represents the results, including the most recent ones, reported by IG-SBRT studies on unresectable pulmonary cancers and spine lesions having as endpoints local control rate and treatment-related side effects.

The above presented studies have demonstrated the efficacy of image-guided SBRT for unresectable early stage non-small cell lung cancers achieving, with minimal invasiveness, high tumour conformality and safe dose escalation. SBRT was also shown to be effective when employed with palliative intent for spinal metastases. Furthermore, Choi *et al.* (2010) performed a retrospective study on 42 patients treated for recurrent spinal tumours within previously irradiated spinal fields showing the feasibility of SBRT using CyberKnife on this difficult patient group.

7.7 THE FUTURE OF IGRT: BIOLOGIC IMAGE-GUIDED RADIOTHERAPY

Biologic image-guided radiotherapy is now achievable via functional imaging such as positron emission tomography (PET) or the more complex PET/CT and functional magnetic resonance imaging (fMRI). These new techniques are very appealing because of their non-invasiveness and highly valuable molecular information offered prior, during and post treatment. The fusion of functional PET with anatomic CT images allows improvement of tumour localisation and delineation reducing possible misinterpretations and increasing therefore normal tissue sparing.

With the development of new radiotracers for PET imaging able to illustrate tumour response during treatment and to identify tumour sub-volumes which are critical for achieving better outcome, a new perspective for IGRT has opened. The newest trend in radiotherapy is to integrate PET/CT and cone beam CT in order to provide higher diagnostic value for anatomic delineation and tissue metabolism as well as excellent verification of position set-up errors (Wu 2009).

^{18}F-FDG PET (fluoro-deoxyglucose) is the most commonly used radiotracer, because of its great sensitivity and specificity for disease detection. The reason this radiolabelled glucose-analogue is the key player in PET imaging is attributable to the fact that tumours have higher metabolic rates for glucose than normal tissue. Consequently, tumour-specific radiotracers can add valuable metabolic information to the anatomical data supplied by CT which leads to a more accurate diagnostic, implying an optimised treatment plan through PET-guided radiotherapy. Clinical information regarding tumour staging, metabolic changes and tissue physiology has a great impact on radiotherapy treatment design. PET/CT can also assist in more accurate GTV definition as reported by various studies that have altered target volumes which were based solely on CT images (Schechter *et al.* 2001; Erdi *et al.* 2002; Bradley *et al.* 2004; Nestle *et al.* 2006). Target volumes were either expanded to include tumour mass which was not discernible on CT or reduced to exclude those regions which were not metabolically active on PET scans. It was shown (see Chapter 17) that PET/CT plays an important role in

Table 7.7. IG-SBRT treatment outcome for pulmonary cancers and spine lesions.

Study/trial	Treatment protocol	Tumour control	Normal tissue toxicity
Pulmonary lesions – curative			
Early stage unresectable NSCLC 70 patients (van der Voort van Zyp 2009)	45 or 60 Gy in 3 fractions using CyberKnife with real-time tumour tracking	96% 2-year local control rate (60 Gy) 78% 2-year local control rate (45 Gy)	3% acute grade 3 10% late grade 3 no grade 3+ toxicity
Early stage unresectable NSCLC 20 patients (Collins 2009)	42–60 Gy delivered in 3 equal fractions <2 weeks using CyberKnife with tumour tracking	87% overall survival estimate at 2 years	5% acute grade 3 radiation pneumonitis
Stage I lung cancer 59 patients (Brown 2007)	15 Gy to 67.5 Gy delivered in 1–5 fractions with image-guided robotic radiosurgery (CyberKnife)	86% overall survival rate at 33 months follow up	limited toxicity
Primary & metastatic lung cancer 45 patients (Onimaru 2003)	48 or 60 Gy in 8 fractions over 2 weeks with IGRT	100% 3-year local control rate (60 Gy) 69.6% 3-year local control rate (48 Gy)	1 patient (2.2%) – grade 2 chest pain 1 patient – treatment-related death
Stage I NSCLC 22 patients (Fukumoto 2002)	48 or 60 Gy in 8 fractions over 2 weeks with IGRT	73% survival rate at 2 years	asymptomatic radiation pneumonitis in all patients
Spine lesions - palliative			
Lesions of the spine and paraspinal region 32 patients (Nelson 2009)	14–30 Gy in 1–4 fractions with SBRT using linear accelerator and on-board imaging	13.5 months 1-year overall survival 40.6% patients – reported complete pain relief 53.1% patients – reported substantial /partial pain relief	21.8% – grade 1 nausea well tolerated treatment
Spinal metastases 74 patients (Gibbs 2007)	16–25 Gy in 1–5 fractions with image-guided robotic radiosurgery CyberKnife	46.3% – 1 year actuarial survival	4% – treatment-related spinal injury
Spinal lesions 115 patients (108 metastatic lesions) (Gerszten 2004)	12–20 Gy single dose image-guided CyberKnife	pain relief was reported by 74 of 79 patients who were symptomatic before treatment	no acute radiation toxicity or added neurological symptoms during follow up period
Spinal lesions 16 patients (Ryu 2001)	11–25 Gy in 1–5 fractions with image-guided radiosurgery using CyberKnife	no progression of disease at 6 months follow up	no complications at 6 months follow up

the management of highly hypoxic tumours via hypoxia-specific radiotracers also being efficient for treatment guidance in tumours with high proliferative ability which often constitute the reason for treatment failure. PET was successfully integrated in radiosurgery due to the critical reliance of radiosurgery on imaging methods for tumour targeting and also for a better understanding of metabolic changes following specialised treatment (Levivier et al. 2007). All these clinical aspects regarding PET/CT bring us

Table 7.8. Advantages of PET/CT-guided radiotherapy over CT or MRI alone.

Advantages	Outcome	References
Greater sensitivity and tumour-specificity than CT or MRI alone	More accurate disease staging and tumour characterisation	Ford 2009 Guha 2008
Allows the *incorporation of biologic information* into radiotherapy targets	The fusion of functional imaging (PET) with anatomic imaging (CT) offers a more accurate diagnostic and planning	Zaidi 2009 Guha 2008 Bradley 2004
More *accurate definition of target volume*	Results in either target volume expansion to include additional tumour mass or reduction to exclude non-active regions. Allows dose escalation without added toxicity to normal tissue	Wang 2006 Bradley 2004 Erdi 2002 Giraud 2001 Schechter 2001
Reduced intra- and inter-observer variability in tumour delineation	More uniform tumour conformality and planning among clinicians	Breen 2007 van Baardwijk 2007 Riegel 2006
High tumour control with favourable toxicity profile	Better overall clinical outcome	Vernon 2008 Wang 2006

closer to the ultimate goal of modern oncology which is individualised treatment.

Several new tracers have been developed for better tumour-specificity and many others are underway to be clinically validated. Still, ^{18}F-FDG remains the most popular among the PET tracers, fact demonstrated by several recent clinical studies using PET/CT for radiotherapy treatment guidance. Further clinical advantages of PET/CT-guided radiotherapy over CT or MRI-only are summarised in Table 7.8.

The last decade has validated the efficacy of PET/CT imaging as part of radiotherapy treatment planning and follow up for a wide variety of tumours. Other multi-modality image fusion techniques such as PET and MRI further aim to complement the functional imaging data with anatomical details. While the role of molecular imaging is quite well established, there is room for further developments and broader integration of biologic image guidance in radiotherapy.

7.8 CONCLUSION

Further technical advances can be expected for all forms of image guidance and adaptive radiation therapy. As for the cone beam CT, the heavy linac gantry limits the rotational speed of the X-ray source and the detector and therefore there is a limit to how fast a

volumetric CT image can be acquired. The integration of cone beam CT and the linac into one device has overcome the separation of imaging and treatment. Similar to Tomotherapy, in-room CT and EPI, cone beam CT is capable of imaging the patient in the treatment position. Tumour and patient position on the couch can be verified immediately before and possibly during treatment, providing truly volumetric anatomical information.

Even though image guidance has the potential to substantially eliminate set-up and organ motion errors, biological uncertainties (i.e. definition of gross tumour volume and clinical target volume) will remain. Further development of adaptive radiotherapy will lead towards more accurate patient-specific PTVs and 'on-the-flight' treatment modification, meaning that treatment replanning and treatment can happen only minutes after cone beam CT images are taken. This is much faster than daily conventional CT planning (Geinitz *et al.* 2000). Cone beam CT imaging for IGRT and ART is expected to yield better tumour control, but increases clinical workload and short-term treatment costs.

Some of the basic questions of treatment planning, like: 'Where is the tumour? What is the disease extent? Where are the tumour areas requiring more radiation dose during radiation treatment?' cannot be answered using CT imaging which is the essential foundation of modern radiation therapy. Functional imaging may give us a tool to solve this problem for at least some clinical situations (Ashamalla *et al.* 2007). Instead of simply identifying tumour volumes on CT scans, it will be possible to identify biological differences within a tumour and between tumour and normal tissues, using the information from functional imaging studies.

For example, while ^{18}F-FDG positron emission tomography (PET) has been crucial for staging and treatment of many cancers, it can also provide a new means for treatment targeting by utilising metabolic information in addition to the anatomic information obtained from CT imaging. Incorporation of this functional information is essential to better define dose objectives and dose limits within the treated volume, leading to so-called painting of the dose across the planning target volume (Tepper 2000) and delivering non-homogenous dose distributions, with different doses delivered to tumour regions of different biological properties (e.g. area of hypoxia or proliferation).

7.9   REFERENCES

Al-Haddad M and Eloubeidi MA (2010) Interventional EUS for the diagnosis and treatment of locally advanced pancreatic cancer. *Journal of the Pancreas* **11**(1): 1–7.

Amer A, Marchant T, Sykes J. *et al.* (2007) Imaging doses from the Elekta Synergy X-ray cone beam CT system. *British Journal of Radiology* **80**(954): 476–482.

Ashamalla H, Guirguis A, Bieniek E, Rafla S *et al.* (2007) The impact of positron emission tomography/computed tomography in edge delineation of gross tumor volume for head & neck cancers. *International Journal of Radiation Oncology Biology and Physics* **68**(2): 388–395.

Ashida R and Chang KJ (2009) Interventional EUS for the treatment of pancreatic cancer. *Journal of Hepato-Biliary-Pancreatic Surgery* **16**(5): 592–597.

Balter JM, Wright JN, Newell LJ, Friemel B, Dimmer S, Cheng Y et al. (2005) Accuracy of a wireless localization system for radiotherapy. *International Journal of Radiation Oncology Biology and Physics* **61**(3): 933–937.

Baumann M, Holscher T and Zips D (2008) The future of IGRT – cost benefit analysis. *Acta Oncologica* **47**(7): 1188–1192.

Berrang TS, Truong PT, Popescu C, Drever L *et al.* (2009) 3D ultrasound can contribute to planning CT to define the target for partial breast radiotherapy. *International Journal of Radiation Oncology Biology and Physics* **73**(2): 375–383.

Bijdekerke P, Verellen D, Tournel K *et al.* (2008) Tomo-Therapy: implications on daily workload and scheduling patients. *Radiotherapy and Oncology* **86**(2): 224–230.

Bradley JD, Perez CA, Dehdashti F and Siegel BA (2004) Implementing biologic target volumes in radiation treatment planning for non-small cell lung cancer. *Journal of Nuclear Medicine* **45**(suppl 1): 96S–101S.

Breen SL, Publicover J, De Silva S *et al.* (2007) Intraobserver and interobserver variability in GTV delineation on FDG-PET-CT images of head & neck cancers. *International Journal of Radiation Oncology Biology and Physics* **68**(3): 763–770.

Brown WT, Wu X, Fayad F, Fowler JF *et al.* (2007) CyberKnife radiosurgery for stage I lung cancer: results at 36 months. *Clinical Lung Cancer* **8**(8): 488–492.

Burridge N, Amer A, Marchant T, Sykes J *et al.* (2006) Online adaptive radiotherapy of the bladder: small bowel irradiated-volume reduction. *International Journal of Radiation Oncology Biology and Physics* **66**(3): 892–897.

Chang JY and Roth JA (2007) Stereotactic body radiation therapy for stage I non-small cell lung cancer. *Thoracic Surgery Clinics* **17**(2): 251–259.

Choi CY, Adler JR, Gibbs IC, Chang SD *et al.* (2010) Stereotactic radiosurgery for treatment of spinal metastases recurring in close proximity to previously irradiated spinal cord. *International Journal of Radiation Oncology Biology and Physics* Feb 2. [Epub ahead of print]

Collins BT, Vahdat S, Erickson K, Collins SP *et al.* (2009) Radical cyberknife radiosurgery with tumor tracking: an effective treatment for inoperable small peripheral stage I non-small cell lung cancer. *Journal of Hematology and Oncology* **2**: 1.

de Crevoisier R, Garcia R, Louvel G, Marguet M *et al.* (2009) Cone beam CT based image guided radiotherapy: implementation and clinical use. *Cancer Radiotherapy* **13**(6–7): 482–489.

De Jean P, Beaulieu L and Fenster A (2009) Three-dimensional ultrasound system for guided breast brachytherapy. *Medical Physics* **36**(11): 5099–5106.

Engels B, De Ridder M, Tournel K, Sermeus A *et al.* (2009) Preoperative helical tomotherapy and megavoltage computed tomography for rectal cancer: impact on the irradiated volume of small bowel. *International Journal of Radiation Oncology Biology and Physics* **74**(5): 1476–1480.

Erdi Y, Rosenzweig K, Erdi A *et al.* (2002) Radiotherapy treatment planning for patients with non-small cell lung cancer using positron emission tomography (PET). *Radiotherapy and Oncology* **62**(1): 51–60.

Ford E, Mageras G, Yorke E *et al.* (2002) Evaluation of respiratory movement during gated radiotherapy using film and electronic portal imaging. *International Journal of Radiation Oncology Biology and Physics* **52**(2): 522–531.

Ford E, Herman J, Yorke H and Wahl L (2009) ^{18}F-FDG PET/CT for image-guided and intensity-modulated radiotherapy. *Journal of Nuclear Medicine* **50**(10): 1655–1665.

Fukumoto S, Shirato H, Shimzu S, Ogura S *et al.* (2002) Small-volume image-guided radiotherapy using hypofractionated, coplanar, and noncoplanar multiple fields for patients with inoperable Stage I nonsmall cell lung carcinomas. *Cancer* **95**(7): 1546–1553.

Geinitz H, Zimmermann F, Kuzmany A *et al.* (2000) Daily CT planning during boost irradiation of prostate cancer. *Strahlentherapie und Onkologie* **176**(9): 429–432.

Gerszten PC, Ozhasoglu C, Burton SA, Vogel WJ *et al.* (2004) CyberKnife frameless stereotactic radiosurgery for spinal lesions: clinical experience in 125 cases. *Neurosurgery* **55**(1): 89–98.

Gibbs IC, Kamnerdsupaphon P, Ryu MR, Dodd R *et al.* (2007) Image-guided robotic radiosurgery for spinal metastases. *Radiotherapy and Oncology* **82**(2): 185–190.

Giraud P, Grahek D, Montravers F *et al.* (2001) CT and ^{18}F-deoxyglucose (FDG) image fusion or optimization on conformal radiotherapy in lung cancers. *International Journal of Radiation Oncology Biology and Physics* **49**(5): 1249–1257.

Groh B, Siewerdsen J, Dranke D *et al.* (2002) A performance comparison of flat-panel imager-based MV and kV cone-beam CT. *Medical Physics* **29**(6): 967–975.

Guckenberger M, Krieger T, Richter A, Baier K *et al.* (2009) Potential of image-guidance, gating and real-time tracking to improve accuracy in pulmonary stereotactic body radiotherapy. *Radiotherapy and Oncology* **91**(3): 288–295.

Guha C, Alfieri A, Blaufox MD and Kalnicki S (2008) Tumor biology-guided radiotherapy treatment planning: gross tumor volume versus functional tumor volume. *Seminars in Nuclear Medicine* **38**(2): 105–113.

Harsolia A, Hugo GD, Kestin LL, Grills IS *et al.* (2008) Dosimetric advantages of four-dimensional adaptive image-guided radiotherapy for lung tumors using online cone-beam computed tomography. *International Journal of Radiation Oncology Biology and Physics* **70**(2): 582–589.

Hoyer M (2008) Improved accuracy and outcome in radiotherapy of lung cancer. *Radiotherapy and Oncology* **87**(1): 1–2.

Huntzinger C (2003) Every breath you take – the image-guided motion management story. *The Journal of Oncology Management* **12**(1): 16–20.

Huntzinger C, Munro P, Johnson S, Miettinen M, Zankowski C, Ahlstrom G, Glettig R, Filliberti R, Kaissl W, Kamber M, Amstutz M, Bouchet L, Klebanov D, Mostafavi H and Stark R (2006) Dynamic targeting image-guided radiotherapy. *Medical Dosimetry* **31**(2): 113–125.

ICRU Report 50 (1993) 'Prescribing, recording and reporting photon beam therapy'. International Commission on Radiation Units and Measurements, Bethesda, MD.

ICRU Report 62 (1999) 'Prescribing, recording and reporting photon beam therapy (supplement to ICRU Report. 50)'. International Commission on Radiation Units and Measurements, Bethesda, MD.

Jaffray D, Siewerdsen J, Wong J *et al.* (2002) Flat-panel cone-beam computed tomography for image-guided radiation therapy. *International Journal of Radiation Oncology Biology and Physics* **53**(5): 1337–1349.

Jaffray D, Kupelian P, Djemil T *et al.* (2007) Review of image-guided radiation therapy. *Expert Reviews in Anticancer Therapy* 7(1): 89–103.

Jereczek-Fossa BA, Zerini D, Fodor C, Santoro L *et al.* (2010) Acute toxicity of image-guided hypofractionated radiotherapy for prostate cancer: nonrandomized comparison with conventional fractionation. *Urologic Oncology* [Epub ahead of print]

Kalender W (2006) X-ray computed tomography. *Physics in Medicine and Biology* 51(13): R29–R43.

Kan M, Leung L, Wong W *et al.* (2008) Radiation dose from cone beam computed tomography for image-guided radiation therapy. *International Journal of Radiation Oncology Biology and Physics* 70(1): 272–279.

Keall P (2004) 4-Dimensional computed tomography imaging and treatment planning. *Seminars in Radiation Oncology* 14(1): 81–90.

Kuriyama K, Onishi H, Sano N *et al.* (2003) A new irradiation unit constructed of self-moving gantry-CT and LINAC. *International Journal of Radiation Oncology Biology and Physics* 55(2): 428–435.

Leonard C, Harlow CL, Coffin C, Drose J *et al.* (1993) Use of ultrasound to guide radiation boost planning following lumpectomy for carcinoma of the breast. *International Journal of Radiation Oncology Biology and Physics* 27(5): 1193–1197.

Levivier M, Massager N, Wikler D, Devriendt D *et al.* (2007) Integration of functional imaging in radiosurgery: the example of PET scan. *Progress in Neurological Surgery* 20: 68–81.

Mackie T (2006) History of tomotherapy. *Physics in Medicine and Biology* 51(13): R427–R453.

Mackie T, Balog J, Ruchala K *et al.* (1999) Tomotherapy. *Seminars in Radiation Oncology* 9(1): 108–117.

Martin JM, Bayley A, Bristow R, Chung P *et al.* (2009) Image guided dose escalated prostate radiotherapy: still room to improve. *Radiation Oncology* 4: 50.

Miften M, Leicher B, Parda D *et al.* (2007) IMRT planning and delivery incorporating daily dose from mega-voltage cone-beam computed tomography imaging. *Medical Physics* 34(10): 3760–3767.

Morin O, Gillis A, Descovich M *et al.* (2007) Patient dose considerations for routine megavoltage cone-beam CT imaging. *Medical Physics* 34(5): 1819–1827.

Muren LP, Redpath AT, Lord H and McLaren D (2007) Image-guided radiotherapy of bladder cancer: bladder volume variation and its relation to margins. *Radiotherapy and Oncology* 84(3): 307–313.

Nelson JW, Yoo DS, Sampson JH, Isaacs RE *et al.* (2009) Stereotactic body radiotherapy for lesions of the spine and paraspinal regions. *International Journal of Radiation Oncology Biology and Physics* 73(5): 1369–1375.

Nestle U, Kremp S and Grosu A (2006) Practical integration of [^{18}F]-FDG-PET and PET-CT in the planning of radiotherapy for non-small cell lung cancer (NSCLC): the technical basis, ICRU-target volumes, problems, perspectives. *Radiotherapy and Oncology* 81(2): 209–225.

Onimaru R, Shirato H, Shimizu S, Kitamura K *et al.* (2003) Tolerance of organs at risk in small-volume, hypofractionated, image-guided radiotherapy for primary and metastatic lung cancers. *International Journal of Radiation Oncology Biology and Physics* 56(1): 126–135.

Park WG, Yan BM, Schellenberg D and Kim J (2010) EUS-guided gold fiducial insertion for image-guided radiation therapy of pancreatic cancer: 50 successful cases without fluoroscopy. *Gastrointestinal Endoscopy* 71(3): 513–518.

Peignaux K, Truc G, Barillot I, Ammor A *et al.* (2006) Clinical assessment of the use of the Sonarray system for daily prostate localization. *Radiotherapy and Oncology* 81(2): 176–178.

Perks JR, Lehmann J, Chen AM, Yang CC *et al.* (2008) Comparison of peripheral dose from image-guided radiation therapy (IGRT) using kV cone beam CT to intensity-modulated radiation therapy (IMRT). *Radiotherapy and Oncology* 89(3): 304–310.

Pouliot J, Bani-Hashemi A, Chen J *et al.* (2005) Low-dose megavoltage cone-beam CT for radiation therapy. *International Journal of Radiation Oncology Biology and Physics* 61(2): 552–569.

Prokop M and Galanski M (2003) *Spiral and Multislice CT of the Body.* Thieme, New York.

Ramsey C, Seibert R, Mahan S *et al.* (2006) Out-of-field dosimetry measurements for a helical tomotherapy system. *Journal of Applied Clinical Medical Physics* 7(3): 1–11.

Redpath AT and Muren LP (2006) CT-guided intensity-modulated radiotherapy for bladder cancer: isocentre shifts, margins and their impact on target dose. *Radiotherapy and Oncology* **81**(3): 276–278.

Riegel AC, Berson AM, Destian S et al. (2006) Variability of gross tumor volume delineation in head-and-neck cancer using CT and PET/CT fusion. *International Journal of Radiation Oncology Biology and Physics* **65**(3): 726–732.

Ryu SI, Chang SD, Kim DH, Murphy MJ et al. (2001) Image-guided hypo-fractionated stereotactic radiosurgery to spinal lesions. *Neurosurgery* **49**(4): 838–846.

Sandhu A, Sethi R, Rice R, Wang JZ et al. (2008) Prostate bed localization with image-guided approach using on-board imaging: reporting acute toxicity and implications for radiation therapy planning following prostatectomy. *Radiotherapy and Oncology* **88**(1): 20–25.

Sandler HM, Liu PY, Dunn RL, Khan DC, Tropper SE, Sanda MG et al. (2010) Reduction in patient-reported acute morbidity in prostate cancer patients treated with 81-Gy Intensity-modulated radiotherapy using reduced planning target volume margins and electromagnetic tracking: assessing the impact of margin reduction study. *Urology* **75**(5): 1004–1008.

Schechter NR, Gillenwater AM, Byers RM et al. (2001) Can positron emission tomography improve the quality of care for head-and-neck cancer patients? *International Journal of Radiation Oncology Biology and Physics* **51**(1): 4–9.

Schulze D, Liang J, Yan D and Zhang T (2009) Comparison of various online IGRT strategies: the benefits of online treatment plan re-optimization. *Radiotherapy and Oncology* **90**(3): 367–376.

Shah A, Langen K, Ruchala K et al. (2007) Patient-specific dose from megavoltage CT imaging with a helical tomotherapy unit. *International Journal of Radiation Oncology Biology and Physics* **69**(3): S193–S194.

Steinke MF and Bezak E (2008) Use of cone-beam computed tomography in image-guided radiation therapy. *Australasian Physical and Engineering Sciences in Medicine* **31**(3): 167–179.

Takayama K, Nagano K, Mizowaki T et al. (2007) Application of a newly developed high-accuracy image guided radiation therapy system to stereotactic radiosurgery. *International Journal of Radiation Oncology Biology and Physics* **69**(3): S627–S628.

Tanyi JA, He T, Summers PA, Mburu RG, Kato CM, Rhodes SM et al. (2010) Assessment of planning target volume margins for intensity-modulated radiotherapy of the prostate gland: role of daily inter- and intrafraction motion. *International Journal of Radiation Oncology Biology and Physics* **78**(5): 1579–1585.

Tepper J (2000) Form and function: the integration of physics and biology. *International Journal of Radiation Oncology Biology and Physics* **47**(3): 547–548.

Thieke C, Malsch U, Schlegel W et al. (2006) Kilovoltage CT using a linac-CT scanner combination. *British Journal of Radiology* **79**: S79–S86.

Thongphiew D, Wu QJ, Lee WR, Chankong V et al. (2009) Comparison of online IGRT techniques for prostate IMRT treatment: adaptive vs repositioning correction. *Medical Physics* **36**(5): 1651–1662.

Timmerman RD, Kavanagh BD, Cho LC et al. (2007) Stereotactic body radiation therapy in multiple organ sites. *Journal of Clinical Oncology* **25**: 947–952.

Tücking T (2007) Development and realization of the IGRT inline concept. Dissertation, Universität Heidelberg.

Uematsu M, Fukui T, Shioda A et al. (1996) A dual computed tomography linear accelearator unit for stereotactic radiation therapy: a new approach without cranically fixated stereotactic frames. *International Journal of Radiation Oncology Biology and Physics* **35**(3): 587–592.

Valentin J (2001) Radiation and your patient: a guide for medical practitioners: ICRP Supporting Guidance 2. *Annals ICRP* **31**(4): 1–52.

van Baardwijk A, Bosmans G, Boersma L et al. (2007) PET-CT-based auto-contouring in non-small-cell lung cancer correlates with pathology and reduces interobserver variability in the delineation of the primary tumor and involved nodal volumes. *International Journal of Radiation Oncology Biology and Physics* **68**(3): 771–778.

van der Voort van Zyp N, Prévost JB, Hoogeman MS, Praag J *et al.* (2009) Stereotactic radiotherapy with real-time tumor tracking for non-small cell lung cancer: clinical outcome. *Radiotherapy and Oncology* **91**(3): 296–300.

Van Dyk J (1999) *The Modern Technology of Radiation Oncology.* Medical Physics Publishing, Madison, WI.

Varadarajulu S, Trevino JM, Shen S and Jacob R (2010) The use of endoscopic ultrasound-guided gold markers in image-guided radiation therapy of pancreatic cancers: a case series. *Endoscopy* **42**(5): 423–425.

Verellen D, De Ridder M, Tournel K, Duchateau M *et al.* (2008) An overview of volumetric imaging technologies and their quality assurance for IGRT. *Acta Oncologica* **47**(7): 1271–1278.

Vernon MR, Maheshwari M, Schultz CJ, Michel MA *et al.* (2008) Clinical outcomes of patients receiving integrated PET/CT-guided radiotherapy for head & neck carcinoma. *International Journal of Radiation Oncology Biology and Physics* **70**(3): 678–684.

Wang D, Schultz CJ, Jursinic PA, Bialkowski M *et al.* (2006) Initial experience of FDG-PET/CT guided IMRT of head-and-neck carcinoma. *International Journal of Radiation Oncology Biology and Physics* **65**(1): 143–151.

Wu TH, Liang CH, Wu JK, Lien CY *et al.* (2009) Integration of PET-CT and cone-beam CT for image-guided radiotherapy with high image quality and registration accuracy. *Journal of Instrumentation* **4**: P07006.

Yan D, Vicini F, Wong J *et al.* (1997) Adaptive radiation therapy. *Physics in Medicine and Biology* **42**(1): 52–64.

Yan D, Lockman D, Brabbins D *et al.* (2000) An off-line strategy for constructing a patient-specific planning target volume in adaptive treatment process for prostate cancer. *International Journal of Radiation Oncology Biology and Physics* **48**(1): 289–302.

Yan BM and Van Dam J (2008) Endoscopic ultrasound-guided intratumoural therapy for pancreatic cancer. *Canadian Journal of Gastroenterology* **22**(4): 405–410.

Yang W and Dempsey PJ (2007) Diagnostic breast ultrasound: current status and future directions. *Radiologic Clinics of North America* **45**(5): 845–861.

Zaidi H, Vees H and Wissmeyer M (2009) Molecular PET/CT imaging-guided radiation therapy treatment planning. *Academic Radiology* **16**(9): 1108–1133.

8 Intensity modulated radiotherapy: radiobiology and physics aspects of treatment

8.1 INTRODUCTION

In Chapter 6 the so-called 3D conformal radiation therapy technique was discussed. This technique uses *fixed radiation field shapes* for each gantry angle and the dose is delivered uniformly across the whole treatment field. From the treatment planning point of view, *forward treatment planning* is used, where optimisation of 3D CRT plans is performed iteratively by manually varying individual treatment beam parameters until a satisfactorily target dose is achieved while sparing adjacent healthy tissues. This process, however, can be time consuming and it may not be possible at all to produce satisfactory plans for unusual target shapes especially when encircling a highly critical structure (e.g. horse shoe shaped target volume). As a result further development of radiation therapy delivery techniques was needed.

In fact the first concepts leading to modern delivery techniques were investigated by Takahashi et al in the sixties of the last century (Takahashi 1965). In their work, dynamic treatments were planned and delivered with a device working in principle as a multileaf collimator. This collimator was connected to a mechanical control unit that allowed the radiation beam aperture to change shape as the beam was rotated around the patient in order to match the projected target shape. Similar pioneering work on radiation beam shaping of the target volume during radiation delivery was performed at the Massachusetts Institute of Technology (MIT) (Wright et al. 1959; Proimos 1960). In 1982 Brahme et al. of the Karolinska Institute, Sweden proposed a novel concept of protecting a critical structure inside a target volume using non-uniform (inhomogeneous) radiation intensity distributions. This led to the development and clinical implementation in the 1990s of a new radiation delivery method known as the *Intensity Modulated Radiation Therapy* (IMRT). The technique is considered to be one of the most significant breakthroughs to have occurred in radiation therapy.

Intensity modulated radiation therapy is an advanced high-precision radiation delivery method using modern computer controlled X-ray linear accelerators. During irradiation, highly conformal and non-uniform radiation dose distributions are produced by modulating the intensity of the radiation beam within the radiation field (aperture) itself. As a result of superior dose conformity, the volume of normal tissues irradiated is smaller and therefore higher radiation doses can be delivered to the target volume (or specific regions only within the target volume) while minimising the dose to surrounding healthy tissues, increasing

L. Marcu et al., *Biomedical Physics in Radiotherapy for Cancer*,
DOI 10.1007/978-0-85729-733-4_8, © CSIRO 2012

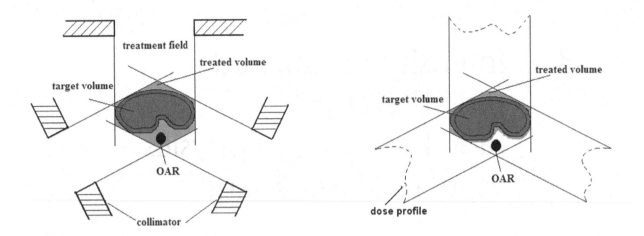

A. Conventional tumour conformality   B. Intensity-modulated tumour conformality

Figure 8.1. Schematic diagram of radiation delivery principle of the conformal radiation therapy (A) based on conformal radiation field apertures (defined by multileaf collimators) within which the radiation dose is delivered uniformly, and intensity modulated radiation radiotherapy (B) where additional dose conformity is achieved using inhomogeneous radiation intensities, sparing thus the organ at risk (OAR).

thus the therapeutic ratio and reducing side effects compared with conventional radiotherapy techniques (Figure 8.1, and Figure 8.2 on p. 211).

Similarly to 3D CRT, combinations of several intensity-modulated fields coming from different beam directions (gantry angles) are used to produce the desired dose pattern (see Figure 8.1). However, the number of beams is generally larger than that used for 3D CRT. Typically around 5 to 9 beams are used, however many more can be used depending on the complexity of the dose pattern desired. In addition, each treatment field consists of smaller areas called segments (also called beamlets or subfields), with specific dose delivered within each segment (Figure 8.3). The dose per segment will be large if it passes through the tumour and will be small (or zero) when passing through an organ at risk (Figure 8.1B). The segments can vary in shape and size and their number can vary between three to several hundreds per field (Xia 2002). Techniques for generation of patient specific intensity modulated radiation fields will be discussed in the following sections.

Currently, IMRT is being used for treatment of cancers of the prostate, central nervous system, head & neck, breast, lungs, gynaecologic malignancies and others. IMRT may also be beneficial for treatment of some paediatric cancers. However, IMRT requires longer treatment times per fraction, therefore the number of fields and segments within must be carefully evaluated so that the impact of IMRT on patient throughput is minimised. The energy of the radiation beam must also be considered so as to minimise its impact on *the integral dose* to a patient. Typically beam energies between 6 and 10 MV are used, as the production of X-ray beams of energies above 10 MV is associated with generation of leakage neutrons increasing thus the integral dose even further (d'Errico *et al.* 1998).

In order to implement IMRT into a clinical practice, its technical requirements, planning concepts/strategies and relevant Quality Assurance (QA) must be understood and implemented (Ezzell *et al.* 2003). In addition, due to increased complexity of dose delivery, pre-treatment as well as *in vivo* dose verification protocols need to be established to monitor the dose delivered to patients treated with intensity modulated radiation therapy.

8.2   PRINCIPLES OF IMRT – DELIVERY METHODS

There are certain minimum technical and staff prerequisites in order to perform intensity modulated

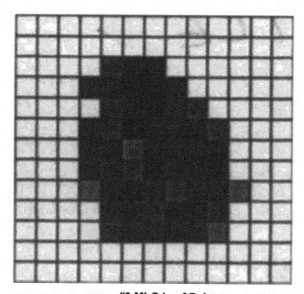

#8 MLC Leaf Pair

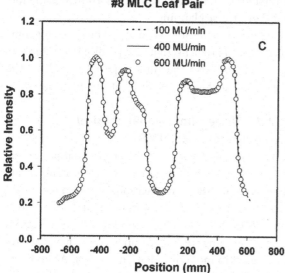

Figure 8.3. An example of segments of different radiation intensities (top) and an example of a radiation beam profile (bottom) of plausible intensity modulated radiotherapy fields. (Reproduced from Xia *et al.* 2002. Copyright (2002), with permission from the American Association of Physicists in Medicine)

radiation therapy. Similar to conventional 3D conformal radiotherapy, IMRT uses CT scans for treatment planning as three dimensional visualisation of patient anatomy is absolutely essential. As a result, CT simulator and software to determine patient positioning are required. Other instrumentation includes 3D planning system with IMRT capability (using *forward*

and *inverse* planning), IMRT capable linear accelerator with corresponding field shaping and/or dose modulating devices and systems to achieve variation in radiation fluence (e.g. compensators, multileaf collimators, dynamic dose rate variation) as well as an adjustable patient couch and on-line imaging apparatus and software for patient set-up verification. In addition, unique quality assurance and dosimetry verification tools including specially designed IMRT phantoms, 2- or 3D detector arrays, and secondary verification software must be available. The IMRT team needs to include trained staff of radiation oncologists, medical physicists, radiation therapists and other technical staff.

As mentioned previously, IMRT uses variation in radiation fluence (i.e. intensity/number of X-rays reaching the patient at a given direction) resulting in variation/modulation of absorbed dose across different parts of the target volume. It needs to be however emphasised here that while the dose from individual fields is non-uniform, the final combined dose distribution within the target volume can be uniform but better conformed to the shape of the planning target volume (Figure 8.1B). Simple dose modulation can be described as follows: Each radiation field consists of two or more subfields or segments. The shape of each subfield is defined by a multileaf collimator (Figure 8.4). Radiation is delivered for each subfield. Relative radiation intensities of all subfields are determined by iteration during the treatment planning process until the planning objectives/goals are achieved. The objectives can include dose conformity, dose boost or normal tissue sparing. Not every treatment site is appropriate for IMRT and it should be used only when 3D CRT plans are not adequate. Immobilisation and position verification are even more important for IMRT than for 3D CRT since only a portion of target is being irradiated at a time and since the margins are reduced and the target dose increased.

There are several techniques that can be considered a form of IMRT. These are:

- Compensator (Metal attenuator) based dose modulation
- 'Stop-and-shoot' or 'Step-and-shoot' static IMRT using multiple MLC shapes per field (sMLC-IMRT); this is also known as segmented IMRT

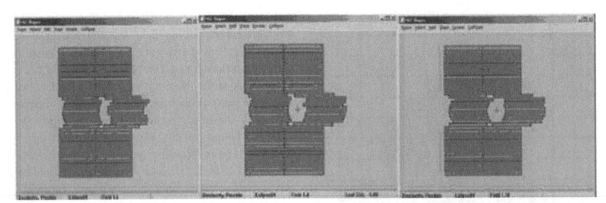

Figure 8.4. An example of subfields/segments generated with a multileaf collimator. The segments form the radiation field for a given beam (gantry) angle.

- 'Dynamic sliding window' IMRT with fixed gantry and moving MLC leaves (dMLC-IMRT)
- Intensity-modulated arc therapy using MLC (IMAT).

8.2.1 Step-and-shoot or segmented IMRT

Step-and-Shoot or segmented IMRT technique uses a number of discreet MLC shapes (segments/subfields) per field with radiation beam turned off between segments (Williams 2003). In other words, the radiation field at a given gantry angle is divided into several sub-fields that are sequentially irradiated using planned amounts of radiation. After each subfield irradiation, the MLC will move to a position for the next segment (see Figures 8.5 and 8.6).

Since sIMRT is quite straightforward in principle, it is simple to understand clinically and individual radiation fluence (or dose) intensity patterns can be verified easily with 2D detector systems (e.g. films, EPIDs, diode or ion chamber arrays). Only a relatively simple accelerator control system is required and the

treatment can be resumed easily if interrupted. The required radiation beam-on-time (so-called Monitor Units) for each segment can be determined using forward or inverse planning.

This technique however may not be suited for complex clinical problems that may require large numbers of segments. Also the time required to deliver the treatment can be quite significant (15–30 minutes).

8.2.2 Three-dimensional physical compensator-based IMRT

Compensators are primary beam attenuators (generally made of metal) used to counteract/compensate the lack of beam attenuation in the anatomical regions of tissue deficiency in particular due to body curvature, for example in the head & neck region. These 'missing tissue' compensators have always been used in modern radiation therapy. As an alternative development, compensators have also been applied in a special case of segmented IMRT (Bartrum *et al.* 2007; Chang *et al.* 2004). Compensator-

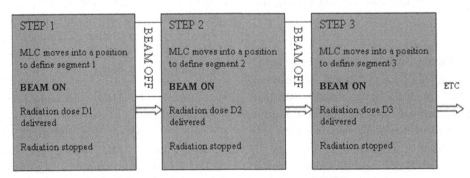

Figure 8.5. Time sequence of dose delivery in a step-and-shoot (or segmented) IMRT.

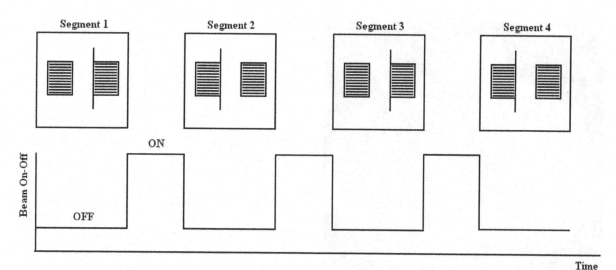

Figure 8.6. Schematic diagram of the step-and-shoot IMRT showing the Beam-off time in relation to MLC moving into the next segment.

based IMRT employs a single compensating metal filter of modulated/varying thickness-segments (Figure 8.7) inserted into the accelerator treatment head. They are generally precisely milled to the patient's tumor size and shape from brass, aluminum, cerrobend, tin and others. The radiation beam passing through the compensator is attenuated differentially depending on the thickness of the compensating material at a given irradiation point, resulting in a modulated radiation fluence. The treatment field is delivered using a single constant beam. There are no moving parts or time variations in the radiation output (beam on, beam off), resulting in a reduced treatment time as there is no beam-off time like in the step-and-shoot IMRT. Spatial resolution of compensator IMRT delivery is sub millimetre (precision of the compensator milling procedure) along both radiation field axes (Bartrum *et al.* 2007). The spatial resolution can be better than that of MLC based IMRT where the resolution is given by the thickness of the leaf end. Since the delivery is faster, patient movement during a treatment fraction can be minimised as well.

This method represents a simple IMRT technique that has good treatment delivery efficiency, while requiring simpler fabrication and a QA verification procedure (Weber and Laursen 2002). It can be performed using any linear accelerator, even a cobalt-60 machine. However, other instrumentation such as a

three-dimensional block cutter or a milling machine and moulding room facilities are required. In addition, compensators will result in the hardening of the radiation beam (i.e. the mean energy of the X-ray spectrum will increase after passing through a compensator) and in production of scattered radiation. Thorough commissioning process of the compensating system must be performed before using clinically.

8.2.3 Dynamic or 'sliding-window' IMRT

Dynamic IMRT (dIMRT) or sliding-window IMRT uses modulated leaf velocity and constant beam intensity during continuous irradiation. In other words, dose delivery is performed without switching the radiation beam off between segments. Individual leaves move according to pre-calculated trajectories yielding the required radiation dose modulation by changing the velocity of their movement. The radiation dose is delivered into an opened space between two opposing MLC leaves; i.e. between the leading leaf and the trailing leaf (Figure 8.8). A point will become irradiated when it stops being shielded by the passing leading leaf and it will cease being irradiated when it is shielded again by the trailing leaf. The separation between the leaves and the leaf velocity will determine the dose delivered at a given point. Both MLC leaf banks move in the same direction. Time sequence of dynamic IMRT is outlined in Figure 8.9.

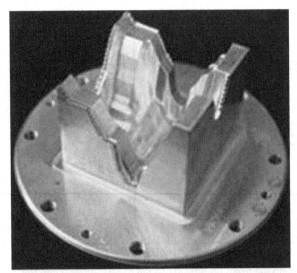

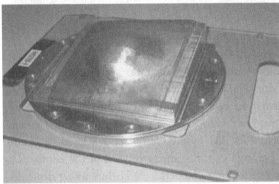

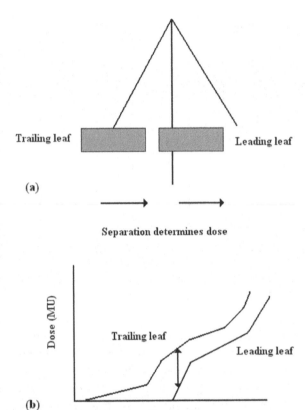

Figure 8.8. Beam modulation using the sliding window multileaf collimation technique: a) leaf separation; b) beam modulation. (Courtesy Convery and Rosenbloom 1992)

Figure 8.7. Picture of a brass compensator (top) (courtesy Decimal®, Inc) and aluminium compensator (bottom) (courtesy Bartrum *et al.* 2007).

Dynamic IMRT is a faster delivery method compared to static technique. It produces smoothly varying radiation intensities compared to step like intensities of the segmented IMRT. In addition, dIMRT can produce more complex dose distributions. On the other hand, this is a more complex technique requiring a complex MLC control system and inverse planning system to calculate the leaf trajectories. Leaf edge effects can produce dosimetric errors when the leaf gaps are small. It is also more difficult to verify/measure the dose patterns.

8.3 IMRT TREATMENT PLANNING – DOSE CALCULATION ALGORITHMS

General planning techniques in IMRT require the use of 'inverse' treatment planning processes. In conven-

tional 3D CRT, therapists or physicists set the linac beams and define MLC positions (i.e. they input delivery patterns into the treatment planning computer). In contrast, in IMRT, the radiation oncologist stipulates specific radiation doses that the tumour and normal surrounding tissues should receive (goals or objectives) or should not exceed (constraints). The physicist/therapist then defines the number of beams, beam directions, delivery method as well as the maximum acceptable complexity of intensity pattern (e.g. minimum size of the segments or minimum monitor units). The program then optimises the plan and calculates an intensity pattern of each beam required to deliver the desired dose distribution and determines the MLC positions and/or leaf sequences (Figure 8.10). This process, whereby clinical objectives are defined first and radiation beam parameters are determined using a computer-based optimisation algorithm, is known as 'inverse treatment planning.'

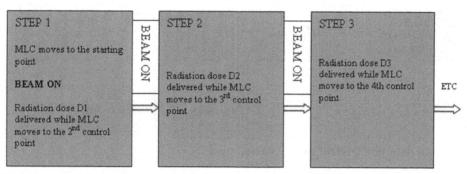

Figure 8.9. Time sequence of dose delivery in a dynamic (or sliding-window) IMRT.

At the beginning of the process, the radiation oncologist or other responsible clinician must carefully delineate the target volume and all relevant critical structures. Accurate contouring is essential as this information will be used by the treatment planning system (TPS) to calculate and optimise the treatment plan and to fine-tune the beam directions and segment intensities. All volumes that need to be kept below certain dose limits must also be defined (Boyer *et al.* 2001a). Failure to outline a structure or to define the dose limit may result in a high dose delivery planned for a given tissue volume by the TPS. The constraints and objectives, defined by the clinician, can also be weighted in order of their importance. The system then needs to determine the particular beam weights and radiation fluence distribution patterns that will fulfil these criteria during the so-called *optimisation* process. From a mathematical point view, the plan objectives are converted into a cost function (also called objective function) and the minimum of this function is sought through computer iterations during optimisation. The results of the optimisation routine (i.e. when the minimum of the cost function has been found) are in the form of radiation fluence that if delivered would best satisfy the clinical criteria/objectives.

Several mathematical algorithms have been developed and implemented in commercially available treatment planning systems to perform IMRT optimisation. The basic of these will be discussed in section 8.3.1. The clinical objectives must be realistic, or the planning computer may not be able to produce clinically acceptable treatment plan. Also, complex mathematical functions with several variables may have more than one local minimum and ideally a global minimum (Figure 8.11) should be found during the optimisation process to best satisfy the objectives. However not all optimisation routines can identify the global minimum. As a result, the physicist or the therapist may need to run several calculation trials before an acceptable solution is found.

As mentioned, the optimisation process yields the radiation fluence/intensity map only and not a deliverable plan as physical limitations of a given MLC systems (e.g. leaves positions and configuration, leaf radiation scatter and transmission) are not taken into account. Consequently, another calculation process, called *leaf sequencing* needs to take place that will calculate a combination of MLC defined segments that will produce the desired dose distribution. Monitor units (beam-on-time) for individual segments are often calculated during this routine as leaf sequence

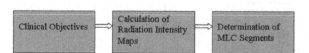

Figure 8.10. Schematic diagram of IMRT inverse planning process sequence.

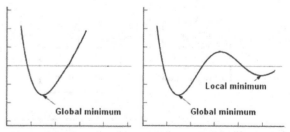

Figure 8.11. Schematic diagram of a function with a single minimum (left) and a function with a local and a global minimum (right).

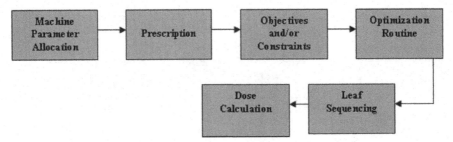

Figure 8.12. Schematic diagram of the IMRT inverse planning process.

corrections may depend on the number of monitor units (Boyer *et al.* 2001b).

Finally, last calculation script is run to calculate the dose distribution representing the dose distribution delivered to a patient for a given MLC segment sequence. Schematic diagram of the IMRT inverse planning process is shown in Figure 8.12.

Once a dose distribution has been calculated it must be evaluated. The dose distribution can be assessed by evaluating the isodose plots, or dose volume histograms. If the dose distribution needs to be improved, another optimisation must be performed with adjusted input parameters. Once the plan is approved by the radiation oncologist, it can be used for treatment delivery, subject to satisfactory QA

verification. Schematic diagram of IMRT workflow is shown in Figure 8.13.

8.3.1   Traditional IMRT optimisation

As mentioned previously, optimisation in IMRT is a process through which the optimum beamlet weights or fluence distribution is determined that can best satisfy the cost function specified by the radiation oncologist. In a simple case, the function, $F(\tau)$, to be minimised is the sum of user-defined objectives, F^k:

$$F(\tau) = \sum_{k=1}^{n} F^k \ (k= 1...n) \tag{8.1}$$

The objectives generally represent a combination of dose and volume limits (e.g. minimum dose,

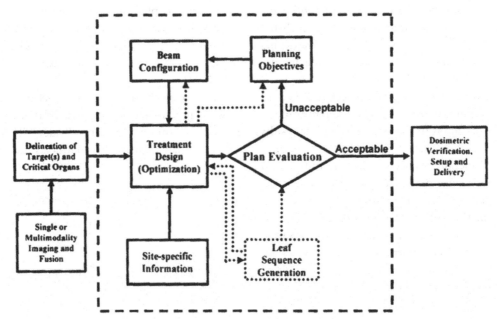

Figure 8.13. Schematic diagram of IMRT planning and delivery process. Dashed box showing the main optimisation process. (Reprinted from Chao, Ozyigit *et al.* 2004. Copyright (2004), with permission from Elsevier)

maximum dose, minimum dose to a given volume, maximum dose to a given volume, and dose uniformity) (Löf 2003). The IMRT optimisation problem can be expressed mathematically as:

$$\min_{\tau} F(\tau) = \begin{cases} C(\tau) \leq 0 \\ \tau \geq 0 \end{cases} \qquad (8.2)$$

where $C(\tau)$ is the constraints vector function, and τ the parameters to be optimised. The condition $\tau \geq 0$ ensures that all negative fluences will be discarded (Hårdemark *et al.* 2004). The resultant fluence distribution produced by the optimisation routine requires further processing by the leaf sequencing and dose calculation algorithms.

8.3.2 Direct machine parameter optimisation

Another approach uses so-called direct machine parameter optimisation, which, given a linac radiation beam model, beamlets can be calculated for radiation fluence, τ, from the actual leaf positions, x, and the weight of each segment, w.

The optimisation problem stated in 8.2 can therefore be expressed as:

$$\min_{x, w} F(x, w) = \begin{cases} C(x, w) \leq 0 \\ Ax \leq b \\ w \geq 0 \end{cases} \qquad (8.3)$$

where Ax represents the machine-specific and user defined leaf position requirements and b is a particular set constraint that could be, amongst others, minimum leaf gap, interdigitation, maximum tip differences, or segment areas (Hårdemark 2004). The condition for segment weight constraint of $w \geq 0$ again ensures that negative fluences are discarded.

As mentioned above, following the optimisation, the fluence distribution needs to be converted into a deliverable radiation fluence applying the leaf sequencing algorithm that takes into account MLC leaf transmission, head scatter and the physical limitations of the MLC. The deliverable fluence is then converted into a so-called *'multilevel approximation distribution using the K-means Clustering method'* (Wu *et al.* 2001). This approach is a non-hierarchal method that takes the intensity of individual beam segments and organises them into a fixed number of predefined intensity levels enabling a large amount of

data to be grouped into clusters of smaller sets of similar data, resulting in a smaller final number of segments (and therefore faster treatment delivery). This sorting of intensity levels into clusters is determined by a set error tolerance between intensity levels (Hartigan 1975). Finally, from the clustered intensity levels, MLC segments are formed to accurately deliver the dose to the target volume.

For step-and-shoot IMRT, MLC leaf trajectory (segment definition) can be set up through two main techniques: *Close in* and *Leaf sweep* (Bortfeld *et al.* 1994). The *Close in* technique produces a profile with a single maximum through the movement of the leaves either towards or from a single point (Convery and Rosenbloom 1992), and the *Leaf sweep* technique is a more simple approach, whereby leaf positions are sorted regarding magnitude (Bortfeld *et al.* 1994) as shown in Figure 8.14.

8.3.3 Dose calculation algorithms

The main dose calculation algorithms employed in IMRT include correction-based pencil beam dose calculation algorithms (Jelen and Alber 2007), superposition-convolution algorithms and Monte Carlo algorithms (Krieger and Sauer 2005). The convolution/superposition-based algorithms are standardly applied in most modern radiotherapy treatment planning systems. While Monte Carlo calculations are considered to be the most accurate, they are often quite complex and time consuming in order to calculate the dose within a desired level of accuracy and as a result are often used as a research tool only. However, with the continual development of computer hardware and software, routine clinical use of Monte Carlo calculation techniques is only a matter of time (Chetty *et al.* 2007).

8.4 QUALITY ASSURANCE IN IMRT

Quality assurance (QA) in IMRT is essential due to high complexity of both treatment planning and treatment delivery. QA for 3D CRT concentrates on the evaluation and monitoring of individual parameters of the whole system (e.g. linac or treatment planning system) and patient specific verification is generally not required. This is not the case for IMRT.

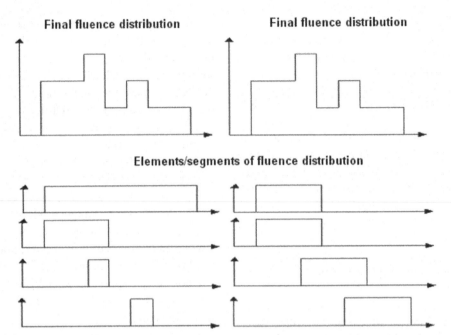

Figure 8.14. Techniques for decomposition of fluences into deliverable segments (left) *Close in* technique (right) *Leaf sweep* technique.

Since there is little correlation between a Monitor Unit and the delivered dose, patient plans (despite similar planning approaches) may vary significantly one from another (especially in regards to optimised leaf sequencing). As a result patient specific QA is necessary (IAEA, TECDOC 1588, 2008) and IMRT QA has two components: a) equipment specific QA and b) patient specific QA.

Equipment specific QA includes: QA of the planning system, overall linac QA, absolute dosimetry, QA of the MLC functionality and positioning, QA of imaging devices as well as data transfer.

Patient specific QA includes pre-treatment verification of the IMRT treatment plan (performed using a geometric phantom), patient set-up verification and *in vivo* dosimetry during delivery.

Equipment specific QA checks the accuracy and constancy of the dose calculation and radiation delivery systems (e.g. TPS, linac, MLC). However, the accuracy of the treatment itself is also related to patient specific parameters like patient set-up, organ motion, and changes in the anatomy (e.g. the presence of a gas bubble in a bowel). Initially, every patient should have the IMRT plan validated prior to the first treatment fraction by delivering the planned irradiation onto a phantom. Once the departments develop 'class solutions' (standard treatment plans and set-ups) for particular treatment areas and a large cohort of patient plans has been verified, the individual patient measurements may be omitted (Budgell *et al.* 2005). However, for any new treatment approaches, individual patient verification is necessary.

The sources of errors in IMRT can come from any stage of the planning and delivery process and are result of:

- uncertainties in patient set-up (caused by couch calibration, changes in patient anatomy during and between treatment fractions, calibration and accuracy of the portal verification systems and position determination algorithms)
- uncertainties in the treatment planning system (caused by uncertainties in the radiation beam model and the dose calculation algorithm, including optimisation routines; and uncertainties in the 3D image acquisition, contours and PTV definition based on imaging information)
- dosimetric uncertainties (dose verification in a phantom, quality of beam data)

- uncertainties in dose delivery (accuracy of MLC positioning, leaf speed and dose modulation during dynamic IMRT, constancy of dose per MU).

8.4.1 Patient set-up verification

Verification of patient set-up in IMRT is essential. The PTV margins in IMRT are smaller compared to standard radiation therapy in order to be able to increase the total tumour dose. This however means that patient position must be verified daily and with high precision as small errors in patient position might lead to large dosimetric errors (geometrical miss). Techniques for patient set-up verification and image guidance have been discussed in Chapters 6 and 7.

8.4.2 Treatment planning system QA

The quality of IMRT starts with the quality of tumour and organs-at-risk delineation. Contouring on CT (or MR) images is the basis of any treatment planning system. With inverse planning, the IMRT optimisation is based on the targets defined by a clinician, so careful and accurate contouring is essential. All outlined organs should be checked from slice to slice to ensure that structures have smooth realistic volumes.

The uncertainties in contours depend on the image quality and type, accuracy of algorithms used to create auto-contours using the gradient in CT image pixel values and on the experience of the clinician performing the task. Differences in contoured volumes were found between individual specialists (Leunens et al. 1993) and contouring represents a weak link in the IMRT workflow. It is a must that clinicians receive training in organ segmentation (delineation) using cross-sectional images (IAEA, TECDOC 1588, 2008). Inaccurate contouring may result in overdosing the healthy tissue or not delivering enough dose to a tumour.

Accuracy of a dose calculation algorithm, employed by a particular treatment planning system, is another critical factor. Routinely, the dose calculation accuracy is evaluated starting from simple homogeneous geometric phantoms to phantoms containing inhomogeneities and more complex geometries. The MLC must be accurately modelled in the TPS, including shape (e.g. rounded leaf end, radiation transmission, penumbra, tongue and groove effect, etc.). Accuracy

of motion algorithm should also be checked in order to ensure that the calculated dose distribution for planned MLC segments or for planned MLC leaf movement in dMLC are in agreement with that delivered during treatment performed using a computer-controlled system (Low et al. 2001).

8.4.3 Multileaf collimator QA

Multileaf collimator QA, especially accuracy of leaf positioning is particularly important in IMRT. Tolerance limits for leaf position accuracy and reproducibility are more stringent than for conventional radiation therapy. While in conventional 3D CRT, leaf position uncertainty of about 1 mm is acceptable, sub-millimetre accuracy is required in IMRT as uncertainties of a fraction of a millimetre in leaf positioning can lead to radiation dose delivery variations of several percent. It was found that the relationship between the relative dose difference and MLC leaf spatial displacement is linear and variation of 0.2 mm in leaf position leads to approximately 1–4% change in the relative dose values for typical IMRT fields (Luo et al. 2006; Mohammadi and Bezak 2007). In addition, the location of the radiation field edge must be identified with respect to the location of the MLC leaf end. For MLCs with rounded leaf ends, there is an offset between the beam edge as defined by the light field and that defined by the 50% relative dose value of the radiation profile/field. This is typically 0.4 to 1.1 mm from the tip of the leaf end. This offset value also needs to be included into the treatment planning system.

The regular MLC QA tests should include (Boyer et al. 2001a; Ezzell 2003): leaf positioning accuracy and isocentricity, light and radiation congruence, radiation leakage between and through the leaves, variation in the width of the radiation field penumbra (i.e. dose fall-off between 80 and 20% isodose line) as a function of leaf position, reproducibility of MLC leaves speed during acceleration and de-acceleration for dynamic IMRT, positional accuracy of generated leaf apertures (segments) and of data file transfer, and evaluation of dose undulation due to stepped field edges generated by MLC leaves, back-up jaw movement and interlocks.

Several techniques have been developed to evaluate MLC positioning accuracy. Evaluation of line profiles

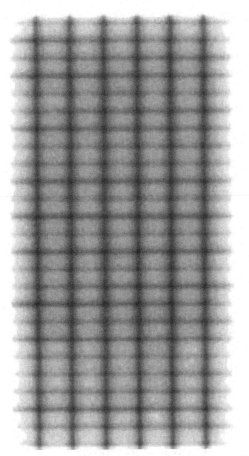

Figure 8.15. QA film produced by moving the 1 mm wide MLC pattern in 2 cm intervals. (Reproduced from Ezzell *et al.* 2003. Copyright (2003), with permission from the American Association of Physicists in Medicine)

measured with radiographic films is generally used to verify relative leaf position and gap width accuracy with the so-called 'picket fence' (LoSasso 2003). In this test an MLC leaf sequence is generated consisting of abutting leaves or narrow strips (e.g. 1 mm wide). The segments are irradiated at regular intervals (e.g. 2 cm) across the whole range of leaf carriage motion. Uniform dose patterns are generated along the match lines (see Figure 8.15) that are sensitive to small differences in individual leave positions. The test allows to assess the positioning of each MLC leaf individually relative to the alignment of the other leaves. A visual inspection can detect improper positioning to a precision of about 0.5 mm (Ezzell *et al.* 2003). The test should also be performed at different gantry and collimator angles.

In case of dynamic IMRT, the ability of the MLC leaves to sustain their specified speed is important. The optimum leaf speed of 1.5 cm/sec at isocentre is recommended for dIMRT deliveries (Galvin *et al.* 1992). Slow leaf movement indicates excessive wear of the motor or other MLC components. Accelerator monitoring system should identify or even interlock the radiation delivery if the leaf speed is below the specified. Radiation engineers must include into the regular preventative linac maintenance program MLC service as well and replace motors as required.

Similar to leaf positioning accuracy, radiographic film can be used to test the constancy of leaf speed, using a sequence of leaf apertures. If the leaf speed is constant then the measured dose profiles will be uniform, otherwise fluctuations will emerge in the delivered profiles. Another way to quantitatively evaluate dMLC leaf positions is by checking the MLC log files recorded during delivery. This is certainly an option for multileaf collimators made by Varian that provides users with software for evaluation of leaf position, called Dynalog File Viewer (Varian Associates, Inc 2001). The software records deviations of monitored and actual leaf positions for individual leaves in terms of root mean square deviation. QA files for various dynamic deliveries (and also step and shoot) are also provided and, once delivered, can be evaluated with the Dynalog File Viewer to pin-point faulty leaf movement (LoSasso 2003). Once again, leaf speed tests should be performed at different gantry angles to test the MLC performance in all difficult gravitational conditions.

Frequency of tests needs to be identified by each department performing IMRT. Generally, accuracy of MLC positioning should be checked weekly, using the picket fence test. Dynamic output as well as dynamic properties (leaf speed, acceleration, de-acceleration) should be checked monthly.

8.4.4   IMRT dose delivery QA

Linear accelerators need to be commissioned for IMRT delivery. As it is possible to plan segments with few or even fractional monitor units (i.e. delivering very small doses), the dose-per-MU constancy must be verified throughout the range used in IMRT. Similarly, the flatness and symmetry of the radiation beam should be confirmed under these conditions (Ezzell *et al.* 2003).

As a consequence of non-uniform radiation fluence use in IMRT, the dose delivery is not intuitive, and it is important to verify the magnitude of dose delivered. It is possible to measure the dose at a suitably located prescription point with the use of a calibrated ionisation chamber. However, ideally the entire dose distribution should be verified. This is usually done using a 'hybrid plan' or QA plan (IAEA, TECDOC 1588, 2008) in which the patient specific modulated IMRT fields are translated onto a flat geometric phantom and the dose in a phantom is computed at normal incidence to the phantom service. On the linac, the same plan is delivered using a flat phantom containing a measuring device (e.g. film, diode or ionisation chamber arrays, and electronic portal imaging devices). The measured and calculated doses are then compared (Figure 8.16 on p. 212). The agreement between the calculated and measured planar dose distributions is then quantified using parameters like the Gamma index (Low *et al.* 1998), percentage dose difference or distance-to-agreement (i.e. how many mm the measured and calculated dose maps/profiles/points need to be shifted by to reach an agreement (same dose within tolerance)). This method allows evaluating both low and high gradient dose regions.

Some modern phantoms contain perpendicular detector arrays and enable measurements in three planes. Gel dosimetry is the only technique that can provide true 3D verification.

8.5 VOLUMETRIC IMRT – INTENSITY MODULATED ARC THERAPY (IMAT)

Next generation arc therapy techniques have established new standards in radiation planning and delivery, both in the view of technical advancements and clinical radiobiology. While the pioneering work on rotational techniques applied to radiotherapy of cancer using conformal radiation delivery originates from 1965 (Takahashi 1965), the idea of intensity modulated arc therapy (IMAT) was first described by Yu three decades later (Yu 1995). To optimise arc therapy algorithms through highly conformal dose delivery in a single arc, Otto (2008) has introduced the volumetric arc therapy (VMAT). The principles of VMAT have been further developed and clinically implemented by three manufacturers under the name of **RapidArc** (Varian Medical Systems, Palo Alto, CA, USA), **VMAT** (Elekta AB, Stockholm, Sweden) and **SmartArc** (Philips Medical Systems, Fitchburg, WI, USA) which represent the latest generation of arc therapy technology.

Volumetric arc therapy delivery with RapidArc is a dynamic treatment achieved with a single 360 degree rotation of the gantry around the patient (similar to tomotherapy) due to a complex treatment planning algorithm which simultaneously changes the rotation speed of the gantry, the dose rate and the shape of the treatment field conformal to the tumour volume, using multileaf collimators. The uninterrupted rotation of the gantry during treatment together with the simultaneous aperture changes, considerably decrease overall treatment time as compared to conventional IMRT, improving therefore patient throughput (Otto 2008; Mayo *et al.* 2010; Verbakel *et al.* 2009a).

Beside the reduction of treatment time with RapidArc the radiobiological advantages of the volumetric arc therapy are the reduction of dose without compromising target coverage and also better sparing of the organs at risk (the RapidArc plan in Figure 8.17, on p. 212, was delivered in less than 80 seconds, which is about 70% time reduction compared to sliding window IMRT).

The above advantages of volumetric arc therapy over IMRT are achieved by combining advanced treatment optimisation algorithms with new linac technology that allows for simultaneous gantry and MLC movement. The optimisation algorithm used in VMAT is based on Otto's concept in developing a treatment plan optimisation and delivery platform which fulfils the following main requirements (Otto 2008):

1. high treatment time efficiency;
2. dose delivery with superior accuracy as compared to existing treatment techniques; and
3. attainment of highly conformal dose distribution.

One aspect of the VMAT algorithm refers to optimisation constraints in terms of efficiency, constraints which are placed on MLC leaf motion and MU variation for a continuous treatment delivery. These constraints have been defined in terms of gantry rotation angle as follows (Otto 2008):

$$\frac{\Delta x}{\Delta \theta} \leq \left(\frac{dx}{d\theta}\right)_{max}$$
$$\frac{\Delta MU}{\Delta \theta} \leq \left(\frac{dMU}{d\theta}\right)_{max} \quad (8.4)$$

where x represents the MLC leaf position, MU is the monitor unit weight, θ is the gantry angle and $(dx/d\theta)_{max} = 0.5$ cm/degree (i.e. 0.5 cm maximum leaf displacement per degree of gantry rotation). The maximum MU weight is also constrained to ensure that the maximum dose rate is not exceeded.

The VMAT optimisation algorithm is based on a progressive sampling of the dynamic source motion of both gantry and MLC leaf positions. The advantage of starting with a small number of source position samples and progressively introducing new ones results in a high-quality plan which can be achieved over a short time period. To begin with, VMAT optimisation uses a course sampling of the gantry positions to model the gantry rotation range, with samples (control points) being incorporated at the start and end of the range with evenly distributed control points in between. After a number of iterations on MLC leaf position and MU weight, additional samples are added as such that they are included midway between the first two existing samples, so the sampling interval between two consecutive control points is reduced. The MLC position for the new sample is linearly interpolated from the positions of the adjacent points and the MU weight is adjusted to result in a uniform MU per degree rotation. With each new sample added, the optimisation progresses until the required sampling frequency is achieved (Otto 2008).

For maximising dosimetric accuracy with the VMAT optimisation algorithm the minimum sampling frequency for both gantry and MLC leaf positions are required. This is achievable by generating VMAT plans with different sampling resolution, and comparing the plans with the same ones when re-sampled at high frequency.

This optimisation technique has led to a delivery time as short as 1.5–3 minutes for a 2 Gy fraction.

Several treatment planning studies have been published comparing VMAT with IMRT and other treatment techniques for various tumour sites such as head & neck (Vanetti et al. 2009), prostate (Shaffer et al. 2009), brain (Fogliata et al. 2008), breast (Popescu et al. 2010), anal carcinoma (Clivio et al. 2009) and cervix (Cozzi et al. 2008). The general conclusions of the aforementioned studies consisted of: shorter treatment times with increased patient tolerance, reduction in monitor units and better sparing of the organs at risk.

For **stereotactic body radiotherapy** (SBRT) the **volumetric arc therapy** is a welcome technological innovation which has been rapidly and widely implemented in clinics (Matuszak et al. 2010; Mayo et al. 2010; Verbakel et al. 2009b). It was demonstrated that while VMAT offers similar dosimetric quality to conformal SBRT for lung and spine, target coverage is improved and treatment delivery time significantly decreased, an important aspect when considering the large single-doses delivered during SRS or SBRT (Matuszak et al. 2010). For these reasons, SBRT with VMAT is considered to be a suitable treatment choice for paediatric cancer patients.

A new VMAT concept has been recently developed and trialled for paraspinal SBRT, under the name of Coll-VMAT, which besides the synchronised gantry rotation, multileaf collimator motion and dose rate modulation, integrates collimator rotation for an additional degree of freedom towards optimum target coverage (Zhang et al. 2010). This collimator trajectory optimisation is based on collimator angle alignment, at each gantry angle, conformal to the spinal cord orientation, so that MLC movement is parallel to the cord direction. The technique eliminates the challenge of obtaining a steep dose gradient between the spinal cord and PTV when treating paraspinal lesions, limiting, therefore, the maximum dose delivered to the cord.

Three treatment techniques: (1) volumetric arc therapy, (2) fixed beam IMRT and (3) conformal radiotherapy with multiple static fields have been compared in a series of patients treated with SBRT for metastases to abdominal lymph nodes (Bignardi et al. 2009). The main parameters compared in the study were CTV and PTV dose coverage and also maximum doses delivered to the organs at risk. Volumetric arc therapy has been shown to improve PTV coverage by about 8% compared to conformal radiotherapy and by 6% when compared to IMRT. While conformal radiotherapy planning has exceeded the dose/volume constraints for the organs at risk in some patients, the objectives have been fulfilled by volumetric arc therapy planning. The study showed clear indication for improved treatment outcome with VMAT with shorter effective treatment times being needed to complete the therapy. Another study comparing volumetric arc IMRT with static intensity modulated treatment for spine body radiotherapy has found similar dose conformity with VMAT and IMRT, while for cord sparing IMRT achieved the best dosimetric results (Wu *et al.* 2009). The only noticeable advantage of VMAT reported by this study was the treatment efficiency which was considerably improved when compared to IMRT. While generally the results are encouraging, there is certainly need for more studies to warrant the wide implementation of volumetric arc therapy into clinics. Furthermore, as with any novel technology, to achieve highly efficient outcome with volumetric arc therapy, it is important to accurately identify those patient groups that are most likely to benefit.

8.6 THE RADIOBIOLOGY OF IMRT

Novel treatment techniques are built upon radiobiological principles evolved over the years which undoubtedly include the 5 R's of radiobiology in the lead towards increased therapeutic ratio: repair of normal tissue damage, repopulation of normal tissue through cells which have survived irradiation, redistribution of cancer cells along the cell cycle, reoxygenation of hypoxic tumours and intrinsic radiosensitivity.

The advent of fractionated radiotherapy was based on the above principles and managed to increase therapeutic ratio compared to single-dose treatment, mainly due to normal tissue sparing. There were, however, certain cancers, which did necessitate alterations to the fractionation regimen, due to their proliferation characteristics. Consequently, head & neck cancers which are known for their ability to undergo accelerated repopulation during radiotherapy, had to be treated with hyperfractionated and/or accelerated fractionation schedules, an aggressive measure for an aggressive tumour. On the other hand, slowly proliferating prostate cancers were shown to respond better to hypofractionated schedules, similar changes of increased dose/fraction also being made to breast cancer protocols.

More insights into the radiobiology of tumours demonstrated that alongside proliferation, the lack of oxygenation in its various forms (perfusion or diffusion-limited hypoxia) creates serious challenges in radio and chemotherapy. The unpredictable pattern of acute hypoxia, both spatially and temporally and added challenges imposed by other tumour non-homogeneities lead to the development of image-guided therapies and delivery of intensity modulated radiation.

Dose delivery and distribution in IMRT is highly variable, both spatially and temporally. The non-uniform dose distribution is intended to compensate for tumour non-homogeneities whereas overall treatment time designed for IMRT (which is significantly longer than for conventional radiotherapy to allow for movement of the multileaf collimators) has important effects upon cell survival. Studies have shown that prolonged fraction treatment time facilitates cellular damage repair. While this is a positive consequence for normal tissue needing cellular recovery after radiation injury, it is negative for the tumour which has to be controlled via irreparable cellular damage. Mu and colleagues (2003) showed that the most effective delivery times for cell killing are those less than 10 minutes. Furthermore, they demonstrated that the cell kill effect increases with faster dose delivery. These observations are supported by more recent work reporting on the strong dependence between reduction of fraction time and the efficiency of IMRT on tumour cells (Bewes *et al.* 2008). The effect of both average dose rate and instantaneous dose rate (pulse amplitude) were investigated on two cell lines with different radiosensitivity: a melanoma and a non-small cell lung cancer cell line. While the instantaneous dose rate did not have an impact on surviving fraction, the average dose rate strongly influenced cell survival: an increase in cell survival was observed with a decreased dose rate, for the same total dose. The results suggest that a longer delivery time should convey a larger radiation dose in order to compensate for cell repair therefore decreased cell kill.

A considerable advantage of IMRT is the possibility to partially boost tumour volumes in spatially non-uniform tumours, thus targeting radioresistant subvolumes due to high hypoxic content.

Beside the highly conformal dose distribution with sharp dose gradient between the planning target

Table 8.1.   Radiobiological advantages and drawbacks of IMRT.

Advantages		Possible drawbacks
protracted fraction treatment time allows for normal tissue repair	$\Longrightarrow$	protracted fraction treatment time allows for repair of damaged tumour cell
sharp dose gradient high conformality	$\Longrightarrow$	miss of tumour margins
MLC-given tumour conformality	$\Longrightarrow$	high total body dose due to leakage through the collimators
reduced early toxicity	$\Longrightarrow$	uncertain long term toxicity

volume and planning organ at risk volume, IMRT has the disadvantage of potentially missing tumour margins. Also the increase in treatment time and machine on-time as well as the leakage through the collimators and gantry head scatter, all contribute to a higher total body dose (Goffman and Glatstein 2002; Mendenhall *et al.* 2006). It was shown that in head & neck IMRT, which is, probably, the most common treatment site using this technology, total-body dose using a standard 6 MV beam IMRT increased over 8 times compared to conventional radiotherapy (1.97 Sv compared to 0.242 Sv) (Verellen and Vanhavere 1999). Consequently, estimates of the risk of second malignancies induced by radiation 10 years after IMRT treatment show an increase from 1% (from 3D-conformal radiotherapy) to 1.75% (Hall and Wuu 2003). The advantages and possible disadvantages of the IMRT technique from a radiobiological perspective are summarised in Table 8.1.

Lately, IMRT is delivered using simultaneously integrated boost (SIB), which consists of delivering different dose to different target volume simultaneously (Mohan *et al.* 2000). The boost dose is therefore integrated into the IMRT dose fractions for a more efficient treatment, delivering high dose to the primary disease and lower dose to the subclinical disease. While incorporating SIB into the treatment confers IMRT better dose distribution conformality, late toxicities could be a problem which remains to be evaluated by well designed clinical trials.

8.7   IMRT IN CLINICAL TRIALS

Intensity-modulated radiotherapy has been implemented in several clinical trials for the management of various tumour sites including head & neck, prostate, brain, lung, rectum, cervix and breast. While tumour control was not always improved with IMRT, majority of trials reported decreased normal tissue toxicity due to superior critical organ sparing compared to other treatment techniques.

A randomised controlled trial on forward-planned IMRT for early breast cancer was designed to assess the impact of IMRT in correcting dose inhomogeneities upon late toxicities and standard of life (Barnett *et al.* 2009). The trial confirmed that IMRT has not only dosimetric advantage but can increase the therapeutic ratio by reducing treatment-related side effects. The management of lung cancer has been improved by the recent advances in IMRT using respiratory-gated radiotherapy. This technique allows for reduction in intrafraction motion for mobile tumours (Keall *et al.* 2006) and offers the possibility to further optimise treatment via better tumour conformality and decreased normal tissue damage. The efficiency of respiratory gated IMRT in reducing clinical target volume to planning target volume margins was also confirmed by breast cancer studies (George *et al.* 2003). These promising results need more confirmation from randomised clinical trials to justify the use of IMRT with gating techniques for other moving targets.

Further details on clinical trials for tumour sites more commonly treated with IMRT are presented as follows.

8.7.1   Head & neck cancer

Due to their location, head & neck cancers are difficult to treat without normal tissue sequelae. The sharp dose gradients delivered with the IMRT technology

Table 8.2. IMRT clinical trials on head & neck cancer.

Trial/# patients	IMRT delivery approach	Dose	Clinical endpoints	Toxicity
Phase II nasopharynx 67 patients (Lee *et al.* 2002)	– manually cut partial transmission blocks – computer-controlled auto-sequencing segmental multileaf collimator – sequential tomotherapy using a dynamic multivane intensity modulating collimator	60 Gy to *clinical target volume*	*4-year:* 88% overall survival 98% loco-regional progression free survival	worst late toxicity grade 3 – 10.4% grade 4 – 1.5%
Phase II oropharynx 74 patients (Chao *et al.* 2004b)	inverse planning IMRT with parotid sparing protocol	66–70 Gy mean prescribed dose	*4-year:* 87% overall survival 87% loco-regional progression free survival	Worst xerostomia grade 1 – 42% grade 2 – 12%
Phase II non-nasopharynx 133 patients (Eisbruch *et al.* 2004)	multisegmental static IMRT	70 Gy to *planning target volume*	*3-year:* 81% loco-regional progression free survival	substantial sparing of parotid gland
Phase II nasopharynx 33 patients (Kwong *et al.* 2004)	inverse planning IMRT	68–70 Gy dose to *gross target volume*	*3-year:* 100% overall survival 100% loco-regional progression free survival	main focus: on salivary function (xerostomia assessment) superior recovery compared to conventional RT
Phase II oropharynx 50 patients (Arruda *et al.* 2006)	– 76% dose painting, – 18% concomitant boost with IMRT in both am and pm deliveries, – 6% concomitant boost with IMRT only in pm delivery	70 Gy average dose to *gross target volume*	*2-year:* 98% overall survival 98% loco-regional progression free survival	Worst mucositis grade 2 – 54% grade 3 – 38%
Phase II IMRT-SIB 115 patients (Studer *et al.* 2006a)	IMRT using simultaneously integrated boost (SIB-IMRT)	60–70 Gy mean prescribed dose (2.0, 2.11 or 2.2 Gy per session)	*2-year:* 77% loco-regional progression free survival	worst toxicity: xerostomia grade 3 – 10% mucositis: grade 3 – 15%
Phase II post-operative IMRT 71 patients (Studer *et al.* 2006b)	IMRT using simultaneously integrated boost (SIB-IMRT)	66.3 Gy mean prescribed dose	*2-year:* 83% overall survival 95% loco-regional progression free survival	worst late toxicity grade 3 – 2.4%

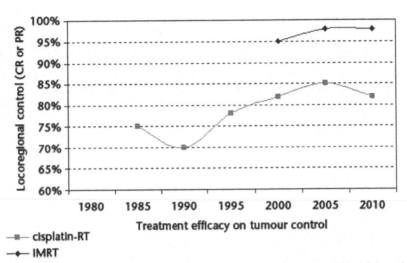

Figure 8.18. The superiority of IMRT over cisplatin-radiotherapy regarding tumour control in head & neck cancer.

lead to a better sparing of the normal tissue (such as parotid glands) making head & neck cancer the ideal candidate for IMRT. Also IMRT using simultaneously integrated boost (SIB) adds to the organ sparing effect of IMRT in head & neck cancers in order to reduce xerostomia, the most common side effect in this patient category. The high dose conformality of IMRT offers the potential for improved tumour control, which the hard-to-manage advanced head & neck cancers can benefit from.

The large number of clinical studies and trials on head & neck tumours demonstrate the high potential of IMRT in increasing the therapeutic ratio by both elevating TCP and reducing NTCP. Clinical trial results illustrate high percentage overall survival and loco-regional progression free survival, both superior to conventional radiotherapy. Some of these results are presented in Table 8.2. All trials which have employed IMRT in parallel with conventional radiotherapy observed significantly reduced mucositis and xerostomia in the IMRT-treated group.

As reported by Studer and colleagues, IMRT using simultaneously integrated boost (IMRT-SIB) has several advantages for head and cancer management: better target conformality, decreased dose to surrounding critical structures, possibility for dose escalation in the gross tumour volume and reduced overall treatment time by moderate treatment acceleration (Studer *et al.* 2006a).

The efficacy of IMRT over other treatment methods for head & neck cancer, such as the most common combination of cisplatin-radiotherapy is illustrated in Figure 8.18. A previously published review has shown the high potential of cisplatin when combined with radiation in managing locally advanced head & neck cancers (Marcu and Yeoh 2009). Here, the superiority of IMRT regarding tumour control is illustrated over the last decade, explaining the preference among clinicians towards this technique.

8.7.2   Brain cancer

The dose limiting potential of IMRT to the surrounding tissues makes intensity-modulated radiotherapy a suitable treatment for brain tumours, both benign and malignant. Sparing of brainstem, optic nerve, eye lenses and chiasm are achievable with sequential arc IMRT which was shown to give similarly good results to stereotactic radiosurgery. IMRT for high-grade gliomas was shown to allow for improved target conformity and better critical tissue sparing than 3D-CRT, without increasing the integral dose to normal brain (Hermanto *et al.* 2007). Similar results were reported by Chan *et al.* (2003) after comparing IMRT using simultaneous boost to the gross tumour volume with 3D-CRT. An added advantage of IMRT consists of treatment planning efficiency, this technique being less labour intensive and less time consuming than 3D conformal radiotherapy planning.

Table 8.3. Latest IMRT clinical trials on prostate cancer with focus on toxicity assessment.

Trial/study design	Radiation dose	Toxicity	Observations
Hypofractionated IMRT (5 field) (Coote *et al.* 2009)	57–60 Gy to prostate in 19–20 fractions	*2-years post treatment:* no grade 4 toxicity; 1 patient – grade 3 bladder toxicity 4% – grade 2 bowel toxicity 4.25% – grade 2 bladder toxicity	patients receiving 60 Gy were more likely to develop bowel toxicity than those receiving 57 Gy generally well tolerated
IMRT-SIB (retrospective toxicity analysis) (McCammon *et al.* 2009)	70 Gy in 28 fractions (2.5 Gy/fraction) to the prostate *with simultaneous delivery* of 50.4 Gy in 28 fractions (1.8 Gy/fraction) to the pelvic lymph nodes	*acute toxicity:* 36.7% – grade 2 cystitis 26.7% – grade 2 urinary frequency *2-years post treatment:* 6.6% – grade 3 toxicity 3.3% – grade 4 toxicity	acute or late bladder and rectal toxicity did not correlate with any of the dosimetric parameters
Hypofractionated Intensity Modulated Arc Therapy (with androgen suppression) (Fonteyne *et al.* 2009)	69.3 Gy (median dose) in 25 fractions to the prostate *and* 50 Gy in 25 fractions to the pelvic lymph nodes	*3-months follow up:* 45% – grade 2 lower gastrointestinal toxicity 45% – grade 2 genitourinary toxicity 6.45% – grade 3 genitourinary toxicity	feasible treatment with low toxicity
IMRT (single institution trial) (Liauw *et al.* 2009)	76 Gy median dose to the planning target volume	*56-months follow up:* 2% – grade 3 genitourinary toxicity 2% – grade 3 gastrointestinal toxicity	IMRT lead to low rates of severe toxicity and excellent biochemical control
IMRT-SIB (Al-Mamgani *et al.* 2009)	78 Gy 3D-conformal radiotherapy technique with a sequential boost (SEQ) versus 78 Gy simultaneous integrated boost using intensity-modulated radiotherapy (SIB-IMRT)	*56-months follow up:* maximum toxicity 20% – grade 2 gastrointestinal toxicity	5-years follow up shows that SIB-IMRT reduced the toxicity without compromising the outcome
Hypofractionated IMRT (with androgen suppression) (Pervez *et al.* 2010)	68 Gy in 25 fractions (2.72 Gy/fraction) to the prostate *with simultaneous delivery of* 45 Gy in 25 fractions to the pelvic lymph nodes	*3-months follow up:* 13.6% – grade 1 gastrointestinal toxicity 18.97% – grade 1 genitourinary toxicity 8.62% – grade 2 genitourinary toxicity	acutely well tolerated longer follow up needed for late toxicity and outcome assessment

While some studies/clinical trials on malignant gliomas showed superior tumour control with IMRT compared to other treatment methods (Hermanto *et al.* 2007), there are also opposing results reported by other groups showing no survival benefits of IMRT (Fuller *et al.* 2007). Albeit tumour control is not improved without dose escalation, there is clinical evidence that IMRT decreases the dose to critical

Table 8.4. IMRT versus other prostate treatment modalities: comparative studies for toxicity and tumour control.

IMRT technique	Comparative treatment technique(s)	Outcome	Reference
IMRT (74–78 Gy)	*I-125 permanent seed implant* (145 Gy)	*normal tissue toxicity:* IMRT lead to less acute and late toxicity *tumour control:* no significant difference	Eade *et al.* 2008
IMRT (75.6 Gy median dose)	*3D-CRT* (68.4 Gy median dose) *I-125 or Pd-103 (BRT)* (144 Gy with I-125 120 Gy with Pd-103) *external beam radiotherapy + brachytherapy boost* (45 Gy external beam + 110 Gy I-125 or 90 Gy Pd-103)	*normal tissue toxicity:* IMRT caused the least acute toxicity *tumour control:* 5-year biochemical control rates 74% for 3D-CRT, 87% for IMRT, 94% for BRT, 94% for EBRT + BRT	Wong *et al.* 2009
IMRT-SIB (78 Gy)	*3D-conformal radiotherapy* with a sequential boost (SEQ) (78 Gy)	*normal tissue toxicity:* IMRT better tolerated *tumour control:* no significant difference	Al-Mamgani *et al.* 2009
IMRT-SIB (60.75 Gy of 2.43 Gy/ fraction to prostate and 45 Gy of 1.8 Gy/ fraction to pelvic nodes	*four-field box technique + 3DCRT boost* (45 Gy in 25 fractions + 27 Gy in 15 fractions) *four-field box technique + IMRT boost* (45 Gy in 25 fractions + 27 Gy in 15 fractions) *IMRT + IMRT boost* (45 Gy in 25 fractions + 27 Gy in 15 fractions)	*normal tissue toxicity:* IMRT-SIB produced the least normal tissue complication and better dose distribution *tumour control:* similar to the other 2 phase treatments *added advantage:* reduced treatment time with IMRT-SIB (with about 3 weeks)	Basu *et al.* 2009

organs due to high dose conformality which might confer this technique an advantage over other treatment methods (Narayana *et al.* 2006).

Next to primary brain tumours, IMRT shows promising results in the management of brain metastases. Edwards *et al.* (2010) reported on a recent study where 11 patients with bulky brain metastatic disease were treated with a standard whole brain radiotherapy (30 Gy, 3 Gy/fraction) and an IMRT boost to the gross tumour volume (to 40 Gy) showing good early control and no acute toxicity. A currently recruiting trial (Thomas Jefferson University Hospital) aims to focus on dose escalation studies during IMRT for patients

with brain metastases. Acute and late CNS toxicities as well as tumour control will be assessed as clinical endpoints.

8.7.3 Prostate cancer

The low alpha/beta ratio of prostate cancer, though with a still debated value, confers eligibility for hypofractionated radiotherapy. Hypofractionated IMRT enables dose escalation to the prostate gland while decreasing normal tissue toxicity. In prostate cancer, as in any other cancer treated with the IMRT technique, late toxicity remains an unresolved challenge imposed by dose intensity modulation. As a consequence, several studies/trials have been designed in order to investigate the extent of dose escalation which can be tolerated without added side effects and also to analyse toxicity-related parameters which influence treatment outcome. Clinical studies have demonstrated the efficiency of the IMRT-SIB technique in prostate cancer management which simultaneously delivers high dose to the prostate and lower dose to the pelvic nodes (Dogan *et al.* 2003). Some recent clinical trial/study results are presented in Table 8.3.

While the usual doses prescribed for prostate IMRT are below 80 Gy (as also seen from Table 8.3), Cahlon and colleagues have trialled an ultra-high dose IMRT, of 86.4 Gy, for localised cancer resulting in excellent biochemical control rates (98% relapse-free survival after 5 years for the low-risk prostate cancer patients and 70% for the high risk prognostic group) and well tolerated treatment (Cahlon *et al.* 2008). Dose volume histogram data indicated a mean D95 of 83 Gy and V100 of 87%. IMRT enables, therefore, dose escalation without added normal tissue toxicity if treatment parameters adhere to normal tissue constraints.

With new technological advances there are multiple treatment options available for the radiotherapy of prostate cancer including, beside IMRT, techniques such as: three dimensional conformal radiotherapy, proton therapy, brachytherapy (either LDR or HDR) and neutron beam-based therapy. The decision upon the optimal treatment can, therefore, be a challenging task, reason why several research groups have comparatively trialled various radiotherapy treatment techniques assessing both normal tissue toxicity and tumour control (see Table 8.4 for the latest results).

Due to major achievements obtained over the last decade in the field of IMRT, the management of treatment related acute and late toxicity has considerably improved among cancer patients. However, as with any other new technology, long term toxicity and clinical outcome remain uncertain.

REFERENCES

Al-Mamgani A, Heemsbergen WD, Peeters ST and Lebesque JV (2009) Role of intensity-modulated radiotherapy in reducing toxicity in dose escalation for localized prostate cancer. *International Journal of Radiation Oncology Biology and Physics* **73**(3): 685–691.

Arruda F, Puri D, Zhung J, Narayana A *et al.* (2006) Intensity-modulated radiation therapy for the treatment of oropharyngeal carcinoma: The Memorial Sloan-Kettering Cancer Center experience. *International Journal of Radiation Oncology Biology and Physics* **64**(2): 363–373.

Barnett GC, Wilkinson J, Moody AM, Wilson CB *et al.* (2009) A randomised controlled trial of forward-planned radiotherapy (IMRT) for early breast cancer: baseline characteristics and dosimetry results. *Radiotherapy and Oncology* **92**(1): 34–41.

Bartrum T, Bailey M, Nelson V and Grace M (2007) Linear attenuation coefficients for compensator based IMRT. *Australasian Physical and Engineering Sciences in Medicine* **30**(4): 281–287.

Basu KS, Bahl A, Subramani V, Sharma DN *et al.* (2009) Normal tissue complication probability: does simultaneous integrated boost intensity-modulated radiotherapy score over other techniques in treatment of prostate adenocarcinoma. *Journal of Cancer Research and Therapeutics* **5**(2): 78–84.

Bewes JM, Suchowerska N, Jackson M, Zhang M *et al.* (2008) The radiobiological effect of intra-fraction dose-rate modulation in intensity modulated radiation therapy (IMRT). *Physics in Medicine and Biology* **53**(13): 3567–3578.

Bignardi M, Cozzi L, Fogliata A, Lattuada P *et al.* (2009) Critical appraisal of volumetric modulated arc therapy in stereotactic body radiation therapy for metastases to abdominal lymph nodes. *International Journal of Radiation Oncology Biology and Physics* **75**(5): 1570–1577.

Bortfeld TR, Kahler DL, Waldron TJ and Boyer A (1994) X-ray field compensation with multileaf collimators. *International Journal of Radiation Oncology Biology and Physics* **28**(3): 723–730.

Boyer A, Biggs P, Galvin J, Klein E *et al.* (2001a) 'Basic applications of multileaf collimators'. Report of Task Group No. 50 Radiation Therapy Committee, AAPM Report No. 72. American Association of Physicists in Medicine by Medical Physics Publishing.

Boyer A, Butler EB, DiPetrillo TA, Engler M *et al.* (2001b) Intensity-modulated radiotherapy: current status and issues of interest. *International Journal of Radiation Oncology Biology and Physics* **51**(4): 880–914.

Brahme A, Roos JE and Lax I (1982) Solution of an integral equation encountered in rotation therapy. *Physics in Medicine and Biology* **27**(10): 1221–1229.

Budgell GJ, Perrin BA, Mott JH, Fairfoul J and Mackay RI (2005) Quantitative analysis of patient-specific dosimetric IMRT verification. *Physics in Medicine and Biology* **50**(1): 103–119.

Cahlon O, Zelefsky MJ, Shippy A, Chan H *et al.* (2008) Ultra-high dose (86.4 Gy) IMRT for localized prostate cancer: toxicity and biochemical outcomes. *International Journal of Radiation Oncology Biology and Physics* **71**(2): 330–337.

Chang S, Cullip T, Deschesne K, Miller E and Rosenman J (2004) Compensators: an alternative IMRT delivery technique. *Journal of Applied Clinical Medical Physics* **5**(3): 15–36.

Chao KS, Apisarnthanarax S and Ozyigit G (2004a) *Practical Essentials of Intensity Modulated Radiation Therapy.* 2nd edn. Lippincott Williams & Wilkins, Philadelphia.

Chao KS, Ozyigit G, Blanco AI, Thorstad WL *et al.* (2004b) Intensity-modulated radiation therapy for oropharyngeal carcinoma: impact of tumor volume. *International Journal of Radiation Oncology Biology and Physics* **59**(1): 43–50.

Chan MF, Schupak K, Burman C, Chui CS *et al.* (2003) Comparison of intensity-modulated radiotherapy with three-dimensional conformal radiation therapy planning for glioblastoma multiforme. *Medical Dosimetry* **28**(4): 261–265.

Chetty IJ, Curran B, Cygler JE, DeMarco JJ *et al.* (2007) Report of the AAPM Task Group No. 105: issues associated with clinical implementation of Monte Carlo-based photon and electron external beam treatment planning. *Medical Physics* **34**(12): 4818–4853.

Clivio A, Fogliata A, Franzetti-Pellanda A, Nicolini G *et al.* (2009) Volumetric-modulated arc radiotherapy for carcinomas of the anal canal: a treatment planning comparison with fixed field IMRT. *Radiotherapy and Oncology* **92**(1): 118–124.

Convery DJ and Rosenbloom ME (1992) The generation of intensity-modulated fields for conformal radiotherapy by dynamic collimation. *Physics in Medicine and Biology* **37**(6): 1359–1374.

Coote JH, Wylie JP, Cowan RA, Logue JP *et al.* (2009) Hypofractionated intensity-modulated radiotherapy for carcinoma of the prostate: analysis of toxicity. *International Journal of Radiation Oncology Biology and Physics* **74**(4): 1121–1127.

Cozzi L, Dinshaw KA, Shrivastava SK, Mahantshetty U *et al.* (2008) A treatment planning study comparing volumetric arc modulation with RapidArc and fixed field IMRT for cervix uteri radiotherapy. *Radiotherapy and Oncology* **89**(2): 180–191.

d'Errico F, Nath R, Tana L *et al.* (1998) In-phantom dosimetry and spectrometry of photoneutrons from an 18 MV linear accelerator. *Medical Physics* **25**(9): 1717–1724.

Dogan N, King S, Emami B, Mohideen N *et al.* (2003) Assessment of different IMRT boost delivery methods on target coverage and normal-tissue sparing. *International Journal of Radiation Oncology Biology and Physics* **57**(5): 1480–1491.

Eade TN, Horwitz EM, Ruth K, Buyyounouski MK *et al.* (2008) A comparison of acute and chronic toxicity for men with low-risk prostate cancer treated with intensity-modulated radiation therapy or (125) I permanent implant. *International Journal of Radiation Oncology Biology and Physics* **71**(2): 338–345.

Edwards AA, Keggin E and Plowman PN (2010) The developing role for intensity-modulated radiation therapy (IMRT) in the non-surgical treatment of brain metastases. *British Journal of Radiology* **83**: 133–136.

Eisbruch A, Marsh LH, Dawson LA, Bradford CR *et al.* (2004) Recurrences near base of skull after IMRT for head-and-neck cancer: implications for target delineation in high neck and for parotid gland sparing. *International Journal of Radiation Oncology Biology and Physics* **59**(1): 28–42.

Ezzell GA, Galvin JM, Low D, Palta JR *et al.* (2003) Guidance document on delivery, treatment planning, and clinical implementation of IMRT: report of the IMRT Subcommittee of the AAPM Radiation Therapy Committee. *Medical Physics* **30**(8): 2089–2115.

Fogliata A, Clivio A, Nicolini G, Vanetti E *et al.* (2008) Intensity modulation with photons for benign intracranial tumours: a planning comparison of volumetric single arc, helical arc and fixed gantry techniques. *Radiotherapy and Oncology* **89**(3): 254–262.

Fonteyne V, De Gersem W, De Neve W, Jacobs F *et al.* (2009) Hypofractionated intensity-modulated arc therapy for lymph node metastasized prostate cancer. *International Journal of Radiation Oncology Biology and Physics* **75**(4): 1013–1020.

Fraass B, Doppke K, Hunt M, Kutcher G, Starkschall G, Stern R and Van Dyk J (1998) American Association of Physicists in Medicine Radiation Therapy Committee Task Group 53: quality assurance for clinical radiotherapy treatment planning. *Medical Physics* **25**(10): 1773–1828.

Fuller C, Choi M, Forthuber B, Wang S *et al.* (2007) Standard fractionation intensity modulated radiation therapy (IMRT) of primary and recurrent glioblastoma multiforme. *Radiation Oncology* **2**: 26.

Galvin JM, Smith AR, Moeller RD, Goodman RL, Powlis WD, Rubenstein J, Solin LJ, Michael B, Needham M and Huntzinger CJ (1992) Evaluation of multileaf collimator design for a photon beam. *International Journal of Radiation Oncology Biology and Physics* **23**(4): 789–801.

George R, Keall PJ, Kini VR, Vedam SS *et al.* (2003) Quantifying the effect of intrafraction motion during breast IMRT planning and dose delivery. *Medical Physics* **30**(4): 552–562.

Goffman TE and Glatstein E (2002) Intensity-modulated radiation therapy. *Radiation Research* **158**(1): 115–117.

Hall E and Wuu C (2003) Radiation-induced second cancers: the impact of 3D-CRT and IMRT. *International Journal of Radiation Oncology Biology and Physics* **56**(1): 83–88.

Hårdemark B, Liander A, Rehbinder H and Lof J (2004) 'P3 direct machine parameter optimisation'. Pinnacle3 White Paper, Philips Medical Systems.

Hartigan JA (1975) *Clustering Algorithms*. John Wiley and Sons, New York.

Helyer S and Heisig S (1995) Multileaf collimation versus conventional shielding blocks: a time and motion study of beam shaping in radiotherapy. *Radiotherapy and Oncology* **37**(1): 61–64.

Hermanto U, Frija EK, Lii MJ, Chang EL *et al.* (2007) Intensity-modulated radiotherapy (IMRT) and conventional three-dimensional conformal radiotherapy for high-grade gliomas: does IMRT increase the integral dose to normal brain? *International Journal of Radiation Oncology Biology and Physics* **67**(4): 1135–1144.

International Atomic Energy Agency (2008) 'Transition from 2-D radiotherapy to 3-D conformal and intensity modulated radiotherapy'. IAEA-TEC-DOC-1588. IAEA, Vienna, Austria.

Jelen U and Alber M (2007) A finite size pencil beam algorithm for IMRT dose optimization: density corrections. *Physics in Medicine and Biology* **52**(3): 617–633.

Keall P, Vedam S, George R, Bartee C *et al.* (2006) The clinical implementation of respiratory-gated intensity-modulated radiotherapy. *Medical Dosimetry* **31**(2): 152–162.

Krieger T and Sauer OA (2005) Monte Carlo- versus pencil-beam-/collapsed-cone-dose calculation in a heterogeneous multi-layer phantom. *Physics in Medicine and Biology* **50**(5): 859–868.

Kwong DL, Pow EH, Sham JS, McMillan AS *et al.* (2004) Intensity-modulated radiotherapy for early-stage nasopharyngeal carcinoma: a prospective study on disease control and preservation of salivary function. *Cancer* **101**(7): 1584–1593.

Lee N, Xia P, Quivey J, Sultanem K *et al.* (2002) Intensity-modulated radiotherapy in the treatment of nasopharyngeal carcinoma: an update of the UCSF experience. *International Journal of Radiation Oncology Biology and Physics* **53**(1): 12–22.

Leunens G, Menten J, Weltens C, Verstraete J and Van Der Schueren E (1993) Quality assessment of medical decision making in radiation oncology: variability in target volume delineation for brain tumours. *Radiotherapy and Oncology* **29**(2): 169–175.

Liauw SL, Weichselbaum RR, Rash C, Correa D *et al.* (2009) Biochemical control and toxicity after intensity-modulated radiation therapy for prostate cancer. *Technology in Cancer Research and Treatment* **8**(3): 201–206.

Lof J and McNutt T (2003) 'P3IMRT inverse planning optimisation'. Pinnacle3 White Paper, Philips Medical Systems.

LoSasso TJ (2003) IMRT delivery system QA. In: *Intensity-modulated Radiation Therapy. The State of the Art.* (Eds JR Palta and TR Mackie) pp. 561–591. Medical Physics Publishing, Colorado Springs, CO.

Low DA, Harms WB, Mutic S and Purdy JA (1998) A technique for the quantitative evaluation of dose distributions. *Medical Physics* **25**(5): 656–661.

Low DA, Sohn JW, Klein EE, Markman J, Mutic S and Dempsey JF (2001) Characterization of a commercial multileaf collimator used for intensity modulated radiation therapy. *Medical Physics* **28**(5): 752–756.

Luo W, Li J, Price RA Jr, Chen L, Yang J, Fan J, Chen Z, McNeeley S, Xu X and Ma CM (2006) Monte Carlo based IMRT dose verification using MLC log files and R/V outputs. *Medical Physics* **33**(7): 2557–2564.

Marks LB and Ma J (2007) Challenges in the clinical application of advanced technologies to reduce radiation-associated normal tissue injury. *International Journal of Radiation Oncology Biology and Physics* **69**(1): 4–11.

Marcu L and Yeoh E (2009) A review of risk factors and genetic alterations in head & neck carcinogenesis and implications for current and future approaches to treatment. *Journal of Cancer Research and Clinical Oncology* **135**(10): 1303–1314.

Matuszak MM, Yan D, Grills I and Martinez A (2010) Clinical applications of volumetric modulated arc therapy. *International Journal of Radiation Oncology Biology and Physics* **77**(2): 608–616.

Mayo CS, Ding L, Addesa A, Kadish S, Fitzgerald TJ and Moser R (2010) Initial experience with volumetric IMRT (RapidArc) for intracranial stereotactic radiosurgery. *International Journal of Radiation Oncology Biology and Physics* **78**(5): 1457–1466.

McCammon R, Rusthoven KE, Kavanagh B, Newell S et al. (2009) Toxicity assessment of pelvic intensity-modulated radiotherapy with hypofractionated simultaneous integrated boost to prostate for inter-mediate- and high-risk prostate cancer. *International Journal of Radiation Oncology Biology and Physics* **75**(2): 413–420.

Mendenhall WM, Amdur RJ and Palta JR (2006) Intensity-modulated radiotherapy in the standard management of head & neck cancer: promises and pitfalls. *Journal of Clinical Oncology* **24**(17): 2618–2623.

Mohammadi M and Bezak E (2007) Evaluation of MLC leaf positioning using a scanning liquid ionization chamber EPID. *Physics in Medicine and Biology* **52**(1): N21–N33.

Mohan R, Wu Q, Manning M and Schmidt-Ullrich R (2000) Radiobiological considerations in the design of fractionation strategies for intensity-modulated radiation therapy of head & neck cancers. *International Journal of Radiation Oncology Biology and Physics* **46**(3): 619–630.

Mu X, Löfroth PO, Karlsson M and Zackrisson B (2003) The effect of fraction time in intensity modulated radiotherapy: theoretical and experimental evaluation of an optimisation problem. *Radiotherapy and Oncology* **68**(2): 181–187.

Narayana A, Yamada J, Berry S, Shah P et al. (2006) Intensity-modulated radiotherapy in high-grade gliomas: clinical and dosimetric results. *International Journal of Radiation Oncology Biology and Physics* **64**(3): 892–897.

Otto K (2008) Volumetric modulated arc therapy: IMRT in a single gantry arc. *Medical Physics* **35**(1): 310–317.

Pervez N, Small C, MacKenzie M, Yee D et al. (2010) Acute toxicity in high-risk prostate cancer patients treated with androgen suppression and hypofractionated intensity-modulated radiotherapy. *International Journal of Radiation Oncology Biology and Physics* **76**(1): 57–64.

Popescu CC, Olivotto IA, Beckham WA, Ansbacher W et al. (2010) Volumetric modulated arc therapy improves dosimetry and reduces treatment time compared to conventional intensity-modulated radiotherapy for locoregional radiotherapy of left-sided breast cancer and internal mammary nodes. *International Journal of Radiation Oncology Biology and Physics* **76**(1): 287–295.

Proimos BS (1960) Synchronous field shaping in rotational megavoltage therapy. *Radiology* **74**: 753–757.

Purdy J (1996) Defining our goals: volume and dose specification foe 3-D conformal radiation therapy. *Frontiers of Radiation Therapy and Oncology* **29**: 24–30.

Purdy JA (2008) Dose to normal tissues outside the radiation therapy patient's treated volume: a review of different radiation therapy techniques. *Health Physics* **95**(5): 666–676.

Shaffer R, Morris WJ, Moiseenko V, Welsh M *et al.* (2009) Volumetric modulated arc therapy and conventional intensity-modulated radiotherapy for simultaneous maximal intraprostatic boost: a planning comparison study. *Clinical Oncology* **21**(5): 401–407.

Studer G, Huguenin P, Davis BJ, Kunz G *et al.* (2006a) IMRT using simultaneously integrated boost (SIB) in head & neck cancer patients. *Radiation Oncology* **1**: 7.

Studer G, Furrer K, Davis BJ, Stoeckly S *et al.* (2006b) Postoperative IMRT in head & neck cancer. *Radiation Oncology* **1**: 40.

Takahashi S (1965) Conformation radiotherapy. Rotation techniques as applied to radiography and radiotherapy of cancer. *Acta Radiologica: Diagnosis (Stockholm)* **Suppl 242**: 1.

Vanetti E, Clivio A, Nicolini G, Fogliata A *et al.* (2009) Volumetric modulated arc radiotherapy for carcinomas of the oro-pharynx, hypo-pharynx and larynx: a treatment planning comparison with fixed field IMRT. *Radiotherapy and Oncology* **92**(1): 111–117.

Varian Associates, Inc (2001) *Dynalog File Viewer, Reference Guide*. Varian Oncology Systems, Palo Alto, CA.

Verbakel WF, Cuijpers JP, Hoffmans D, Bieker M *et al.* (2009a) Volumetric intensity-modulated arc therapy vs. conventional IMRT in head-and-neck cancer: a comparative planning and dosimetric study. *International Journal of Radiation Oncology Biology and Physics* **74**(1): 252–259.

Verbakel WF, Senan S, Cuijpers JP, Slotman BJ *et al.* (2009b) Rapid delivery of stereotactic radiotherapy for peripheral lung tumors using volumetric intensity-modulated arcs. *Radiotherapy and Oncology* **93**(1): 122–124.

Verellen D and Vanhavere F (1999) Risk assessment of radiation-induced malignancies based on whole-body equivalent dose estimates for IMRT treatment in the head & neck region. *Radiotherapy and Oncology* **53**(3): 199–203.

Webb S (1997) Megavoltage portal imaging, transit dosimetry and tissue compensators. In: *The Physics of Conformal Radiotherapy: Advances in Technology*. 1st edn. Medical Sciences. (Eds R Mould, C Orton, J Spaan *et al.*) pp. 221–249. Institute of Physics Publishing, Bristol.

Weber L and Laursen F (2002) Dosimetric verification of modulated photon fields by means of compensators for a kernel model. *Radiotherapy and Oncology* **62**(1): 87–93.

Williams P (2003) IMRT: delivery techniques and quality assurance. *British Journal of Radiology* **76**: 766–776.

Wong WW, Vora SA, Schild SE, Ezzell GA *et al.* (2009) Radiation dose escalation for localized prostate cancer: intensity-modulated radiotherapy versus permanent transperineal brachytherapy. *Cancer* **115**(23): 5596–5606.

Wright KA, Proimos BS, Trump JG *et al.* (1959) Field shaping and selective protection in megavoltage therapy. *Radiology* **72**: 101.

Wu XR, Yan D, Sharpe MB, Miller B *et al.* (2001) Implementing multiple field delivery for intensity modulation beams. *Medical Physics* **28**(11): 2188–2197.

Wu QJ, Yoo S, Kirkpatrick JP, Thongphiew D *et al.* (2009) Volumetric arc intensity-modulated therapy for spine body radiotherapy: comparison with static intensity-modulated treatment. *International Journal of Radiation Oncology Biology and Physics* **75**(5): 1596–1604.

Xia P, Chuang CF and Verhey LJ (2002) Communication and sampling rate limitations in IMRT delivery with a dynamic multileaf collimator system. *Medical Physics* **29**(3): 412–423.

Yu CX (1995) Intensity-modulated arc therapy with dynamic multileaf collimation: an alternative to tomotherapy. *Physics in Medicine and Biology* **40**(9): 1435–1449.

Zelefsky MJ, Fuks Z, Happersett L, Lee HJ *et al.* (2000) Clinical experience with intensity modulated radiation therapy (IMRT) in prostate cancer. *Radiotherapy and Oncology* **55**(3): 241–249.

Zhang P, Happersett L, Yang Y, Yamada Y *et al.* (2010) Optimization of collimator trajectory in volumetric modulated arc therapy: development and evaluation for paraspinal SBRT. *International Journal of Radiation Oncology Biology and Physics* 77(2): 591–599.

http://www.clinicaltrial.gov/ct2/show/NCT00328575 (accessed on 2/02/2010)

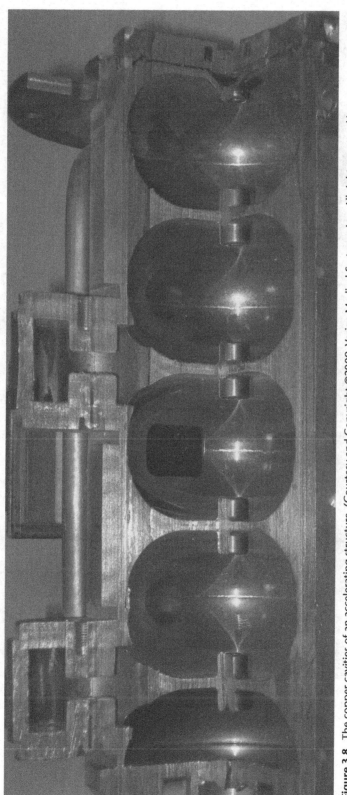

Figure 3.8. The copper cavities of an accelerating structure. (Courtesy and Copyright ©2009, Varian Medical Systems, Inc. All rights reserved.)

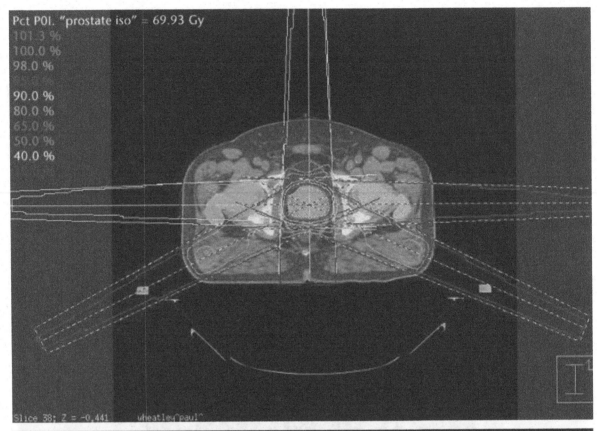

Pct POI. "prostate iso" = 69.93 Gy

101.3 %
100.0 %
98.0 %

90.0 %
80.0 %
65.0 %
50.0 %
40.0 %

Slice 38; Z = -0.441   wheatley^paul"

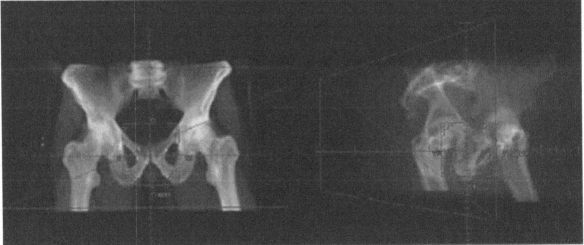

Figure 6.5. A single CT slice (top) showing contoured anatomy and the planning target volume (prostate in yellow) as well as position of the treatment beams and the resulting dose distribution. Digitally reconstructed radiographs (bottom) with corresponding radiation field projections, shaped with multileaf collimators) at a given gantry angle. (Courtesy the Royal Adelaide Hospital)

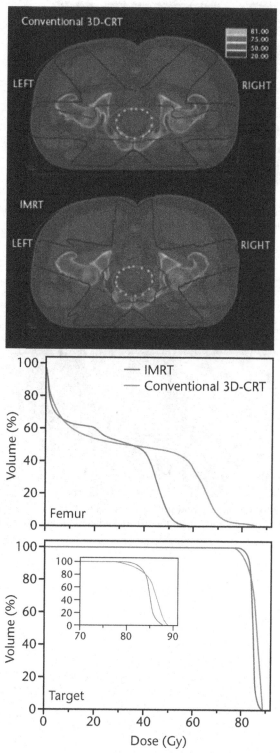

Figure 8.2. Comparison of 3D CRT and IMRT plans for prostate with isodose distribution (top) and dose volume histograms (bottom). The IMRT plan shows improved PTV coverage as well as significant sparing of femoral heads. (Reprinted from Zelefsky *et al*. 2000. Copyright (2000), with permission from Elsevier)

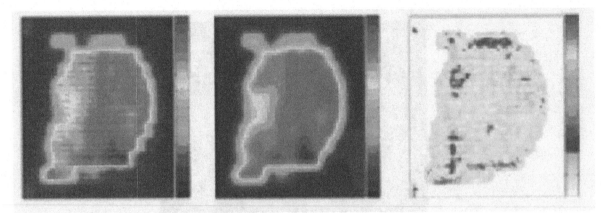

Figure 8.16. Example of measured (using EPID) and calculated dose maps for one IMRT field. A dose difference map is shown on the right (arbitrary units). (Courtesy Royal Adelaide Hospital)

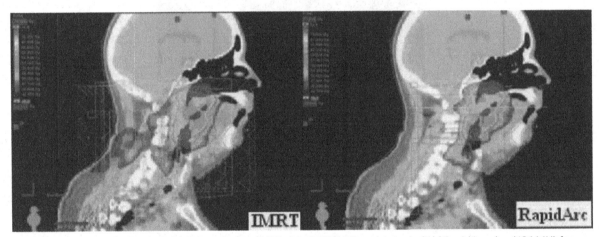

Figure 8.17. Comparison of a 7-field sliding window IMRT plan (1685 MU) and a single-field RapidArc plan (496 MU) for head & neck cancer treatment. (Courtesy and Copyright ©2010, Varian Medical Systems, Inc. All rights reserved.)

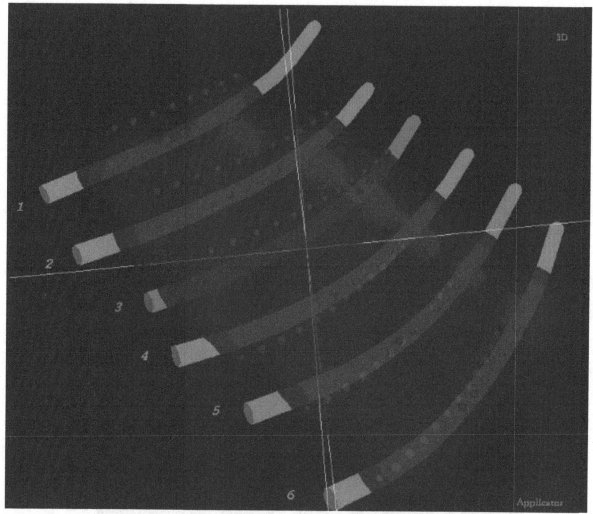

Figure 9.3. A three dimensional dose distribution given by ^{192}Ir in an interstitial head & neck cancer treatment with 6 channels. (Courtesy of Radiation Oncology Department, Royal Adelaide Hospital, Australia)

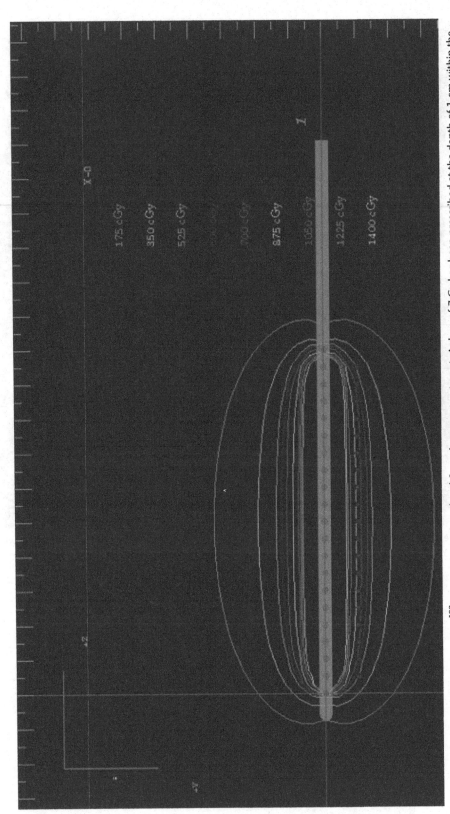

Figure 9.4. Dose distribution given by ^{192}Ir in an intracavitary head & neck cancer treatment. A dose of 7 Gy has been prescribed at the depth of 1 cm within the tissue (red isodose line). (Courtesy of Radiation Oncology Department, Royal Adelaide Hospital, Australia)

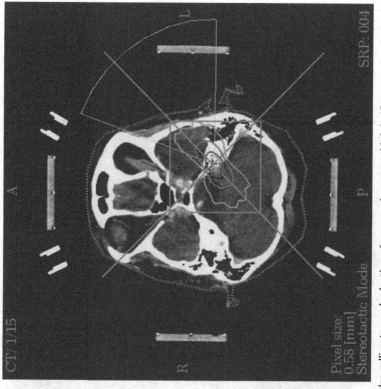

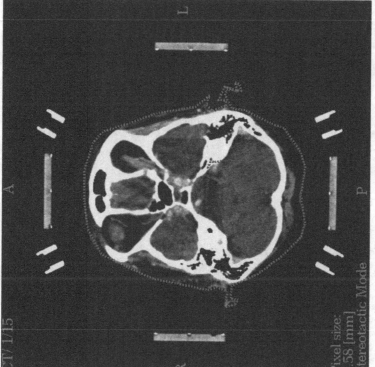

Figure 10.2. Acoustic neuroma: tumour outline (left); dose distribution with a circular collimator and selection of non-coplanar arcs (right). (Courtesy Royal Adelaide Hospital)

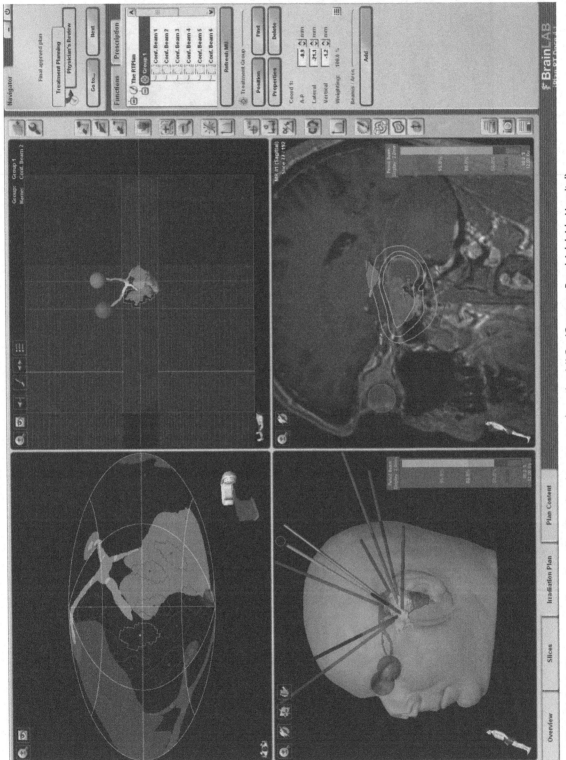

Figure 10.3. Brainlab 3D reconstruction of a patient head and treatment plan using MLCs. (Courtesy Royal Adelaide Hospital)

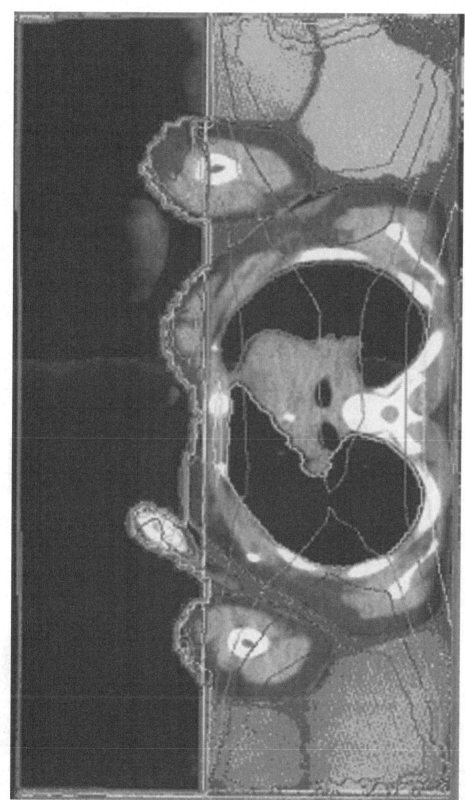

Figure 11.8. TBI treatment plan with isodose lines illustrating the inclusion of lung bolus. The thickness of the bolus can be adjusted until satisfactory lung dose is achieved. (Courtesy Royal Adelaide Hospital)

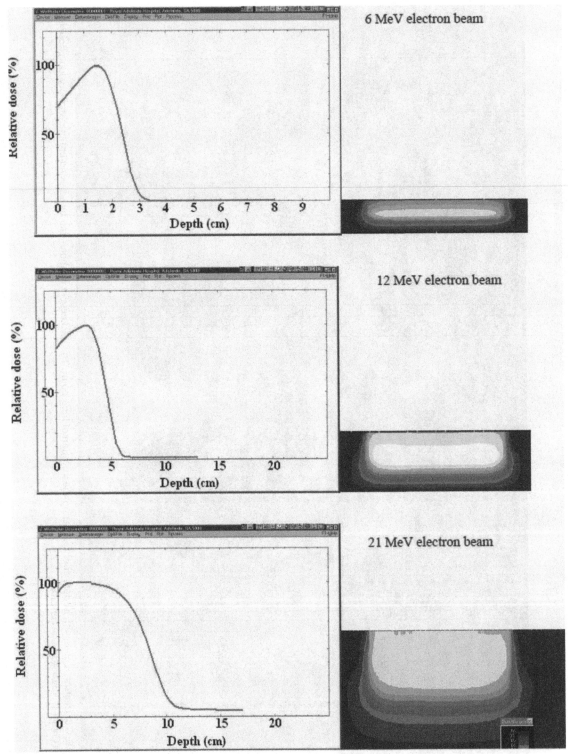

Figure 12.12. Percentage depth dose curves and corresponding isodose distributions for 6, 9 and 21 MeV electron beams produced by a Siemens KD2 accelerator. The phenomena of bulging and constricting of isodose curves can be seen. (Courtesy Royal Adelaide Hospital)

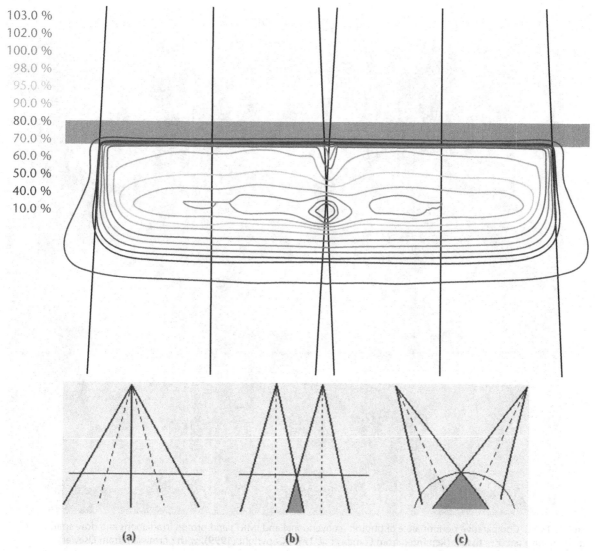

103.0 %
102.0 %
100.0 %
98.0 %
95.0 %
90.0 %
80.0 %
70.0 %
60.0 %
50.0 %
40.0 %
10.0 %

(a)   (b)   (c)

Figure 12.15. Combined isodose distribution from two abutting electron fields (top). Dose hot spot in the overlap between the two fields can be seen (courtesy Royal Adelaide Hospital). Schematic diagram of dose overlap (bottom) depending on the position of the central axes for both beams: a) diverging, b) parallel and c) converging.

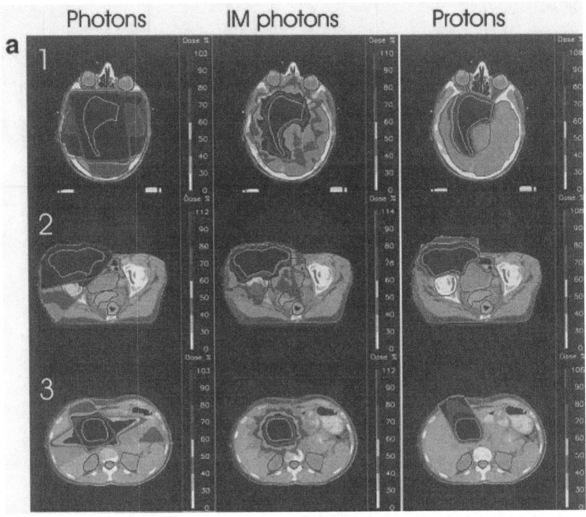

Figure 13.11. Comparative performance of photon (conventional and IMRT) and proton irradiations and dose sparing of dose limiting sensitive tissue. (Reprinted from Lomax *et al.* 1999. Copyright (1999), with permission from Elsevier)

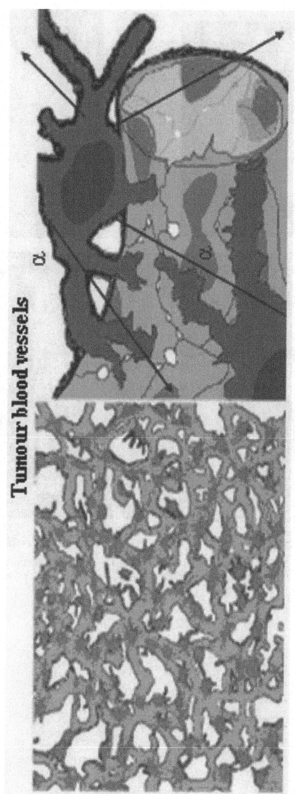

Figure 15.5. Tumour vascular structure, capillary fenestrations and effect of alpha radiation. (Reprinted from Baluk *et al.* 2005. Copyright (2005), with permission from Elsevier)

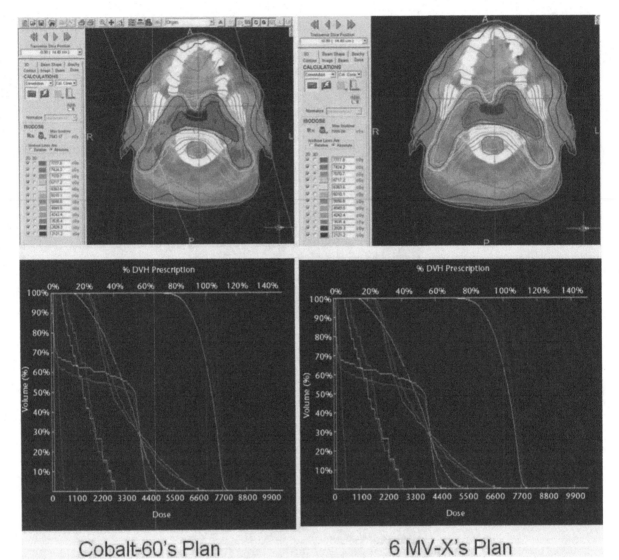

Figure 16.3. Co-60 plan versus 6 MV plan for nasopharynx cancer (9 beam IMRT plan). (Reproduced from Workshop on Palliative Radiotherapy for Developing Countries, Workshop Proceedings, November 2008, editors B. Allen and M. Rahman with permission)

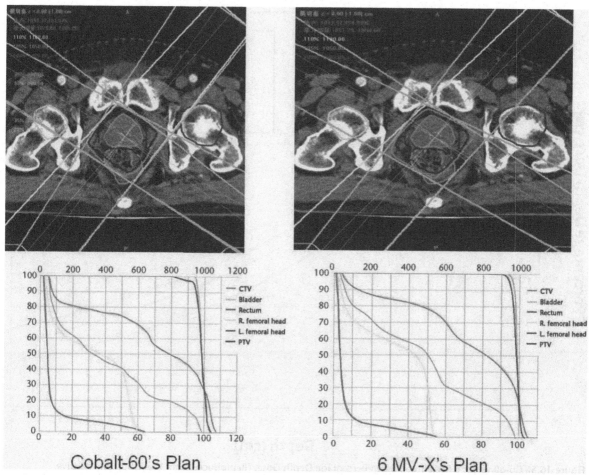

Figure 16.4. Co-60 plan versus 6 MV plan for Prostate Cancer (4 beam 3D-CRT plan). (Reproduced from Workshop on Palliative Radiotherapy for Developing Countries, Workshop Proceedings, November 2008, editors B. Allen and M. Rahman with permission)

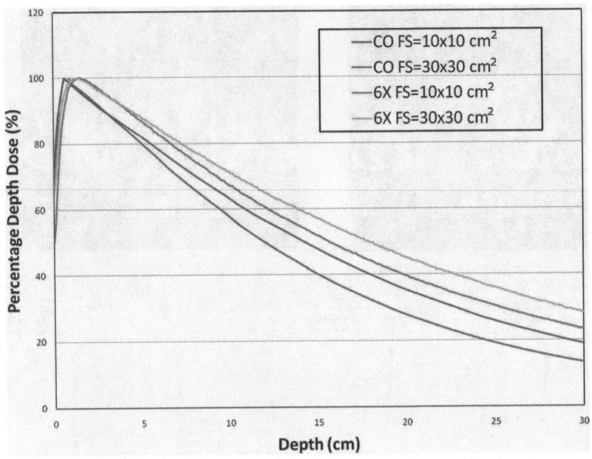

Figure 16.5. Co-60 versus 6 MV Photon Beam Percentage Depth Dose. (Reproduced from Workshop on Palliative Radiotherapy for Developing Countries, Workshop Proceedings, November 2008, editors B. Allen and M. Rahman with permission)

9   Brachytherapy: radiobiology and physics aspects of treatment

9.1   SHORT HISTORY OF BRACHYTHERAPY

Brachytherapy is a terminology used to illustrate short distance treatment ('brachy' originates from Greek and it means short). This type of treatment is also referred to as curietherapy or endocurietherapy. The effect of brachytherapy is timely localised because the radioactive source used for treatment is placed near the tumour and quite often within the tumour mass.

The most popular source employed to treat various cancers in the early days of brachytherapy was Radium-226. Despite its several limitations, radium was used until the 1970s in several countries (Nickers et al. 1997). The fixed shape of the radium source did not allow conformal tumour treatment, a limitation which was overcome with the development of linear accelerators in the 1950s. Another drawback of the radium source was radiation safety-related, namely the heavy lead shielding needed for radioprotection against high energy beams and also the radiation hazard caused by radon-222, one of radium's decay products, today known as the second risk factor, after smoking, for lung cancer.

The very first brachytherapy treatment for cancer was conducted by Goldberg and London, in 1903 (Mould 1995). The patient had a successful therapy for a basal cell carcinoma, and it was immediately followed by another patient treated for the same clinical condition. Brachytherapy treatment in the first three decades of the 20th century was administered without any physics-based dosimetric calculations or dosimetry system. Brachytherapy planning in this period was guided by biological dosimetry, materialised by the amount of radium contained in the source. The early radium plaques used in brachytherapy all had a uniform distribution of radium content, until 1930 when the Manchester System developed by Paterson and Parker brought the knowledge of non-uniform radium content distribution on the plaque in order to achieve a homogenous dose distribution on the skin surface (Meredith 1967). The Paris dosimetric system was developed in the 1960s based on the principle of equidistant parallel linear sources of uniform activity, with the delivered dose being specified along an isodose line (Mould 1995). This dosimetric system is preferred to the Manchester one since today's planning computers allow for computations of volumetric dose distribution for any source arrangement.

The most common treatment site in the early period of brachytherapy, due to its high incidence and also clinical accessibility, was the cervix. The first centres to treat gynaecological cancers were established around

L. Marcu et al., *Biomedical Physics in Radiotherapy for Cancer*,
DOI 10.1007/978-0-85729-733-4_9, © CSIRO 2012

1910 in a few notable locations around the world: Munich (1908), Baltimore (1908), Stockholm (1910) and later in Paris (1919) (Mould 1995). After the successful clinical results obtained with radium as surface applicators or intracavitary sources, it was proposed to use radium for interstitial brachytherapy. Breast, lung, oesophagus and prostate are among the tumour sites treated with interstitial brachytherapy technique. As the scientific community became more aware of the radiation protection issues around radium sources, there were attempts to develop afterloading devices. While the idea of afterloading applicators originates from the 1900s, the first remotely controlled afterloading device was created in the 1960s for gynaecological applications (Henschke et al. 1964; Walstam 1962).

For the prostate gland, the first cases of brachytherapy treatments were reported in 1911 by Pasteau and Degrais (Pasteau 1911; Pasteau and Degrais 1914) who used radium to treat prostate cancer via a transurethral catheter. Other treatments with Ra-226 were reported about the same time by Barringer, who applied the radioisotope insertion technique to deliver radiation to the prostate and bladder (Barringer 1917). These early brachytherapy treatments preceded the use of external beam for the management of prostate carcinoma. Gold-198 in a colloidal form was introduced in the 1950s by Flocks as a post operative treatment for prostate cancer (Flocks et al. 1952). In the 1970s the colloidal gold was replaced by gold seeds used for implantation of the pedicles after radical prostatectomy. Around the same period, Felix Mick has designed iodine pellets encapsulated in titanium tubing using low energy iodine-125 for permanent implant. After I-125 became commercially available, seed implantation with iodine started to gain ground. The first treatment employing I-125 seeds was conducted by Whitmore et al. (1972). His pioneering procedure consisted of a retropubic I-125 implantation into the prostate, a technique that became a standard in prostate brachytherapy for the following 20 years. The first generation of Mick applicators was developed in 1973 to achieve a better control on loose seeds and also to increase radioprotection (Mick Radionuclear Instruments, Mount Vernon, NY).

For head & neck carcinomas, successful treatment reports using surface moulds date back to the 1920s.

For deep seated head & neck cancer interstitial brachytherapy was developed to overcome the side effects of X-ray treatment because much healthy tissue has to be traversed in order to deliver cancericidal doses to the tumour target volume. In 1903, the German physician H. Strebel reported the first interstitial treatment technique with radium (Mould 1995). More sophisticated treatments followed during the second half of the 20th century with the employment of the afterloading applicators in brachytherapy, and high dose rate (HDR) treatments now widely available for intracavitary and interstitial brachytherapy.

While in the 1920s radical mastectomy was the first choice of treatment for women with breast cancer, the poor outcome lead the British physician G. Keynes to initiate a different approach in the management of this malignancy. The pioneering work of Keynes consisted of radium needles inserted into the breast and adjacent lymph nodes achieving excellent outcome (Kuske 1999). Brachytherapy for breast cancer was abandoned over the war and the method was rejuvenated much later but again, with great success.

Ocular malignancies have been treated with radioactive applicators (plaques) since the 1960s. One of the most commonly used radioisotopes for the management of ophthalmic tumours is ruthenium (Ru-106) which was introduced in clinics by Lommatzsch and Vollmar in 1966 (Lommatzsch and Vollmar 1966).

The advances in brachytherapy over the last century are impressive, whether considering the history of radioactive sources, the development of clinical procedures or the evolution of dosimetric systems from biological to physical dosimetry. This chapter presents the main aspects of modern brachytherapy from both physical and radiobiological perspectives as well as treatment methods using brachytherapy techniques for various tumour sites.

9.2 PHYSICAL AND RADIOBIOLOGICAL ASPECTS OF BRACHYTHERAPY

The aim of radiation therapy is to deliver a cancericidal dose to the tumour whilst sparing or limiting damage to the surrounding normal tissue. One of the advantages of brachytherapy over external beam radiotherapy is the limited volume of normal tissue irradiated achieved through the geometrical configuration of the implanted (inserted) source. Not only is tumour dose delivery and the dose distribution superior for brachytherapy versus external beam treatment, but the normal tissue exposure is also reduced when the radioactive source is inserted or implanted into the tumour. The isotropic dose distribution around the source decreases very rapidly in intensity (with the square of the distance from the source). Therefore, while the tumour which is in close contact with the radioisotope receives the full or higher treatment dose resulting in higher cell kill, damage in the surrounding normal tissue is minimised.

9.2.1   Classification of brachytherapy

Brachytherapy can be classified as a function of source placement in the following categories:

- intracavitary (using radioactive sources placed in body cavities close to the tumour);
- intraluminal (using radioactive sources inserted into a lumen, such as oesophagus or bile duct);
- interstitial (either using radioactive sources located within fine needle catheters inserted in the tumour or implanting radioactive seeds directly into the tumour); and
- intravascular (using radioactive sources placed in arteries).

9.2.2   Dose rate classification

There are also three ways of delivering brachytherapy based on the dose-rate of the radioactive source used in the treatment (see Table 9.1), as established by The International Commission on Radiation Units & Measurements (ICRU 38, 1985). High dose rate (HDR) and low dose rate (LDR) brachytherapy are the most commonly used local treatments.

Low dose rate brachytherapy employs sources of low activity and therefore long irradiation times. The prescribed dose is delivered to the patient during several hours or days. A special case of LDR is the permanent interstitial brachytherapy. *High dose rate* brachytherapy involves radionuclides with high activity, leading to short treatment times per fraction. The prescribed total dose is delivered in several fractions, with at least 24 hours interfraction time to allow for

Table 9.1.   Classification of brachytherapy based on dose-rate.

Type of brachytherapy	Dose rate range (Gy/h)
Low dose rate (LDR)	0.4–2
Medium dose rate (MDR)	2–12
High dose rate (HDR)	>12

normal tissue repair. Now, HDR is delivered using modern afterloading machines capable of multichannel treatment. *Medium dose rate* brachytherapy employs sources with activities in between LDR and HDR: thus, treatment times are also reduced compared to LDR (usually a few hours). *Pulsed dose rate* (PDR) brachytherapy is a technique whereby radiation is delivered in pulses, at high dose rates. The radiation pulses are usually delivered for about 10–15 minutes and they are repeated in hourly intervals. This treatment is preferred by those clinicians who would like to obtain the radiobiological effects of a low dose rate therapy delivered with a high dose rate machine (Hall and Brenner 1996). For increased therapeutic ratios the fraction size (pulse duration) and the time interval between fractions can be adjusted for each treatment site. PDR therefore offers therefore a favourable ground for the development of new fractionation schedules in brachytherapy (Polo 2008).

Intracavitary therapy at low dose rate (50 cGy/h) lasts between 1–4 days. When high dose rate is used, the whole dose is delivered within minutes for each of several fractions, in order to spare the surrounding normal tissue. Although late effects on normal tissue are potentially worse with HDR versus LDR brachytherapy, a careful choice of the source, accurate localisation of the catheter and the ability to optimise dose have been used to overcome its potential for increased normal tissue complications. In view of this, HDR brachytherapy is now preferred as it is more convenient for the patient.

When interstitial treatment is applied via LDR brachytherapy, in the majority of cases the radioisotope is inserted permanently into the tumour. Depending on the tumour volume, isotopes with different half-lives are chosen. Iodine 125 is one of the most commonly used isotopes for permanent implant (particularly for prostate cancer) having a 60 days half-life. The LDR brachytherapy gives a cell survival curve similar to an infinite number of small fractions; therefore it is almost ideal as far as the radiobiology of a slowly proliferating tumour, such as prostate cancer, is concerned.

9.2.3 Radioisotopes used in brachytherapy: physical and biological characteristics

There is a large variety of radioactive sources clinically implemented in brachytherapy for the treatment of various tumours whether benign or malignant. The choice for a particular radioisotope is made as a function of treatment type, tumour volume and radiobiological properties, tumour localisation, and the energy, half-life and size of the radionuclide. Table 9.2 presents some physical characteristics of various radioisotopes used in brachytherapy. While the list is far from being exhaustive, the presented radionuclides are those that are the most commonly used, as they fulfil the basic requirements for a source to be employed in brachytherapy:

- the energy of the radioactive source should be high enough to control the tumour but low enough not to require difficult radioprotection measures;
- the half-life of the isotope should be short for permanent implants (a few days) and longer for temporary implants (a few weeks);
- the radionuclide intended for permanent implant should allow for encapsulation to avoid dispersion of the radioactive material; and
- the source should be commercially available at reasonable cost.

The most common sourced used in brachytherapy are gamma emitters (see Table 9.2). However, for specialised treatments, such as ocular malignancies, beta emitting sources in the form of eye plaques are employed. Below is a short description of the physical characteristics and mechanical presentation of the most common isotopes in the history of brachytherapy.

Ruthenium-106 (Ru-106) is a β emitting radioisotope, commonly used as surface applicator in the management of ocular carcinomas. It has recently replaced Sr - 90 as it emits higher energy beta rays. Ruthenium is a transition metal of the platinum group and is obtained as fission product. The most stable of ruthenium radioisotopes is Ru-106, which decays to Rhodium-106:

$$^{106}_{44}\text{Ru} \rightarrow {}^{106}_{45}\text{Rh} + \beta^-$$

Ruthenium is used in the form of a plaque, with a diameter of 12–14 mm, with the active part encapsulated in a silver sheet.

Strontium-90 is also a fission product and is used in brachytherapy for a similar purpose to Ru-106 due to its beta emitting property:

$$^{90}_{38}\text{Sr} \rightarrow {}^{90}_{39}\text{T} + \beta^-$$

The beta energy resulting from strontium decay is too low to be used in brachytherapy. However, the daughter product, Y-90, decays to Zr-90 emitting high-energy betas (2.27 MeV), therefore the nomenclature Sr/Y-90. This radioisotope was also used in intravascular brachytherapy to prevent or treat restenosis.

Table 9.2. Some physical characteristics of the most commonly used radioisotopes in brachytherapy.

Radioisotope			Mean energy (MeV)	Half-life	Half value layer in lead (mm)
HDR	β *emitters*	Ru/Rh – 106	3.54	1.02 y	–
		Sr/Y – 90	2.27	28.7 y	–
	γ *emitters*	Co – 60	1.25	5.26 y	11
		Ra – 226	0.83	1620 y	14
		Cs – 137	0.66	30 y	5.5
		Ir – 192	0.38	73.8 d	3
LDR		Au – 198	0.41	2.7 d	2.5
		I – 125	0.028	60 d	0.02
		Pd – 103	0.021	17 d	0.01

Cobalt-60 is produced in nuclear reactors by bombarding Co-59 with thermal neutrons (nuclear activation):

$$^{59}_{27}\text{Co} + n \rightarrow {}^{60}_{27}\text{Co} + \gamma$$

Co-60 beta decays to Ni-60 with an emission of high energy gamma rays:

$$^{60}_{27}\text{Co} \rightarrow {}^{60}_{28}\text{Ni}^* + \beta^- + \gamma$$

In brachytherapy, Co-60 is used in the form of pellets in remote afterloading devices with a usual activity of 0.5 Ci per pellet.

Radium-226 has a long history in cancer management. Ra-226 and radon-222 were the first and only radioisotopes used in the early days of brachytherapy. Ra-226 is a naturally occurring isotope that decays to Rn-222 by alpha emission:

$$^{226}_{88}\text{Ra} \rightarrow {}^{222}_{86}\text{Rn} + {}^{4}_{2}\alpha + \gamma$$

Ra-226 presents with a complex decay series that end with a stable isotope of Pb-206. The average energy of gamma rays emitted by Ra-226 and its decay products is about 0.8 MeV and the maximum beta energy is 3.26 MeV. Radium sourced are presented in the form of radium salt cells (radium sulphate powder) placed in tubes or needles with platinum walls to absorb unwanted beta rays. The potential damage to the source capsule and the emission of hazardous Rn-222 gas led to the abandonment of Ra-226 in the modern days. This pioneering isotope has only historical significance.

Caesium-137 is a fission product of uranium-238 and it beta decays to Ba-137 with the emission of gamma rays with an average energy of 0.66 MeV:

$$^{137}_{55}\text{Cs} \rightarrow {}^{137}_{56}\text{Ba} + \beta^- + \gamma$$

With a half-life of 30 years and low photon energy, caesium-137 is recommended for low dose rate brachytherapy. It is widely used in the treatment of cervical carcinoma. The radioisotope is usually distributed within a ceramic matrix encapsulated in stainless steel sheaths, to avoid radiochemical hazards. Caesium-137 is available for brachytherapy treatment in various forms, such as needles, pellets or tubes. Another isotope of caesium, Cs-131, is currently used in the form of seeds for permanent prostate implants.

Iridium-192 is produced by the neutron activation of iridium-191 and it decays to platinum-192 via beta decay:

$$^{192}_{77}\text{Ir} \rightarrow {}^{192}_{78}\text{Pt} + \beta^- + \gamma$$

The radiotherapeutic dose comes from photons, which are emitted via Ir-192 decay with an average energy of 0.38 MeV. The average beta energy emitted is 0.2 MeV, which is taken into account for capsule design. For low dose rate brachytherapy, manual implants, Ir-192 is used in the form of a wire with an iridium/platinum alloy core surrounded by a 0.1 mm thick platinum sheath. Ir-192 is also used for HDR brachytherapy: the afterloaders employing specially designed sources. The HDR iridium source is encapsulated in a 5 mm long and 1.1 mm thick stainless steel cylinder and has a usual activity of 10 Ci.

Iridium-192 is probably the most commonly employed radioactive nuclide in high dose rate brachytherapy worldwide.

Gold-198 is produced by the neutron activation of Au-197 and it decays to Mercury-198 by beta emission:

$$^{198}_{79}\text{Au} \rightarrow {}^{198}_{80}\text{Hg} + \beta^- + \gamma$$

The main energy emitted consists of gamma photons with an average energy of 0.41 MeV. Au-198 is mainly presented in a grain/seed form, with the active material being encapsulated in platinum. Due to the medium energy emitted, gold seeds were used for permanent implants, in particular for squamous carcinomas of the head & neck. They were employed in prostate implants as well, but due to the higher energy as compared to Pd-103 or I-125 seeds, Au-198 did not gain wide acceptance.

Iodine-125 is a daughter product of Xenon-125 and it decays by electron capture to Tellurium-125:

$$^{125}_{53}\text{I} + e^- \rightarrow {}^{125}_{52}\text{Te} + \gamma$$

Iodine-125 is manufactured in a seed form that is used preponderantly in permanent prostate implants. The low energy gamma photons (28 keV average energy) and the 60 days half-life make iodine-125 an ideal candidate for permanent interstitial brachytherapy. Consequently, several manufacturers produce I-125 in various seed types. Usually I-125 is absorbed on to a silver rod, which is further encapsulated in a titanium case, but it can also be absorbed on to resin. In the latter, there is need for an X-ray marker to be also incorporated within the capsule. The average length of the I-125 seed is 4.5 mm with a diameter of approximately 0.8 mm.

Palladium-103 is the I-125 competitor for permanent interstitial brachytherapy. Pd-103 can be obtained through the neutron activation of Pd-102 and it decays by electron capture to Rhenium-103:

$$^{103}_{46}Pd + e^- \rightarrow ^{103}_{45}Rh$$

Palladium seeds are manufactured similarly to iodine seeds, by absorbing Pd on to resin beads with two inactive gold beads serving as X-ray markers indicative of source location. Due to the low energies emitted by both Pd-103 and I-125, radioprotection is more easily achieved than with Au-198 seeds; therefore, they are more widely accepted and implemented in clinics worldwide.

9.3   RADIOBIOLOGICAL MODELS IN BRACHYTHERAPY (THE LQ MODEL)

The linear quadratic model applied for fractionated external beam radiotherapy was presented in Chapter 5. It was demonstrated that the Biologically Effective Dose (BED) is the parameter by which different fractionation regimens can be compared. Further, BED is a useful tool when inter-comparing different types of radiation therapy, such as external beam and brachytherapy, or LDR versus HDR brachytherapy. Thus:

$$BED = D\left[1 + \frac{d}{(\alpha/\beta)}\right] = nd\left[1 + \frac{d}{(\alpha/\beta)}\right] \quad (9.1)$$

When tumour repopulation is considered, the above expression of BED becomes (Dale and Deehan 2007):

$$BED = nd\left[1 + \frac{d}{(\alpha/\beta)}\right] - K(T - T_k) \quad (9.2)$$

The parameter K is equivalent to daily BED needed to be delivered in order to compensate for tumour repopulation. Equation (9.2) is a quantitative representation of the LQ model for external beam radiotherapy delivered in 'n' fractions as well as for fractionated high dose rate brachytherapy.

The effectiveness of radiation on proliferating cells is illustrated by the sublethal damage that is created when a radiation-induced single strand break occurs. The sublethal damage (SLD) becomes lethal if a subsequent dose of radiation creates another strand break before the first one has been restored. Therefore, sublethal damage repair can take place if there is sufficient time between consecutive fractions for the DNA to mend the damaged strand. Repair half-times ($T_{1/2}$) for mammalian cells range between 0.5 and 3 hours (Bentzen *et al.* 1999). If it is considered that the repair process is exponential in form then the relationship between the repair rate (μ) and repair half-time can be expressed as (Dale and Deehan 2007):

$$\mu = \frac{\ln 2}{T_{1/2}} \quad (9.3)$$

For low dose rate brachytherapy, when the treatment is administered over a longer period of time (a few days) radiation delivery is considered to be continuous; therefore, there is no possibility for the tumour to repopulate during treatment (or repopulation is negligible). BED for continuous LDR brachytherapy is expressed as a function of cellular repair rate (μ) and dose rate ($R = D/T$):

$$BED = D\left[1 + \frac{2D}{\mu T(\alpha/\beta)}\right] \Leftrightarrow BED = RT\left[1 + \frac{2R}{\mu(\alpha/\beta)}\right]$$
$$(9.4)$$

When employing radioactive seeds for permanent interstitial implant, an important parameter that directly influences the rate of damage is the activity of the source or the physical decay. BED for permanent implants is dependent on the radioactive decay constant (λ) of the radionuclide and the initial dose rate (R_0) (Dale 1985):

$$BED = \frac{R_0}{\lambda}\left[1 + \frac{R_0}{(\mu + \lambda)(\alpha/\beta)}\right] \quad (9.5)$$

It is important to note that all of the above relations for biologically effective doses are specified at single points and they do not consider the influence of high dose gradients that are characteristic for brachytherapy treatment. These models should be used carefully when treatments involving different source geometries are compared.

9.4 DOSE PRESCRIPTION AND DOSE CALCULATION IN BRACHYTHERAPY

The evolution of brachytherapy depended on the expansion of knowledge of the spatial dosimetry and dose distribution of individual radioactive sources as well as of the combined dose distributions of source arrays. Reporting of absorbed dose distributions was minimal in the early days or none at all. The first computer algorithms were developed in 1960s to calculate in 2D the approximate dosimetry of individual sources (point and linear) and to sum doses resulting from arrangement of sources. Source-end effects, medium scatter and attenuation, tissue heterogeneities and shield effects have since all been subject to thorough investigations and are at present modelled using computer calculations. In the latest development, CT/MRI compatible applicators and advances in computational techniques allow for image guided 3D (volume) based treatment planning of dose distributions.

In brachytherapy, the dose distributions are non-homogeneous within the treated volume around a radioactive implant, characterised by steep dose gradients and pockets of high dose surrounding each source. There are also regions of minimum dose between the sources. Prior to availability of computerised dose calculations, several systems have been used over the years to calculate and describe dose distributions of brachytherapy implants, taking into account geometry and the spacing of the source positions and detailing how the dose calculations should be made. In addition, the dose was prescribed according to systems which were linked to a particular applicator design (e.g. for intra-uterine treatments). In these systems as well as in some of the brachytherapy treatment planning models, usually no contours of organs or the patient surface are considered, no inhomogeneity corrections are applied and generally no correction is made for different applicator

materials and shielding incorporated in some applicators. However, clinical experience related to patient outcomes was gained using these systems and modern recommendations originated from them. Some of the commonly used systems are the Manchester system and the Paris system.

9.4.1 Manchester system

The Manchester system is the most commonly used prescription method for brachytherapy of cervical cancer. It was designed by Tod and Meredith in the 1950s (Tod and Meredith 1953) with three objectives in mind:

- Definition of the treatment in terms of dose to a point that is comparable from patient to patient, in a region where the dosage is not very sensitive to small alterations in applicator position and that allows for correlation of the prescribed dose with the clinical effects.
- Design and Development of a set of applicators and determination of their loading using a given amount of radium source, that would give the same dose rate irrespective of the combination of applicators used.
- Design a prescription convention for the activity, relationship and positioning of the radium sources in the uterine tumours and the vaginal ovoids, that will give rise to the desired dose rates.

The concept of the dosage prescription to a single point made this system the most acceptable and widespread brachytherapy technique for the treatment of cervical cancer. A cervix applicator designed (and used with modifications to these days) consists of a central intrauterine tube (tandem) and lateral pods (ovoids or colpostats). The source loading rules were such that the point received the same dose rate regardless of which ovoid and intrauterine combination was used. The prescription point, generally known as point 'A' is located 2 cm lateral to the uterine canal and 2 cm from the mucous membrane of the lateral superior fornix of the vagina in the plane of the uterus. Limiting radiation dose was found to be the dose to the Paracervical Triangle, a region in the medial edge of the broad ligament where uterine vessels cross the urethra. The bladder and rectum were considered critical structures. In order to maintain the sufficient width of the dose distribution, considering sharp lateral dose gradient, reference point 'B' was also defined at a distance of 5 cm from the mid-line and 2 cm up from the mucus membrane of the lateral fornix. The dose at point B is nearly independent of the geometrical distribution of radium sources in the ovoids and intrauterine tandems, but it depends primarily on the total number of the radium sources used.

Currently, the high doserate remote afterloading systems use dwell time optimisation (DTO), which can be used to determine loading of intracavitary applicator and vaginal ovoids optimally to deliver dose to either prescription points or to a target volume. The dose to critical organs (bladder and rectum) can also be reduced using DTO.

9.4.2   Paris system

This is a more recent system of prescribing for interstitial implants. It has been developed by Pierquin *et al.* (1978) and by large replaced some of the older systems like Patterson-Parker or Quimby, that were based on tables of total dose delivered as a function of area or volume to be treated (Podgorsak 2005). The Paris system is designed for single and double plane implants, especially removable/temporary implants of longer line sources, e.g. 192 Ir wires. It is not valid for other types of volume implants. In order to achieve the desired dose distributions, the following set of general rules for the selection and placement of the sources must be adhered to:

- all sources must be linear, positioned in parallel, uniformly spaced, and of equal length, source strength/linear activity;
- the centres of all sources must be located in a single plane (central plane);
- spacing between sources should be wider when using long sources;
- the average of the minimum dose between sources inside implanted volume is called basal dose; and
- dose prescription is based on a reference isodose, fixed at 85% of the basal dose.

If these guidelines are applied, then the whole treated target volume will be encompassed the reference isodose surface. For planar and curved surfaces the basal dose rate is calculated midway between each pair of sources and averaged. For triangular or square source arrangement, the basal dose rates are calculated equidistant from each of the adjacent sources (e.g. in the centre of the square).

9.4.3   Present reporting

With the increased utilisation of brachytherapy irradiation in radiation oncology practice, a need evolved to set up guidelines for the prescription of the treatment dose and the reporting of the delivered dose in brachytherapy. As a result, the International Commission on Radiation Units and Measurements published two reports (No. 38 and No. 58) with the objective to develop a standardised approach for centres around the world and to identify the minimum dosimetric information required to be provided by each facility conducting brachytherapy procedures. *'The intent was to provide a means for specifying dose and volume in a way that can be closely related to the outcome of treatment and that can be generally understood'* (ICRU report no. 58). The reports provide guidelines for the definition of the treated volumes, description of the implants and specification of delivered dose. According to these reports, the reference air kerma rate in air (cGy/h at 1 m) is the recommended quantity for specifying source strength.

9.4.4   Intracavitary treatments

The absorbed dose level of 60 Gy was identified as the appropriate reference dose for LDR gynaecological brachytherapy. If the treatment also includes external beam radiotherapy, the reference isodose for brachytherapy is determined by subtracting the external beam dose from a total dose of 60 Gy. In addition, the dimensions (width, height and thickness) of the pear shaped 60 Gy isodose reference volume need to be specified.

ICRU Report No. 38 recommends the following data for reporting of gynaecological brachytherapy:

- description of the technique (source, applicator)
- the source strength (i.e. total reference air kerma rate)
- description of the reference volume
- the time and dose fractionation pattern

- the dose at reference points (bladder, rectum, paracervical triangle, pelvic wall).

9.4.5   Interstitial treatments

The report provides guidelines for temporary implants, permanent implants, single stationary source line, moving sources and surface applicators. In addition to the total reference air kerma, the high dose regions, the low dose regions, prescription dose (or the mean central dose) and peripheral dose must be evaluated in order to comprehensively characterise the implant procedure. Together with dose volume histograms, these data is essential in estimates of tumour control or normal tissue toxicities. Generally, high dose regions (>150% of the mean central dose) and low dose regions (<90% of the peripheral dose) should be reported.

In summary, ICRU Report No. 58 recommends the following data for reporting of interstitial brachytherapy implants:

- definition of clinical target volumes
- the sources, technique (temporary and permanent implants) and implant time
- the source strength (i.e. the total reference air kerma)
- reference doses in the central plane, mean central dose and peripheral dose
- dose reporting: prescription to a point/surface, prescription dose
- reporting of the high and low dose regions and dose uniformity indices
- dose–volume histograms (DVHs).

9.4.6   Dose calculations

In 1995 the American Association of Physicists in Medicine (AAPM) published the report of Task Group (TG) 43 that had been established to develop a dose calculation formalism to determine 2D dose distributions around cylindrically symmetric sources (AAPM report no. 51, 1995). The American APM TG 43 formalism is considered to be the most complete formalism available today and provides a comprehensive description of brachytherapy dose calculations. Its approach is used in modern computer based Treatment Planning Systems (TPS) and is also suitable as a method for TPS commissioning.

The TG 43 report was revised in 2004. The updated report 'recognised that both the utilisation of permanent source implantation and the number of low-energy interstitial brachytherapy source models commercially available have dramatically increased' (AAPM report 84, 2004). This, in addition to introduction of new primary standard of air-kerma strength provided by national laboratories, plethora of published brachytherapy dosimetry reports, improvement in dosimetry techniques and dosimetric characterisation of particular source models, warranted that the TG-43 protocol for calculation of doserate distributions around photon-emitting brachytherapy sources be updated.

Full details of the mathematical formalism will not be discussed here and can be found in the corresponding AAPM reports as well as in (Glasgow 1998). Briefly, both reports use the 2D doserate equation presented in the 1995 TG-43 protocol. According to this protocol, the dose rate $\dot{D}(r, \theta)$ at the point of interest $P(r, \theta)$ in water due to a line radioactive source in polar coordinate system is then written as:

$$\dot{D}(r, \theta) = S_K \Lambda \frac{G_L(r, \theta)}{G_L(r_0, \theta_0)} g_L(r) F(r, \theta) \qquad (9.6)$$

where r is the distance in cm from the centre of the active source to the point of interest, r_0 is the reference distance (1 cm in this protocol), and θ is the polar angle between the direction to the point-of interest, $P(r, \theta)$, and the source longitudinal axis. The reference angle, θ_0, defines the source transverse plane, and is specified to be 90° or $\pi/2$ radians (see Figure 9.1).

$G(r, \theta)$ is the geometry function, $g(r)$ is the radial dose function and $F(r, \theta)$ is the anisotropy function.

Air-kerma strength, S_K, is the air-kerma rate, $\dot{K}_\delta(d)$, *in vacuo* and due to photons of energy greater than δ, at distance d, multiplied by the square of this distance:

$$S_K = \dot{K}_\delta(d) d^2 \qquad (9.7)$$

The definition of the dose-rate constant in water, Λ, is the ratio of dose rate at the reference position, $P(r_0, \theta_0)$, and S_K:

$$\Lambda = \frac{\dot{D}(r_0, \theta_0)}{S_K} \qquad (9.8)$$

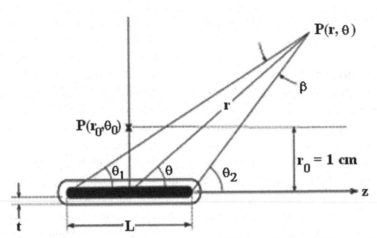

Figure 9.1. Coordinate system used for brachytherapy dosimetry calculations. (Courtesy AAPM report no. 84)

The dose-rate constant depends on both the radio-nuclide and source model, and is influenced by both the source internal design.

The purpose of the geometry function, $G(r, \theta)$, is to improve the accuracy with which dose rates can be calculated by interpolation from data tabulated at discrete points. The geometry function neglects scattering and attenuation, and provides an effective inverse square-law correction. The protocol recommends use of different geometry functions for point- and line-source models. The radial dose function, $g(r)$, accounts for dose fall-off on the transverse-plane due to photon scattering and attenuation and the 2D anisotropy function, $F(r, \theta)$, describes the variation in dose as a function of polar angle relative to the transverse plane.

9.5 BRACHYTHERAPY FOR VARIOUS TUMOUR SITES

9.5.1 Brachytherapy for prostate cancer

The last decade of prostate cancer treatment was a remarkable learning experience for both the scientific and medical communities throughout the world. New concepts such as bystander effects and adaptive response, as well as the push towards hypofractionation have changed the image of prostate treatment significantly. The controversial α/β ratio of prostate tumours debated in the literature led to the vast variety of treatments for this malignancy, such as: conventional external beam therapy; intensity modulated

radiotherapy; three-dimensional conformal radiotherapy; low dose rate (LDR) brachytherapy (permanent implants with either Iodine-125 or Palladium-103 cased in titanium shells) and high dose rate (HDR) brachytherapy with Iridium-192. LDR brachytherapy employing radioactive seeds for permanent implantation and HDR brachytherapy are competitive procedures for localised prostate carcinomas and they will be described below.

A. HDR brachytherapy

The low α/β value(s) indicated by the literature ($\alpha/\beta = 1.5$) (Bentzen and Ritter 2005) makes the prostate more sensitive to dose rate than the rectum ($\alpha/\beta = 6$) or bladder ($\alpha/\beta = 8$). Therefore, higher doses than 2 Gy/fraction could offer a therapeutic advantage. This can be achieved with either external beam radiotherapy or with high dose rate brachytherapy. HDR brachytherapy is administered either as a boost following external beam radiotherapy, usually delivering a 45 Gy dose, or as monotherapy which varies from two to four fractions with an overall dose of 26–36 Gy.

Both HDR and LDR procedures use the transperineal transrectal ultrasound guided approach. The catheters (HDR) or the needles (LDR) are evenly spaced and inserted through a template that is fixed to the perineum. Treatment planning is realised with commercially available softwares and adjustments to the initial plan are achievable before fractions if the scans indicate discrepancies between initial images and subsequent images due to post-implant prostatic

Table 9.3.   Target – Dose Volume Histogram (DVH) requirements.

	Definition	Value
D80	The dose received by 80% of the target volume	>180 Gy
D90	The dose received by 90% of the target volume	>165 Gy
V100	The relative volume to receive 100% of reference dose	≥97%
V150	The relative volume to receive 150% of reference dose	<65%
V200	The relative volume to receive 200% of reference dose	<25%

oedema. HDR dosimetry is based on defined dwell time positions. Treatment plan optimisation is possible for each catheter, even after insertion (but before any radiation is delivered) using either 2.5 or 5 mm dwell positions. Therefore, the possibility of delivering an optimal treatment with HDR is highly achievable.

B. LDR brachytherapy

Low dose rate brachytherapy represented by permanent interstitial implant is the most conformal radiation therapy for the prostate. However, patient selection must be carried out carefully, since pre-treatment factors predict long-term results. For early stage prostate carcinoma, permanent implants of I-125 radioactive seeds are an effective treatment (Grimm and Sylvester 2004). There are three major considerations involved in the selection of patients for permanent seed implantation: the stage of cancer; treatment eligibility; and risk factor/toxicity issues. Once the staging of cancer and the corresponding risk factors are assessed, the next step in the process is the assessment of treatment eligibility. This is determined through the volume study, by measuring the volume of the prostate using a transrectal ultrasound-guided image. A series of transverse ultrasound images of the prostate are taken, which form the basis for organ reconstruction, and later, for planning. The image obtained is used for organ outlining where both target and critical organs are delineated. The eligibility criteria for I-125 implants restrict the volume of the prostate to a value within the range of (20cc–55cc). Patients with larger prostate volumes usually undergo hormone therapy before being reconsidered for the implant.

The aim of brachytherapy is to increase therapeutic ratio by both increasing tumour control and decreasing normal tissue complications, therefore the target constraints are strictly met during planning and implant. Consequently, when 0.4 mCi iodine 125 seeds are used (with a reference dose of 145 Gy), no part of the urethra should receive more than 130% relative dose and the dose to 2cc of rectum should be limited to 110 Gy. Table 9.3 presents various dose volume histogram requirements for the prostate (target) to be met for optimal tumour control.

The implant is completed after the volume study through a template-guided procedure. On average, the number of I-125 seeds implanted during a prostate treatment is around 70 when seeds with 0.4 mCi activity are used (Marcu and Quach 2006) (see Figure 9.2). Usually, one month after the procedure a CT scan of the pelvic area is taken to assess the post-implant dosimetry. Post-implant dosimetry provides feedback on prostate coverage, which correlates with tumour control, on dose to critical organs (rectum, urethra, bladder, penile bulb) correlated with risk of side effects, and on the effects of the implantation technique upon both tumour control and normal tissue toxicity. In other words, the quality of an implant can be assessed by post-implant dosimetry (Stock and Stone 2002). If the dosimetric parameters are not optimal, extra seeds can be implanted to achieve the desired therapeutic ratio.

Another choice for permanent implant in prostate brachytherapy is Pd-103 seeds. While the mean energy emitted by Pd-103 is similar to the mean energy of I-125 (Table 9.2), the half-life of 17 days for Pd-103 gives a higher dose rate than I-125 ($t_{1/2}$ = 60). Consequently, it would be expected that the two treatments would produce different late normal tissue morbidities. This hypothesis was tested by Herstein et al. (2005) and it was observed that patients treated with Pd-103 had more intense radiation prostatitis shortly after implant than patients treated with I-125.

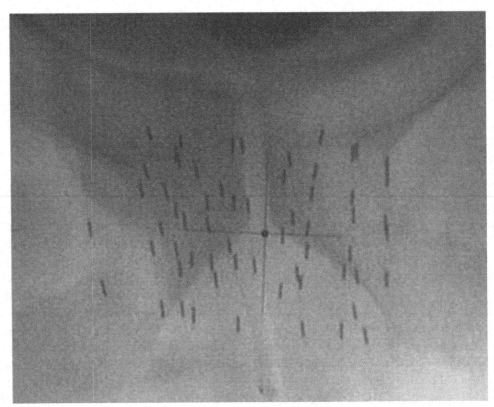

Figure 9.2. Fluoroscopic image of I-125 seeds implanted in the prostate.

However, the recovery after Pd-103 implant also occurred faster, consistent with Pd-103 shorter half-life. Other studies comparing clinical outcome after I-125 and Pd-103 implant concluded that the two radionuclides gave similar tumour response regarding disease-free survival (Wallner *et al.* 2003; Peschel *et al.* 2004). However, normal tissue complication rates were higher for those patients treated with I-125 (Peschel *et al.* 2004). This might also be because while the minimum tumour dose for Pd-103 is 120 Gy, for I-125 implants the reference dose is 145 Gy.

Although first used in 1965 for permanent implants, Cs-131 has not been a commonly applied radionuclide in clinics in the past decades. Recently, with the growing interest in interstitial implants several medical centres are now employing Cs-131 instead of I-125 due to its shorter half-life (10.7 days) reducing the duration of side effects. The photon energy emitted by Cs-131 peaks in the 29–34 keV region. In 2008, the Cesium Advisory Group has established certain recommendations for permanent

prostate brachytherapy with Cs-131 (Bice *et al.* 2008). Since the published literature on the clinical safety of Cs-131 is limited, the group recommends that Cs-131 implant should be performed differently from I-125 or Pd-103. The source should be placed further from the urethra and rectum, V150 for the prostate should be kept ≤45 Gy and sufficient margins should be left by limiting seed placement to the capsule. In addition, the prescribed dose for monotherapy should be 115 Gy and when delivered as a boost to external beam should not be more than 85 Gy. There is need for clinical trials to establish the role of Cs-131 in the management of prostate cancer and to rank its efficacy among the other radionuclides used for the same purpose.

LDR versus HDR for prostate brachytherapy

The LDR gives a cell survival curve similar to an infinite number of small fractions, therefore it is almost ideal as far as radiobiology is concerned. The great advantage of the infinite number of small fractions in the treatment of prostate cancers delivered via LDR is to offer a better organ sparing compared to external beam, when organs at risk receive the same dose as the tumour. For example, the urethra receives 2 Gy dose with each fraction during external beam treatment, while with LDR, the radioactive seeds are inserted further from the urethra, keeping strict dose constraints for this organ.

The latest studies on the α/β ratio of the prostate showed that, unlike other tumours with a α/β ratio of around 10 Gy, prostate cancers present with an unusually small value, of about 1.5 Gy. This would make the tumour more responsive to hypofractionated treatment than to hyperfractionated regimen. Therefore, HDR brachytherapy, which is the equivalent of hypofractionated radiotherapy, should lead to a higher therapeutic ratio than LDR. In addition, HDR in the management of localised prostate cancer offers some practical and physical advantages over LDR (Koukourakis *et al.* 2009):

- There are no free (or loose) radioisotopes during the procedure.
- There is no risk of seed movement within the prostate gland or seed loss during or after implant.
- After patient discharge there are no radioprotection issues as the patients leave free of radioactive isotopes.
- There is no intraoperative radiation exposure to the personnel.
- It is a cost effective procedure, since many clinical centres already have an HDR theatre with an iridium afterloading machine to treat other-than-prostate tumour sites.
- Besides the prostate gland it is possible to place catheters in the extra-prostatic tissue, allowing for the treatment of more advanced cases.
- HDR provides a greater dosimetric accuracy than LDR.

More randomised studies are still needed to investigate the effectiveness of one or the other brachytherapy treatment.

9.5.2 Brachytherapy for head & neck cancers

The vast majority of squamous cell carcinomas of the head & neck are difficult to manage clinically due to their location in relation to critical organs, advanced status when detected, high hypoxic content and rapid regrowth during treatment. The clinical literature published in recent decades has shown that high doses are needed to achieve loco-regional control. Furthermore, while external beam radiotherapy can deliver high doses to the tumour, the sparing of the surrounding normal tissue is very difficult. Consequently, head & neck cancers can benefit from brachytherapy as the dose is delivered locally via radionuclides with rapid fall-off, leading to better organ sparing.

Brachytherapy can be delivered as a sole treatment, as a local boost after external beam therapy or as complementary treatment to surgery. Irrespective of the treatment choice, the overall treatment time should be as short as reasonably achievable to overcome tumour repopulation. Ideally, a combined radiation therapy for head & neck carcinomas (external beam + brachytherapy) should be completed within 8 weeks (Mazeron *et al.* 2009).

Brachytherapy for head & neck cancers is delivered either intracavitary or interstitially. In interstitial implants, the catheters are inserted through tumour tissue and its vicinity to encompass any microscopic extensions. The most common sites treated with interstitial implants are the following: lip, tongue, floor of mouth, tonsil, cheek, soft palate and neck nodes (see Figure 9.3 on p. 213).

With intracavitary treatment, the catheters are inserted into the oral or nasal cavities to reach the tumour (see Figure 9.4 on p. 214). For head & neck cancers, intracavitary treatment is less common than interstitial implant.

Brachytherapy in head & neck cancers therefore offers several advantages over other modalities of treatment:

- local tumour control as good as from external radiotherapy if not better is achieved with appropriate case selection
- better preservation of the structure and function of the treated organ
- avoidance of surgical disfigurement
- better sparing of critical structures situated in the proximity of the treated area, such as brain, spinal cord and eyes from unwanted radiation dose

- potential of HDR brachytherapy to salvage in patients with previously irradiated tumours where no further external radiation can be given

- potential for overcoming radioresistance of hypoxic cells in advanced head & neck cancers through delivery of high doses of radiation locally

- potential for overcoming accelerated repopulation, another characteristic of head & neck cancers, through the use of HDR brachytherapy.

While interstitial brachytherapy for head & neck carcinomas is considered a highly effective treatment, especially due to the better sparing of the normal tissue and the very conformal radiation delivery, randomised trials are needed to confirm the advantage of brachytherapy over external beam radiotherapy, which employs an altered fractionation schedule.

9.5.3 Brachytherapy for breast cancer – MammoSite

Breast Conserving Therapy (BCT) involving Accelerated Partial Breast Irradiation (APBI) is currently being used as an alternative treatment method to mastectomy for patients with early stage breast cancer (Baglan et al. 2001; Lawenda 2003). One form of APBI uses a traditional interstitial brachytherapy implant technique (Athas et al. 2000; Baglan et al. 2001; King et al. 2000; Perera et al. 1997; Polgar et al. 2002; Vicini et al. 1997, 1998, 1999a, 2001, 2002; Wazer et al. 2002), enabling the delivery of a large dose per fraction to a limited portion of breast tissue adjacent to the lumpectomy cavity in a shorter treatment time. However, interstitial brachytherapy is not trivial to deliver and only provided by a limited number of cancer centres (Fentiman et al. 1996; Kestin et al. 2000; Vicini et al. 1999b). Moreover, the treatment planning with this technique is time-consuming and needs experienced staff (Major et al. 2006).

In response, a new approach of breast brachytherapy technique has been developed recently (Edmundson et al. 2002). This technique uses the so-called MammoSite brachytherapy system (Hologic, Inc., Bedford, MA, USA) as a sole radiation treatment for patients with early stage breast cancer following lumpectomy. It consists of a small balloon connected to a catheter with an inflation channel and a catheter for the passage of a high dose rate brachytherapy source (Ir-192) shown in

Figure 9.5. The device is placed in the lumpectomy cavity during or following breast surgery (Edmundson et al. 2002). The MammoSite balloon is inflated with the sterile saline with a small amount of radiographic contrast to a size that both completely fills the cavity and ensures conformance of the tissue to the balloon (Borg et al. 2007; Dickler et al. 2004). A Computed Tomography (CT) scan is obtained to assess the balloon conformance to the lumpectomy cavity and to determine the distance from the surface of the balloon to the skin, the symmetry, diameter of the inflated balloon, the planning target volume and the dose distribution (Edmundson et al. 2002), see Figure 9.6. If used as monotherapy, the treatment with the MammoSite device is generally 34 Gy delivered in 10 fractions (3.4 Gy/fraction twice daily) at 1.0 cm from the balloon surface with minimum of 6 hours between fractions on the same day (Edmundson et al. 2002; Weed et al. 2005). There are recommendations regarding the patient selection criteria for the MammoSite treatment. Generally, the MammoSite is used for treatment of patients diagnosed with ductal carcinoma in situ (DCIS), invasive ductal carcinoma (IDC) and a primary tumour of size $\leq$ 3 cm.

The MammoSite brachytherapy device has been commercially available since 2002. The first published study on the use of the MammoSite demonstrated that both device insertion and performance are simple and efficient (Edmundson et al. 2002). Recently, Borg et al. (2007) reported that the treatment planning time with this device may be decreased to 25 minutes. Other advantages of the MammoSite technique include better dose homogeneity, sparing of normal tissues, less radiation exposure to the staff and potential reduction in acute and late side effects.

In the past five years a number of publications investigated various aspects of MammoSite treatment. A few studies have investigated the volume of breast tissue treated with the MammoSite applicator in comparison with interstitial brachytherapy and external beam radiotherapy techniques. Recently, clinical results have appeared reporting the cosmetic outcome of patients who were treated with the MammoSite as a sole radiation method.

Several publications have evaluated the dosimetry achieved with the MammoSite technique (Major et al. 2006; Edmundson et al. 2002; Dickler et al. 2004;

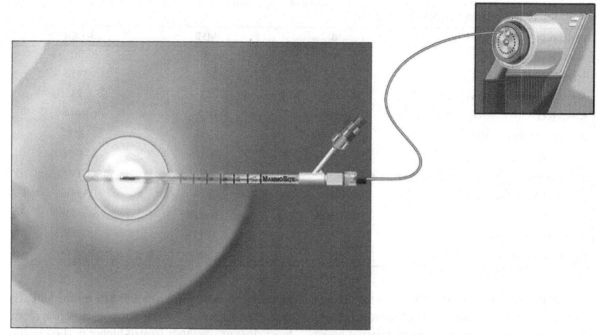

Figure 9.5. MammoSite® Radiation Therapy System. (Courtesy of Hologic, Inc., MA, USA)

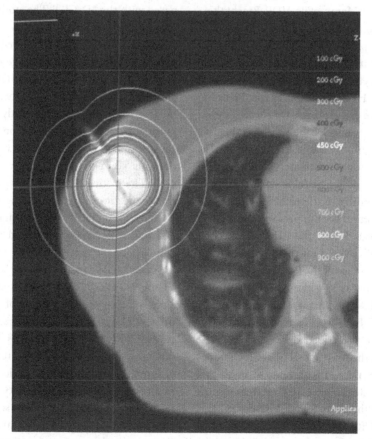

Figure 9.6. Example of a calculated dose distribution for mammosite brachytherapy. (Courtesy Royal Adelaide Hospital)

Table 9.4. Patient characteristics including total dose, volume of lumpectomy cavity, volume of ipsilateral breast, volume of ipsilateral lung and heart volume (Weed *et al.* 2005).

Variables	IB	MSB	3D-CRT
Number of patients	10	10	10
Total dose (cGy)	3200	3400	3850
Average lumpectomy cavity (cc)	38	53	24
Range (cc)	5–101	37–70	8–44
Average PTV volume (cc)	192	107	237
Range (cc)	97–357	83–125	104–380
PTV expansion (cm)	1.5	1	1 + CTV (1.5)
Average breast volume (cc)	1920	1628	1568
Range (cc)	1059–2654	1147–2729	633–2569
Average lung volume (cc)	1116	1404	1355
Average heart volume (cc)	563	568	584

Khan *et al.* 2006). Weed *et al.* (2005) reported the first single-institutional dosimetric comparison of patients treated with three forms of accelerated partial breast irradiation techniques: Interstitial High Dose Rate Brachtherapy (IB), the MammoSite HDR Brachytherapy (MSB) and 3D Conformal Radiation Therapy (3D-CRT). The 3D-CRT plans were performed using 3D planning system, Pinnacle 6.0. For the MammoSite and interstitial brachytherapy patients, the plans were generated using the HDR Plato Nucletron Planning System. Dose Volume Histograms (DVHs) were used to evaluate the dose coverage of the PTV and the normal structures including the ipsilateral breast, ipsilateral lung, and heart for all patients. A summary of patient information is shown in Table 9.4. Coverage of the PTV varied according to the technique used and the margin drawn around the lumpectomy cavity.

The results indicated that the 3D-CRT method offered the best PTV coverage of the three treatment techniques. The percentage of the PTV receiving 100% of the prescribed dose was 58% in the IB method compared with 76% and 94% with the MSB and 3D-CRT techniques respectively. The percentage of the PTV receiving 90% of the prescribed dose was 68%, 91% and 100% for the IB, the MSB and 3D-CRT techniques respectively. Furthermore, the results showed that both brachytherapy techniques delivered a significantly lower dose to the normal breast tissue, as compared with the 3D-CRT. For example, the percentage volume of the ipsilateral breast receiving 100% of the

prescribed dose was 5%, 10% and 24% for the MSB, IB and 3D-CRT patients, respectively. However, both brachytherapy methods treated higher portion of the breast volume above 115% of the prescribed dose compared with the 3D-CRT. The study concluded that the MammoSite device consistently provided better dose coverage of the PTV as compared to IB. However, the 3D-CRT offered better coverage of the PTV in comparison to either of the brachytherapy techniques. However, this resulted in a higher dose to the normal breast tissues and lung. The study highlighted that the optimal partial breast irradiation technique is a clinical decision. The shortcoming of the study is that it does not compare dosimetry in identical patient data sets. The patients representing the three different treatment groups were different which can make the dosimetric comparison less straightforward.

Khan *et al.* (2006) presented results of dosimetric comparison of three different methods of PBI: the MSB, 3D-CRT and Intensity Modulated Radiation Therapy (IMRT). The results of the study are summarised in Table 9.5. The volume of the PTV was smaller in MSB plans than in 3D-CRT and IMRT plans. The study highlighted that both 3D-CRT and IMRT methods have the advantage of not requiring a placement of foreign object inside the patient. However, the difficulty of identifying the cavity in certain patients, respiratory motion and patient set-up are of the main concerns when using 3D-CRT and IMRT techniques. Conversely, these issues are not significant with the

Table 9.5. Summary of dosimetric comparison (Khan *et al.* 2006).

Variables	MSB	3DCRT	IMRT
PTV volume (cc)	94.3	184.3	184.3
V_{110} (%)	84.2	0.99	0.8
V_{100} (%)	94.9	92.3	93.7
V_{95} (%)	97.9	910.9	910.9
V_{90} (%)	910.3	910.9	100.0
Ipsilateral breast V_{50} (%)	210.2	55.8	46.2
Ipsilateral lung V_{30} (%)	5.4	6.7	1.9
Heart V_5 (%)	11.6	4.1	1.2

use of the MammoSite device. The study concluded that the choice of optimal PBI method is complex and requires both doctor decision and patient selection.

Balloon contrast concentration

Once in place, The MammoSite device is inflated to a size that would fill the surgical cavity using saline and an amount of radiographic contrast. A computed tomography scans are obtained and the treatment plan is developed. At present, the commercially available brachytherapy treatment planning systems (for example, Plato and Nucletron) perform dosimetry calculations according to the recommendations of the AAPM TG-43 protocol (Nath *et al.* 1995). The dosimetry is based the assumption that the high dose rate brachytherapy source is located in water medium. As the contrast medium contains elements with high atomic number (iodine with Z=53), the balloon is no longer equivalent to tissue or water. Thus, the treatment planning system does not accurately predict the effect of the radiographic contrast medium inside the balloon on the prescribed dose.

Several studies have investigated the effects of radiographic contrast on the delivered dose in the MammoSite breast brachytherapy technique. Mitra *et al.* (2003) investigated the dose perturbation due to the contrast medium of various concentrations ranging from 5–25%. The study found that 25% contrast concentration produces up to 6% in dose perturbation at the surface of the balloon as compared to balloon filled with saline only. It was also found from this study that the brachytherapy planning system (Plato) predicts about 9% higher dose near the balloon surface compared with measured values. This is because

of the lack of inhomogeneity corrections in brachytherapy planning system. Ye *et al.* (2004) used Monte Carlo (MC) simulations to evaluate dose errors in the MammoSite balloon due to various contrast concentrations. The results showed that a 25% contrast concentration in the balloon resulted in up to 5% dose reduction at the surface of the balloon. The study concluded that the effect of contrast medium attenuation can be taken into account by increasing the dwell time in clinical practice.

MammoSite and cosmetic outcomes

The important factors for achieving optimal cosmetic results are balloon cavity conformance and skin-to-balloon surface distance. The conformance of the balloon to the cavity is essential for accurate dosimetry. As the dose with the MammoSite brachytherapy applicator is prescribed at 1 cm from the balloon surface, if the cavity is within that distance, the skin will be exposed to at least the prescribed dose. A minimum distance of 5 mm was chosen to keep the skin dose less than 150% of the prescribed dose (Keisch *et al.* 2003; Dragun *et al.* 2007). However, recent publications have reported that a balloon-to-skin distance of larger than 7 mm is recommended to optimise the probability of excellent cosmetic results (Niehoff *et al.* 2006; Dragun *et al.* 2007). Dragun *et al.* (2007) reported excellent cosmetic results in 68.9%, good in 21.1%, fair in 8.9% and poor in 1.1% of 100 patients treated with the MammoSite device at a median fellow up of 2 years. No breast tumour recurrence was reported. Overall, the excellent cosmetic results were associated with a balloon to skin distance larger than 7 mm.

Summary

The endpoint of the MammoSite treatment technique as with any other radiotherapy, modality is to achieve high tumour control probability and minimal normal tissue complications. Existing clinical findings have demonstrated highly acceptable outcomes with the MammoSite breast brachytherapy device regarding tumour control, acute complications and cosmetic results. The data coming from the presented clinical trials with an average follow up of 16 months have neither reported tumour recurrence nor normal tissue complications among the treated patients. This indicates that smaller PTV coverage in MammoSite brachytherapy does not represent a significant reduction in the treatment outcomes while offering better patient comfort (shorter treatment time) and cosmesis.

9.5.4 Brachytherapy for gynaecological malignancies

One of the primary applications of brachytherapy is the treatment of gynaecological cancers, often applied as a boost to the external beam radiotherapy. Traditionally, for cervical cancer the treatment is performed as intracavitary brachytherapy using tandem ovoid applicators, tandem rings, moulds, or vaginal cylinders with intrauterine tubes. Several prescription methods have been developed but in most cases, a typical pear-shaped dose distribution is achieved when the intravaginal and intrauterine applicators and sources are applied.

However, for patients with extensive pelvic and/or vaginal disease interstitial brachytherapy, using interstitial implants/needles, is required to improve local control. This technique might also be used when a patient's anatomy does not allow for intracavitary treatment with standard applicators. The radiation dose can be planned in such a way that a better coverage of the planning target volume is achieved that is at the same time conformal to the patient anatomy. Initially, interstitial implants were performed with free-hand placement of radioactive needles containing radium, cobalt or iridium sources/wires. With the recent development of transperineal and transvaginal templates, a more accurate needle positioning can be achieved and when combined with the current imaging techniques including transrectal ultrasound, computed tomography, fluoroscopy

and others, 3D planning and even live planning (tracking the actual needle insertion and updating the dose distribution accordingly) are possible.

A combined intracavitary and interstitial brachytherapy applicator, known as Vienna Ring Applicator Set (tandem/ring applicator), has been developed recently for larger cervical tumours (Kirisits *et al.* 2006). This CT/MR applicator makes use of a ring with nine holes (see Figure 9.7) which is also used as a template for interstitial titanium needles, so it offers a dual solution for both intracavitary and interstitial techniques. The interstitial needles can be inserted directly into the tumour spread (for example, in the parametria). Depending on the individual patient, different lengths of the pre-bent titanium needles are available.

Treatment planning can still be based on X-ray simulation but at present, there is a move towards using 3D CT/MRI image sets. The dose distribution is calculated and optimised according to prescribed dose at fixed dose points, target dimensions, and tolerance doses to organs at risk (OARs) (Dimopoulos *et al.* 2006). The final dose distribution is always limited by OARs (the anterior bladder wall, the posterior rectal wall, and the sigmoid/intestines proximal to the vaginal part of the applicator). The 3D imaging approach allows for better dose optimisation resulting in better target coverage, increases in treated volume and total dose plausible without increasing the dose to critical structures.

The feasibility study of the Vienna group (Dimopoulos *et al.* 2006) showed that a combined intracavitary and interstitial brachytherapy treatment using the Vienna Ring Applicator in conjunction with MRI based treatment planning is feasible, safe, accurate and reproducible, resulting in appropriate target coverage in combination with low side effects. The improvement gained by using interstitial needles is not limited to extension of the treated volume but also allows for dose shaping in case of unfavourable topography, where a standard dose distribution leads to high exposure for bladder or rectum, but the lateral extension remains within 20 mm from the tandem axis.

9.5.5 Ophthalmic brachytherapy (eye plaques)

Brachytherapy and external irradiation are widely employed in the management of ophthalmic tumours

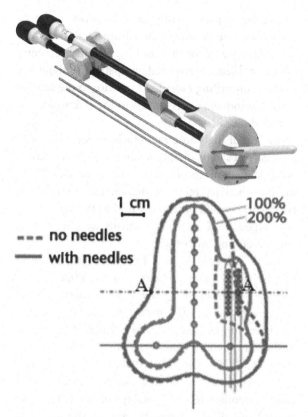

Figure 9.7. The new interstitial/intracavitary applicator for gynaecological brachytherapy and an example of typical dose distribution. (Reproduced with the kind permission of Nucletron, the Netherlands)

daughter product, rhodium (Rh-106) emits high energy beta rays (3.54 MeV) used in ophthalmic implants to treat small and medium sized ocular tumours (with a width of about 5 mm). The advantage of using Ru/Rh-106 for ocular applicators is the rapid dose fall-off and reduced risk of cataract formation. The eye plaque consists of a thin Ru-106 film, which is encapsulated within a sheet of silver, with a total thickness of the plaque of 1 mm. Due to its long half-life, the plaque is reused several times during a year, after sterilisation. The spherical shape of the plaque allows comfortable handling while the minimal side scatter and the backing of the plaque offers radioprotection as it absorbs about 95% of the emitted beta radiation.

In a uveal melanoma treatment study conducted by Georgopoulos *et al.* (2003), the authors reported on tumour regression as a result of one of the three radiotherapy treatments employed: Ru-106, stereotactic radiotherapy with gamma knife or linear accelerators. They concluded that brachytherapy with Ru-106 resulted in a faster tumour regression than with external radiation and, additionally, they observed an increased internal reflectivity, which is an important indicator of a successful treatment. A representative study conducted by Shields and colleagues (Shields *et al.* 2002) on 354 patients with large uveal melanomas (>8 mm) indicated that plaque radiotherapy employing Ru-106 resulted in tumour control at 10 years in 87% of the patients. The effectiveness of Ru-106 in ophthalmic brachytherapy has led to its popularity among other radioisotopes.

Strontium is another radionuclide that contributes towards brachytherapy treatments. While it has a long half-life of 27.8 years (Table 9.2), it emits only low-energy beta particles (546 keV). Conversely, the daughter product of Sr-90 is yttrium (Y-90) and emits high-energy beta particles (2.27 MeV), having a short half-life of 64 hours. Since the activity of Y-90 is maintained by the decay of Sr-90, the short half-life enabled the use of Sr/Y-90 as components of ophthalmic applicators. Attention is always paid to Sr/Y dosimetry as dose-rate measurements from these sources are complex. Several papers reported on dosimetric measurements of beta-ray ophthalmic applicators. Soares *et al.* (2001) undertook a study in which they compared

and inflammatory disease. Brachytherapy is used either as a standalone treatment or as a boost to radiation therapy. One of the greatest advantages of brachytherapy is the highly conformal localisation of the treatment which implies reduced normal tissue damage. Precise localisation of radiation is crucial, particularly with ophthalmic malignancies that generally are surrounded by several critical organs. Radioactive applicators (eye plaques) are generally used for the treatment of retinoblastoma, melanoma of the iris and uveal melanoma.

The most common radioisotopes employed for the treatment of ocular pathologies are Ru-106 and Sr/Y-90. Ru-106 is one of the 9 (known) radioisotopes of ruthenium that are successfully used in clinics due to their physical properties. Ru-106 is formed in the fission of uranium-235 and has a half-life of 1.02 years. It decays via low-energy beta emission however, its

different dosimetry measurement methods employed internationally, such as: radiochromic film; thermoluminescence dosimeters (TLDs); alanine pellets; plastic scintillators; extrapolation ionisation chambers; a small fixed-volume ionisation chambers, a diode detector; and a diamond detector. Their findings indicated that the above listed methods led to consistent absolute dosimetry results at the level of one standard deviation when measurements were determined at 1 mm from the source surface in water.

In the last few decades, palladium-103 seeds have found their role in the treatment of intraocular malignant melanomas as well. A clinical study comparing the effectiveness of Pd-103 and I-125 in both tumour control and normal tissue toxicity showed that the lower energy photons generated by Pd-103 were more rapidly absorbed in the tissue than the photons originating from I-125 and they were less likely to reach critical structures within the treated area (Finger *et al.* 1993). The same group has undertaken a 7-year follow-up of a phase I clinical trial for patients treated with Pd-103 plaque radiation therapy for macular degeneration (Finger *et al.* 2003). Patients were treated with a mean radiation dose of 17.62 Gy over 34 hours. The results showed no sight limiting radiation complications during the follow-up period, illustrating the efficacy of Pd-103 in ophthalmic brachytherapy.

9.6   RADIATION PROTECTION AND QUALITY ASSURANCE

The medical use of radioactive material is subject to national codes of practice in each country and generally, a quality management program needs to be established at each brachytherapy facility to satisfy radiation protection regulations. A Medical Physicist is usually in charge of the development of such a program.

Everyone involved in brachytherapy procedures will work with radioactive sources and as such should be trained in the principles of radiation safety. Protective measures should always be in place to keep the doses as low as practically achievable (ALARA). Appropriate protocols must be in place for source storage, manipulation, disposal and transport as well as for patient care while undergoing brachytherapy. Different radiation safety rules will apply for manu-

ally loaded or permanently loaded sources compared to remote afterloaders, that eliminate unnecessary radiation dose to hospital staff (e.g. a nurse can enter the room whenever required by a patient, without any worries concerning radiation exposure, as the sources will be automatically retracted to the safe inside the afterloader unit).

In case of high dose rate brachytherapy, the need for rigorous safety, quality assurance (QA) and treatment delivery protocols is even more pressing due to the high activity of the radiation sources used, as emergencies could potentially lead to the high radiation exposure of staff and patients in a very short amount of time (minutes).

Good reference sources for quality assurance in brachytherapy include: *Code of practice for brachytherapy physics: Report of the AAPM Radiation Therapy Committee Task Group No. 56* and *High dose-rate brachytherapy treatment delivery: Report of the AAPM Radiation Therapy Committee Task Group No. 59* (Nath *et al.* 1995; Kubo *et al.* 1998).

In accordance with these internationally recognised recommendations, suitably qualified and experienced Medical Physicists are responsible for ensuring that the high dose rate unit is used safely, that it functions correctly prior to any treatment on any treatment day, and for taking a leading role in the recovery of the radioactive source should control of it be lost. The Medical Physicist attending the HDR procedure must ensure that all of the required safety equipment is present and functional prior to the first treatment on any treatment day. The Medical Physicist will also ensure that the QA procedure has been completed and a certified record is available showing that the unit is in a state that it can be safely used. A sample of a possible pre-treatment QA tests is provided in Appendix A1.

A treatment should not proceed unless the Radiation Oncologist, Radiation Therapist and Medical Physicist have signed the pre-treatment form. In signing the form these persons take joint responsibility for ensuring: a) the correct person is about to receive treatment; b) the plan made on the planning computer will deliver the intended prescription; c) the dwell times and positions printed on the pre-treatment form are identical (within the limit of rounding error) to the dwell times and position of the computer plan; and d) the catheters are connected to the respective channels on the after loader.

A source calibration, in terms of dose rate or exposure rate, must be performed as part of the commissioning process before the first medical use of the brachytherapy unit and then following a source change or any major repair. For example, an iridium-192 source is typically replaced four times per annum in order to keep dose rates and treatment times at a reasonable level. That means that the source calibration should be performed at least four times a year.

For brachytherapy, the independent check of the dose calculation (for example, source dwell times) is desired, but there is no generally recommended method for this. Physicists may develop their own spreadsheets; however, some commercial products are now appearing on the market (for example, Radcalc, LifeLine Software inc, TX, USA), that can perform HDR, LDR, and permanent implant calculations, import plans via DICOM RT, visualise sources in 3D, and create a treatment schedule.

The Prescribing Radiation Oncologist, the Radiation Therapist and the Medical Physicist must be present for the duration of the HDR exposure. It is of primary importance that all personnel have practised the Emergency Procedure in the previous 6 months. The expiry date of their Emergency Practice Certification should be recorded. Emergency training covers the proper response to a radiation emergency, for example, the failure of the source to be retracted into the afterloader safely at the completion of treatment.

During exposure, the Medical Physicist, who generally fulfils the role of a Radiation Safety Officer, will ensure that each person who is expected to be involved in the potential emergency procedure to regain control of the source is given an electronic direct reading dosimeter. The attending physicist needs to remain vigilant during treatment to ensure that the unit is behaving normally, keeping constant note of the channel and position of the source, so that in the event of the loss of control of the source, the Medical Physicist (with the added information from the Error Message on the Screen) will know where to expect the uncontrolled source to be. In this way, the Medical Physicist will be in a position to be able to ensure that the recovery procedure will be achieved in minimal time, and will result in minimal dosage to all concerned.

Under normal circumstances, immediately after a treatment is complete, the Medical Physicist must ensure that no radiation hazard exists before allowing medical, therapy and nursing staff into the room to tend the patient.

9.7   REFERENCES

AAPM Report No. 51, Nath R, Anderson LL, Luxton G, Weaver KA, Williamson JF and Meigooni AS (1995) Dosimetry of interstitial brachytherapy source, report of AAPM Radiation Therapy Committee Task Group 43. *Medical Physics* **22**(2): 209–234.

AAPM Report No. 84, Rivard MJ, Coursey BM, DeWerd LA,. Hanson WF, Huq MS, Ibbott GS, Mitch MG, Nath R and Williamson JF (2004) Update of AAPM Task Group No. 43 Report: a revised AAPM protocol for brachytherapy dose calculations. *Medical Physics* **31**(3): 633–642.

Athas WF, Adams-Cameron M, Hunt WC, Amir-Fazli A and Key CR (2000) Travel distance to radiation therapy and receipt of radiotherapy following breast-conserving surgery. *Journal of the National Cancer Institute* **92**(3): 269–271.

Baglan KL, Martinez AA, Frazier RC, Kini VR, Kestin LL, Chen PY *et al.* (2001) The use of high-dose-rate brachytherapy alone after lumpectomy in patients with early-stage breast cancer treated with breast-conserving therapy. *International Journal of Radiation Oncology Biology Physics* **50**(4): 1003–1011.

Barringer B (1917) Radium in the treatment of carcinoma of the bladder and prostate: review of one year's work. *Journal of the American Medical Association* **68**: 1227–1230.

Bentzen SM, Saunders MI and Dische S (1999) Repair halftimes estimated from observations of treatment-related morbidity after CHART or conventional radiotherapy in head & neck cancer. *Radiotherapy and Oncology* **53**(3): 219–226.

Bentzen S and Ritter M (2005) The α/β ratio for prostate cancer: what is it, really? *Radiotherapy and Oncology* **76**: 1–3.

Bice WS, Prestidge BR, Kurtzman SM, Beriwal S *et al.* (2008) Recommendations for permanent prostate brachytherapy with (131)Cs: a consensus report from the Cesium Advisory Group. *Brachytherapy* 7: 290–296.

Borg M, Yeoh E, Bochner M, Butters J, Van Doorn T, Farshid G *et al.* (2007) Feasibility study on the MammoSite in early-stage breast cancer: initial experience. *Australasian Radiology* **51**(1): 53–61.

Dale R (1985) The application of the linear quadratic theory to fractionated and protracted radiotherapy. *British Journal of Radiology* **58**: 515–528.

Dale R and Deehan C (2007) Brachytherapy. In: *Radiobiological Modelling in Radiation Oncology*. (Eds R Dale and B Jones) pp. 113–137. The British Institute of Radiology, London.

Dickler A, Kirk M, Choo J, His WC, Chu J, Dowlatshahi K *et al.* (2004) Treatment volume and dose optimization of MammoSite breast brachytherapy applicator. *International Journal of Radiation Oncology Biology Physics* **59**(2): 469–474.

Dimopoulos J, Kirisits C, Petric P, Georg P, Lang S, Berger D and Pötter R (2006) The Vienna Ring Applicator for combined intracavitary and interstitial brachytherapy of cervical cancer: clinical feasibility and preliminary results. *International Journal of Radiation Oncology Biology Physics* **66**(1): 83–90.

Dragun AE, Harper JL, Jenrette JM, Sinha D and Cole DJ (2007) Predictors of cosmetic outcome following MammoSite breast brachytherapy: a single-institution experience of 100 patients with two years of follow-up. *International Journal of Radiation Oncology Biology Physics* **68**(2): 354–358.

Edmundson GK, Vicini FA, Chen PY, Mitchell C and Martinez AA (2002) Dosimetric characteristics of the MammoSite RTS, a new breast brachytherapy applicator. *International Journal of Radiation Oncology Biology Physics* **52**(4): 1132–1139.

Fentiman IS, Poole C, Tong D, Winter PJ, Gregory WM, Mayles HM *et al.* (1996) Inadequacy of iridium implant as sole radiation treatment for operable breast cancer. *European Journal of Cancer* **32A**: 608–611.

Finger PT, Lu D, Buffa A, DeBlasio D and Bosworth J (1993) Palladium-103 versus iodine-125 for ophthalmic plaque radiotherapy. *International Journal of Radiation Oncology Biology Physics* **27**: 849–854.

Finger PT, Gelman YP, Berson AM and Szechter A (2003) Palladium-103 plaque radiation therapy for macular degeneration: results of a 7 year study. *British Journal of Ophthalmology* **87**: 1497–1503.

Flocks R, Kerr D, Elkins H and Culp D (1952) Treatment of carcinoma of the prostate by interstitial radiation with radioactive gold 198: a preliminary report. *Journal of Urology* **68**: 510–522.

Georgopoulos M, Zehetmayer M, Ruhswurm I, Toma-Bstaendig S *et al.* (2003) Tumour regression of uveal melanoma after Ruthenium-106 brachytherapy or stereotactic radiotherapy with gamma knife or linear accelerator. *Ophthalmologica* **217**: 315–319.

Glasgow GP (1998) Isodose planning: brachytherapy. In: *Treatment Planning in Radiation Oncology*. (Eds FM Khan and RA Potish) pp. 243–280. Williams and Wilkins, Baltimore, USA.

Grimm P and Sylvester J (2004) Advances in brachytherapy. *Reviews in Urology* **6**: S37–S48.

Hall EJ and Brenner DJ (1996) Pulsed dose rate brachytherapy: can we take advantage of new technology? *International Journal of Radiation Oncology Biology Physics* **34**: 511–512.

Henschke UK, Hilaris BS and Mahan DG (1964) Remote afterloading with intracavitary applicators. *Radiology* **83**: 344.

Herstein A, Wallner K, Merrick G, Mitsuyama H, Armstrong J, True L *et al.* (2005) I-125 versus Pd-103 for low-risk prostate cancer: long-term morbidity outcomes from a prospective randomized multicenter controlled trial. *Cancer* **11**: 385–389.

International Commission on Radiation Units and Measurements (ICRU) report 38 (1985) 'Dose and volume specification for reporting intracavitary therapy in gynecology'. International Commission on Radiation Units and Measurements, Bethesda, Maryland, USA.

International Commission on Radiation Units and Measurements (ICRU) report 58 (1998) 'Dose and volume specification for reporting interstitial brachytherapy'. International Commission on Radiation Units and Measurements, Bethesda, Maryland, USA.

Keisch M, Vicini F, Kuske RR, Hebert M, White J, Quiet C *et al.* (2003) Initial clinical experience with the MammoSite breast brachytherapy applicator in women with early-stage breast cancer treated with breast-conserving therapy. *International Journal of Radiation Oncology Biology Physics* 55: 289–293, 2003.

Kestin LL, Jaffray DA, Edmundson GK, Martinez AA, Wong JW, Kini VR *et al.* (2000) Improving the dosimetric coverage of interstitial high-dose-rate breast implants. *International Journal of Radiation Oncology Biology Physics* 46: 35–43.

Khan FM and Potish RA (1998) *Treatment Planning in Radiation Oncology.* Williams and Wilkins, Baltimore, USA.

Khan AJ, Kirk MC, Mehta PS, Seif NS, Griem KL, Bernard DA *et al.* (2006) A dosimetric comparison of three-dimensional conformal, intensity-modulated radiation therapy, and MammoSite partial-breast irradiation. *Brachytherapy* 5(3): 183–188.

King TA, Bolton JS, Kuske RR, Fuhrman GM, Scroggins TG and Jiang XZ (2000) Long-term results of wide-field brachytherapy as the sole method of radiation therapy after segmental mastectomy for T(is,1,2) breast cancer. *American Journal of Surgery* 180(4): 299–304.

Kirisits C, Lang S, Dimopoulos J, Berger D, Georg D and Pötter R (2006) The Vienna applicator for combined intracavitary and interstitial brachytherapy of cervical cancer: design, application, treatment planning, and dosimetric results. *International Journal of Radiation Oncology Biology Physics* 65(2): 624–630.

Koukourakis G, Kelekis N, Armonis V and Kouloulias V (2009) Brachytherapy for prostate cancer: a systematic review. *Advances in Urology*, 327945, doi:10.1155/2009/32.

Kubo HD, Glasgow GP, Pethel TD, Thomadsen BR and Williamson JF (1998) High dose brachytherapy treatment delivery: report of the AAPM radiation therapy committee task group No 510. *Medical Physics* 25: 375–403.

Kuske R (1999) Breast brachytherapy. *Hematology/Oncology Clinics of North America* 13: 543–558.

Lawenda BD, Taghian AG, Kachinic LA, Hamdi H, Smith BL, Gadd MA *et al.* (2003) Dose-volume analysis of radiotherapy for T1N0 invasive breast cancer treated by local excision and partial breast irradiation by low-dose-rate interstitial implant. *International Journal of Radiation Oncology Biology Physics* 56(3): 671–680.

Lommatzsch P and Vollmar R (1966) [A new way in the conservative therapy of intraocular tumors by means of beta-irradiation (Ruthenium-106)][Article in German]. *Klinische Monatsblätter für* **Augenheilkunde** 148: 682–699.

Major T, Niehoff P, Kovacs G, Fodor J and Polgar C (2006) Dosimetric comparisons between high dose rate interstitial and MammoSite balloon brachytherapy for breast cancer. *Radiotherapy and Oncology* 79(3): 321–328.

Marcu L and Quach K (2006) The role of post-implant dosimetry in the quality assessment of prostate cancer. The RAH experience. *Australasian Physical and Engineering Sciences in Medicine* 29: 310–314.

Mazeron JJ, Ardiet JM, Haie-Meder C, Kovacs Gy *et al.* (2009) GEC-ESTRO recommendations for brachytherapy for head & neck squamous cell carcinomas. *Radiotherapy and Oncology* 91: 150–156.

Meredith WJ (Ed.) (1967) *Radium Dosage: The Manchester System.* 2nd edn. Livingstone, Edinburgh.

Mitra RC, Cheng C and Das I (2003) Dose perturbation due to contrast medium in MammoSite: Dosimetric investigation of dose calculation accuracy. *Medical Physics* 30: 1388.

Mould RF (1995) *A Century of X-rays and Radioactivity in Medicine.* 2nd edn. Institute of Physics Publishing, Bristol.

Nath R, Anderson LL, Luxton G, Weaver KA, Williamson JF and Meigooni AS (1995) Dosimetry of interstitial brachytherapy sources: recommendations of the AAPM Radiation Therapy Committee Task Group No. 43. American Association of Physicists in Medicine. *Medical Physics* 22(2): 209–234.

Nickers P, Kunkler I and Scalliet P (1997) Modern brachytherapy: current state and future prospects. *European Journal of Cancer* 33: 1747, 1751.

Niehoff P, Polgar C, Ostertag H, Major T, Sulyok Z, Kimmig B *et al.* (2006) Clinical experience with the MammoSite radiation therapy system for brachytherapy of breast cancer: results from an international phase II trial. *Radiotherapy and Oncology* **79**(3): 316–320.

Pasteau O (1911) Traitment du cancer de la prostate par le Radium. *Rev. Malad. Nutr.* 363–367.

Pasteau O and Degrais P (1914) The radium treatment of cancer of the prostate. *Arch Roentgen Ray* **18**: 396–410.

Perera F, Engel J, Holliday R, Scott L, Girotti M, Girvan D *et al.* (1997) Local resection and brachytherapy confined to the lumpectomy site for early breast cancer: a pilot study. *Journal of Surgical Oncology* **65**(4): 263–267.

Peschel R, Colberg JW, Chen Z, Nath R and Wilson L (2004) Iodine 125 versus palladium 103 implants for prostate cancer: clinical outcomes and complications. *Cancer* **10**: 170–174.

Pierquin B, Dutreix A, Paine CH, Chassagne D, Marinello G and Ash D (1978) The Paris system in interstitial radiation therapy. *Acta Oncologica* **17**(1): 33–48.

Podgorsak EB (Ed.) (2005) *Review of Radiation Oncology Physics: A Handbook for Teachers and Students*. Chapter 13. International Atomic Energy Agency, Vienna, Austria.

Polgar C, Sulyok Z, Fodor J, Orosz Z, Major T, Takacsi-Nagy Z *et al.* (2002) Sole brachytherapy of the tumor bed after conservative surgery for T1 breast cancer: five-year results of a phase I-II study and initial findings of a randomized phase III trial. *Journal of Surgical Oncology* **80**(3): 121–128.

Polo A (2008) Pulsed dose rate brachytherapy. *Clinical Translational Oncology* **10**: 324–333.

Shields CL, Naseripour M, Cater J, Shields JA *et al.* (2002) Plaque radiotherapy for large posterior uveal melanomas (> or =8-mm thick) in 354 consecutive patients. *Ophthalmology* **109**: 1838–1849.

Soares CG, Vynckier S, Järvinen H, Cross WG *et al.* (2001) Dosimetry of beta-ray ophthalmic applicators: comparison of different measurement methods. *Medical Physics* **28**: 1373–1384.

Stock R and Stone N (2002) Importance of post-implant dosimetry in permanent prostate brachytherapy. *European Urology* **41**: 434–439.

Tod M and Meredith W (1953) Treatment of cancer of the cervix uteri – a revised 'Manchester method'. *British Journal of Radiology* **26**: 252–257.

Vicini FA, Horwitz EM, Lacerna MD, Dmuchowski CF, Brown DM, White J *et al.* (1997) Long-term outcome with interstitial brachytherapy in the management of patients with early-stage breast cancer treated with breast-conserving therapy. *International Journal of Radiation Oncology Biology Physics* **37**(4): 845–852.

Vicini FA, Jaffray DA, Horwitz EM, Edmundson GK, DeBiose DA, Kini VR *et al.* (1998) Implementation of 3D-virtual brachytherapy in the management of breast cancer: a description of a new method of interstitial brachytherapy. *International Journal of Radiation Oncology Biology Physics* **40**(3): 629–635.

Vicini F, Kini VR, Chen P, Horwitz E, Gustafson G, Benitez P *et al.* (1999a) Irradiation of the tumor bed alone after lumpectomy in selected patients with early-stage breast cancer treated with breast conserving therapy. *Journal of Surgical Oncology* **70**(1): 33–40.

Vicini FA, Kestin LL, Edmundson GK, Jaffray DA, Wong JW, Kini VR *et al.* (1999b) Dose-volume analysis for quality assurance of interstitial brachytherapy for breast cancer. *International Journal of Radiation Oncology Biology Physics* **45**: 803–810.

Vicini FA, Baglan KL, Kestin LL, Mitchell C, Chen PY, Frazier RC *et al.* (2001) Accelerated treatment of breast cancer. *Journal of Clinical Oncology* **19**(7): 1993–2001.

Vicini F, Baglan K, Kestin L, Chen P, Edmundson G and Martinez A (2002) The emerging role of brachytherapy in the management of patients with breast cancer. *Seminars in Radiation Oncology* **12**(1): 31–39.

Wallner K, Merrick G, True L, Sutlief S, Cavanagh W and Butler W (2003) 125I versus 103Pd for low-risk prostate cancer: preliminary PSA outcomes from a prospective randomized multicenter trial. *International Journal of Radiation Oncology Biology Physics* **57**: 1297–1303.

Walstam R (1962) Remotely-controlled afterloading radiotherapy apparatus. *Physics in Medicine and Biology* **7**: 225.

Wazer DE, Berle L, Graham R, Chung M, Rothschild J, Graves T *et al.* (2002) Preliminary results of a phase I/II study of HDR brachytherapy alone for T1/T2 breast cancer. *International Journal of Radiation Oncology Biology Physics* **53**(4): 889–897.

Weed DW, Edmundson GK, Vicini FA, Chen PY and Martinez AA (2005) Accelerated partial breast irradiation: a dosimetric comparison of three different techniques. *Brachytherapy* **4**(2): 121–129.

Whitmore WF, Hilaris B and Grabstald H (1972) Retropubic implantation of iodine-125 in the treatment of prostate cancer. *Journal of Urology* **108**: 918–920.

Ye SJ, Brezovich IA, Shen S and Kim S (2004) Dose errors due to inhomogeneities in balloon catheter brachytherapy for breast cancer. *International Journal of Radiation Oncology Biology Physics* **60**(2): 672–677.

APPENDIX A1

Treatment Day Quality Assurance Procedure on HDR Brachytherapy Unit

One day prior to the treatment the following Q.A. shall be performed

Date _____   Treatment Day Date _____

Check of Activity

(1a)   Record the current Activity from System Information   _____Ci

(1b)   Calculated activity today (from print-out, half life = 73.83 days)   _____Ci. Decay Factor(DF) _____

(1c)   Agreement within 1%   Pass ☐   Fail ☐

Connect Well Chamber (do not lock indexer yet), call standard plan 'QA CONSTANCY, WELL CHAMBER' to deliver 5 Gy.

Measure Pressure _____   Temperature _____

$$PT = \frac{1013}{P} \cdot \frac{273.15 + T}{293.15} = \underline{\hspace{3cm}}$$

In treatment mode, set up for a treatment and try to initiate the exposure with everything correct BUT:

(2)   key in OFF position in HDR unit   Treatment does not Start   Pass ☐   Fail ☐

(3)   Door open   Treatment does not Start   Pass ☐   Fail ☐

(4)   Indexer is not locked on a Catheter   Treatment does not Start   Pass ☐   Fail ☐

(5)   Key in 'Standby' position in Console   Treatment does not Start   Pass ☐   Fail ☐

With Afterloader idle (ie not treating)...

(6)   Press STOP on Console 'Emergency Stop' window comes up and treatment stops   **Pass** ☐   **Fail** ☐

(6a)   'Reset' is needed to complete the treatment   **Pass** ☐   **Fail** ☐

Initiate a treatment, check the time of the second dwell using a stop watch, and then make interruptions during the following active dwell positions

(7a)   Dwell time set _____ secs.   Dwell time actual _____ secs.   **Pass** ☐   **Fail** ☐

Press INTERRUPT on Console: Active returns, system reports interruption   **Pass** ☐   **Fail** ☐

Initiate a treatment With the Well Chamber connected. (Electrometer at +100%, charge).

Reading _____, PT corrected: _____

Calibrated at source replacement _____ (difference <2%)   **Pass** ☐   **Fail** ☐

Check 'check cable' distance readout by comparing with the reading on the ruler   **Pass** ☐   **Fail** ☐

Check 'check cable retraction' on **Power Fail** situation (wall socket)   **Pass** ☐   **Fail** ☐

Check that emergency light is working: **Pass** ☐   **Fail** ☐

Treatment should not start unless the HDR Console and Afterloader Unit pass all of the above tests.

Signature of person doing the Tests _____

Pre-Treatment Safety Equipment Check on HDR Brachytherapy Unit

Check that the following Equipment is present and in proper working order.

(1)   In room radiation monitor   present ☐   working ☐
        reading _____ counts

(2)   Door radiation monitor   present ☐   working ☐
        reading _____ counts

(3)   Hand held monitor   present ☐   working ☐
        reading on top of Unit _____ μSv/hr

(4)   C.C. Television   Unit 1   present ☐   working ☐
                                   Unit 2   present ☐   working ☐

(5)   3 personal monitors for:
      Oncologist/Registrar   present ☐   working ☐   zeroed ☐

      Medical Physicist   present ☐   working ☐   zeroed ☐

      Medical Physicist   present ☐   working ☐   zeroed ☐

(6)   Safety Screen   present ☐   working ☐

(7)   Wire cutters   present ☐

(8)   Long forceps   present ☐

(9)   Emergency container   present ☐

      installed in front of HDR unit (lid open)   ☐

(10) Intercom   present ☐   working ☐

(11) Paper in Printer   present ☐

Date _____   Checked by _____

10 Stereotactic radiosurgery: radiobiology and physics aspects of treatment

10.1 INTRODUCTION

Stereotactic radiosurgery (SRS) is the treatment involving a precise delivery of a single, high dose of radiation in a one-day session. This therapy is usually limited to the brain and also head & neck area, because of the possibility for immobilisation with devices that completely restrict the head's movement, permitting therefore a highly precise and accurate treatment. Stereotactic radiosurgery often implies a single high precision fraction of high dose radiation (typically 12–24 Gy in a one day treatment and even up to 140 Gy for radiosurgical thalamotomy) delivered to a target localised in three dimensions (3D) based on CT and/or MRI imaging (Sahgal 2009). Stereotactic radiotherapy (SRT) is a fractionated stereotactic radiation treatment delivered in a fractionated manner, over a period of days or weeks. The treatment is delivered with the assistance of removable masks and frames with a lesser degree of immobilisation than SRS.

The term radiosurgery was coined in 1951 by the Swedish neurosurgeon Lars Leksell (Leksell 1951) with the procedure being initially designed for the treatment of benign brain lesions and functional disorders (Sven-nilson et al. 1960; Leksell et al. 1972). Most of Leksell's pioneering work was centred on the isotope-based Gamma knife unit, rather than particle accelerators. However, the limited availability of the Gamma Knife restricted radiosurgery to only a few institutions in the world until the mid 1980s. A more widespread application of radiosurgery consisted of the linac-based units with several radiotherapy centres around the world purchasing the required hardware and software to upgrade their linacs and making them equipped for radiosurgery. New generation linear accelerators designed for image-guided radiotherapy have been specifically adapted for radiosurgery treatments and there has been increasing interest in applying this procedure not only for benign conditions but also for small malignant lesions, either primary or brain metastases.

The most common sites treated in radiotherapy clinics with SRS/SRT are the following:

- Arteriovenous malformations (AVM)
- Benign brain tumours:
  - Acoustic neuromas
  - Meningiomas
  - Pituitary tumours

L. Marcu et al., *Biomedical Physics in Radiotherapy for Cancer*,
DOI 10.1007/978-0-85729-733-4_10, © CSIRO 2012

Table 10.1.   Estimated acute and late neurological toxicity after radiosurgery (RTOG 90-05 report).

Diameter of the lesion	Maximum tolerated dose	Total toxicity (acute + late)
<20 mm	24 Gy	16%
21–30 mm	18 Gy	21%
31–40 mm	15 Gy	22%

- Malignant brain tumours:
  - Astrocytomas
  - Gliomas
- Metastatic brain tumours
- Functional disorders:
  - Trigeminal neuralgia
  - Parkinson's
  - Epilepsy

Lately, radiosurgery is also being used to treat cancer in other parts of the body in a procedure called stereotactic body radiotherapy (SBRT), such as lung and spinal cord. Rapid advances in imaging and computer technologies in the last decade have resulted in development of a variety of different radiosurgery techniques and their wider applications. Currently, linac-based radiosurgery, the Gamma Knife, the CyberKnife robotic arm and proton beam therapy represent the main radiosurgery systems implemented into clinical use.

10.2   TREATMENT PLANNING AND DOSE PRESCRIPTION

Very important aspects of treatment planning and delivery in radiosurgery or stereotactic radiotherapy are target dose conformity and the effect of dose inhomogeneity inside the target volume on treatment outcome. While hot spots within a well-defined target area do not, usually, lead to normal tissue sequelae,

dose inhomogeneity with high dose areas will increase complications in a poorly delineated treatment volume. Most linac-based radiosurgeries prescribe treatment dose to 80% isodose lines whereas Gamma Knife users traditionally treat with the 50% isodose as the treatment volume, enabling multiple isocentre treatment plans with a sharp dose fall-off outside this isodose line (Flickinger 2002).

Dose selection in radiosurgery also imposes a therapeutic challenge, as larger doses which usually result in a better tumour control lead to higher normal tissue complication rates. Finding the optimal TCP/NTCP ratio as well as the appropriate patient selection are key factors influencing treatment outcome.

When treating large lesions (>35 mm) the radiation gradient into surrounding normal tissues is not as large as for smaller diameter lesions, therefore the risk of radiation-induced late effects increases. The Radiation Therapy Oncology Group dose escalation study (90-05) has estimated the total normal tissue toxicity (acute and late) following radiosurgery at the RTOG maximum tolerated dose levels (see Table 10.1) (Shaw *et al.* 2000).

Field shaping and dose conformity in SRS is achieved either with circular cones (Figure 10.1, and Figure 10.2 on p. 215) or using multileaf collimator system (Figure 10.3 on p. 216). Table 10.2 presents some of the advantages and drawbacks of the two collimation systems.

Convergent beam stereotactic radiosurgery (SRS) has been used extensively for irradiation of small

Table 10.2.   Comparative table between circular cone and multileaf collimators for SRS.

Collimation	Advantages	Disadvantages
Circular cone	Good collimation, no leakage Small penumbra Easy to implement for any linear accelerator	Limited field shaping
Multileaf collimators	Easily conformed to irregular shapes	Leakage Penumbra

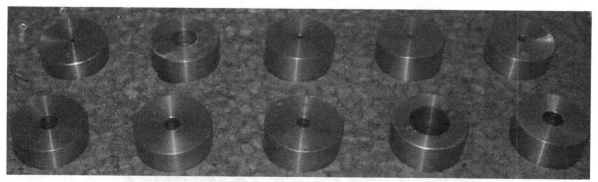

Figure 10.1. Circular cones for beam shaping. (Courtesy Royal Adelaide Hospital)

intracranial lesions with the high dose. A near spherical distribution around a focal spot (isocentre) results from using standard arcs combination obtained with circular collimators. However, a substantial number of clinically treated lesions are not spherical. Therefore the use of standard arc technique would result in excessively high radiation dose delivered to the normal tissues adjacent to the target. Irregular shaped or elongated dose distributions can be produced through applying multiple isocentres. One of the disadvantages of multiisocentre treatments with linac-based systems is the significant increase in the treatment time. Furthermore, the multiisocentre technique results in inhomogeneous dose distribution which is believed to be associated with higher complication rates (Nedzi *et al.* 1991). Another approach to achieving uniform distributions conformed to the target shape is based on computer optimisation techniques.

10.3 TREATMENT DELIVERY

10.3.1 Treatment delivery techniques

The **linear accelerator**-based radiosurgery equipment is prevalent throughout the world. One benefit of this technology is its ability to easily treat large tumour volumes (over 3.5 cm) by treating over several sessions (fractionated stereotactic radiotherapy) or in a one-session treatment (stereotactic radiosurgery).

For linac-based treatments, pre-treatment quality assurance is part of the SRS treatment protocol, and is substantiated by checking the correct alignment of laser beams. The aim of the pre-treatment QA is to provide a precise indication of **laser alignment**, and

also of the laser and **radiation isocentre coincidence**. This would ensure an accurate patient set-up.

While there are various QA tests designed for different SRS systems, for linac-delivered SRS the standard pre-treatment quality assurance and isocentre verification is based upon the Winston-Lutz test (Winston and Lutz 1988). Beside the planning system which has to meet the requirements for an optimal treatment plan, the hardware involved in the SRS technology has to be specially designed and reliable. Therefore, special collimators are needed in order to replace the suboptimal (for stereotactic purpose) linac collimation achieved by the jaw movements which give a rectangular beam, difficult to be adjusted to an exact size and treat at higher SSD resulting in large penumbra.

Winston and Lutz have proposed a new collimator assembly consisting of a cylindrically shaped cone holder, to decrease the distance to the isocentre thus to minimise penumbra and better focalise the primary beam. The cylindrical collimator can be mounted to the gantry head in a reproducible manner and the circular cones of various openings are inserted inside the cone holder (see Figure 10.1). An added advantage of the circular collimators compared to rectangular ones is the sharper dose gradient achieved when radiation is delivered over a hemisphere. Laser and radiation isocentre coincidence verification is achieved by using the smallest collimator size (usually with the 2 mm SRS collimator in the collimator slot on the treatment head) and making both anterior-posterior (gantry at 0°) and lateral (gantry at 90°) radiographic exposures of a film fixed inside the QA board and pricked with a needle at the laser intersection point (Figure 10.4). The shift (if any) in laser and radiation isocentre coinci-

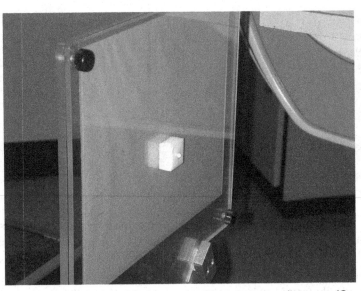

Figure 10.4. Pre-treatment quality assurance board for laser and radiation isocentre alignment. (Courtesy Royal Adelaide Hospital)

dence indicates the adjustment(s) required for accurate patient positioning.

One of the highly successful technologies developed for the treatment of brain tumours is **Gamma Knife®**. The cobalt-60 based machines can provide extremely accurate targeting and precise treatment for brain cancers. They are dedicated to treating only brain tumours and dysfunctions in a one-day treatment. The operation involves 201 accurately focused beams of radiation from cobalt-60 sources (gamma rays) that are contained in the Gamma Knife unit (Figure 10.5).

The energy emitted by the Co-60 sources is focused into intersecting beams by collimators that have a highly intense focal point. The Gamma Knife is a dedicated cranial SRS unit through its geometric design, and requires an invasive stereotactic head frame for localisation and immobilisation. The most recently introduced model is the Perfexion® (Elekta, AB) – Figure 10.6. The accuracy of the treatment is within less than a millimeter; therefore, the adjacent healthy tissues are well spared.

The CyberKnife® Stereotactic Radiosurgery System is a frameless robotic radiosurgery technology which incorporates a compact 6 MV linear accelerator (Figure 10.7). The two main elements of the CyberKnife are (1) the small linear particle accelerator which pro-

duces a narrow radiation beam collimated using fixed tungsten circular collimators from 5 to 60 mm and (2) a computer-controlled robotic arm with six degrees of freedom which allows the energy to be directed at any part of the body from any direction.

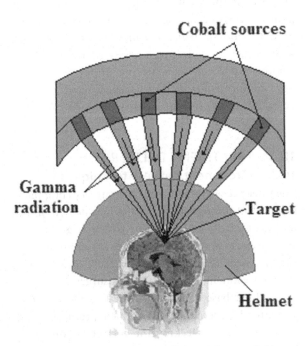

Figure 10.5. Schematic representation of Gamma Knife treatment.

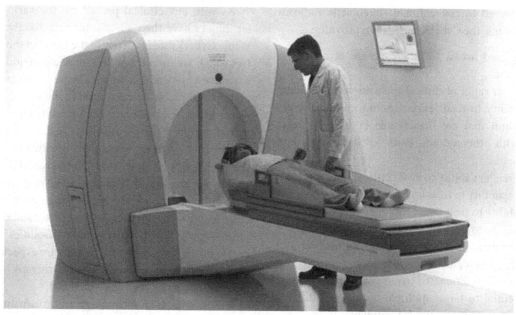

Figure 10.6. Leksell Gamma Knife Perfexion. (Copyright 2010 Elekta AB)

The small linear accelerator is mounted on a robotic arm which manoeuvres with ease around the patient. Image-guidance utilises X-ray imaging cameras that are located on supports around the patient and track the tumour through small body movements. The image-guidance technology thus eliminates the need for a rigid stereotactic frame and, as an added advantage, enables treatment of extra-cranial sites.

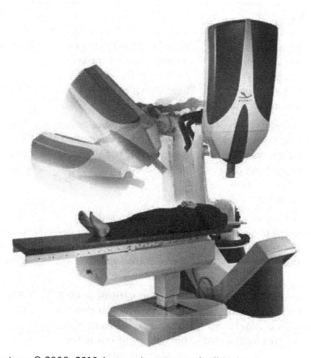

Figure 10.7. CyberKnife. (Courtesy: © 2008–2010 Accuray Incorporated. All Rights Reserved)

Compared to conventional stereotactic radiosurgery systems, the CyberKnife system provides:

- increased access to and coverage of any target volume
- broader range of clinical applications including:
  - ability to treat lesions in and around the cranium that are inaccessible or hard to access with other systems (such as the low posterior fossa);
  - excellent ability to avoid critical structures;
  - capability to treat lesions in the neck and spine;
  - ability to treat larger tumours;
  - ability to treat tumours that are inoperable;
  - ability to treat lesions throughout the body.
- delivery of highly conformal doses
- option of fractionated treatment
- potential to target multiple tumours at different locations during a single treatment.

However, treatment times are generally longer and the system represents a more expensive SRS equipment solution.

As with any clinical procedure, the various SRS techniques have their advantages and disadvantages. While CyberKnife is currently the trend in those centres which are in quest of SRS implementation, linac-based systems have a longer history and are still preferred for convenience and financial advantage where linacs are available. The role of Gamma Knife in radiosurgery has greatly increased since its first implementation at the Karolinska Institute in Sweden (1967) although it is restricted to intracranial tumours. Proton therapy is still limited to a few centres worldwide although the well localised Bragg peak and the close-to-zero exit dose makes it a great candidate for radiosurgery. With more proton facilities under development further clinical reports are expected and possibly trials to compare proton therapy against other dedicated radiosurgery methods.

Advancements in technology and treatment planning algorithms have increased the geometric accuracy and the overall quality of all SRS treatment techniques. Table 10.3 presents some of the main characteristics of the clinically used SRS systems.

Table 10.3. Main characteristics of various SRS treatment techniques.

Technology	Clinical application	Dose delivery	General characteristics
Linac-based radiosurgery	Used for the treatment of both smaller tumours (single fraction) and larger tumours (fractionated therapy). Stereotactic treatment via Linac is used only for brain.	Radiation is delivered through collimators (one at a time) having various diameters to conform to the size of the tumour (not an ideal tumour conformality).	The head frame prevents movement during treatment and enables accurate positioning and reproducibility of patient set-up between CT and Linac. Commonly used system.
Co-60 (photon) GammaKnife	Ideal for smaller tumours (less than 3.5cm diameter) and functional disorders of the brain. Dedicated only for brain disorders in single-session treatments.	Highly accurate dose delivery achieved by superimposing a large number of photon beams at the isocentre.	Gamma knife is successfully used in several clinics for its high precision. Commonly used system.
CyberKnife	Used to treat lesions throughout the body, even in the difficult-to-reach or sensitive areas.	Highly conformal doses produced by a compact linac are delivered using a robotic arm with six degrees of freedom.	Frameless, image-guided procedure which eliminates invasiveness. Commonly used system.
Protons	Used for the treatment of both brain disorders and body tumours outside the cranial cavity in a fractionated regimen.	Good normal tissue sparing due to rapid fall off after the target is reached and high tumour control due to the possibility to accurately localise the Bragg peak.	Not as common as Linac or Co-60 treatments.

Stereotactic radiosurgery relies on stereotaxy for target localisation/delineation and dose delivery which is achieved by superimposing the fixed 3D-coordinates upon the treated organ or lesion. The procedure is built on the following levels:

- *Imaging and planning*: three-dimensional imaging that determines the exact coordinates of the target within the body;
- *Set-up and immobilisation*: systems to immobilise and carefully position the patient;
- *SRS treatment*: highly focused gamma-ray, X-ray or proton beams that converge on a tumour or abnormality.

Image-guided radiation therapy (IGRT) which uses medical imaging to confirm the location of a tumour immediately before or during the delivery of radiation can also be employed to further improve the precision and accuracy of the treatment.

10.3.2 Frame-based procedures

Patient immobilisation plays an imperative role in delivering the prescribed dose to the target area with high accuracy. While in stereotactic radiosurgery a single large dose of radiation is delivered with high precision, in a multi-fraction treatment regimen immobilisation is important for patient set-up and treatment reproducibility. Therefore, rigid stereotactic frames are used as fixed reference systems which are applied to the patients' skull (Figure 10.8). The frame is kept in place during patient set-up, verification and treatment as it correlates the intracranial anatomy with the fixed coordinate system which also served as reference for treatment planning. For better immobilisation during fractionated radiotherapy, a personalised head mould is made and fitted to the head ring, thus minimising target movements and increasing treatment reproducibility.

A linac-based treatment using head frame for patient immobilisation can be outlined as follows (see Figure 10.9a–d):

1. A series of CT images of the head with the head ring are acquired (for AVMs the CT is preceded by angiography).
2. The CT images are transferred to the planning computer where reconstruction of the skull rela-

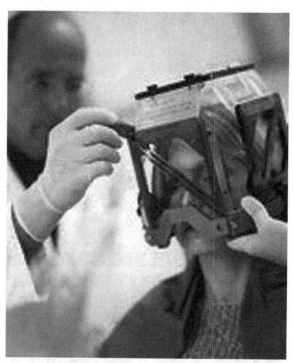

Figure 10.8. Leksell Gamma Knife frame. (Courtesy: © Copyright 2010 Elekta)

tive to the frame (fiducial plates) is employed. Treatment plan is designed.

3. Patient positioning with mm accuracy is undertaken using the planned target coordinates. A head ring with inbuilt micrometers along the three directions (x, y and z) assists in positioning. Four fiducial plates (Anterior, Posterior, Left, Right) are placed on the ring, to allow reconstruction of tumour position.

4. One anterior-posterior and one lateral film are taken and digitised using the reconstruction software. If tumour isocentre is within 1.2 mm the patient is treated with current set-up. Otherwise, repositioning is necessary along the required directions (as indicated by the films).

10.3.3 Frameless procedures

Until recently, rigid patient immobilisation was considered the gold standard for high-precision target localisation and accurate delivery in stereotactic radiosurgery (SRS). Rigid patient immobilisation can, however, result in patient discomfort, which is exacerbated by the long duration of SRS treatments. The risk of

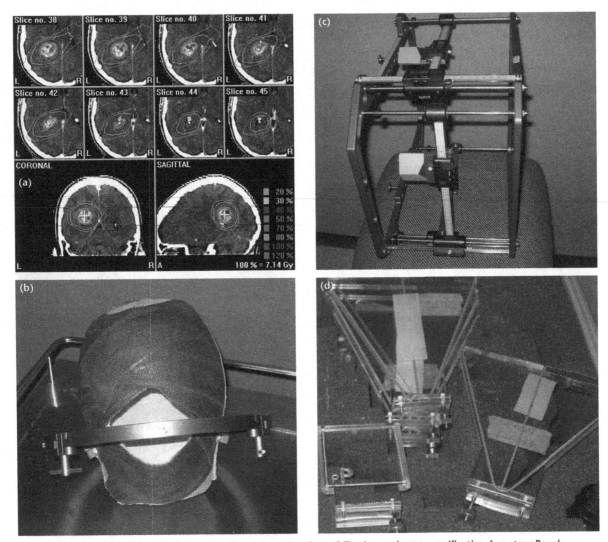

Figure 10.9. Elements of SRS/SRT treatment planning, patient immobilisation and set-up verification (courtesy Royal Adelaide Hospital). (a) CT-image reconstruction and treatment planning. (b) Head mould with ring for stereotactic radiotherapy (fractionated treatment) for immobilisation and set-up reproducibility. (c) Head frame for patient set-up verification. (d) Large fiducial plates used for CT imaging and set-up; small fiducial plates used for linac set-up and positioning.

bleeding and infection requires extra medical support and supervision. Also, with the frame-based radiosurgery, treatment planning must be completed after frame placement and imaging to avoid frame movement and minimise patient discomfort, which eliminates the possibility of a more advanced planning technique such as IMRT (Ramakrishna *et al.* 2010).

With the advent of image-guided treatment systems such as CyberKnife, the procedure involving invasive head frame can be replaced by a frameless technique with the advantage of improving patient comfort. The

pioneer of this frameless stereotactic system is Dr. JR Adler whose vision of advanced radiosurgery technology was put into practice in the late 1990s (Adler *et al.* 1997). The complex computer-guidance system allows for navigational targeting, without the involvement of a head frame. The frameless technique makes SRS available in those clinical centres where neurological support cannot be offered. In frameless settings, similarly to CyberKnife, target localisation and patient set-up are achieved via image guidance inside the treatment room (such as X-ray or ultrasound) or using optical tracking technology (such as stereoscopically mounted cameras) monitoring surgically placed internal fiducials or light emitting markers mounted on the patient's skin (Bova *et al.* 2006).

10.4 STEREOTACTIC BODY RADIOTHERAPY (SBRT)

The possibility to focalise radiation beams to treat intracranial lesions with a precision which leads to high therapeutic ratio has opened an avenue towards extracranial stereotactic radiotherapy. Stereotactic body radiotherapy employs the same treatment principles as SRT and delivers, to the extracranial sites, a single or very few high-dose fractions. The most common sites treated with SBRT are lung, spine, prostate, liver and pancreas, with other sites being trialled currently.

One of the initial impediments for an earlier implementation of stereotactic body radiotherapy was the challenge of rigid immobilisation outside the skull. While immobilising frames were successfully used in SRT, their implementation for SBRT was more complex. Extracranial body frames for spinal immobilisation have been devised in the mid-1990s with associated three-dimensional coordinate systems for tumour location relative to bony anatomy (Hamilton *et al.* 1995). Although the treatment accuracy of 2 mm was an indication of good patient set-up, the technique was time-consuming and too troublesome to be widely implemented. This challenge was later overcome by the use of fiducial markers and by the technological advances of image-guided radiotherapy.

Gamma knife was shown to be very effective for intracranial lesions but its applicability cannot reach outside the head because of the skull-limiting design of this Co-60-based treatment. A system which enables, beside intracranial treatment, also extracranial therapy, is the CyberKnife. This frameless, single-source linear accelerator with robotic arm system which employs real-time X-ray images for treatment guidance compensates for organ movement during treatment. The classic linac-based SBRT has significantly developed along with the implementation of electronic portal imaging devices which allowed for patient set-up assessment and correction (Martin and Gaya 2010). Volumetric imaging methods such as cone beam CT have further improved the accuracy of patient positioning and tumour localisation, thus minimising inter-fraction movements.

The increasing role of SBRT in the management of unresectable tumours or lesions located close to critical structures brings CyberKnife among the emerging technologies in modern oncology (Gibbs 2006; Hara *et al.* 2007; Calcerrada *et al.* 2008). A comprehensive review on SBRT published by Martin and Gaya (2010) which has included phase I/II clinical trials for various treatment sites has highlighted the potential of extracranial radiosurgery in achieving excellent local tumour control rates for well-designed patient groups. Randomised phase III trials to compare SBRT with surgery or other treatment modalities are therefore warranted.

The AAPM Task Group 101 has recently published a report on clinical findings and expected outcomes for stereotactic body radiotherapy including equipment, resources and quality assurance procedures (Benedict *et al.* 2010). While clinical findings are promising, patient selection (tumour spread, size and location) plays an important role regarding treatment outcome.

10.5 RADIOBIOLOGICAL ASPECTS OF SRS/SRT

The major radiobiological advantages of stereotactic radiosurgery rely on (1) the steep dose gradient between the target and the surrounding normal tissue and (2) the ability to deliver a high dose to a spatially confined tumour mass.

While the radiobiology of normal tissue indicates that single-dose radiation treatment can successfully manage benign lesions (such as AVMs) it was suggested that for malignant tumours, single-dose irradiation results in suboptimal therapeutic ratio due to increased late toxicity (Hall and Brenner 1993). Based on biologically effective dose calculations, Shigematsu *et al.* (1998) arrived at the same conclusion, recommending SRS for AVMs and benign tumours having well-defined margins which separate them from the surrounding healthy tissue. Fractionated radiotherapy should be employed in the treatment of malignant lesions (tumours without well-defined boundaries) but, on the other hand, would not be effective for arteriovenous malformations.

Table 10.4. Treatment parameters and outcome in External beam radiotherapy (EBRT) versus Stereotactic radiosurgery.

Treatment parameter	EBRT	SRS
Treatment field size	Large field RT	Small field
Dose administration	Small doses in multiple fractions (based on the 5R's)	High dose in a single fraction
Dose gradient	Broad dose gradient to large tissue volume	Sharp dose gradient to small volume of tissue
Radiobiological outcome	Effective in killing rapidly dividing cells	Effective in arresting cells irrespective of their mitotic activity
		Vascular injury is characteristic to high doses of radiation
Clinical outcome	Latency period between irradiation and detection of pathological alterations shorter for SRS than conventional RT (depends also on total dose delivered and biological end-point).	
Clinical advantages	Less invasive than surgery, requires less recovery time; may not require a hospital stay	Less invasive than surgery, requires less recovery time; may not require a hospital stay
		Offers high tumour control with very low risk of post-operative complications
		Suitable for small sites (tumours and various functional disorders) and for tumours situated in the vicinity of critical structures, due to its high accuracy

Regardless of the radiobiological principle that fractionation is preferable for rapidly proliferating tumours, the efficacy of radiosurgery in the management of metastatic tumours has been trialled over the years and eventually validated.

Specialised treatments for difficult tumours, such as stereotactic radiosurgery/therapy for malignant brain lesions, always offer advantages over conventional external beam radiotherapy as a result of better focalisation of the beam in reaching the target and also enhanced sparing of adjacent critical organs. Table 10.4 presents, in a comparative manner, various treatment-related parameters for external beam radiotherapy and stereotactic radiosurgery.

10.5.1   The radiosensitivity of the brain

The three main brain cell categories which have radiobiological relevance for SRS or SRT are neurons (non-proliferating end-cells in adults), glial cells (slow cell-turnover) and endothelial cells (slow cell-turnover but able to proliferate rapidly after injury). Stereotactic radiosurgery affects brain lesions through early cytotoxic effects (apoptotic and necrotic death) and

late vascular changes. *Brain metastases* and *malignant gliomas* are rapidly proliferating, so they show the effect of radiation early. *Arteriovenous malformations* react with a prolonged latency period as they do not undergo spontaneous proliferating activity. Stereotactic radiosurgery differs from open surgery insofar as stereotactic radiosurgery has no immediate cytoreductive role. The goal of radiosurgery is, therefore, to alter the biology of tumour cells so as to hinder their proliferative potential.

The failure of certain brain cancer treatments implies that the management of brain tumours raises particular challenges. To date, there is still lack of understanding of the mechanisms responsible for tumour resistance as well as the role of the 'neural environment' in tumour radioresistance. Furthermore, one of the reasons for treatment failure is attributable to the evidence that malignant brain tumours (especially gliomas) 'escape' apoptosis. Other pathological characteristics of malignant brain tumours such as active invasiveness and the special form of angiogenesis known as microvascular hyperplasia lead to rapid progression (Oliver *et al.* 2009). Since

Table 10.5. Median pO_2 values measured in brain tumours versus normal brain.

Brain lesion	Median pO_2 [mmHg]	References
Low-grade gliomas	17	Collingridge *et al.* 1999
	15	Lally *et al.* 2004, 2006
High-grade gliomas	6	Collingridge *et al.* 1999
	13	Clavo *et al.* 2002
	3	Lally *et al.* 2004, 2006
Glioblastomas	7	Rampling *et al.* 1994
	9	Beppu *et al.* 2002
Normal brain	24	Rampling *et al.* 1994
	27	Clavo *et al.* 2002
	24	Vaupel *et al.* 2003

local tumour control can be achieved via different physiological processes including apoptosis, vascular damage and necrosis, the above-named challenges have to be elucidated for a successful clinical outcome.

Hypoxia in brain tumours is a long-known but still hard to manage clinical issue. The main reasons for tumour hypoxia in brain lesions are commonly found in other tumour sites as well and they are: the functional and structural abnormalities of tumour vasculature, limitation in oxygen diffusion and therapy-induced anaemia. To illustrate the high hypoxic content of certain brain tumours Table 10.5 presents median partial oxygen pressure values measured in brain tumours and, comparatively, in normal brain. The measurements were done directly, using the polarographic oxygen electrode.

It was demonstrated by recent studies that a transcription factor that upregulates the target genes under hypoxic conditions, known as the hypoxia-inducible factor-1 (HIF-1) plays a critical role in determining tumour radioresistance. Hypoxia-inducible factor-1 modulates over 100 genes which are involved in the regulation of proliferation, apoptosis and angiogenesis (Semenza 2003). Clinical studies have shown that HIF-1 expression levels increase under the effect of radiation as early as 24 hours after the start of radiotherapy and last up to 1 week (Moeller and Dewhirst 2006). The mechanism behind this process was shown to be radiation-induced tumour reoxygenation (Moeller *et al.* 2004). After irradiation, when radiosensitive cells are killed and they free up space and oxygen to be delivered to the previously hypoxic

regions, the process of reoxygenation of hypoxic cells takes place. The oxidative stress generated during reoxygenation (the free radical species created) causes the activation of the HIF-1 pathway. Therefore, in a paradoxical way, reoxygenation causes activation of HIF-1 pathway, which is usually responsive to decreased oxygen levels. Because of its active role in tumour radioresistance, HIF-1 may constitute a therapeutic target for hypoxic tumours.

The most common methods employed in order to overcome tumour radioresistance and hypoxia are radiation dose fractionation (based on the 5 R's of radiobiology), the use of high LET particles in the management of brain lesions and also the implementation of bio-reductive drugs as adjuvant treatment.

High LET particles are advantageous over low LET due to their high radiobiological effectiveness and low oxygen enhancement ratio (close to 1) compared to the OER of three for low LET radiation. Therefore, hypoxic tumours, such as several types of brain lesion, could benefit from high LET treatment if it is delivered with high focalisation and accurate patient set-up.

Though stereotactic treatment is effective on small lesions without affecting the organs at risk, the question arises whether large cranial tumours are safe to be treated with high single doses of radiation. It is known that the sensitivity of CNS (central nervous system) to radiation damage increases with the treatment volume (volume effect) which limits the radiation dose used in treating large intracranial tumours. The answer to the question: *are particular regions of the brain less sensitive to radiation damage (so they*

Table 10.6. Radiosurgery results for radiation-induced intracranial tumours.

Treatment type	Radiation dose	Tumour control	Normal tissue toxicity
Gamma knife radiosurgery of radiation-induced intracranial tumours 19 patients with meningiomas (24 tumours) (*Kondziolka 2009*)	Median tumour margin dose 13 Gy	94.1% 3-year overall survival 80.7% 5-year overall survival	5.3% overall morbidity rate (optic neuropathy)
Stereotactic radiation for nonbenign meningiomas (recurrent and radiation-induced) 25 patients (52 tumours) (*Mattozo 2007*)	**SRS**: peripheral dose 12 to 18 Gy (median 15.5 Gy) **SRT**: 25 to 54 Gy (median 49.3 Gy) delivered in 25 to 28 daily fractions	3-year survival rates: grade I – 100% grade II – 100% malignant progression – 57%	8% patients – radiation-induced edema
Gamma knife radiosurgery of radiation-induced intracranial tumours 19 patients with meningiomas 1 patient schwannoma (*Jensen 2005*)	Median tumour margin dose 16 Gy (12–20 Gy)	92% 3-year overall survival 80% 5-year overall survival	6% patients – increased seizure activity

could be treated more aggressively)? would probably solve the dilemma. Until these challenges are overcome, the near future of SRS rests in the adoption of additional strategies to increase TCP (through tumour radiosensitisation) and to decrease NTCP (through normal tissue radioprotection).

10.6 RADIOSURGERY OF RADIATION-INDUCED SECONDARY (INTRACRANIAL) TUMOURS

Although radiosurgery is effective for the treatment of intracranial tumours, studies have shown the downside of irradiation resulting in the initiation of secondary intracranial tumours. Radiation-induced intracranial tumours are usually meningiomas or schwannomas which are typically managed with surgery resection though clinical results show that they respond effectively to radiation treatment. It was shown that radiation-induced meningiomas have a different molecular genetic pattern from sporadic meningiomas therefore they can take a malignant form and they are likely to be multiple (Shoshan *et al.* 2000). Table 10.6 presents clinical outcome for the latest three studies which have employed radiosurgery for the treatment of secondary

brain tumours induced by previous radiotherapy. The paradox of radiation treatment is that radiotherapy-induced tumours, which are either unresectable or partially resectable, are treated yet again with radiation. This fact shows that specialised radiotherapy, such as radiosurgery or stereotactic radiotherapy, remains the treatment of choice for both benign and malignant tumours which are poor candidates for resection and often as an adjuvant treatment to surgery.

In a recent study of 19 patients with radiation-induced meningiomas, Kondziolka *et al.* (2009) concluded that gamma knife radiosurgery has a decisive role for patients who are poor candidates for resection (Table 10.6). Both tumour control and normal tissue toxicity were very similar to the study outcome conducted by Jensen *et al.* (2005) indicating that radiosurgery is a viable treatment for these tumours. The literature also reports on the situations, though rare ones, when previous intracranial irradiation has induced malignant gliomas (Prasad and Haas-Kogan 2009). As demonstrated by retrospective studies in paediatric population the initiation of malignant gliomas after intracranial radiation treatment is both age and radiation dose/volume dependent, with the incidence decreasing in the adult population.

The number of studies and cases reported on radiation-induced intracranial lesions strengthen the evidence that radiotherapy has important delayed effects on the central nervous system. These delayed effects are materialised either through benign or malignant lesions. Radiosurgery was shown to be a viable treatment for radiation-induced intracranial tumours, especially for non-resectable lesions. However, paediatric cases need extra attention when planning initial radiation therapy since young patients showed an increase in the incidence of second tumours later in life.

The major advantages presented by stereotactic radiosurgery techniques are:

- Accurate targeting and delivery of single fraction of high dose by multiple beams, intersecting at the target;
- Highly conformal dose to spare sensitive surrounding tissue (e.g. brain);
- Alternative treatment option to surgery for smaller (<35 mm) lesions with critical surroundings or non-resectable lesions.

Stereotactic radiosurgery has undergone rapid growth in the last two decades due to computing and imaging advances, and increase of indications for SRS and SBRT treatment.

10.7 REFERENCES

Alder JR, Chang SD, Murphy MJ et al. (1997) The CyberKnife: a frameless robotic system for radiosurgery. *Stereotactic Functional Neurosurgery* **69**: 124–128.

Benedict SH, Yenice KM, Followill D, Galvin JM et al. (2010) Stereotactic body radiation therapy: the report of AAPM Task Group 101. *Medical Physics* **37**(8): 4078–4101.

Beppu T, Kamada K, Yoshida Y, Arai H et al. (2002) Change of oxygen pressure in glioblastoma tissue under various conditions. *Journal of Neuro-Oncology* **58**(1): 47–52.

Bova F, Meeks S, Friedman W and Wagner T (2006) Linac radiosurgery: system requirements, procedures, and testing. In: *Treatment Planning in Radiation Oncology*. 2nd edn. (Ed. F Khan) pp. 215–243. Lippincott Williams & Wilkins, Philadelphia.

Calcerrada Díaz-Santos N, Blasco Amaro JA, Cardiel GA and Andradas Aragonés E (2008) The safety and efficacy of robotic image-guided radiosurgery system treatment for intra- and extracranial lesions: a systematic review of the literature. *Radiotherapy and Oncology* **89**(3): 245–253.

Clavo B, Robaina F, Morera J, Ruiz-Egea E et al. (2002) Increase of brain tumor oxygenation during cervical spinal cord stimulation: report of three cases. *Journal of Neurosurgery* **96**(1): 94–100.

Collingridge DR, Piepmeier JM, Rockwell S and Knisely JP (1999) Polarographic measurements of oxygen tension in human glioma and surrounding peritumoural brain tissue. *Radiotherapy and Oncology* **53**(2): 127–131.

Colombo F, Benedetti A, Pozza F et al. (1985) External stereotactic irradiation by linear accelerator. *Neurosurgery* **16**(2): 154–160.

Emami B, Lyman J, Brown A, Coia L, Goiten M et al. (1991) Tolerance of normal tissue to therapeutic radiation. *International Journal of Radiation Oncology Biology and Physics* **21**: 109–122.

Evans RG (1983) Radiobiological considerations in magna-field irradiation. *International Journal of Radiation Oncology Biology and Physics* **9**(12): 1907–1911.

Flickinger J (2002) Radiobiological and dosimetric considerations in stereotactic radiosurgery. In: *Contemporary Stereotactic Radiosurgery Technique and Evaluation*. (Ed. BE Pollock) pp. 37–52. Futura Publishing Company, New York.

Gibbs IC (2006) Frameless image-guided intracranial and extracranial radiosurgery using the Cyberknife robotic system. *Cancer Radiotherapy* **10**(5): 283–287.

Hall EJ and Brenner DJ (1993) The radiobiology of radiosurgery: rationale for different treatment regimes for AVMs and malignancies. *International Journal of Radiation Oncology Biology and Physics* **25**(2): 381–385.

Hamilton AJ, Lulu BA, Fosmire H, Stea B et al. (1995) Preliminary clinical experience with linear accelerator-based spinal stereotactic radiosurgery. *Neurosurgery* **36**(2): 311–319.

Hara W, Soltys SG and Gibbs IC (2007) CyberKnife robotic radiosurgery system for tumor treatment.

Expert Review of Anticancer Therapy **7**(11): 1507–1515.

Jensen AW, Brown PD, Pollock BE, Stafford SL *et al.* (2005) Gamma knife radiosurgery of radiation-induced intracranial tumors: local control, outcomes, and complications. *International Journal of Radiation Oncology Biology and Physics* **62**(1): 32–37.

Kondziolka D, Kano H, Kanaan H, Madhok R *et al.* (2009) Stereotactic radiosurgery for radiation-induced meningiomas. *Neurosurgery* **64**(3): 463–469.

Lally BE, Colasanto JM, Fischer JJ and Knisely JP (2004) Is there an optimal hemoglobin level for patients with glioblastoma multiforme? *The Cancer Journal* **10**(6): 391–396.

Lally BE, Rockwell S, Fischer DB, Collingridge DR *et al.* (2006) The interactions of polarographic measurements of oxygen tension and histological grade in human glioma. *The Cancer Journal* **12**(6): 461–466.

Leksell L (1951) The stereotaxic method and radiosurgery of the brain. *Acta Chirurgica Scandinavica* **102**: 316–319.

Leksell L, Meyerson BA and Forster DM (1972) Radiosurgical thalamotomy for intractable pain. *Confin Neurology* **34**: 264.

Leksell L, Lindquist C, Adler JR, Leksell D *et al.* (1987) A new fixation device for the Leksell stereotaxic system. Technical note. *Journal of Neurosurgery* **66**: 626–629.

Martin A and Gaya A (2010) Stereotactic body radiotherapy: a review. *Clinical Oncology* **22**(3): 157–172.

Mattozo C, De Salles AA, Klement IA, Gorgulho A *et al.* (2007) Stereotactic radiation treatment for recurrent nonbenign meningiomas. *Journal of Neurosurgery* **106**(5): 846–854.

Moeller BJ, Cao Y, Li CY and Dewhirst MW (2004) Radiation activates HIF-1 to regulate vascular radiosensitivity in tumors: role of reoxygenation, free radicals, and stress granules. *Cancer Cell* **5**: 429–441.

Moeller BJ and Dewhirst MW (2006) HIF-1 and tumour radiosensitivity. *British Journal of Cancer* **95**(1): 1–5.

Nedzi LA, Kooy H, Alexander E, Gelman RS and Loefler JS (1991) Variables associated with the development of complications from radiosurgery of intracranial tumours. *International Journal of Radiation Oncology Biology and Physics* **21**(3): 591–599.

Oliver L, Olivier C, Marhuenda FB, Campone M *et al.* (2009) Hypoxia and the malignant glioma microenvironment: regulation and implications for therapy. *Current Molecular Pharmacology* **2**(3): 263–284.

Prasad G and Haas-Kogan DA (2009) Radiation-induced gliomas. *Expert Review of Neurotherapeutics* **9**(10): 1511–1517.

Ramakrishna N, Rosca F, Friesen S, Tezcanli E *et al.* (2010) A clinical comparison of patient setup and intra-fraction motion using frame-based radiosurgery versus a frameless image-guided radiosurgery system for intracranial lesions. *Radiotherapy and Oncology* **95**: 109–115.

Rampling R, Cruickshank G, Lewis AD, Fitzsimmons SA *et al.* (1994) Direct measurement of pO2 distribution and bioreductive enzymes in human malignant brain tumors. *International Journal of Radiation Oncology Biology and Physics* **29**(3): 427–431.

Sahgal A, Ma L, Chang E, Shiu A, Larson DA, Laperriere N *et al.* (2009) Advances in technology for intracranial stereotactic radiosurgery. *Technology in Cancer Research and Treatment* **8**(4): 271–280.

Schneider R, Schultze J, Jensen JM, Hebbinghaus D *et al.* (2008) Long-term outcome after static intensity-modulated total body radiotherapy using compensators stratified by pediatric and adult cohorts. *International Journal of Radiation Oncology Biology and Physics* **70**(1): 194–202.

Semenza GL (2003) Targeting HIF-1 for cancer therapy. *Nature Reviews Cancer* **3**: 721–732.

Shaw E, Scott C, Souhami L, Dinapoli R *et al.* (2000) Single dose radiosurgical treatment of recurrent previously irradiated primary brain tumors and brain metastases: final report of RTOG protocol 90-05. *International Journal of Radiation Oncology Biology and Physics* **47**(2): 291–298.

Shigematsu N, Kunieda E, Kawada T, Kitamura M *et al.* (1998) Radiobiological considerations for stereotactic irradiation. *Nippon Acta Radiologica* **58**(6): 281–286.

Shoshan Y, Chernova O, Juen SS, Somerville RP *et al.* (2000) Radiation-induced meningioma: a distinct molecular genetic pattern? *Journal of Neuropathology & Experimental Neurology* **59**(7): 614–620.

Steel GG and Weldon TE (1991) The radiation biology of paediatric tumours. In: *Paediatric Oncology.* (Eds R Pinkerton and N Plowman) pp. 73–86. John Wiley, London.

Svennilson E, Torvik A, Lowe R and Leksell L (1960) Treatment of parkinsonism by stereotatic thermolesions in the pallidal region. A clinical evaluation of 81 cases. *Acta Psychiatrica Scandinavica* **35**: 358–377.

Vaupel P, Thews O, Kelleher DK and Konerding MA (2003) O(2) extraction is a key parameter determining the oxygenation status of malignant tumors and normal tissues. *International Journal of Oncology* **22**(4): 795–798.

Winston K and Lutz W (1988) Linear accelerator as a neurosurgical tool for stereotactic radiosurgery. *Neurosurgery* **22**(3): 454–464.

http://clinicaltrials.gov/ct2/show/NCT00576979 accessed on 3/03/2010.

http://clinicaltrials.gov/ct2/show/NCT00988013 accessed on 3/03/2010.

11 Total body irradiation: radiobiology and physics aspects of treatment

11.1 INTRODUCTION

Total body irradiation (TBI) is systemic radiotherapy treatment in which a relatively small number of widely dispersed/circulating radiosensitive cells are sterilised (killed). It is used as part of the preparative and conditioning schedule for hematopoietic stem cell (i.e. bone marrow) transplantation used for the treatment or prevention of leukemic relapse and multiple myeloma. Total body irradiation is generally used in conjunction with high-dose cytotoxic drugs to destroy a patient's bone marrow and leukemic cells. Killing a patient's lymphohemopoietic stem cells and lymphoid cells also prevents rejection of donor cells when allogeneic (i.e. genetically non-identical) bone marrow transplantation is used. In addition, killing of lymphohemopoietic stem cells creates spaces in bone marrow for donor cells to establish themselves and grow (Lin and Drzymala 2003). The patients treated with TBI can vary in age from months to adults and elderly. The majority of patients are diagnosed with various types of leukaemia (acute non-lymphoblastic, acute lymphoblastic and chronic myelogenous), malignant lymphoma and anaplastic anaemia. Some patients can also be treated for multiple myeloma, although the results for this group are not very good.

The 'conditioning' schedule consists of firstly isolating the patient, administering antibiotics and anti-fungal agents. The patient then undergoes a course of cytotoxic drugs and then immediately prior to transplantation is given a short course (3–4 days) of radiation to the total body. The transplantation can be a) autologous, using patient's own stem cells, b) syngeneic, using stem cells from an identical twin or c) allogeneic, using stem cells from HLA (human leukocyte antigen) matched relatives (Lin and Drzymala 2003).

While the main objective of TBI treatment is to kill tumour cells, the radiotherapy complications must be minimised at the same time. The whole treatment procedure is particularly risky as the patient's hemopoietic (i.e. blood cell producing) system is totally destroyed and then generated anew from the transplanted cells. While the advances of modern pharmacology have reduced many risks and improved the probability of stem cell seeding, patients may succumb to infection, engraftment failure, pneumonitis, graft-versus-host disease (i.e. the donor's bone marrow attacks the patient's organs and tissues), metabolic failure or disease relapse.

Total body irradiation is generally considered to be a special procedure as it differs significantly from more standard radiation treatment techniques. Firstly, the treatment fields for TBI are larger than the size of the scattering volume in all directions (i.e. the entire body is within the radiation field), and secondly the

L. Marcu et al., *Biomedical Physics in Radiotherapy for Cancer*,
DOI 10.1007/978-0-85729-733-4_11, © CSIRO 2012

irradiated volume has highly irregular shape of vary-ing dimensions and containing many inhomogenei-ties. The aim is to deliver a dose uniform to within ±10% of the prescribed dose to the patient's whole body. Megavoltage photon beams, either ^{60}Co gamma rays or megavoltage bremsstrahlung photons are used for this purpose. The beams can either be stationary, with field sizes of the order of 70 × 200 cm^2 (or even 150 × 150 cm^2) covering the whole patient, or moving in translational or rotational motion, using smaller radiation field sizes to irradiate the whole patient. Usu-ally, parallel opposed radiation fields of equal weights are used to deliver the dose for each fraction and the patient's position is rotated between the two fields.

In a broader sense, the treatment concepts of whole body irradiation also encompass other irradiations with large photon fields, such as:

- half body irradiation;
- total nodal (also known as lymphoid) irradiation; and
- irradiation of the whole body except for a few spe-cific organs, which are partially or fully shielded from the prescribed dose.

Half body irradiation (HBI) is generally a palliative therapy used to reduce symptoms of disseminated metastatic disease (Fitzpatrick 1976). For example, HBI of lower body can be used for ovarian ablation (i.e. to stop ovaries from producing hormones like estrogen) in metastatic breast cancer (Fitzpatrick and Garrett 1981).

Total nodal (or lymphoid) irradiation is used for treatment of Hodgkin's disease (Poussin-Rosillo et al. 1978) but as it results in immunosuppressive effects it has also been used for management of autoimmune diseases such as rheumatoid arthritis, aplastic anemia, multiple sclerosis and others (Strober et al. 1981).

Depending on the specific clinical situation, indi-vidual TBI techniques can use a variety of dose deliv-ery schedules (Van Dyk et al. 1986):

- high dose TBI; using between one and six frac-tions of 2 Gy each in three days (up to total dose of 12 Gy)
- low dose TBI; delivering 10–15 fractions of 10–15 cGy each

- half-body irradiation; dose of 8 Gy is delivered to the upper or lower half body in a single session
- total nodal irradiation; for example treatment using 16 fractions and total dose of 3600 cGy was used for patients with rheumatoid arthritis (Strober et al. 1981).

Alternative TBI schedules can also include a single dose of 7.0 to 8.5 Gy or treatment to a total dose of 13.2 Gy in 8 fractions of 1.65 Gy/fraction (Bhat et al. 2002). Often two fractions per day are delivered with mini-mum of 6 hours between fractions to allow for the repair of healthy tissues.

11.2 PHYSICS AND TECHNICAL ASPECTS OF TBI

Large radiation fields required for total body irradia-tion can be produced using:

- dedicated irradiators specifically designed for TBI
- conventional radiotherapy apparatus (e.g. teleco-balt units) modified to produce large fields
- conventional radiotherapy apparatus (e.g. linacs) in combination with non-standard irradiation set-ups to achieve irradiation of the patient's whole body.

Not many radiation oncology departments can jus-tify (based on patient numbers treated) the purchase, installation and maintenance of a dedicated TBI irra-diator. Figure 11.1 shows a ceiling-mounted Co-60 based unit dedicated to TBI (Podgorsak and Podgor-sak 2005). The distance between the unit and the patient lying on a floor mattress is 250 cm, thus achieving an adequate radiation field size. The patient is treated with two beams, while lying alternately in prone and supine positions.

Total body irradiation is more commonly delivered using modified conventional megavoltage radiother-apy equipment and/or with non-standard set-ups and radiation delivery. The approaches to changes/modifi-cations depend on the apparatus itself and on local conditions (e.g. the bunker size); therefore several TBI techniques have been established at present.

The methods with modified conventional radio-therapy equipment include (Podgorsak and Podgor-sak 1999):

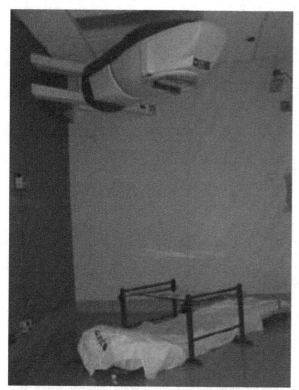

Figure 11.1. A picture of ceiling mounted Co-60 dedicated total body irradiator. The source to floor distance is 250 cm. (Reproduced after Figure 15.5 on p. 519 of International Atomic Energy Agency, *Radiation Oncology Physics: A Handbook for Teachers and Students*, IAEA, Vienna (2005), copyright IAEA)

- *Standard source-to-surface distance (SSD) treatment*; after the collimator from a Co-60 teletherapy unit is removed (utilising the fact that the radiation from a radioisotope is emitted into a 360° spatial angle, so the removal of the beam limiting device (collimator) increases the radiation field size available by increasing the aperture for the radiation source emission). The radiation beam is static.

- *Extended SSD treatment*; delivered with a conventional megavoltage linac and with patient positioned at the extended source-to-surface distance (Figure 11.2). Due to radiation beam divergence, the patient's whole body can be irradiated simultaneously. The radiation beam is static.

- *Moving beam treatment*; using a conventional megavoltage linac and translational or sweeping beams. As the radiation field size does not encompass the whole body of a patient, the total body irradiation is achieved by translating/moving the patient on a couch through the radiation beam or moving the gantry so that the radiation beam sweeps across the patient's whole body (Figure 11.3).

The treatment with moving beams seems to be more challenging as the details of delivery and dosimetry will have to be carefully determined, including

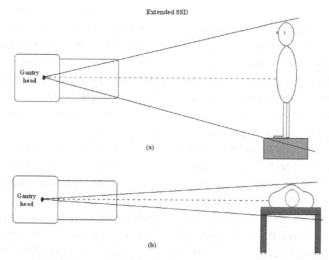

Figure 11.2. Schematic diagram of TBI treatment delivered with conventional megavoltage linac and with patient positioned at the extended source-to-surface distance. Due to radiation beam divergence, the patient's whole body can be irradiated simultaneously. The radiation beam is static. Patient position is rotated between 2 beams to achieve irradiation with parallel opposed beams.

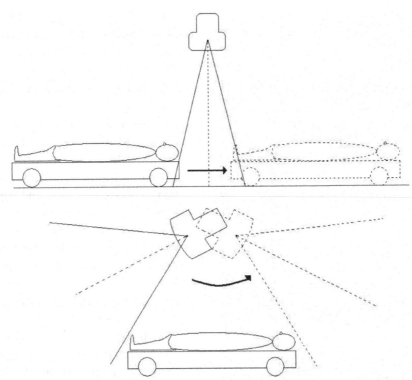

Figure 11.3. Schematic diagram of TBI treatment using a conventional megavoltage linac and moving radiation beams. As the radiation field size does not encompass the whole body of a patient, the total body irradiation is achieved by translating/ moving the patient on a couch through the radiation beam (top) or moving the gantry so that the radiation beam sweeps across the patient's whole body (bottom).

the speed of all movements involved as well as determination of dose accumulation at a given point while moving through the beam.

Two radiation beams are generally used. Patient position is rotated between the two beams to achieve irradiation with parallel opposed beams. Anterior-to-Posterior (AP) and Posterior-to- Anterior (PA) parallel opposed fields are preferred due to smaller patient thickness in that dimension (Figure 11.3 top). However if radiation beams of high enough energies are used, then ±10% uniformity can be achieved with bilateral (left-to-right and right-to-left) fields (Figure 11.3 bottom). Figure 11.4 shows a percentage depth dose curve (yellow) for an 18 MV linac X-ray beam as measured in water. Attenuation of the dose as a function of depth is evident. However, if parallel opposed beams are used, the combined depth dose curve is fairly flat and within ±10%.

Typical photon energy range used in total body irradiation varies between cobalt-60 gamma ray energies (i.e. 1.17 and 1.33 MeV) and 25 MV X-rays. The

higher energies will give a more uniform dose distribution (excluding the build-up region). Ratio of maximum/peak dose to midplane dose on the central beam axis versus patient thickness is shown in Figure 11.5 adopted from the AAPM report no. 17 (Van Dyk *et al.* 1986). The shaded region represents a 15% range of this ratio. Better dose uniformity achieved for higher energy beams is apparent. Percentage depth dose curves for stationary and sweeping beams are shown in Figure 11.6.

While dose build-up region is advantageous in conventional radiation therapy (generally involving smaller target volumes compared to TBI) as it results in skin sparing effect, it may be undesired in total body irradiation. Bone marrow and hemopoietic stem cells can be present in regions/tissues close to the body surface (e.g. shoulder blades, ribs). If a megavoltage photon beam is used with depth of maximum dose of several centimeters (e.g. around 3 cm for 18 MV photon beam), not all cells will be destroyed. As a result, so-called 'beam spoilers' (i.e. screens)

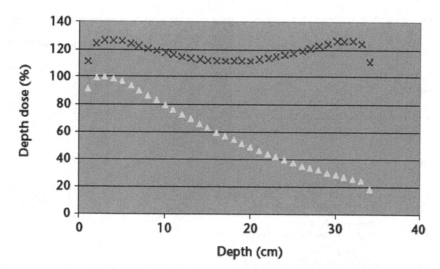

Figure 11.4. Percentage depth dose curve (▲) for an 18 MV linac X-ray beam as measured in water. The combined depth dose curve (✕) from two parallel opposed beams is fairly flat and within ±10%.

made of tissue equivalent material (e.g. perspex) should be positioned in the beam path, close to a patient to boost the low body surface dose using the electrons scattered from the spoiler. In other words, radiation dose will build up in the beam spoiler

screen, ensuring that maximum dose is reached at the patient's body surface.

Dose horns seen on the blue curve (i.e. the combined percentage depth dose curve for parallel opposed beams) in Figure 11.4 can be further reduced by using

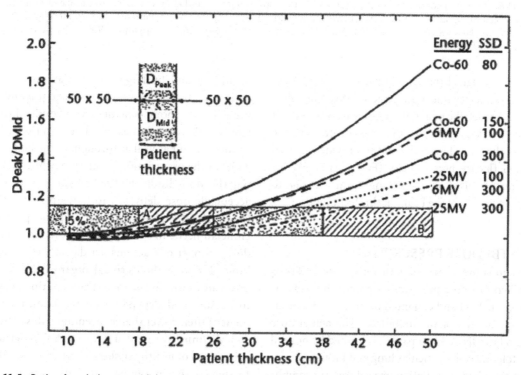

Figure 11.5. Ratio of peak dose to midplane dose on the central beam axis versus patient thickness. The shaded region represents a 15% range of this ratio. Better uniformity of higher energy beams is evident. (Courtesy Van Dyk *et al.* 1986)

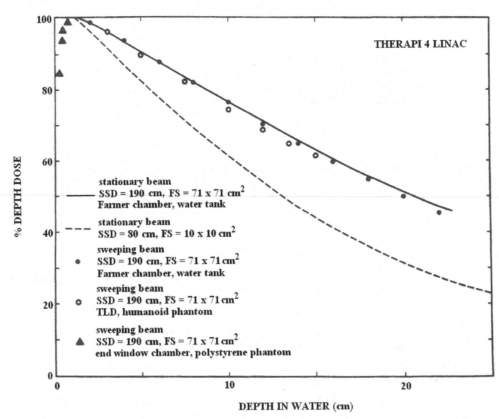

Figure 11.6. Percentage depth dose curves for a 4 MV photon beam measured at 80 cm source to surface distance (dashed curve) and at 190 cm SSD for stationary and sweeping beams (full curve). The beam hardening at the extended SSD is clearly demonstrated. (Reprinted from Podgorsak and Podgorsak 1999. Fig. 17A.10, Copyright (1999), with permission from Medical Physics Publishing)

a specially designed flattening filter inserted into the treatment head of a linear accelerator. Flattening filters are made of metallic materials and consist of a series of concentric circles of varying thickness to attenuate the radiation beam differentially and to provide required radiation fluence homogeneity (Figure 11.7). Wedge filters may be used in a sweeping beam TBI due to oblique incidence of the beam in this technique.

11.3   TBI DOSE PRESCRIPTION

Similar to conventional radiotherapy, dose in TBI is prescribed to a dose prescription point. This point is inside the patient and can often be placed at the midpoint at the level of the umbilicus. The actual dose that can be delivered to a patient is limited by normal tissue tolerance, in particular lung and kidneys.

The total body irradiation procedures are complicated by complexity and uncertainty in absolute

dosimetry and by large dose variations across the patient body due to varying patient thickness and presence of inhomogeneities. As a result, the objective is to deliver the prescribed dose to the dose prescription point as well as throughout the body within ±10% of the prescription point dose (while maintaining the dose limits to the critical structures; e.g. acceptable dose delivered to lungs may need to be lower that the dose at the prescription point). The clinician needs to specify dose per fraction and total dose, number of fractions per day as well as all dose limits for individual critical organs. The radiation dose rate as well as the total treatment time may need to be specified depending on the clinical requirements. Often, lower than conventional dose rates (e.g. 100 MU/min) are applied due to radiobiological considerations of healthy tissues. There is some evidence to suggest that pulmonary toxicity as well as bone marrow killing are dose rate dependent (Van Dyk *et*

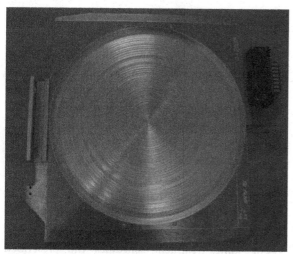

Figure 11.7. A photograph of an aluminium flattening filter. (Courtesy Royal Adelaide Hospital)

al. 1986). If the patient is treated at an extended distance (300–400 cm) then the dose rate at the patient midline will be even lower (e.g. ~0.09 Gy/min (Bhat *et al.* 2002)).

CT based planning with a commercial treatment planning system can be used to determine relative dose distribution in a patient. If the specially designed TBI treatment couch allows the patient to be treated in the supine position then CT scanning, treatment planning and treatment can be all performed in nearly the same position. Once the dose distribution has been calculated, the peak lung dose volume should be inspected. Lung bolus can be included (see section 11.3.1) into the treatment planning process in the form of manually added regions on interest of water density (Figure 11.8 on p. 217). Their thickness can be adjusted until a desired lung dose is achieved. This would then be the thickness of lung bolus used during treatment delivery.

While a treatment planning system can provide the 3D dose distribution, the beam-on-time or linac monitor units may need to be determined from measurements using real TBI set-up as planning systems are generally not designed to perform calculations at extremely extended SSDs.

11.3.1 Inhomogeneity compensation in TBI

Apart from the specifically stated dose limits to critical structures (e.g. lungs), all other parts of the body should receive a uniform TBI dose within ±10%. In order to achieve this, the influence of irregular body contours and tissue inhomogeneities has to be estimated and compensated for. This influence is larger if bilateral fields are used as the patient thickness varies considerably between head, neck, torso and legs.

There are several methods available to compensate for contour variation and missing tissue. The lead compensators/attenuators and tissue equivalent bolus are most commonly used for this purpose. The objective is to 'convert' patient's irregular body contour to an approximately rectangular box. This will ensure that the radiation beam undergoes the same effective attenuation (i.e. the effective path length is the same) along any ray within the treatment field, whether at the patient's head or patient's waist or ankles.

Tissue-equivalent bolus material is positioned directly on the patient's skin. Rice flower or sodium bicarbonate are often used, filled into small bags. The use of powder material means that the bags are flexible and can be easily moulded around a patient and assembled rapidly as required. Achieving exactly the desired thickness of bolus may though be difficult. Semi-flexible materials such as Superflab (Radiation Products Design, Inc) may provide easier thickness control. This material is a synthetic oil gel with a specific density of 1.02 g/cm^3. The density of any material used as bolus needs to be checked for its tissue-equivalency.

In the second approach, lead attenuators are used as tissue compensators to achieve uniform dose distribution at mid-lateral separation of head, neck, knees and ankles. While the bolus is placed directly onto the patient skin, the Pb attenuators are generally attached to an accessory tray in the accelerator treatment head. The particular thickness of the attenuator needs to be calculated for each patient's specific dimensions. Figure 11.9 shows a schematic diagram of the principle of Pb attenuators used as tissue compensators (please note that the real dimensions of the lead attenuators are much smaller when positioned in the linac head).

In order to calculate the thickness of the Pb attenuators required, the total effective thicknesses/separations of the patient at the prescription point (e.g. umbilicus level) and at the head, neck, knees and ankles have to be determined from the treatment planning system. Physical measurements of patient separations at these sites can be used as well; however, the impact of inhomogeneities contained within the body will not be accounted for. The required *Dose*

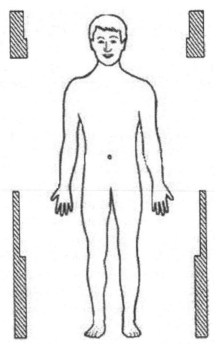

Figure 11.9. The principle of application of lead attenuators of varying thickness compensating for different amount of missing tissue at the head, neck and lower limb regions and 'converting' thus a patient's irregular body contour roughly into a square box.

Reduction Factor for the given site can be then calculated using the central percentage dose values, measured in water:

$$\text{Dose Reduction Factor (\%)} = \left(\frac{CPD_R}{CPD_C}\right) \times 100 \qquad (11.1)$$

where CPD_R is the central (midpoint) percentage dose at the prescription point level and CPD_C is the central percentage dose at the level where compensation is required (e.g. head). The Dose Reduction Factor is then matched to the same amount of lead transmission, where lead transmission must be measured for the linac beam used for TBI and a range of lead attenuators of varying thicknesses and tabulated. The thickness of lead required for compensation of missing tissue thickness at the given site can then be determined from the tabulated data.

For some treatment schedules the prescribed tumour dose is well above the lung tolerance (e.g. 12 Gy total dose versus 10 Gy lung dose limit). In this case the dose to lung has to be reduced to minimise the probability of lung complications. Commonly, bolus is added to the chest wall to reduce the lung dose. Partial transmission lung blocks have been used as well. Similarly, in case of AP-PA TBI, tissue equivalent bolus material should also be positioned in front of the neck to limit the dose to larynx.

11.3.2 Set-up procedure

An example of a TBI patient set-up is shown in Figure 11.10. For this set-up configuration (TBI Manual,

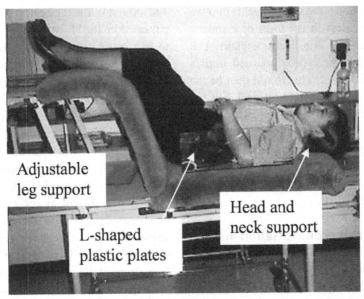

Adjustable leg support

L-shaped plastic plates

Head and neck support

Figure 11.10. Position of the patient on a TBI couch prior to placing chest bolus. (Courtesy Royal Adelaide Hospital)

RAH 2002), patients are treated with two laterally opposing fields applied at a distance of 340 cm between the radiation source and patient midline. At this distance the maximum radiation field size is approximately 1.3 m^2, which covers the patient in a supine position with legs resting on an adjustable leg support as shown in the picture. The purpose-built treatment couch has adjustable leg support and head & neck support to position the patient consistently at each treatment fraction. In addition to this, the two L-shaped plastic plates support the upper limbs and the bolus material consisting of rice flower bags around the chest region (bolus not shown). The patient's upper arms are held by the side of the chest with the hands folded across the anterior abdomen. The antero/lateral chest is bolused according to the treatment plan. A line laser is mounted onto the bunker ceiling at the treatment distance (340 cm) in order to position the patient midline reproducibly at the right distance.

The linac gantry angle of 270° and a collimator angle of 45° are used for treatment and TBI accessory tray is inserted into the linac head. The radiation field size is set to maximum (e.g. 40 × 40 cm^2). The accessory tray needs to contain outlines (e.g. using black paint or masking tape blocking the light field) indicating where the radiation fluence just starts to fall off at the beam edge when the collimator is fully opened, as no part of patient body should be placed in the beam fall-off (penumbra) region. The lead attenuators are taped on to the accessory tray to shield lower legs, neck and head (Figure 11.11). A build-up screen (beam spoiler) is positioned as close as possible to the TBI couch between the machine and the patient to give full build-up. The couch is rotated by 180° between the two beams.

11.3.3 *In vivo* dosimetry in TBI

Potentially lethal total body radiation dose is delivered during TBI in a relatively small number of treatment fractions. Often, non-standard patient and machine set-ups are applied, including highly extended SSD (>300 cm), low dose-rate, non-standard patient positions (see Figure 11.10) and TBI-specific treatment add-ons such as build-up screens or tissue compensators. Moreover, the patient must be turned between the beams and position of some equipment re-adjusted (e.g.

Pb attenuators). Variations in patient position can alter the distributions dramatically. In addition, limitations of the available input data and inherent problems with the calculation schemes make accurate determination of TBI dose distributions very difficult using most computer-generated treatment planning systems.

For these reasons, monitoring of the patient dose during treatment delivery, known as *in vivo* dosimetry, is highly desired and recommended (Yorke *et al.* 2005). Ion chambers, thermoluminescent dosimeters (TLDs), diodes or mosfets have all been used (Planskoy *et al.* 1996), with each detector type having some advantages and disadvantages that must be carefully considered. For example, TLDs require further processing so the results are not known for several hours. Diodes need various corrections to be applied due to their orientation, dose rate and energy dependence. They, however provide instantaneous readout so any remedial action (if required, e.g. due to inaccurate positioning of bolus or attenuators) can be taken immediately.

One method of determining midline doses employs entrance and exit dose measurements using detectors positioned at the head, axilla (to measure lung dose), waist, knee and ankle levels (see Figure 11.12). The detectors can be left on the patient in the same position for both treatment beams. The final result of each detector will then be the sum of doses received from the entrance dose of one field and the exit dose of the other. The central axis (midline) dose is calculated as:

$$D_{\text{centre}} = \left(\frac{D_L + D_R}{2}\right) \times F_{\text{Det}} \qquad (11.2)$$

where D_L is the dose received by a detector positioned on the left side of the patient, D_R is the dose received by a detector positioned on the right side of the patient and F_{Det} is a calibration factor related to patient thickness at the given anatomical site. F_{Det} is determined empirically from measurements for a given TBI set-up and a given detector system.

In addition to empirical measurements of detector calibration factor to determine the midline/midpoint dose from entrance and exit dose information, analytical approaches can be used as well. There are many different algorithms reported for deriving/estimating midpoint dose; however, none produces exact results, especially for inhomogeneous conditions. Some of the

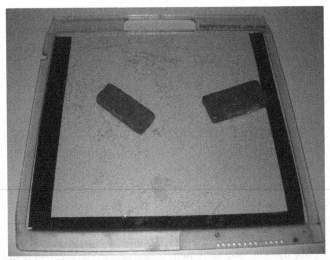

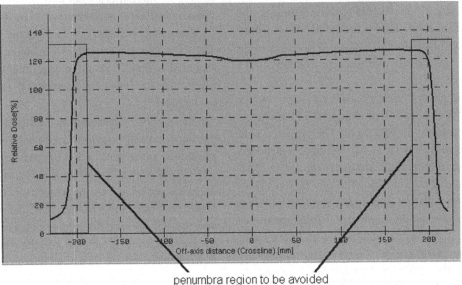

penumbra region to be avoided

Figure 11.11. Lead attenuators placed on an accessory tray ('shadow tray') to compensate for missing tissue in lower legs and head & neck regions (top). The black outline on the accessory tray blocks out the light field corresponding the radiation penumbra region, so that no part of the patient anatomy is positioned in the dose fall-off part of the dose profile (bottom). (Courtesy Royal Adelaide Hospital)

commonly used algorithms were derived by Huyskens *et al.* (1994) and Noel *et al.* (1995). Huyskens' algorithm employs entry and exit dose measurements as well as the measured beam data (tissue maximum ratios, backscatter factors).

Each clinic will have to develop its *in vivo* dosimetry protocol. It is advisable to measure the entrance and exit doses during the first 3 fractions. If the dose readings are consistent, the averaged results will provide accurate estimate of the dose delivered to the

prescription point as well as to the critical structures. If the results are inconsistent, further monitoring may be required for subsequent fractions. The clinician may adjust/reduce the prescription for the final fraction if it seems that dose tolerances (e.g. to lungs) will be exceeded.

11.3.4   Quality assurance in TBI

Quality assurance in TBI includes performance checks of the treatment planning system (including a

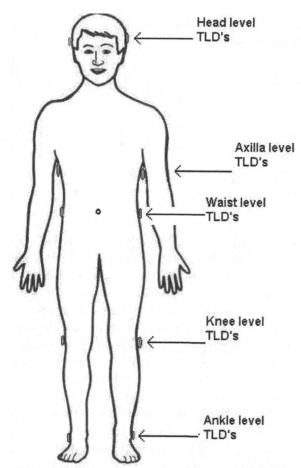

Figure 11.12. Schematic diagram of TLDs position for *in vivo* dosimetry in TBI. (Courtesy Royal Adelaide Hospital)

CT simulator) and the dose delivery apparatus (i.e. linac or Co-60 teletherapy unit). Attenuator and bolus thicknesses must be determined for the patient specific dimensions and manufactured (e.g. Pb attenuators) prior to treatment. The QA protocols need to cover linac dose calibration for the given TBI technique (e.g. extended SSD) and checks of all equipment used for TBI delivery. This includes application and correct positioning of all TBI specific add-ons such as flattening and attenuating filters or bolus and use of correct linac and patient specific treatment and set-up parameters.

Any detectors used for *in vivo* dosimetry need to be carefully calibrated and all correction factors determined. Constancy and reproducibility of detector performance need to be monitored as well.

11.4 RADIOBIOLOGICAL ASPECTS OF TBI

Total body irradiation is the systemic treatment of disseminated disease using external beam radiotherapy. TBI is traditionally employed for the irradiation of the spinal cord of leukemia and lymphoma patients in preparation for bone marrow transplant (BMT). The aim of TBI is to eradicate malignant cells of the spinal cord and also to suppress the immune system of the patients before transplant in order to avoid tissue rejection. Optimised TBI treatment regimens can reduce morbidity and mortality risks after BMT (Vriesendorp *et al.* 1994).

Radiation damage to critical organs and tissues during and after TBI is of major concern since certain radiation toxicities can be life-threatening or lead to long-term sequelae. The most affected organs and tissue systems after total body irradiation are the hematopoietic system, the spinal cord and the lungs. The paragraphs below describe the radiobiological aspects of radiation exposure of these affected tissues.

11.4.1   The hematopoietic system

Hematopoietic tissues are mostly located in the bone marrow, 60% of which reside in the pelvis and vertebrae. A very small fraction of stem cells of the hematopoietic system exist in the circulatory system of blood. Before becoming mature circulating blood cells, stem cells undergo a period of division and maturation, followed by differentiation without division. This transit time for transformation of a stem cell varies as a function of the type of circulatory blood cell (Table 11.1).

A hematopoietic stem cell divides into two daughter stem cells: the myeloid progenitor and the lymphoid progenitor. The myeloid progenitor is also called common myeloid progenitor (CMP) because it gives rise to all cells in the myeloid lineage. The common lymphoid progenitor (CLP) gives rise to all cells in the lymphoid lineage comprising T cells, B cells and natural killer cells. The discovery of the lymphoid progenitor in 1997 (Kondo *et al.* 1997) brought new hope in oncology for identifying the origins of various leukemias. Currently under investigation is whether the cellular events that transform normal cells into cancerous ones occur within the stem or progenitor

Table 11.1.   The hematopoietic system.

Hematopoietic stem cell	Myeloid progenitor	Erythrocyte
		Thrombocyte
		Granulocyte
		Macrophage
		Monocyte
		Dendritic cell
	Lymphoid progenitor	B-lymphocyte
		T-lymphocyte
		Natural killer (NK) cell

cell populations and also whether the leukemias are actually mature blood cells that have reacquired the self-renewal ability of stem cells.

Table 11.2 presents the effect of radiation exposure of various dose levels on blood cells. A dose as small as 30 cGy will reduce the number of lymphocytes, making them one of the most radiosensitive cells in the body.

11.4.2   The spinal cord

The spinal cord is the most typical serially structured organ, consequently large doses of radiation can cause irreversible side effects. The tolerance dose to the spine depends essentially on fraction size, and shows little dependence on overall treatment time. Lower fractional doses therefore reduce the risk of late effects. There is experimental evidence of two components of cell repair: one with a half-time less than 1 hour and one with a half-time of about 4 hours. Thus, in hyperfractionated radiation treatment, the time between two consecutive daily fractions should be kept to at least 6 hours. Late damage

to the spine results in two clinico-pathological syndromes. The first occurs from 6 to 18 months, and involves demyelination (loss of myelin which preserves the function of the axon) and necrosis of the white matter. The second has a longer latency period (from 1 to 4 years) and is based on vasculopathy. Early demyelination may develop after doses as low as 35 Gy, but is usually reversible. The tolerance dose or $TD_{5/5}$ (the dose which leads to 5% incidence of long-term adverse reactions in 5 years) for late vasculopathic damage is about 50 Gy for a 10 cm length of cord, and 55 Gy for a 5 cm irradiated length (Emami *et al.* 1991). For a total dose of 70 Gy using conventional fractions (2 Gy), the incidence of myelopathy increases to 50%.

11.4.3   The lung

Based on discussions on organ architecture (Chapter 5), the lung is considered to be a parallel organ because of the particular arrangement of its functional subunits. Therefore, the lung is dose-limiting only if a large volume is irradiated and also if the non-irradiated

Table 11.2.   The effect of radiation exposure of various dose levels on blood cells.

Radiation dose	Hematopoietic reaction
30 cGy	Reduction in the number of lymphocytes.
>0.3 Gy	Alteration in the number of blood cells, resulting in lymphocytopenia, granulocytopenia, thrombocytopenia, and anemia.
4–6 Gy	Temporal increase in granulocytes (due to mobilisation of the reserve pool) followed by a rapid fall by the end of the first week. Another fall occurs 18–20 days after irradiation.
>30 Gy (partial body irradiation)	Permanent aplasia (the bone marrow ceases to produce sufficient number of blood elements)

lung is not capable of adequate functioning because of pre-existing disease. The lung is also considered to be an intermediate- to late-responding organ because acute pneumonitis can occur at 2 to 6 months after treatment, and fibrosis can develop over a period of several months to years. The severity of radiation injury therefore depends on the volume irradiated, overall dose and fraction size (since fractionation is crucial for late-responding tissues). The lung is particularly sensitive to fractionation, having an α/β ratio of about 3 Gy.

11.4.4   TBI treatment

Among the treatment challenges raised by TBI the following are of major significance: the irregular shape of the irradiated volume (the human body), the extension of the radiation field beyond the treated volume in all directions and the achievement of a uniform dose distribution (for a homogeneously distributed tumour cell population). Shielding of critical organs is therefore required, yet maintaining a uniform dose along the treated area. Fractionation, as demonstrated by the 5R's (see Chapter 5), has crucial importance for both normal tissue repair and repopulation as well as for tumour reoxygenation and rearrangement along the cell cycle, though it is unlikely that hypoxia and repopulation constitute a problem in TBI of leukemia (Weldon 1997). Fractionated TBI, with fraction sizes around 3 Gy, was shown to be more effective than single-dose treatment (Vriesendorp *et al.* 1994) thus fractionated TBI has been commonly trialled in clinics. While bone marrow stem cells, leukemic cells and immunocytes have a limited ability to repair radiation damage, lung tissue cells have a greater capacity of sublethal damage repair (Evans 1983). Fractionation, therefore, represents an advantage for damaged lung cells, allowing them time for repair in between fractions, an added reason to diverge from large single doses of radiation.

A study conducted by Gopal *et al.* (2001) aimed to compare two TBI fractionation regimens with respect to pulmonary toxicity. One protocol consisted of twice-daily fractions of 1.7 Gy for 3 days to a total of 10.2 Gy through lateral fields, without lung shielding and, in the other protocol, the dose was increased to a total of 12 Gy, delivered in fractions of 3 Gy once daily for 4 days through anteroposterior fields, with lung shielding during the third dose. Progression-free survival at 3-years was superior in the higher-dose per fraction group (81%) compared with the lower dose group (31%). Next to superior control of the disease the study showed that dose escalation does not increase pulmonary toxicity, making this protocol feasible for decreasing recurrence rate in patients with hematologic malignancies.

Regarding the optimal fractionation protocol for leukemia, a common consensus is yet to be established as the response of the leukemic cells to radiation was shown to be leukemia type-dependent. Clonogenic surviving fractions after 2 Gy (SF_2) have been determined for various human leukemia cell lines irradiated *in vitro* and the distribution of SF_2 ranged from 0.1 to 0.7 (Weldon 1997). While most leukemic cell lines are radiosensitive, there is a significant percent of leukemic cells which are more radioresistant than typical carcinomas ($SF_2 = 0.5$). Survival curve data indicate that majority of leukemic lines have high α/β ratio (with low β, implying low repair capacity) (Steel and Weldon 1991).

11.5   CLINICAL TRIALS

The large volume of normal tissue irradiated during TBI necessitates new treatment techniques which are able to diminish radiation-induced side effects, without decreasing tumour control. The clinical success of IMRT has enabled the implementation of intensity-modulated treatment in TBI therapy. The role of intensity-modulation is to preferentially focalise the radiation dose on the spine, reducing the dose to the adjacent organs. The scientific literature includes a number of feasibility studies for linac-based intensity modulated total marrow irradiation (Aydogan *et al.* 2006; Wilkie *et al.* 2008) or helical tomotherapy showing substantial dose reduction to critical structures (Hui *et al.* 2005; Wong *et al.* 2006). A three iso-centre technique delivered with linac-based intensity modulation trialled on a Rando phantom showed, using 22 thermoluminescent detectors throughout the phantom, a 29%–65% dose reduction to critical organs compared to conventional TBI (Wilkie *et al.* 2008). An added advantage of helical tomotherapy was the 50% treatment time reduction by increasing the field width in the inferior-superior direction (Hui *et al.* 2005). While presently the number of studies

Table 11.3. Compilation of clinical trials designed for TBI with intensity modulated radiotherapy.

Trial/reference	Treatment protocol	Outcome
Intensity-modulated total marrow irradiation (**IM-TMI**) for advanced hematologic malignancies *Phase I trial – Currently recruiting (University of Illinois 2010 update)* ClinicalTrials.gov Identifier: NCT00988013	Intensity modulated total marrow irradiation with the delivery of 3 Gy per day for either: 1, 2, 3, or 4 days.	*Primary outcome measures:* overall toxicity and day 100 transplant related mortality
IMRT + chemotherapy before donor stem cell transplant for patients with relapsed or refractory acute lymphoblastic leukaemia *Phase I–II trial – Currently recruiting (National Cancer Institute 2009 update)* ClinicalTrials.gov Identifier: NCT00576979	IMRT using helical tomotherapy once or twice daily on days -9 to -6 or -9 to -5 (depending on dose) *(prior to transplant)*. Etoposide IV administered on day -5 or -4 and cyclophosphamide IV on day -3 or -2.	*Primary outcome measures:* - maximum tolerated dose of IMRT - toxicity - overall survival - relapse-free survival - event-free survival - relative risk
Static **IMRT** (intensity modulated therapy with compensators) for hematologic malignancies *257 patients (Schneider 2008)*	12 Gy total dose delivered in 6 fractions within 3 days before transplant	*Tumour control:* 47.9% 5-year overall survival 23% 5-year tumour-related mortality rate *Toxicity:* 10.9% interstitial pneumonitis
Helical tomotherapy **targeting total bone marrow** *dose escalation trial and clinical feasibility study; 1 case study (Hui 2007)*	6 Gy in 3 fractions + chemotherapy possible to escalate dose	*Tumour control:* no evidence of disease 150 days post transplant *Toxicity:* no adverse effects (only early nausea which was managed)
Targeted total marrow irradiation (TMI) using three-dimensional image-guided tomographic IMRT *dosimetric and feasibility study (Wong 2006)*	potential to escalate the dose to the bone (and marrow) to 20 Gy while maintaining doses to normal tissue below conventional TBI doses	*Toxicity:* 1.7- to 7.5-fold reduction in median organ doses was observed with TMI compared with conventional TBI

reporting on clinical outcome after TBI using intensity-modulated radiotherapy is very limited, the promising results have encouraged the development of new trials which are currently recruiting patients (Table 11.3).

To constrain the lung dose and also to homogenise the dose delivered to the whole body Schneider *et al.* (2008) have designed a TBI regimen using intensity-modulated compensators based on total body CT scans. Their report on the long-term outcome after treatment (TBI + transplant) showed very good 5-year survival rates with decreased toxicity for patients with hematologic malignancies (see Table 11.3), suggesting also that dose limitation to other organs (such as

kidneys) using IMRT with compensators could further decrease long-term adverse effects.

The safe delivery of IMRT with helical tomotherapy turns this technique into the most advanced TBI treatment available. Ongoing clinical trials will define the maximum tolerated doses and the potential advantages and limitations of new treatment delivery techniques with intensity modulation and image guidance for total body irradiation.

11.6   REFERENCES

Aydogan B, Mundt AJ and Roeske JC (2006) Linac-based intensity modulated total marrow irradiation (IM-TMI). *Technology in Cancer Research and Treatment* **5**(5): 513–520.

Bhat M, Bezak E and Nicholls R (2002) 'Total body photon irradiation procedure for TS2 (23 MV), RAH TBI manual, March 2002'. Royal Adelaide Hospital, internal report.

Emami B, Lyman J, Brown A, Coia L, Goiten M *et al.* (1991) Tolerance of normal tissue to therapeutic radiation. *International Journal of Radiation Oncology Biology and Physics* **21**: 109–122.

Evans RG (1983) Radiobiological considerations in magna-field irradiation. *International Journal of Radiation Oncology Biology and Physics* **9**(12): 1907–1911.

Fitzpatrick PJ and Garrett PG (1981) Metastatic breast cancer ovarian ablation with lower half-body irradiation. *International Journal of Radiation Oncology Biology and Physics* **7**(1): 1523–1526.

Fitzpatrick PJ and Rider WD (1976) Half body radiotherapy of advanced cancer. *Journal of the Canadian Association of Radiologists* **27**: 75–79.

Galvin JM (n.d.) 'Total body irradiation dosimetry and practical considerations'. http://www.aapm.org/meetings/2001AM/pdf/7233-71758.pdf

Gopal R, Ha CS, Tucker SL, Khouri IF *et al.* (2001) Comparison of two total body irradiation fractionation regimens with respect to acute and late pulmonary toxicity. *Cancer* **92**(7): 1949–1958.

Hui SK, Kapatoes J, Fowler J, Henderson D *et al.* (2005) Feasibility study of helical tomotherapy for total body or total marrow irradiation. *Medical Physics* **32**(10): 3214–3224.

Hui SK, Verneris M, Higgins P, Gerbi B *et al.* (2007) Helical tomotherapy targeting total bone marrow – first clinical experience at the University of Minnesota. *Acta Oncologica* **46**(2): 250–255.

Huyskens D, Van Dam J and Dutreix A (1994) Midplane dose determination using in-vivo dose measurements in combination with portal imaging. *Physics in Medicine and Biology* **39**: 1089–1101.

Kondo M, Weissman IL and Akashi K (1997) Identification of clonogenic common lymphoid progenitors in mouse bone marrow. *Cell* **91**: 661–672.

Lin H and Drzymala RE (2003) Total-body and hemibody irradiation. In: *Principles and Practice of Radiation Oncology*. 4th edn. (Eds C Perez and L Brady) pp. 400–410. J.B. Lippincott company, Philadelphia.

Noel A, Aletti P, Bey P and Malissard L (1995) Detection of errors in individual patients in radiotherapy by systematic in vivo dosimetry. *Radiotherapy and Oncology* **34**: 144–151.

Planskoy B, Bedford AM, Davis FM, Tapper PD *et al.* (1996) Physical aspects of total-body irradiation at the Middlesex Hospital (UCL group of hospitals), London 1988–1993: I. Phantom measurements and planning methods. *Physics in Medicine and Biology* **41**(11): 2327–2343.

Podgorsak EB and Podgorsak MB (1999) Total body irradiation with photon beams. In: *Modern Technology in Radiation Oncology*. (Ed. J Van Dyk) pp. 642–662. Medical Physics Publishing, Wisconsin.

Podgorsak EB and Podgorsak MB (2005) Special procedures and techniques in radiotherapy. In: *Radiation Oncology Physics: A Handbook for Teachers and Students*. (Ed. EB Podgorsak) pp. 516–522. IAEA publication 1196. International Atomic Energy Agency, Vienna.

Poussin-Rosillo H, Nisce LZ and Lee BJ (1978) Complications of total nodal irradiation of Hodgkin's disease stages III and IV. *Cancer* **42**(2): 437–441.

Schneider R, Schultze J, Jensen JM, Hebbinghaus D *et al.* (2008) Long-term outcome after static intensity-modulated total body radiotherapy using compensators stratified by pediatric and adult cohorts. *International Journal of Radiation Oncology Biology and Physics* **70**(1): 194–202.

Steel GG and Weldon TE (1991) The radiation biology of paediatric tumours. In: *Paediatric Oncology*. (Eds R Pinkerton and N Plowman) pp. 73–86. John Wiley, London.

Strober S, Kotzin BL, Hoppe RT, Slavin S *et al.* (1981) The treatment of intractable rheumatoid arthritis with lymphoid irradiation. *International Journal of Radiation Oncology Biology and Physics* **7**: 1–7.

Van Dyk J, Galvin JM, Glasgow GP and Podgorsak EB (1986) 'The physical aspects of total and half body photon irradiation'. A report of Task Group 29 Radiation Therapy Committee, AAPM Report No. 17. American Association of Physicists in Medicine, New York.

Vriesendorp HM, Chu H, Ochran TG, Besa PC *et al.* (1994) Radiobiology of total body radiation. *Bone Marrow Transplant* **14**(Suppl 4): S4–8.

Weldon TE (1997) The radiobiological basis of total body irradiation. *British Journal of Radiology* **70**: 1204–1207.

Wilkie JR, Tiryaki H, Smith BD, Roeske JC *et al.* (2008) Feasibility study for linac-based intensity modulated total marrow irradiation. *Medical Physics* **35**(12): 5609–5618.

Wong JY, Liu A, Schultheiss T, Popplewell L *et al.* (2006) Targeted total marrow irradiation using three-dimensional image-guided tomographic intensity-modulated radiation therapy: an alternative to standard total body irradiation. *Biology of Blood and Marrow Transplantation* **12**(3): 306–315.

Yorke E, Alecu R, Ding L, Fontenla D, Kalend A, Kaurin D, Masterson-McGary ME, Marinello G, Matzen T, Saini A, Shi J, Simon W, Zhu TC and Zhu XR (2005) 'Diode in vivo dosimetry for patients receiving external beam radiation therapy'. Report of Task Group 62 of the Radiation Therapy Committee, AAPM Report no. 87. Published for the American Association of Physicists in Medicine by Medical Physics Publishing.

http://clinicaltrials.gov/ct2/show/NCT00576979 accessed on 3/03/2010.

http://clinicaltrials.gov/ct2/show/NCT00988013 accessed on 3/03/2010.

12   Electron therapy: radiobiology and physics aspects of treatment

12.1   INTRODUCTION

Electron therapy is a form of external beam radiotherapy in which the tumour volume is irradiated with energetic (~4 MeV to 25 MeV) electrons. Due to the relatively short range of the electrons (see Chapter 1), electron therapy is generally used in the treatment of superficial tumours (within 5 cm from the patient's surface). It is also used to boost the radiation dose to cancer node sites. Examples of electron beam therapy include treatment of skin and lip cancers, head & neck cancers, chest-wall cancers, upper respiratory and digestive-tract superficial tumours and as a boost treatment to lymph nodes, operative scars and residual tumour disease, for example after mastectomy (Tapley 1976; Meyer and Vaeth 1991). Electron therapy can be delivered using electron beams only or by combining electron and photon beams and/or interstitial therapy (Tapley 1977).

Radiation dose deposited by an electron beam in a medium initially increases from the surface, until a dose plateau (~90% to 100% of maximum dose on the central axis) is reached. The dose distribution then falls off steeply as the electrons come to a stop by losing all their energy and therefore cannot deposit anymore dose. Typical percentage depth dose curves on the central axis for electron beams of various energies between

6 and 18 MeV are shown in Figure 12.1. The small amount of dose deposited beyond the range of electrons (dose tail) is due to bremsstrahlung photons generated in the interactions of electrons with the medium (mostly with the linac scattering foils, see section 12.2).

Because of the sharp dose fall-off, superficial cancers can be irradiated to required doses while underlying healthy tissues receive minimum dose. This is generally not possible to achieve with X-rays as the exponential character of their dose attenuation and higher penetrating capacity (depending on the X-ray beam energy) lead to much higher doses to underlying anatomy. Figure 12.2 compares percentage depth dose curves for 9 MeV electron and 6 MV photon beams produced by a Varian iX linear accelerator.

The bremsstrahlung photon production increases with the energy of the accelerated electrons. As a result of their contribution to total dose, at electron beam energies around 20 MeV, the depth dose curves lose their sharp fall-off and the dose in tail increases considerably (~10%). Consequently, electron beams of energies higher than ~20 MeV may have only limited clinical value.

The use of electron beam energies between 3 and 6 MeV could clinically compete with 250 kV X-ray orthovoltage irradiation. However, electrons offer the

L. Marcu et al., *Biomedical Physics in Radiotherapy for Cancer*,
DOI 10.1007/978-0-85729-733-4_12, © CSIRO 2012

Central axis distribution

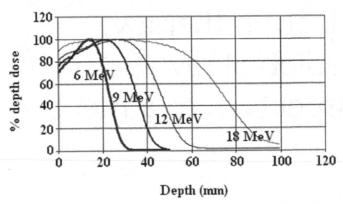

Figure 12.1 Central axis depth dose distributions of electron beams between 6 and 18 MeV from a Siemens KD2 accelerator measured in water for a 10 × 10 cm² field size and 100 cm source-to-surface distance. (Courtesy Royal Adelaide Hospital)

advantages of skin sparing (due to dose build up at the surface) and the increased depth dose penetration compared to 250 kV photon beam. Electrons are particles with low linear energy transfer and therefore the relative biological effectiveness of high-energy electrons is considered to be the same as that of megavoltage photons. As a result, electron beams can be quite straightforwardly combined with photons to achieve a desired dose distribution. The selection of beam energies and the ratio of electron and photon beam doses depend on the location of the tumour and the depth to be treated. The commonly used treatment set-ups use either a single field or parallel opposed fields (Tapley 1977).

12.2 PRODUCTION OF ELECTRON BEAMS

Electrons have been used for radiation treatments since the 1950s and they represent a common treatment modality available in most modern clinics. At present, linear accelerators are mostly used to produce photons. Modern high energy medical linacs can work in so-called dual mode, i.e. they can produce both

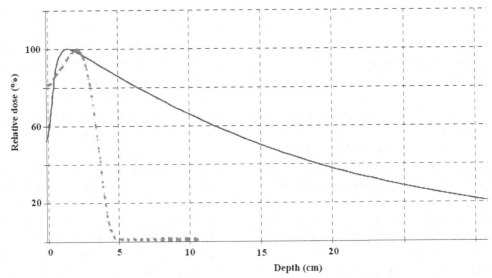

Figure 12.2. Comparison of the percentage depth dose curves for 9 MeV electron beam (dotted line) and 6 MV photon beam (solid line) from Varian iX linear accelerator. (Courtesy Royal Adelaide Hospital)

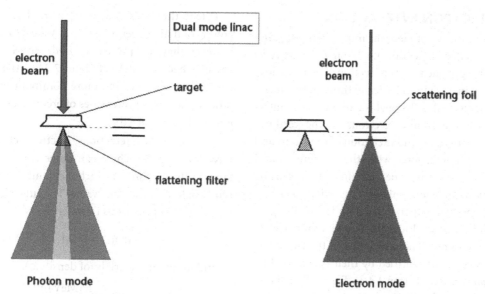

Figure 12.3. Schematic diagram of linac treatment head in an X-ray (left) and in an electron (right) mode. In order to produce an electron beam, the target and the flattening filter are removed from the beam path and scattering foils are inserted instead to broaden up the accelerated electron pencil beam.

clinical X-ray as well as electron beams. The linacs can typically provide two to three megavoltage photon energies, and up to seven electron beam energies in the range from 4 to 22 MeV (Strydom *et al.* 2005).

As medical linear accelerators use (to start with) accelerated electrons to produce bremsstrahlung photons in interactions with the target nuclei after exiting from a waveguide (see Chapter 3), it is an obvious conclusion that the accelerated electron beam itself can be used as the source of therapeutic radiation. In order to deliver a high energy electron beam, electrons are accelerated in the waveguide in the same manner as for X-ray production. The target and the flattening filter are removed from the electron beam path (see Figure 12.3) and the energetic electrons will exit the accelerator. As the waveguide produces a fine pencil-beam of electrons (less than 2 mm in diameter), it cannot cover the treatment area and must be therefore broadened to the desired clinical dimensions. To achieve this, the electrons are scattered by a pair of scattering foils (Figure 12.3). As discussed in Chapter 1, electrons scatter extensively and the scattering power (i.e. the probability of scattering interaction) is proportional to the atomic number, Z, of the foil and inversely proportional to the electron energy. Thin metal foils are generally used (usually a combination of Sn, Au or Pb foils) to scatter electrons as they

provide the advantage of high Z (and therefore high scattering power) and can be rolled to very thin thickness (to minimise the electron energy loss in the foil). A dual foil system is usually applied. The first foil is designed to widen the beam by multiple scattering, while the second foil is designed to make the beam intensity uniform/flat in cross-section. The thickness of the second foil is not the same across the beam to provide required amount of flattening and widening of the beam. Different foil combinations are used for different electron energies produced by a linac. The choice of foil is a compromise between spreading the electron beam while aiming to:

- keeping it flat
- not degrading the energy too much
- not contaminating the spectrum with bremsstrahlung X-rays.

Also of note is the fact, that the electron bunches (produced by an electron gun) entering the waveguide contain many more electrons in the X-ray mode than in the electron mode. Much higher initial electron intensities are required to produce the desired amount of X-rays as bremsstrahlung yield is quite small (only a few percent) and most of the electrons will lose their energy in collision interactions with other electrons of the target material.

12.3 ELECTRON INTERACTIONS

As the basic theory of electron interactions was discussed in Chapter 1 (section 1.4.7), only a short revision will be provided in this section. Electrons lose their energy in a medium basically through two interaction processes: a) collisional (or ionisational) interactions with the atomic electrons of the medium resulting in ionisation and excitation of the atoms and b) Coulomb interactions with the medium nuclei resulting in electrons decelerating and causing bremsstrahlung photon emission (i.e. radiative energy loss). The energy loss per interaction is usually quite small, requiring about 100 000 interactions for an electron to come to rest. The probability of the two interaction processes is quantified by their corresponding *stopping powers* (see section 1.4.3). Figure 12.4 shows the dependence of collisional, S_{col}/ρ, and radiative, S_{rad}/ρ, electron mass stopping powers (normalised to density, ρ, of the material) for water and lead. Collisional energy loss depends on the ratio of the atomic number to the mass number, Z/A, of the atoms of the medium (i.e. S_{col}/ρ is higher for water compared to lead). In addition, it increases as the kinetic energy of the electron gets smaller (*1/E* dependence).

Due to the Z dependence of the radiative stopping power, radiative energy losses in water are minimal, however they are present in lead even for electron energies below 1 MeV; at about 7 MeV the radiative energy loss becomes the more dominant interaction process (i.e. higher intensities of bremsstrahlung photons will be produced).

As a result of interactions, electrons change their directions rapidly. The mean range is the depth/distance in the medium at which the number of electrons is one-half of the original value. The rule of thumb for the range, R, of electrons in water is:

$$R\,(cm) = \frac{E}{2}\,(MeV) \qquad (12.1)$$

and for other materials (of density ρ):

$$R\,(cm) = \frac{E\,(MeV)}{2}\frac{1}{\rho} \qquad (12.2)$$

If the range of electrons is expressed in terms of g/cm², it is independent of the absorbing material and only depends upon energy.

Range straggling for electrons (section 1.4.4) is significant as the total path of energy loss is different for all initially monoenergetic electrons within the

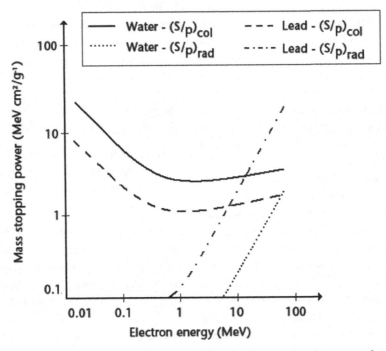

Figure 12.4. Dependence of electron collisional, S_{col}/ρ, and radiative, S_{rad}/ρ, mass stopping powers for water and lead as a function of electron energy.

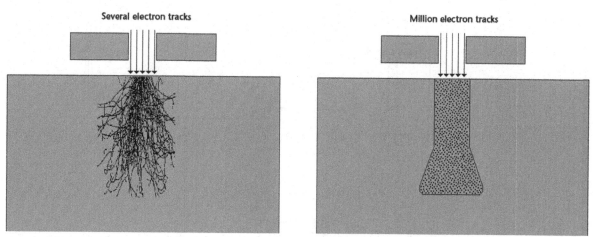

Figure 12.5 Schematic diagram of electron tracks in a medium due to a small number of electrons (left) and the averaging effect of millions of electron tracks. (Courtesy Royal Adelaide Hospital)

beam (see Figure 12.5 left); only large electron intensities will result in smooth/homogenous dose profiles.

While the waveguide produces a monoenergetic electron beam, its interactions with scattering foils and other materials in the linac treatment head mean that the single energy of the initial electron beam is lost in the scattering process; the electron energy is reduced and energy spread occurs (i.e. the beam becomes polyenergetic with the mean energy smaller than that of the initial electron pencil beam). In other words, the energy reduces with depth into the medium and energy spectrum becomes more 'smeared out'. Figure 12.6 shows how the energy spectrum of a 10 MeV electron pencil beam changes during stopping in a carbon attenuator. In a clinical situation, upon exiting the accelerator, further reduction and

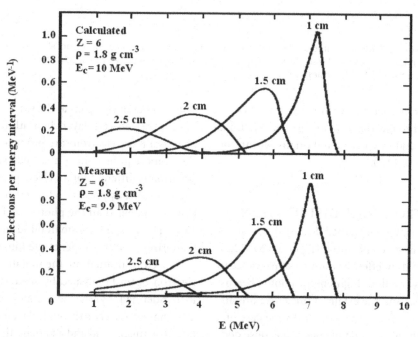

Figure 12.6. Calculated and measured energy fluence spectra for a 10 MeV electron beam stopping in carbon. (With kind permission from Springer Science&Business Media: Symposium on high energy electrons: Energiespektren schneller elektronen in verschiedenen tiefen, 1965, p. 260, Harder D., Copyright Springer-Verlag, Berlin)

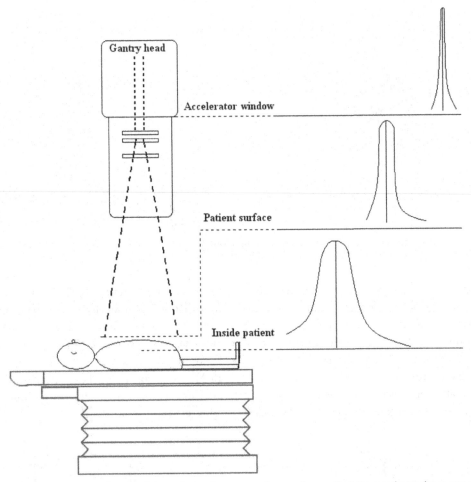

Figure 12.7. Schematic diagram of gradual degradation (i.e. energy loss and spread) of the accelerated monoenergetic electron beam as it passes through the scattering foils, through the air gap between the accelerator window and a patient surface and inside a patient (not to scale).

spread of electron energies within the beam occurs while passing through the air gap between the linac treatment head and the patient and finally within the patient (see Figure 12.7).

12.4   ELECTRON DOSE DISTRIBUTION

Electron beams exhibit absorbed dose build-up effect close to the surface of a phantom (Figures 12.1, 12.2). Though this build-up effect has similar appearance to the build-up observed for high-energy photon beams, the physical basis and the extent of this effect are different for the two types of radiations. In the case of a photon beam, the absorption of energy (i.e. dose deposition) takes place only when secondary electrons are first produced by photon interactions with matter.

The number of electrons at the surface is small. As the beam penetrates the layers beneath the surface of the phantom more electrons are produced until a state of electronic equilibrium is reached (section 3.2). The situation is different for an electron beam. Since electrons are already present in the beam, the surface dose is much higher than the photon surface dose (Figure 12.2). The reason for a small build-up is due to lateral scattering as electrons penetrate into the tissue layers.

In a clinical situation, the radiation field size of an electron beam broadened by scattering foils is collimated/defined by the accelerator jaws. While the electron beam passes through the air gap between the linac treatment head and a patient, the electrons interact with the air molecules and scatter. This results in the loss of sharp radiation field edge definition as the

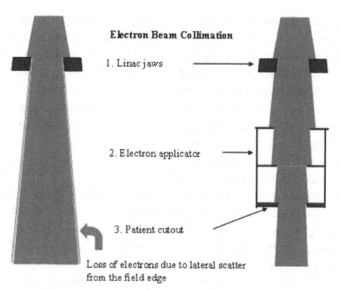

Figure 12.8. Schematic diagram of electron beam collimation on a linear accelerator.

penumbra (i.e. the width of the radiation field edge defined as the distance between the 80% and 20% isodose lines) broadens. Consequently, the electron beam needs to be collimated again closer to the patient surface (~5–15 cm) with the use of so-called electron cones (Figures 12.8, 12.9) that are mounted into the linac head. The cones define square or rectangular fields only. Any personalised field shaping is achieved by inserting a patient specific cutout made of e.g. cerrobend or another high Z material into the applicator. The cutout material will absorb undesired portions of the electron beam and the opening within the cutout will produce a conformal field aperture.

There is some radiation leakage from the electron applicator. According to international standards, the maximum leakage permissible at the applicator surface is 5% of the maximum dose on the central axis.

Once the collimated electron beam hits the patient, the electrons will start scattering far more intensely (compared to scatter in air) resulting in the loss of electrons from the beam's central axis. However, some electrons will also scatter from within the beam towards the central axis; i.e. they compensate the loss of the electrons scattered laterally from the axis. This is observed as the dose build-up on the percentage depth dose curve (Figure 12.10). The dose will stop rising when so-called *lateral electronic equilibrium* is reached; i.e. as many electrons are scattered away from the central axis as are scattered towards it.

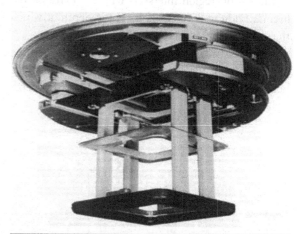

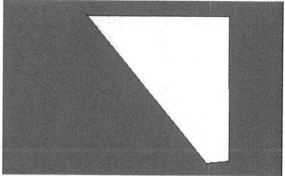

Figure 12.9. An electron applicator (top) mounted to the accelerator treatment head to shape the electron beam (Copyright ©2009, Varian Medical Systems, Inc. All rights reserved.). Schematic diagram of a custom patient cutout (bottom) where the undesired portions of the electron beam will be absorbed by the cutout made of high Z material (shaded region).

12.4.1   Percentage depth dose curve of an electron beam

Specification of the parameters used to characterise the electron beam central axis depth dose curve are based on ICRU report no 35 (ICRU 1984) and relate to description of four distinct regions: skin (surface) dose, build up region, fall-off region and bremsstrahlung tail.

As shown in Figure 12.10, the relative surface dose, D_S, is defined at 0.5 mm depth in a medium (i.e. tissue/water) as it is experimentally difficult to determine the dose exactly at the surface. D_S is expressed in terms of percentage (%) of the maximum dose. Range parameters R_{100}, R_{50} and R_p are the depth of the dose maximum, D_{max}, in water, the depth of the 50% dose level and the practical range respectively (measured in cm or g/cm^2). The practical range R_p is the depth at which the tangent plotted through the steepest portion of the fall-off region intersects with the extrapolated bremsstrahlung dose (D_x). R_q is the depth at which the same tangent meets the level of D_{max}.

The measure of the clinically useful portion of the depth dose profile is usually taken as the distance between the 85% dose levels, R_{85}^* and R_{85} (this value

can vary between the 80% and 90% isodose lines, depending on the local clinical practice). This is also called the therapeutic range. D_x represents the relative dose (% of D_{max}) due to the bremsstrahlung contribution to total dose.

The normalised dose gradient, G_0, quantifies the steepness of the fall-off region of the depth dose curve and is defined as:

$$G_0 = R_p / (R_p - R_q) \qquad (12.3)$$

Rapid fall-off of the dose beyond the therapeutic range is generally desired to avoid irradiation of healthy tissues beyond the tumour volume.

Other parameters are also often used to describe an electron beam. These include the most probable energy $E_{p,0}$ on the phantom surface, the mean energy $\overline{E_0}$ on the phantom surface, and R_{50}, the depth at which the absorbed dose falls to 50% of the maximum dose.

A 2D or 3D deposition of dose within a medium is visualised through the use of isodose curves. An isodose curve is a line on which all points receive the same radiation dose. A series of these curves form a map of relative radiation dose intensities. Isodoses are

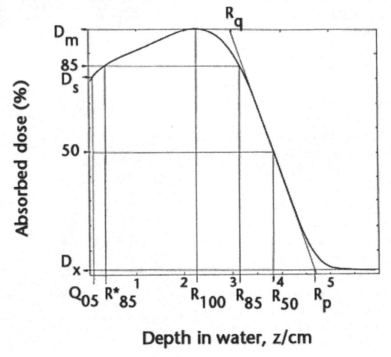

Figure 12.10. Specification of parameters used to characterise electron beam central axis depth dose curve based on ICRU report no 35 (courtesy ICRU 1984). See text for parameter definition.

usually displayed as percentage of the dose delivered to a reference point; usually D_{max} on the central axis. The shape of isodose curves also reflects the scattering of the electron beam. The degree of spread of an isodose curve depends on the isodose level, electron energy, field size and shape.

For the low value isodose curves (<20%) a bulging effect is seen. This is a consequence of the increase in electron scattering angle as the electrons slow down (the scattering angle is inversely proportional to the electron energy). At higher electron energies, the beams display constriction of the higher value isodose curves (>80%) due to the loss of sharp definition of the field edge as electrons penetrate into the tissue layers and scatter laterally (Strydom *et al.* 2005). The effect of isodose bulging and constricting due to electron scattering in air can also be observed as the distance between the electron applicator and the patient surface increases (Figure 12.11). In other words, the useful field size actually shrinks as the source-to-surface distance increases.

Typical percentage depth dose curves and corresponding isodose distributions for 6, 9 and 21 MeV electron beams produced by a Siemens KD2 accelerator are shown in Figure 12.12 (p. 218). The isodose distribution is greatly influenced by the type of electron cones used in the machine. The phenomena of bulging and constricting isodose curves can be seen. Increase in bremsstrahlung dose contribution with the increasing electron energy is also visible.

The shape of the percentage depth dose curve remains the same with increasing field size for field sizes larger than the practical range of the electron beam for a given energy. This is because electrons from the radiation field edge cannot reach the central axis and contribute to the depth dose. On the other hand, if the radiation field size is small, the lateral electronic equilibrium can never be achieved. As a result, the dose rate on the central axis decreases and the depth of maximum dose moves closer to the surface and the surface dose increases. The depth dose curves also lose the dose plateau and the sharp dose gradient in the fall-off region. The isodose curve becomes essentially two penumbral regions and the high dose volume is very constricted in width at depth. The shape of the percentage depth

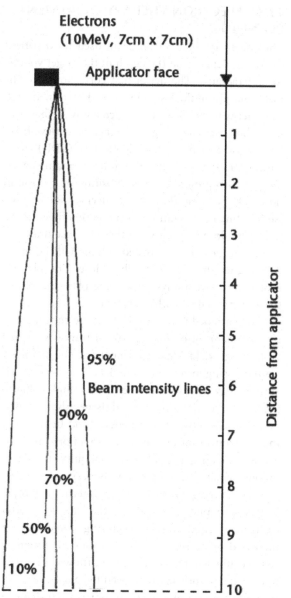

Figure 12.11. Constriction of the 95 and 90% isodose lines and bulging of the 10% isodose line as the distance from the electron applicator increases. This phenomenon is a result of electrons scattering in the air. (Reproduced with permission from Medical Physics Publishing, Madison, WI: Figure 6.29. p. 432, *Physics and Dosimetry of Therapy Electron Beams* by Stanley C. Klevenhagen, 1993)

dose curves for a 12 MeV electron beam produced by a Varian iX linac and 2, 3, 4, 5, 6, 10 cm² field sizes are shown in Figure 12.13. The loss of sharp dose fall-off and movement of D_{max} position can be seen for field sizes below 5 cm².

12.4   ELECTRON THERAPY TREATMENT PLANNING

The energy of the electron beam used for a patient treatment depends on the depth of the target volume to be irradiated. The depth that corresponds to the distal margin of the lesion must be determined first. The energy is then selected in such a way so that relatively homogeneous target coverage is achieved; i.e. the central axis percentage depth dose (PDD) curve parameters are matched to the clinical circumstances. Dose is then prescribed at the position of maximum dose, D_{max}, or at the second (deeper) 80 or 90% isodose line (i.e. within the therapeutic range). If the treatment dose is specified to these isodose lines, the maximum dose to the treated volume will be up to 20% higher than the prescribed dose. The planner should therefore always inspect the plan and report the maximum dose within a patient.

As mentioned in section 12.1 most electron beam treatments are used for superficial tumours treated with a single field. Many treatments may be manually planned using measured beam data. The dose distributions may however become more complex due to presence of uneven surfaces and tissue inhomogeneities. Consequently, once the energy and field size of the electron beam are chosen, corrections must be applied for air gaps and beam obliquity, for tissue inhomogeneities (e.g. lungs and bones), uneven surfaces. Both irregular surfaces and internal heterogeneities generate changes in the lateral scatter electronic equilibrium producing volumes of increased or decreased dose. Add-ons like bolus (a tissue equivalent material like paraffin wax or polysterene) and absorbers might need to be used in order to compensate for missing tissue or irregular shape or to modify skin dose or dose at depth. Irregular surfaces are often encountered when treating nose, eye or ear areas as well as areas affected by surgical interventions/excisions.

Variations in radiation field size of the beam influence the percentage depth dose curve as well as dose rate on the axis (often related to as the dose output). The oblique (non-perpendicular) beam incidence results in the maximum dose, D_{max}, shifting to shallower depths; the larger the incidence angle the shallower the depth of maximum dose and the larger the

dose output at this point. Oblique beam incidence often occurs in treatments of sloped or curved surfaces like chest wall, skull or limbs. Extending the source-to-surface distance produces a large change in the dose output, only a minimal change in the percentage depth dose curve and a significant change in the beam penumbra.

Electrons also produce dose distributions with higher dose gradients than those of photons. This is the result of different interaction processes within an absorbing medium. Thus different modelling algorithms are needed to calculate dose deposition by an electron beam.

Commonly used algorithm, that is implemented in several modern 3D planning systems (e.g. Pinnacle and CMS Focus), is Hogstrom's pencil-beam algorithm (Hogstrom *et al.* 1981) and is based on the Fermi–Eyges pencil beam theory. Square-field central axis depth dose data measured in water are used as input for the model to calculate dose for any field size. It also utilises CT data on a pixel-by-pixel basis and can accurately model variable air gap. It can accurately calculate the effect of irregular surface on dose homogeneity regardless of the air gap between the source and the patient (Hogstrom and Almond 2006).

12.4.1   Lead skin collimation

Apart from custom made cutouts (Figure 12.9) skin collimation may also be used to define the electron beam aperture. This is generally used to reduce the penumbra of the small fields when treating near critical structures. It is usually made of lead or lead alloy material that conforms to and is placed on the patient's surface. The lead thickness needs to be sufficient to absorb the unwanted radiation but not excessive. A rule of thumb can be used to estimate the thickness: use 1 mm of Pb for every 2 MeV of electron energy (i.e. for a 12 MeV electron beam 6 mm lead thickness is required). Radiation scatter from lead will affect the PDD. As a result, the dose output must be measured for each case carefully.

12.4.2   Internal shielding

For some clinical scenarios internal shielding might need to be used to protect critical structures (e.g. gums when treating lip lesions or eyes when treating eyelid

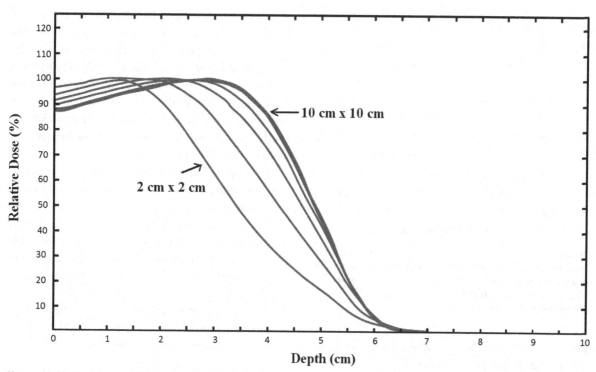

Figure 12.13. The shape of the percentage depth dose curves for a 12 MeV electron beam produced by a Varian iX linac and 2, 3, 4, 5, 6, 10 cm² field sizes. The loss of sharp dose fall-off can be seen for field sizes below 5 cm². The practical range of the beam is ~6 cm. (Courtesy Royal Adelaide Hospital)

lesions). Lead is often used for this purpose. Electron backscatter from lead can however present a problem. As electrons hit the high density, high atomic number material (lead) they also scatter backwards in a direction towards the source. This results in a highly increased dose to patient's surface lying directly 'on top' of the shield. The dose increase at the tissue lead interface can be substantial, up to 30%–70% in the range of 1 to 20 MeV electron energies, having a higher value for the lower-energy beams (see Figure 12.14.). In order to reduce the extra dose due to backscatter, a layer of tin can be placed on top of the lead surface facing the beam. The whole assembly is then covered with paraffin wax. The tin does not cause backscatter of the same magnitude as lead and together with the wax it helps to absorb the backscattered electrons and to reduce the dose to tissues. In the case of a tissue–lead interface, the electron backscatter factor (EBF) is empirically given by (Klevenhagen *et al.* 1982):

$$EBF = 1 + 0.735 \exp(-0.052\overline{E}_d) \qquad (12.4)$$

where $\overline{E}_d$ is the average energy of the electrons incident on the interface.

Paraffin wax is used in the construction of both the lead skin collimation and internal shields. It is used as a barrier from direct contact between lead and skin as lead is poisonous. It is though also used to absorb low energy scattered photons coming from the underside of the lead.

12.4.3 Bolus

As mentioned above, bolus material is used to bring the dose towards the skin surface and to smooth out surface irregularities. This may further reduce the 'skin sparing' (i.e. surface dose). If the tumour lies on the surface (e.g. lip lesion), this may be a desired effect. Source-to-surface distance should be set to the bolus surface not the patient surface for dose calculation purposes. Bolus should be placed over the whole field and air gaps between the bolus and the patient surface should be avoided. The different densities at the bolus-

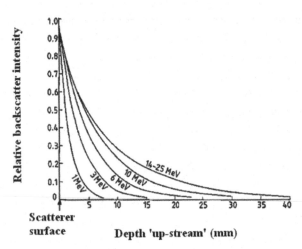

Figure 12.14. Graph of relative ionisation due to electron backscatter from lead versus depth upstream in polystyrene resulting from a broad electron beam incident on lead. (Reproduced from Lambert and Klevenhagen 1982, with permission of IOP Publishing Ltd.)

patient interface will have an effect when using electron beams, resulting in hot or cold spots.

12.4.4   Electron field abutment

When treating large or curved/sloped surfaces, two adjoining (abutting) electron fields may need to be used. Due to bulging and constricting of various isodose lines at depth, dosimetric characteristics at the junction between the two fields need to be investigated. As a result of these effects and increasing field penumbra, hot spots and cold spots will nearly always be present in the target volume. These will have to be checked for volume, magnitude and position within the patient. Some degree of dose inhomogeneity may be acceptable depending on these factors as well as on the clinical scenario. When treating sloped surfaces, the converging central axes will result in the largest overlap. Ideally, the electron beams should be parallel to avoid significant overlap of the high value isodose lines at depth (Figure 12.15 on p. 219). If using abutting fields, some basic 2D dosimetry (e.g. film) should be performed at the junction to verify the dose distribution and the extent of dose inhomogeneity.

12.4.5   Tissue heterogeneities

Tissue heterogeneities represent a major challenge in dosimetry of electron beams. Bone, lung and air cavities within the treatment volume can significantly alter the electron dose distribution. If an electron beam strikes the interface between two materials the resulting scatter perturbation will affect the dose distribution at the interface. The lower density material will receive a higher dose, due to the increased scattering of electrons from the higher density side. In addition increased scatter from the denser material into the less dense one leads to a cold spot beneath the dense material (Figure 12.16).

For large and uniform inhomogeneities the coefficient of equivalent thickness (CET) method can be used to account for their effect (Strydom *et al.* 2005). The CET corrects the thickness of the inhomogeneity by converting it to an equivalent thickness of water of the same attenuating capacity (using the density of electrons in the tissue). Based on this, lung has density of 0.25 g/cm^3 so the corresponding CET is 0.25. Solid bone has a CET of around 1.6. The effective depth in water equivalent tissue, z_{eff}, can be calculated from the following expression (Strydom 2005):

$$z_{eff} = z - t(1 - CET) \qquad (12.5)$$

where z is the depth of the point of interest in a patient and t is the thickness of the inhomogeneity.

The reduced attenuation in lung results in about three-fold increase in electron range. This leads to an increase in dose at depth (relative to a homogenous water phantom), both to lung tissue and to structures beyond the lung. There is a loss of electronic equilibrium at the interface, with reduced dose on the soft tissue side and increased dose on the lung side.

The effect of a small inhomogeneity is predominantly due to changes in scattering of electrons. The effects are most pronounced at the edge itself, but blurs at increasing depth.

The air gap created by the irregularity of curvature of the skin surface also affects the dose distribution. The increased air gap has an effect at the boundaries of the dose distribution and on the build-up. The increased air gap also reduces the dose.

12.5   TOTAL SKIN ELECTRON THERAPY (TSET)

Due to their short range in tissue, electrons are predominantly used for the treatment of superficial lesions. Megavoltage electron beams often represent a unique treatment option for superficial tumours (<5 cm depth in tissue). One such clinical application is **total skin electron therapy** (TSET) used in the management of skin-based T-cell lymphomas. The treatment is delivered to the entire surface of the body, with the patient in a standing position, by exposing the skin to a uniform dose of electrons without causing damage to deep seated tissues and organs (Figure 12.17). A comprehensive description of the techniques and dosimetry considerations in TSET is found in the AAPM Report No. 23 (1988). The most essential physical considerations listed by the task group in the aforementioned report are:

- treatment field size;
- depth of electron beam penetration;
- electron energy and field flatness at treatment plane;
- prescribed dose and dose rate at treatment plane; and
- X-ray background.

The treatment is usually delivered with low energy electrons (4–10 MeV), in sequential two-day treatment cycles, encompassing six dual-fields (day 1: one anterior field and two posterior-angled fields; day 2: one posterior field and two anterior-angled fields, etc). Beam penetration depth ranges from 5 mm to about 15 mm at the 50% isodose line. A typical sched-

ule consists of 9 weeks treatment, with an overall dose of 36 Gy delivered in 1 Gy/fraction, 4 days a week, using three dual fields a day.

For an appropriate total skin dosage the field size delineated by the combined electron beam must have an approximate height of 200 cm and a width of 80 cm. Within this field a ± 8% vertical uniformity and ± 4% horizontal uniformity along the central area of the treatment plane can be achieved (AAPM report 23, 1988).

While the six-field technique is convenient to use, the rotational technique whereby the patient stands on a rotating platform, delivers a more uniform skin dose. Improvement of dose uniformity is attained by placing a scatterer panel (2 m × 1 m) at 20 cm distance from the patient. The role of the panel (also known as 'beam scatterer-energy degrader') is to scatter the emergent electrons thus improving dose uniformity on oblique body surfaces and at the same time reducing beam penetration and depth of dose fall-off (Kumar and Patel 1978; Holt and Perry 1982; Podgorsak *et al.* 1983).

Dosimetry for TSET is a complex process due to the requirement to measure absorbed dose at superficial depths over large treatment areas (Brahme 1981; Berger and Seltzer 1982). It is recommended that the absorbed dose be evaluated at the calibration point (see Figure 12.17) using a parallel-plate

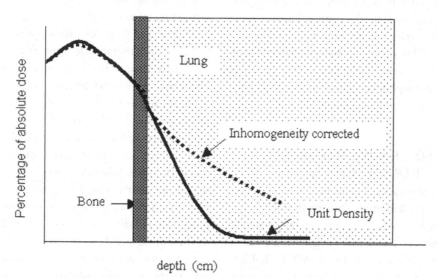

Figure 12.16. The impact of tissue inhomogeneities on dose distribution: dose distribution in water (full line) and dose distribution corrected for inhomogeneities (broken line) – the dose is increased due to smaller lung density. (Courtesy Klevenhagen *et al.* 1982)

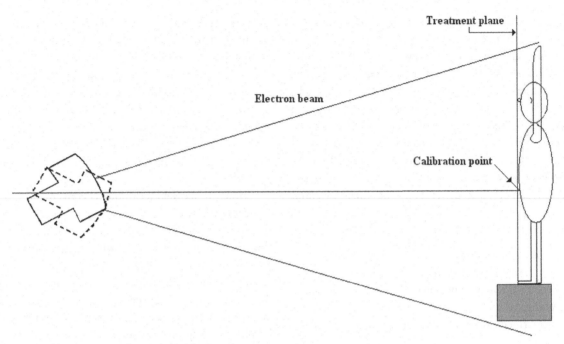

Figure 12.17. Patient set-up for total skin electron therapy.

ionisation chamber, possibly with a gap of 1 mm or less, and having an established N_{gas} value. Thermo-luminescent dosimeters for *in vivo* dosimetry located in different regions along the patient's anatomy can offer valuable data when implementing a TSET technique (AAMP report 23, 1988).

Currently, TSET is not a widespread treatment as retrospective studies indicate that relapse rates are very high even in early stage disease TSET (Jones *et al.* 1995). Higher response and survival rates are associated with greater skin doses (32–36 Gy) delivered with 4–6 MeV electrons (Jones *et al.* 1995). Often, TSET for cutaneous T-cell lymphomas is combined with photo-chemotherapy for better therapeutic outcome.

12.6 INTRAOPERATIVE ELECTRON RADIATION THERAPY (IOERT)

Electrons have been successfully used within Intra-Operative Electron Radiation Therapy (IOERT) since the early 1970s when Abe *et al.* have intraoperatively delivered megavoltage radiation originating from a linear accelerator (Abe *et al.* 1971). Within IOERT, electron radiation treatment is delivered in a single large dose directly into the tumour bed or residual

tumour during surgery. Since the procedure requires both an operating theatre and a linac, it is not cost-effective to have a dedicated linac for IOERT purpose in the operating room. Both US and European manu-facturers managed this logistical problem by design-ing and clinically implementing mobile linacs: Mobetron (Intraop Medical Incorporated of Santa Clara, California) and Novac7 (Hitesys SRL, Latina, Italy) (Beddar *et al.* 2006) (Figure 12.18).

Mobile and stationary linacs present with similar physical and therapeutic properties. Consequently, both deliver superficially penetrating electron radia-tion using applicators to focus the beam within the surgical treatment area. Beam modifiers to reduce penetration and lead absorbers to shield surrounding normal structures are also employed. Mobile linacs offer certain advantages over stationary accelerators due to their flexibility in patient set-up and the ability to deliver an electron beam with a flatter profile. However, a major concern with mobile units is radio-protection of adjoining rooms during beam-on time, as these units are designed to be used in unshielded operating theaters. Therefore, their usage in a theatre is restricted to about 3–4 patients per week, including machine warm-up (Daves and Mills 2001). For

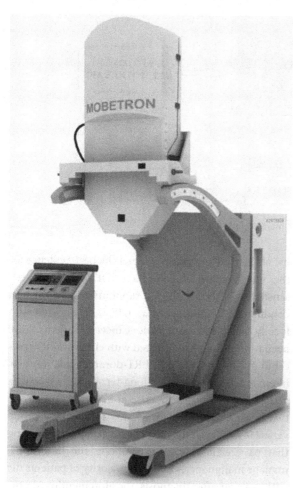

Figure 12.18. Mobetron – Mobile self-shielded linear accelerator designed for IOERT (courtesy IntraOp Medical Corp, California) with the following beam characteristics: energy range 4–12 MeV, dose rate 10 Gy/min, field size 3 cm–10 cm, flatness ±5% (www.intraopmedical.com).

radioprotection purpose mobile units are provided with a beam stopper which is designed to track the gantry movement in all directions and to intercept the primary beam. To surmount excessive exposure to adjacent areas, some departments preferred undertaking their mobile linac commissioning and thereafter the annual quality assurance tests at the manufacturers' facilities (Beddar *et al.* 2006).

Recent improvements to the Mobetron shielding design required an update on the photon leakage and scatter radiation assessment as well as on patient load when considering single fraction doses of up to 20 Gy. Shielding and radiation survey measurements con-

ducted by Krechetov *et al.* (2010) showed that patient load can be increased with a safe delivery up to 250 Gy per week if the areas around the operating theatre are occupied and non-controlled and standard building materials and distances to the walls are considered.

Acceptance testing of a mobile linac consists of the following procedures:

* radiation survey;
* interlocks and safety features testing;
* mechanical testing;
* beam characteristics tuning;
* docking system test; and
* accessories evaluation.

Detailed information on the above procedures, commissioning of mobile IOERT linacs, dose measurements and also on the recommended quality assurance can be found in the AAPM Radiation Therapy Committee Task Group No. 72 Report (Beddar *et al.* 2006).

With mobile linacs, the therapeutic dose is prescribed to the 90% isodose line to ensure adequate target coverage but the dose at d_{max} (depth of maximum dose) is also reported (Palta *et al.* 1995). The IOERT target is defined immediately before irradiation, after the surgical resection, when a clear view of the tumour/tumour bed is assured. Parameters such as tumour margins, target depth, beam energy, field shaping and type of applicator will be established once the target and the surrounding normal tissues are clinically assessed.

While also used as monotherapy, IOERT is often employed as a radiation boosting technique which can be integrated in a multimodality cancer treatment (Calvo *et al.* 1992; del Carmen *et al.* 2003; Merrick *et al.* 2003) (Figure 12.19). IOERT used in combination with external beam radiotherapy (EBRT) results in smaller integral doses and shorter overall treatment times, however chemotherapy and radiosensitising agents can be added to the treatment as well, depending on tumour location and characteristics.

The precise focalisation of the radiation beam inside the tumour and the good visualisation of tumour bed during the procedure confer this irradiation technique feasibility in the management of several tumour types. The most commonly treated

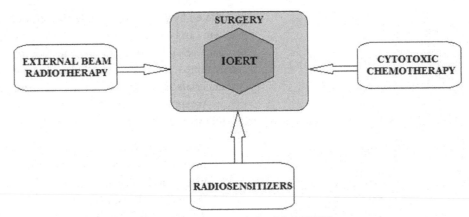

Figure 12.19. Diagram presenting the multidisciplinary approach involving IOERT.

tumour sites with IOERT are: soft tissue sarcomas, gynecological malignancies (cervical, ovarian and uterine tumours), breast cancers (Figure 12.20), gastric cancers (stomach, pancreas), rectal and anal cancers and also prostate and bladder tumours. Due to difficulty in accruing large numbers of patients treated with IOERT for the same histopathological site the likelihood of conducting phase III clinical trials for evaluating the efficacy of the procedure is small. There are, however, single-institution reports on the effectiveness of intraoperative radiotherapy in the management of advanced and also recurrent cancers (Gunderson *et al.* 1993; Mahé *et al.* 1996; Hashiguchi *et al.* 1999; Martinez-Monge *et al.* 2001; Pierie *et al.* 2006; Roeder *et al.* 2010).

Among the radiobiological advantages of IOERT which can lead to improved therapeutic ratio, the following are mentioned:

- higher dose delivered to tumour
- decreased exposure to normal tissue
- shorter overall treatment time
- good conformality with small tumours which might not be well distinguishable with conventional treatment techniques (such as external beam radiotherapy)
- safe to be delivered to tumours located in close vicinity to critical organs.

With an oxygen enhancement ratio of 2.5–3 electrons are not particularly effective on hypoxic tumours. However, IOERT allows the efficient concurrent use of radiation sensitisers with hypoxia-specific-

ity, at the time of surgery. One of the best evidence for the effectiveness of combined IOERT-hypoxic cell sensitisers is the result of a randomised clinical trial conducted by Karasawa *et al.* (2008) on patients with locally advanced pancreatic cancers. Patients have been randomised to be treated with either IOERT (placebo group) or with IOERT-doranidazole (a new hypoxic cell sensitiser) and long-term results showed a significant survival difference at 3 years between the two arms: 23% survival for IOERT-doranidazole group versus 0% survival for the placebo group. Considering that pancreatic cancers are among the hardest-to-manage malignancies and that majority of patients die within a year after diagnosis, the aforementioned procedure shows very promising results in improving long-term survival in this patient group.

An extensive analysis on long-term normal tissue effects of intraoperative electron radiotherapy based on data resulting from 739 IOERT-treated patients has been published by Azinovic *et al.* (2001) underpinning the unique profile of late-toxicity of IOERT derived from the radiobiology of high, single-dose electron beam radiation. The most common normal tissue toxicity was found to be peripheral neuropathy, with higher frequency in those locations in which a peripheral nerve was present in the surgical bed. Considering that 65% of the patients received 15 Gy in a single dose, radiobiological principles imply that the length of the irradiated nerve played an important role in determining the extent of late toxicity.

The biologically effective dose (BED) for the assessment of normal tissue reaction after the combined

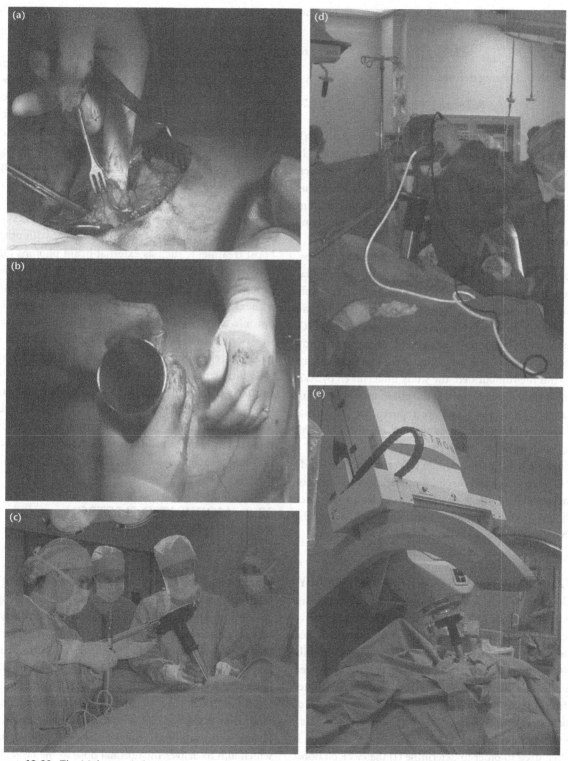

Figure 12.20. The Mobetron in breast cancer treatment (courtesy from Dr Don Goer, IntraOp Medical Corporation, Sunnyvale, CA, USA). (a) Excision of tumour and tumour margins. (b) Selection and installation of the applicator tube. (c) Fixation and positioning of the cone. (d) Checking of the applicator placement. (e) Mobile linac set up for treatment.

IOERT-EBRT is determined as a sum of each treatment-related BED (van der Kogel 1993):

$$BED_{total} = BED_{IOERT} + BED_{EBRT} \qquad (12.6)$$

with BED being defined as:

$$BED = D\left(1 + \frac{d}{\alpha/\beta}\right) \qquad (12.7)$$

In the above relation: D is the total dose delivered, d is the dose per fraction and the α/β ratio has a 3.5 Gy value for late fibrosis. Mean BED values have been estimated in long-term IOERT survivors for various tumour sites and showed to cover a wide range: from 100.5 Gy for bone sarcoma to 141.2 Gy for soft tissue sarcomas (Azinovic et al. 2001).

One of the major concerns with radiation therapy, particularly when delivering single high-dose radiation, is the unwanted sequelae in terms of irreversible complications or even more, the induction of second cancers. While early animal experiments with IOERT suggest the possibility of second cancer induction (Gillette et al. 1990) by high-dose electron beams within the tumour bed, the study undertaken by Azinovic et al. did not confirm the observation in human patients. However, they have reported on 8 patients with second malignancies yet outside the radiation boosted volume. Still, the authors recommend a longer follow-up (the median follow-up in their study was 94 months) and careful monitoring of patients for this unwanted effect of IOERT in order to reinforce the exclusion of second malignancies induced by the abovementioned radiation technique.

12.7 ELECTRON BOOST RADIOTHERAPY

Electrons in radiotherapy are also used as a boost treatment to lymph nodes, residual tumour or operative scars (Hogstrom and Almond 2006). Operative bed electron boost after whole breast irradiation (usually 10 Gy–16 Gy in 2 Gy fractions) is commonly employed in the radiotherapy of early-staged breast cancers after clinical trials revealed its role in reducing the risk of local recurrence (Romestaig et al. 1997; Polgár et al. 2002; Bartelink et al. 2007). Ultrasound guidance is often used in order to determine (1) the electron boost field for the postoperative cavity and (2) the beam energy required for the thickness of breast tissue (Smitt

et al. 2001; Warszawski et al. 2004). Consequently, overdosage of normal tissue and underdosage of the postoperative cavity can be avoided.

Photons were also employed for the management of tumour bed after breast conserving surgery however, the excess doses to the normal tissue delivered with 2D photon boosts hindered their use. Lately, the implementation of more conformal techniques, such as 3DCRT conferred photon planning an advantage over electrons due to superior healthy tissue sparing and better dose coverage (Kovács et al. 2008; Toscas et al. 2010).

Several studies have compared the effectiveness of electron boost in early stage breast cancer with other boost treatments such as external beam photons (3D conformal, IMRT, RapidArc), HDR brachytherapy or proton therapy (Table 12.1). The studies show that while electrons are preferred to 2D photon treatments, optimised external beam photon therapy results in superior treatment outcome when compared to external beam electron boost. The clinical outcome after Ir-192 implants and electrons for boost appears to be similarly efficient in regards to local control and survival (Polgár et al. 2002; Poortmans et al. 2004; Hill-Kayser et al. 2010), however normal tissue effects reported by some studies were found to be more pronounced after brachytherapy (Hill-Kayser et al. 2010).

12.8 MODULATED ELECTRON RADIOTHERAPY (MERT)

Modulated electron radiotherapy (MERT) is a novel approach to technological enhancement of electron beam therapy which was developed along with IMRT, offering superior dose distribution to photons (Hogstrom and Almond 2006) for shallow tumours. The advent of electron MLC technology (eMLC) in the early 2000s was shown to bring certain dosimetric advantages and also convenience in beam shaping and modulation, thus eliminating the need for electron cutouts (Lee et al. 2000; Ma et al. 2000; Ravindran et al. 2002; Hogstrom 2004). MERT employs multiple electron beams with different energies (energy modulation) which aim to deliver the optimal dose to the target by varying the beam intensity (intensity modulation). Dose optimisation along the beam direction is achieved via

Table 12.1. Electron boost versus other boost techniques in the management of post-lumpectomy early stage breast cancer.

Clinical study/trial	Electron boost schedule	Compared boost techniques	Conclusions
Toscas *et al.* 2010 *Planning study* 14 patients *(tumour bed from deep-seated tumours)*	16 Gy boost dose in 2 Gy per fraction	*3D conformal photon* boost either static or dynamic arc, static gantry *IMRT, RapidArc* Or *Intensity modulated proton beam*	The goal to cover 100% of the CTV with 95% of the prescribed dose was not achieved by electrons. Electrons delivered the highest dose to the heart in left-sided breast tumors. Optimised photon or proton beams are preferred as boost to electrons, especially for deep-seated tumours.
Hill-Kayser *et al.* 2010 *Retrospective clinical study* 141 patients	18 Gy median boost dose	*Ir-192 implant* delivering a median boost dose of 15 Gy	Local recurrence and overall survival after 10/20 years was similar for the two groups. Better cosmesis was achieved in the electron boost group. Higher rate of fibrosis in the implant group.
Shah *et al.* 2010 *Dosimetric-analysis study* 15 patients	10–16 Gy in 2 Gy fractions	*MammoSite* brachytherapy applicator 3.4 Gy × 3 fractions normally but 2 Gy per fraction planned for the comparative study with the electron dose	MammoSite offers superior tumour coverage to electrons: Mean PTV V100 95.5% (MammoSite) versus 77.4% (electron boost) Similar doses to normal tissue from the two techniques.
Kovács *et al.* 2008 *Dosimetric-analysis study* 78 patients	10 Gy prescription dose to the 90% isodose line (14 MeV)	*3D conformal photon* boost with two oblique wedged fields; 10 Gy boost dose to the tumour bed	Dosimetric parameters (such as conformality index and coverage index) were in favour of photon boost.
Poortmans *et al.* 2004 *Randomised trial* 2661 patients	16 Gy boost dose in 2 Gy per fraction	*Photon boost* Or *Interstitial brachytherapy*	Local recurrence at 5 years: 4.8% (electrons) versus 4% (photons) versus 2.5% (brachytherapy). Similar normal tissue toxicity (fibrosis) in the three groups.
Reitsamer *et al.* 2004 *Clinical study* 378 patients	12 Gy boost dose	*Intraoperative electron radiotherapy (IOERT)* 9 Gy boost dose	Local recurrence after 55.3 months (external electron boost) 4.3% versus no recurrence (IOERT) after 25.8 months follow up. Distant metastases 7.9% (external electron boost) versus 1.1% (IOERT).
Polgár *et al.* 2002 *Randomised trial* 207 patients	16 Gy boost dose in 2 Gy per fraction	*High dose rate brachytherapy* 12–14.25 Gy Or *No boost*	Boost dose significantly improves outcome: Local recurrences: 6.7% (boost) versus 15.5% (no boost); No difference in local tumour control between HDR boost and electron boost.

energy modulation, whereas lateral dose conformity is attained by intensity modulation or beam shaping using a multileaf collimator (Ma *et al.* 2003).

Several methods of implementing electron-specific multileaf collimators (eMLC) have been reported in the literature. Using photon MLC for electron delivery in a conventional air filled linac treatment head produces wide penumbra and also bremsstrahlung radiation. Therefore, to overcome this inconvenience, the air from the treatment head was replaced with helium and the secondary scattering foil has been moved up higher in the linac head, which has significantly improved the penumbras and has also reduced the unwanted electron scatter (Karlsson *et al.* 1999; Lee *et al.* 2000). Another possible set-up in order to limit the bremsstrahlung contribution to the electron dose delivered is to employ photon MLC in tracking the eMLC with a margin to avoid penumbra widening (Olofsson *et al.* 2005).

While there were attempts to redesign existing treatment heads for electron collimation (Lee *et al.* 2000; du Plessis *et al.* 2006), the implementation of a specific eMLC by mounting it on an electron applicator frame seemed more feasible (Figure 12.21) (Ma *et al.* 2000). Dosimetric characteristics of a manually-driven prototype eMLC consisting of 25 tungsten leaf pairs (2 cm thickness and 0.6 cm width), mounted on a treatment head of a Varian 21EX linac have been investigated and recently reported in the literature (Eldib *et al.* 2010). PDD curves and profiles have been compared between the prototype eMLC and the square electron applicator (matching field sizes), using Monte Carlo codes for accelerator simulation and dose calculations. The comparative study showed no significant differences between the PDDs and beam profiles and, furthermore, the Monte Carlo simulations were found to be able to accurately model the electron beam delivered by the eMLC (Eldib *et al.* 2010).

Salguero *et al.* (2010) have assessed the feasibility of delivering energy- and intensity-modulated electron radiotherapy using a photon multileaf collimator for superficial head & neck cancers (such as parotid glands, oronasal and middle ear tumours). MERT dose-volume histograms were compared to those obtained via conventional photon and electron treatments, including IMRT and the results were found to

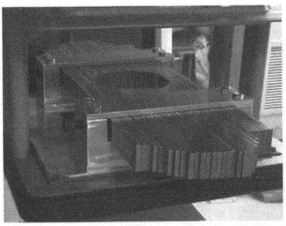

Figure 12.21. Prototype manual-driven eMLC for MERT (Reprinted from Ma *et al.* 2000, with permission of IOP Publishing Ltd.)

be comparable or even superior to conventional techniques. The same group has investigated the feasibility of MERT in the irradiation of post-mastectomy chest wall (Salguero *et al.* 2009) using an in-house planning system based on MC simulations. The MC planning system was designed for MERT when delivered with a double-focused Siemens Primus MLC for electron beam shaping. The group obtained better PTV coverage and considerable reduction of the doses to the organs at risk compared to a conventional chest wall irradiation technique. These results are in agreement with other reported data of dose distributions in superficial tumours or postoperative chest walls treated with modulated electron therapy (Ma *et al.* 2003; Vatanen *et al.* 2009).

While MERT is a promising technology for several treatment sites, there are still some limitations to overcome, such as the MLC location/ positioning uncertainties relative to the patient and the high manufacturing cost of an inbuilt eMLC.

12.9   REFERENCES

AAPM Report No. 23 (1988) 'Total skin electron therapy: technique and dosimetry'. American Institute of Physics, New York.

Abe M, Fukuda M, Yamano K, Matsuda S *et al.* (1971) Intra-operative irradiation in abdominal and cerebral tumours. *Acta Radiologica* **10**: 408–416.

Azinovic I, Calvo FA, Puebla F, Aristu J et al. (2001) Long-term normal tissue effects of intraoperative electron radiation therapy (IOERT): late sequelae, tumor recurrence, and second malignancies. *International Journal of Radiation Oncology Biology and Physics* **49**(2): 597–604.

Bartelink H, Horiot JC, Poortmans PM, Struikmans H et al. (2007) Impact of a higher radiation dose on local control and survival in breast-conserving therapy of early breast cancer: 10-year results of the randomized boost versus no boost EORTC 22881-10882 trial. *Journal of Clinical Oncology* **25**(22): 3259–3265.

Beddar S, Biggs P, Chang S, Ezzell G et al. (2006) Intraoperative radiation therapy using mobile electron linear accelerators: report of AAPM Radiation Therapy Committee Task Group No. 72. *Medical Physics* **33**(5): 1476–1489.

Berger MJ and Seltzer SM (1982) 'Tables of energy-deposition distributions in water phantoms irradiated by point-monodirectional electron beams with energies from 1 to 60 MeV and applications to broad beams'. NBS report, NBSIR 82-2451. National Bureau of Standards, Washington DC.

Brahme A (1981) Physics of electron beam penetration: fluence and absorbed dose. In: *Proceedings of the Symposium on Electron Dosimetry and Arc Therapy*, Madison, Sept. 1981, pp. 45–68.

Calvo FA, Santos M and Brady LW (1992) *Intraoperative Radiotherapy*. Clinical Experiences and Results. Springer Verlag, Heidelberg.

Daves JL and Mills MD (2001) Shielding assessment of a mobile electron accelerator for intraoperative radiotherapy. *Journal of Applied Clinical Medical Physics* **2**: 165–173.

del Carmen MG, Eisner B, Willet CG and Fuller AF (2003) Intraoperative radiation therapy in the management of gynecologic and genitourinary malignancies. *Surgical Oncology Clinics of North America* **12**(4): 1031–1042.

du Plessis FC, Leal A, Stathakis S, Xiong W and Ma CM (2006) Characterization of megavoltage electron beams delivered through a photon multi-leaf collimator (pMLC). *Physics in Medicine and Biology* **51**(8): 2113–2129.

Eldib A, ElGohary M, Fan J, Jin L et al. (2010) Dosimetric characteristics of an electron multileaf collimator for modulated electron radiation therapy. *Journal of Applied Clinical Medical Physics* **11**(2): 5–22.

Gillette SM, Gillette EL, Powers BE and Withrow S (1990) Radiation-induced osteosarcoma in dogs after external beam or intraoperative radiation therapy. *Cancer Research* **50**: 54–57.

Gunderson LL, Nagorney DM, McIlrath DC, Fieck JM et al. (1993) External beam and intraoperative electron irradiation for locally advanced soft tissue sarcomas. *International Journal of Radiation Oncology Biology and Physics* **25**(4): 647–656.

Harder D (1965) Energiespektren schneller elektronen in verschiedenen tiefen. In: *Symposium on High Energy Electrons*. (Eds A Zuppinger and G Poretti) p. 260. Springer-Verlag, Berlin.

Hashiguchi Y, Sekine T, Sakamoto H, Tanaka Y et al. (1999) Intraoperative irradiation after surgery for locally recurrent rectal cancer. *Diseases of the Colon & Rectum* **42**: 886–893.

Hill-Kayser CE, Chacko D, Hwang WT, Vapiwala N et al. (2010) Long-term clinical and cosmetic outcomes after breast conservation treatment for women with early-stage breast carcinoma according to the type of breast boost. *International Journal of Radiation Oncology Biology and Physics* (in print).

Hogstrom KR, Mills MD and Almond PR (1981) Electron beam dose calculation. *Physics in Medicine and Biology* **26**: 445–459.

Hogstrom KR (2004) Electron beam therapy: dosimetry, planning, and techniques. In: *Principles and Practice of Radiation Oncology*. (Eds C Perez et al.) pp. 252–282. Lippincott, Williams & Wilkins, Baltimore, MD.

Hogstrom KR and Almond P (2006) Review of electron beam therapy physics. *Physics in Medicine and Biology* **51**: R455–R489.

Holt JG and Perry DJ (1982) Some physical considerations in whole skin electron beam therapy. *Medical Physics* **9**: 769–776.

International Atomic Energy Agency (IAEA) (1997) 'The use of plane parallel ionization chambers in high energy electron and photon beams'. Technical Reports Series No. 381. IAEA, Vienna.

International Atomic Energy Agency (IAEA) (2000) 'Absorbed dose determination in external beam radiotherapy'. Technical Reports Series No. 398. IAEA, Vienna.

International Commission on Radiation Units and Measurements (ICRU) (1984) 'Radiation dosimetry: electron beams with energies between 1 and 50 MeV'. Rep. 35. ICRU, Bethesda, MD.

Jones GW, Hoppe RT and Glatstein E (1995) Electron beam treatment for cutaneous T-cell lymphoma. *Hematology/Oncology Clinics of North America* **9**: 1057–1076.

Karasawa K, Sunamura M, Okamoto A, Nemoto K *et al.* (2008) Efficacy of novel hypoxic cell sensitiser doranidazole in the treatment of locally advanced pancreatic cancer: long-term results of a placebo-controlled randomised study. *Radiotherapy and Oncology* **87**(3): 326–330.

Karlsson MG, Karlsson M and Ma CM (1999) Treatment head design for multileaf collimated high-energy electrons. *Medical Physics* **26**(10): 2161–2167.

Khan FM (2003) *The Physics of Radiation Therapy.* Lippincott, Williams and Wilkins, Baltimore, MD.

Klevenhagen SC (1985) Physics of electron beam therapy. In: *Medical Physics Handbook vol 13.* pp. 106–136. Hilger, Bristol, UK.

Klevenhagen SC, Lambert GD and Arbari A (1982) Backscattering n electron beam therapy for energies between 3 and 35 MeV. *Physics in Medicine and Biology* **27**: 363–373.

Klevenhagen SC (1993) *Physics and Dosimetry of Therapy Electron Beams.* Medical Physics Publishing, Madison, WI.

Kovács A, Hadjiev J, Lakosi F, Glavak C *et al.* (2008) Comparison of photon with electron boost in treatment of early stage breast cancer. *Pathology and Oncology Research* **14**: 193–197.

Krechetov AS, Goer D, Dikeman K, Daves JL and Mills MD (2010) Shielding assessment of a mobile electron accelerator for intra-operative radiotherapy. *Journal of Applied Clinical Medical Physics* **11**(4): 263–273.

Kumar PP and Patel IS (1978) Rotation technique for superficial total body electron beam irradiation. *Journal of the National Medical Association* **70**: 507–509.

Lambert GD and Klevenhagen SC (1982) Penetration of backscattered electrons in polystyrene for energies between 1 and 25 MeV. *Physics in Medicine and Biology* **27**: 721–725.

Lee MC, Jiang SB and Ma CM (2000) Monte Carlo and experimental investigations of multileaf collimated electron beams for modulated electron radiation therapy. *Medical Physics* **27**: 2708–2718.

Ma CM, Pawlicki T, Lee MC, Jiang SB *et al.* (2000) Energy- and intensity-modulated electron beams for radiotherapy. *Physics in Medicine and Biology* **45**: 2293–2311.

Ma CM, Ding M, Li JS, Lee MC *et al.* (2003) A comparative dosimetric study on tangential photon beams, intensity-modulated radiation therapy (IMRT) and modulated electron radiotherapy (MERT) for breast cancer treatment. *Physics in Medicine and Biology* **48**(7): 909–924.

Mahé MA, Gerard JP, Dubois JB, Roussel A *et al.* (1996) Intraoperative radiation therapy in recurrent carcinoma of the uterine cervix: report of the French intraoperative group on 70 patients. *International Journal of Radiation Oncology Biology and Physics* **34**(1): 21–26.

Martinez-Monge R, Jurado M, Aristu J, Moreno M *et al.* (2001) Intraoperative electron beam radiotherapy during radical surgery for locally advanced and recurrent cervical cancer. *Gynecological Oncology* **82**: 538–543.

Merrick HW 3rd, Gunderson LL and Calvo FA (2003) Future directions in intraoperative radiation therapy. *Surgical Oncology Clinics of North America* **12**(4): 1099–1105.

Meyer JL and Vaeth JM (Eds) (1991) *The Role of High Energy Electrons in the Treatment of Cancer: 25th Annual San Francisco Cancer Symposium*, February 1990, Karger Publishers, Basel, Switzerland.

Olofsson L, Karlsson MG and Karlsson M (2005) Effects on electron beam penumbra using the photon MLC to reduce bremsstrahlung leakage for an add-on electron MLC. *Physics in Medicine and Biology* **50**(6): 1191–1203.

Palta JR, Biggs PJ, Hazle DJ, Huq MS *et al.* (1995) Intraoperative electron beam radiation therapy, technique, dosimetry, and dose specification: report of Task Group 48 of the radiation therapy committee, American Association of Physicists in

Medicine. *International Journal of Radiation Oncology Biology and Physics* **33**(3): 725–746.

Pierie JP, Betensky RA, Choudry U, Willett CG *et al.* (2006) Outcomes in a series of 103 retroperitoneal sarcomas. *European Journal of Surgical Oncology* **32**(10): 1235–1241.

Podgorsak EB, Pla C, Pla M, Lefebvre PY and Heese R (1983) Physical aspects of a rotational total skin electron irradiation. *Medical Physics* **10**: 159–168.

Polgár C, Fodor J, Orosz Z, Major T *et al.* (2002) Electron and high-dose-rate brachytherapy boost in the conservative treatment of stage I-II breast cancer first results of the randomized Budapest boost trial. *Strahlentherapie und Onkologie* **178**(11): 615–623.

Poortmans P, Bartelink H, Horiot JC, Struikmans H *et al.* (2004) The influence of the boost technique on local control in breast conserving treatment in the EORTC 'boost versus no boost' randomised trial. *Radiotherapy and Oncology* **72**(1): 25–33.

Ravindran BP, Singh IR, Brindha S and Sathyan S (2002) Manual multi-leaf collimator for electron beam shaping – a feasibility study. *Physics in Medicine and Biology* **47**: 4389–4396.

Reitsamer R, Peintinger F, Kopp M, Menzel C *et al.* (2004) Local recurrence rates in breast cancer patients treated with intraoperative electron-boost radiotherapy versus postoperative external-beam electron-boost irradiation. A sequential intervention study. *Strahlentherapie und Onkologie* **180**(1): 38–44.

Roeder F, Timke C, Oertel S, Hensley FW *et al.* (2010) Intraoperative electron radiotherapy for the management of aggressive fibromatosis. *International Journal of Radiation Oncology Biology and Physics* **76**(4): 1154–1160.

Romestaig P, Lehingue Y, Carrie C, Coquard R *et al.* (1997) Role of a 10-Gy boost in the conservative treatment of early breast cancer: results of a randomized clinical trial in Lyon, France. *Journal of Clinical Oncology* **15**: 963–968.

Salguero FJ, Palma B, Arrans R, Rosello J *et al.* (2009) Modulated electron radiotherapy treatment planning using a photon multileaf collimator for post-mastectomized chest walls. *Radiotherapy and Oncology* **93**(3): 625–632.

Salguero FJ, Arrans R, Palma BA and Leal A (2010) Intensity- and energy-modulated electron radiotherapy by means of an xMLC for head & neck shallow tumors. *Physics in Medicine and Biology* **55**(5): 1413–1427.

Shah AP, Strauss JB, Kirk MC, Chen SS *et al.* (2010) A dosimetric analysis comparing electron beam with the MammoSite brachytherapy applicator for intact breast boost. *Physica Medica* **26**(2): 80–87.

Smitt M, Birdwell R and Goffinet D (2001) Breast electron boost planning: comparison of CT and US. *Radiology* **219**: 203–206.

Strydom W, Parker W and Olivares M (2005) Special procedures and techniques in radiotherapy. In: *Radiation Oncology Physics: A Handbook for Teachers and Students.* (Ed. EB Podgorsak) pp. 273–300. IAEA publication 1196. International Atomic Energy Agency, Vienna.

Tapley N duV (1976) *Clinical Applications of the Electron Beam.* John Wiley and Sons, New York.

Tapley N duV (1977) High-energy photon and electron beam. *Cancer* **39**: 788–801.

Toscas JI, Linero D, Rubio I, Hidalgo A *et al.* (2010) Boosting the tumor bed from deep-seated tumors in early-stage breast cancer: a planning study between electron, photon, and proton beams. *Radiotherapy and Oncology* **96**(2): 192–198.

van der Kogel AJ and Ruifrok ACC (1993) Calculation of isoeffect relationships. In: *Basic Clinical Radiobiology.* (Ed. GG Steel) pp. 72–80. Arnold Publisher, London.

Vatanen T, Traneus E and Lahtinen T (2009) Comparison of conventional inserts and an add-on electron MLC for chest wall irradiation of left-sided breast cancer. *Acta Oncologica* **48**(3): 446–451.

Warszawski A, Baumann R and Karstens J (2004) Sonographic guidance for electron boost planning after breast-conserving surgery. *Journal of Clinical Ultrasound* **32**(7): 333–337.

www.intraopmedical.com (accessed on the 29/11/2010).

13 External beam hadron radiotherapy

13.1 RADIOBIOLOGY

Radiotherapy is carried out with three types of radiation, i.e. photons, leptons and hadrons. Photons in the form of X-rays, gamma rays and bremsstrahlung have developed to be the most widespread radiation modality over 100 years. Sources are X-ray tubes, radioisotopes and linear accelerators respectively. Electrons belong to the lepton particle group that is characterised by so-called weak interaction; e.g. β-decay is a form of weak interaction. They have a role in the treatment of superficial tumours (see Chapter 12), and are generated by linacs as well.

Hadrons are particles that undergo the strong nuclear interaction; e.g. the force between neutrons and protons inside a nucleus. In recent decades hadrons have spun off from nuclear physics research to be applied to radiotherapy of cancers. They comprise baryons (e.g. neutrons and protons) and mesons. They have masses much greater than that of electrons and as a result are often referred to as heavy particles. If nuclei or ions of masses larger than that of hydrogen (i.e. single proton) are considered then they are referred to as heavy ions. This chapter will address developments in radiotherapy using protons and heavy ions and Chapter 14 will discuss the use of neutrons. Neutrons represent a special case of a nucleon with zero charge. All other hadrons are particles or ions with single or multiple charges, e.g. protons have 1+, alphas 2+, carbon up to 6+.

The advantage in the use of hadrons for radiotherapy lies in two factors: high relative biological effectiveness (RBE) and for ions the Bragg peak. Neutrons have a high RBE but a poor depth-dose profile. Fast neutrons have a similar depth-dose profile to 4 MV photons (Figure 13.1), which is regarded to be inadequate for deep seated tumours. Protons have a low RBE but excellent depth-dose profile (Figure 13.1). Initially, the ions lose energy with depth in tissue (dE/dx) at a relatively constant rate (plateau region) until they slow down to lower kinetic energies when the dE/dx rapidly increases, creating the Bragg peak in the dose deposition. The exact position of the Bragg peak in tissue depends on the energy, the mass and the charge of the accelerated heavy ions. This peak has additional properties of higher LET and a sharp dose cut-off with depth (i.e. charged particles have a definite range in matter, beyond which the delivered dose is zero). Thus the tumour-to-skin dose ratio far exceeds that achievable for a single photon field. Further, the dose cut-off protects dose limiting normal tissues lying beyond the target volume. A single Bragg peak, however, is too narrow to irradiate most of the

L. Marcu et al., *Biomedical Physics in Radiotherapy for Cancer*,
DOI 10.1007/978-0-85729-733-4_13, © CSIRO 2012

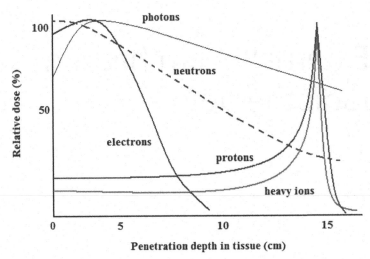

Figure 13.1. Dose deposition with tissue depth for photons, neutrons, electrons, protons and heavy ion beams. Protons and heavy ions have the lowest skin entry doses, the highest tumour doses but heavy ions exhibit a distal dose well above that for protons.

tumours so several beams of closely spaced energies are superimposed to create a range of uniform dose over a depth of the target. These extended regions of uniform dose are called 'Spread-Out Bragg Peaks' (SOBP) (Figure 13.2).

Without a doubt, heavy ions represent the most effective radiation for cancer therapy of small tumours. However, their performance drops off with larger tumours, whereas photon therapy improves with multiple fields and fractionation.

The overall properties of the different radiation modalities are shown in Figure 13.3. Increasing photon energy improves the dose depth profile markedly, but higher energies lead to the photo-production of ions

and increased background doses. Intensity modulated radiotherapy gives high spatial resolution for dose, being comparable to heavy ions. Fast neutrons have a similar dose-depth profile to 4 MV photons, which is regarded to be inadequate for deep seated tumours.

As discussed in Chapter 1, the Coulomb interactions by primary charged particle beams result in ionization and excitation of tissue atoms and molecules, initiating a chain of chemical and biological events. Neutrons, on the other hand cause indirect ionization by nuclear elastic and inelastic scattering with hydrogen atoms (proton knock-on collisions) and neutron capture reactions at higher energies, causing the emission of secondary charged particles. These events cause

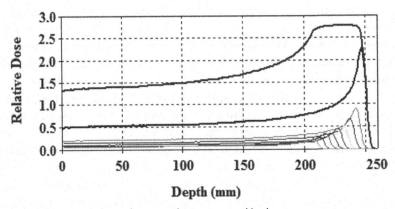

Figure 13.2. Broadening of the target volume decreases the tumour to skin dose.

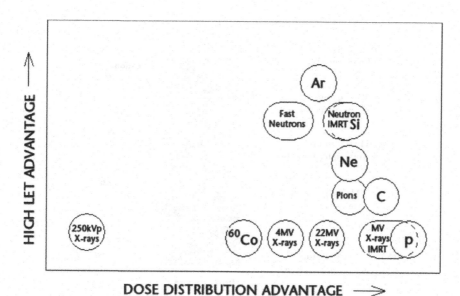

Figure 13.3. Comparative performances of different radiation modalities. Note all points are for external beam therapy with the exception of TAT (targeted alpha therapy) which is a systemic, high LET internal therapy that targets individual cancer cells and tumours (Chapter 15).

the formation of radicals (molecules with unpaired electrons) which cause chemical damage to molecules and subsequent biological effects. The time scale for these events is shown in Figure 13.4.

The biological effect of radiation depends on the wavelength compared with the lateral dimensions of DNA, which is ~2 nm. The average spacing of ionisation events for a 10 keV electron is 13.4 nm. This means that the chance of a DNA hit is relatively low compared with heavy ions with ~4 hits for a 1 MeV proton and many ionisations for lower energy protons, alpha and C-12 ions as shown in Figure 13.5.

The main physical and biophysical properties of ion beams (electrons, protons, alpha particles and carbon-12) of various initial energies are presented in Table 13.1.

If the energy of the heavy ions is high enough, in addition to direct ionization events, nuclear reactions

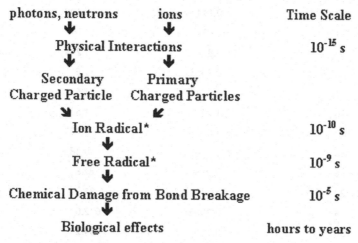

Figure 13.4. Times scale for physical and biological interactions of different radiations. Cancer can arise from molecular damage to genes and can have a latency period of decades before clinical symptoms are observed.

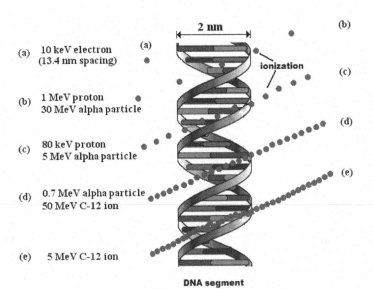

Figure 13.5. Average ionisation spacings for electrons and heavy ions compared with DNA dimensions.

between the heavy ions and nuclei of tissue elements will also take place. The secondary particles produced in these interactions will contribute to radiation dose delivered to tumour as well as to healthy tissue. The larger the treatment/tumour depth, the greater the initial energy of the respective heavy ion beam needs to be to reach this depth and the larger the dose from secondary particles.

It has been demonstrated that as much as 25% of the total physical dose may originate from secondary particles. Common secondary particles when using proton beams are: α-particles, helium-3, neutrons and

Table 13.1. Properties of ion beams.

Particle	Energy (MeV)	Range (mm)	Stopping Power (keV/μm)	Average spacing of ionising events (nm)
e	0.01	0.0022	2.24	13.4
	0.1	0.144	0.408	74
	1.0	4.41	0.184	163
	10	50.3	0.213	141
p	0.08	0.0013	85.6	0.35
	1	0.0246	22.6	1.33
	10	1.24	4.53	6.63
	100	77.8	0.723	41.5
	250	383	0.388	77.4
α	5	0.038	87.8	0.34
	20	0.370	31.2	0.96
C-12	5	0.0095	672.0	0.045
	100	0.350	164.2	0.183
	1000	20.2	26.4	1.14
	4800	292	9.69	3.10

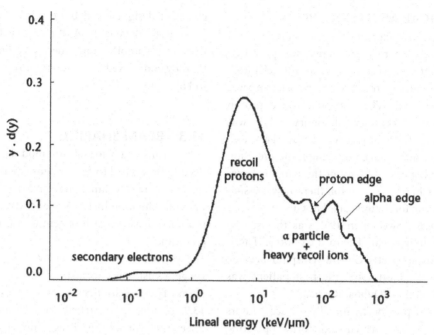

Figure 13.6. LET spectrum resulting from high energy deuterons on a Be target, at 10 cm depth, central axis.

deuterons. Higher mass particles, such as carbon or oxygen nuclei may also undergo fragmentation (or break-up) reactions when colliding with the target nuclei; i.e. the primary nucleus is broken into two or more fragments each carrying away a significant fraction of initial energy. As a result, to calculate the dose deposited by heavy ions, the dose contributions from all particles generated along beam track must be accounted for. Some of this dose is deposited beyond the Bragg peak, partially losing the advantage of the sharp dose drop-off for the primary beam.

The microdosimetry spectrum of secondary particles arising from the bombardment of 48.5 MeV deuterons on a Be target is shown in Figure 13.6 where the lineal energy y keV/μm is plotted as a function of energy deposited (y.dy). The central axis spectrum at 10 cm depth shows the contribution of secondary electrons, recoil protons, alpha particles and heavy

ions arising from the nuclear reaction. The heavy ions contribute most to the high LET component.

This means that the for heavy ions, the same absorbed dose gives a much higher effective dose, tumour hypoxia and cell cycle times are much less of a problem than for low LET radiation (Table 13.2).

However, these important differences can lose their effect if the normal tissues are also just as dependent on high LET. It is the Therapeutic Gain Factor (TGF) that is the ultimate parameter to be optimised. This is the ratio of cancer kill to normal tissue kill, i.e.:

$$TGF = \frac{RBE_{tumour}}{RBE_{tissue}}$$

Conventional radiotherapy uses 30 fractions over six weeks to optimise tumour to normal tissue effects, allowing tissue to repair between dose fractions. Limited studies with high LET radiation suggest that 4 dose fractions are sufficient to optimise this ratio.

Table 13.2. The biological advantages of high LET radiation.

Radiobiological property	High LET	Low LET
Radiobiological effectiveness	3	1
Oxygen enhancement ratio	~1.5	3
Cell cycle effect	uniform radiosensitivity	high sensitivity in G2 and M

13.2   MEDICAL ACCELERATORS

The application of cyclotrons for the production of high energy protons for cancer therapy was proposed by Wilson (1946). At that time proton accelerators were limited to nuclear research laboratories in Sweden, the US and Russia. The first application of proton therapy at Lawrence Berkeley Laboratory in 1954 was with small cross-fired beams for radiosurgery and therapy of uveal melanoma, requiring some precision in beam targeting and stability of the patient. However, this was achieved and proton therapy was a successful application for many years. The Gustav Werner Institute, Uppsala, Sweden in 1957 was the first to spread out the Bragg peak. Harvard Cyclotron Laboratory and Massachusetts General Hospital became operational in 1961. In 1968, the first patient was treated with protons in Dubna, Russia.

As mentioned previously, initially all accelerators were based in physics research laboratories, operating at energies from 160 MeV to 1 GeV. These were dedicated research machines applied to cancer treatments (i.e. these were not accelerators developed for clinical purposes). Fixed beams from these accelerators were used to treat lesions in the head & neck. However, the need for hospital-based facilities was acknowledged in the early 1980s. Projects recognized the need for <250 MeV beams to provide sufficient penetration to treat all sites in the body. Rotating gantries were also developed to allow isocentric radiotherapy techniques.

Two types of accelerators are available to produce high energy heavy charged particle beams: the synchrotron or the cyclotron (see Chapter 3). The synchrotron has variable energy but low intensity whereas the cyclotron has high current but fixed energy. The synchrotron should be the ideal accelerator as it allows for pulse-to-pulse energy variation that is essential to generate the spread-out Bragg peak. However, the cyclotron can produce a variable energy beam using an energy degrader to reduce energy to the desired value and magnetic momentum analysis to remove undesired energy straggling of ions.

It was only with the development of 250 MeV proton synchrotrons that proton therapy became applicable for deep seated tumours in the body. The first commercial, purpose designed proton therapy facility was built at Loma Linda in California. It was a synchrotron designed and built by the Fermi National Laboratory, Batavia, USA. It comprised 3 gantries for isocentric radiotherapy, one fixed beam room for therapy and 1 fixed beam room for research, as shown in Figure 13.7.

13.3   BEAM SHAPING

When using heavy ions, beam modulation techniques need to be applied to achieve dose distribution covering the target volume and sparing organs-at-risk. Beam modulation includes energy (i.e. particle range) modulation as well as broadening of the original pencil beam.

Cyclotrons rely on extensive beam shaping and range adjustments to achieve the desired treatment plans. These techniques are shown in Figures 13.8–13.9. To adjust the particle energy/range (i.e. to produce the spread-out Bragg peak) the so-called modulator wheel (also called the range shifter) made of steps of varying thickness is employed. The wheel rotates within the beam. Some of the heavy ion energy will be absorbed within the wheel. The energy reduction/shift is given by the step height through which the beam has passed.

The range modulation enables to change the position of the Bragg peak as a function of depth in tissue. As the accelerated particle beam is narrow, it needs to be spread out laterally as well. The traditional technique of spreading the beam on to the target volume is called passive scattering. This involves scattering foils made of high Z atoms to give large scattering angles of the protons with little energy loss. Uniformly spread-out Bragg peak will result in the excessive dose to normal tissue. Consequently, custom (patient specific) collimator and compensator are used to correct for patient curvature and to shape/conform the dose to PTV. The collimator shapes the beam aperture (i.e. treatment field) of the broadened particle beam; i.e. it shapes the beam laterally. It is usually made of metal, e.g. brass. A compensator corrects for the patient body contour and for the distal shape of the PTV; it shapes the beam distally (as a function of depth). It is usually made of wax or acrylic (see Figure 13.9 left). It must be mentioned here that secondary neutrons are produced in the scatterers as

(a)

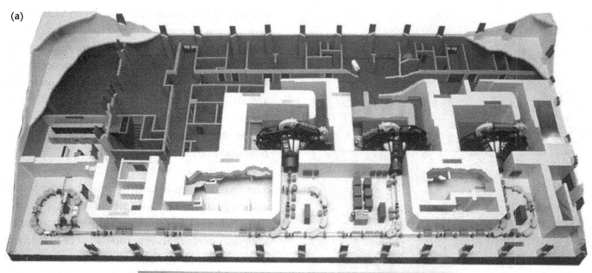

(b)

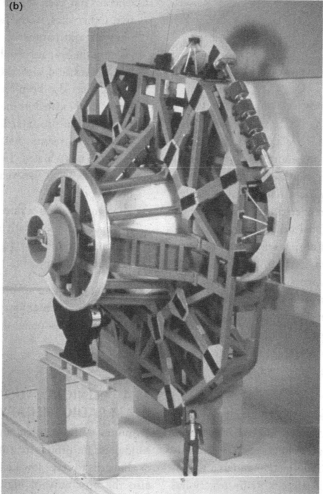

Figure 13.7. (a) Layout of the LLUMC showing the synchrotron at lower left and three treatment rooms with the massive gantries (compared to a man in Figure 13.7b). (Courtesy Loma Linda University Medical Centre)

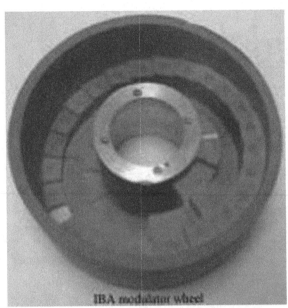

Figure 13.8. The variable thickness of the range modulator wheel reduces the proton energy range according to the requirements of the dose prescription. (Courtesy IBA)

well as in the modulation wheel, contributing to the patient dose.

Beam scanning methods are an alternative to the passive techniques. The procedure involves electromagnetic scanning of a confined, narrow proton beam, producing concentric circles. This is called 'beam wobbling'. Another alternate scanning method is via full three-dimensional beam scanning, sometimes referred to as voxel or spot scanning. The position of the proton beam is controlled by sweeper magnets horizontally, range shifters in depth, and vertically by moving the patient's bed mechanically. This way all three dimensions of the target volume may be given the high dose in the Bragg peak region.

The dose distribution advantage of charged particle beams can be exploited in two ways:

1. Radiosurgery

   These are procedures in which small radiation beams with a relatively pronounced Bragg peak are used to treat small lesions. They are usually delivered as a single dose fraction and as an alternative to conventional surgery. Radiosurgery has been used to treat pituitary lesions and ocular melanomas on the retina of the eye. The use of protons in the treatment of ocular melanomas is now quite widespread. Several specialised centres have been set up for this procedure, since a 60 to 70 MeV beam provides sufficient penetration. Primary brain tumors and metastatic brain lesion are also treated with proton radiosurgery. Some patients with benign diseases such as arteriovenous malformations and macular degeneration have also been shown to benefit.

2. Precision Radiation Therapy

   The proton beam is used to limit the dose to the critical structures in close proximity to the tumor. This technique has been used in the treatment of chondrosarcomas and chordomas close to the base of the skull, the brain stem and the spinal cord, where it has been shown to be particularly effective. Other sites, in the head & neck, are the oropharynx and paranasal sinus. Normal tissues at risk are the spinal cord, brain stem, optic chiasm and nerves and also the eyes. Precision proton therapy has also been applied to the treatment of large, deep-seated tumors such as adenocarcinoma of the prostate. Improved sparing of the bladder and rectum has allowed the dose to the tumor to be escalated. Tumor control probabilities as high as 95%, five years after treatment, have been reported.

   High tumor control rates have also been reported in small groups of patients with inoperable meningioma, craniopharyngioma, rectal carcinoma and soft tissue sarcoma.

Other applications of proton therapy include the paraspinal tumors, maxillary sinus cancer, carcinoma of the tonsils, esophageal carcinoma and cervix cancer.

13.4 CLINICAL STUDIES OF PROTON BEAM RADIOTHERAPY

Tumours of the central nervous system are good candidates for proton treatment due to the properties of glial cells to resist low LET radiation treatment and also the proximity of highly radiosensitive critical structures which need attentive sparing. Optic pathway gliomas in pediatric patients have been treated

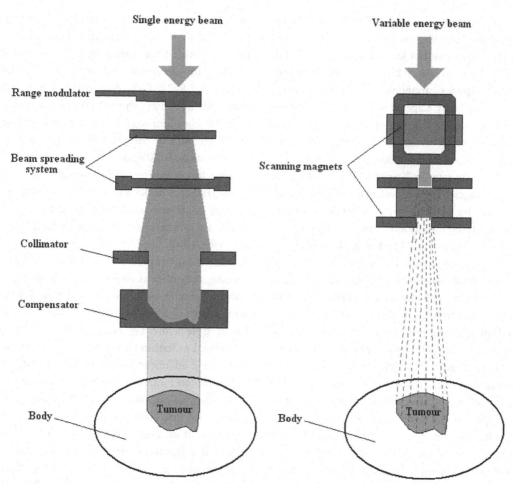

Figure 13.9. The beam delivery arrangement for passive scattering and beam scanning techniques to provide accurate dose distributions.

with proton beams with the aim of increasing therapeutic gain (Fuss *et al.* 1999). Treatment plans have been generated, comparatively, for protons, 3D conventional photons and standard photon techniques (lateral beams). Of utmost importance when treating pediatric patients is the sparing of normal tissue in order to avoid long-term complications. The current study has reported a dose reduction to the contralateral optic nerve with proton therapy by 47% and 77% as compared to 3D photons and standard photon technique, respectively. Similar results have been reported by Lin *et al.* (2000) after a comparative study between proton therapy and 3D photons for pediatric posterior fossa tumours. Organs at risk analysis have shown significant reduction of dose to normal tissue with protons as compared to photons. Consequently,

the cochlea received about only 25% of prescribed dose from protons versus 75% from photons and furthermore, while 40% of the temporal lobe was completely excluded using protons, photon treatment resulted in 31% of the dose to be delivered to 90% of the temporal lobe. Long-term effects of proton radiotherapy studies are just about to be reported enabling the objective comparison with the results of tradisional techniques.

The great value of protons in reducing dose to organs at risk has been underlined by radiotherapy results of advanced **cervical carcinoma** treated with either proton or photon beams. The study conducted by Georg *et al.* (2008) has reported mean dose reductions of 50–80% for colon and small bowel with proton therapy and also intensity modulated proton therapy

(IMPT) as compared to photon-IMRT. Significant reductions have been observed for femoral heads and kidneys and noticeable but less pronounced dose fall-offs for bladder and rectum. Long-term results of proton beam therapy for carcinoma of the uterine cervix have been reported by Kagei *et al.* (2003) demonstrating the effectiveness of the combined photon beam (to the pelvis) and proton therapy (to the primary tumour) delivering a median total tumour dose of 86 Gy. The good local control rates at 5 years (100% for stage IIB and 61% for stages IIIB/IVA patients) make this treatment effective for patients ineligible for intracavitary treatments and who usually have a poor prognosis.

Advanced, unresectable **head & neck cancers** are often a clinical challenge due to radioresistance and proximity of dose limiting normal tissues. Excellent treatment outcome (93% overall survival rate, 84% local progression-free survival rate and 71% relapse-free survival rate at 5-years) has been reported by Nishimura *et al.* (2007) on olfactory neuroblastoma patients treated with 65 GyE proton beam with 2.5 GyE fractions once daily with minimal normal tissue toxicity (Grade 1-2 dermatitis in the acute phase). Combined proton and photon radiotherapy has been employed at Massachusetts General Hospital, Boston, for the treatment of adenoid cystic carcinoma with skull base extension with a median total dose delivered to the tumour of 75.9 GyE achieving a local control at 5-years of 93% (Pommier 2006). The major role of protons was in the reduction of dose to adjacent normal tissue, greatly improving late toxicity compared to results of previous studies involving conventional radiotherapy. Clinical investigations with protons on oropharyngeal tumours have been undertaken at the Loma Linda University Medical Centre employing combined proton-photon radiotherapy (Slater 2005). The increased locoregional control (84% at 5-years) without added normal tissue toxicity warrant further investigations into the optimum time-dose schedule of combined proton-photon radiotherapy for oropharyngeal cancers. Similarly good results by means of treatment outcome have been achieved for nasopharyngeal tumours (Noel *et al.* 2002; Widesott *et al.* 2008). Ares *et al.* (2009) from the Center for Proton Radiation Therapy from Paul Scherrer Institute have reported the long-term results

on the effectiveness and safety of spot scanning proton therapy for chordomas and chondrosarcomas of the skull base. After delivering a median total dose of 73.5 GyE for chordomas and 68.4 GyE for chondrosarcomas at 1.8-2.0 GyE dose per fraction, treatment endpoints at 5-years showed good local control rates (81% for chordomas and 94% for chondrosarcomas) and high rates of disease specific survival (81% for chordomas and 100% for chondrosarcomas).

Due to promising clinical results, multi-institutional trials are underway to define the role of proton therapy in the management of head & neck and also skull base carcinomas (Chan and Liebsch 2008; Frank and Selek 2010).

The efficacy of protons in **prostate cancer** has been investigated either as stand-alone radiotherapy or as a boost to photon treatment since the early 90's. Long-term results of a randomised trial comparing conventional dose (70.2 Gy equivalents) with high-dose conformal radiation therapy (79.2 Gy equivalents) in early-stage adenocarcinoma of the prostate reported by the proton radiation oncology group of the American college of radiology 95-09 show superior cancer control for men receiving high-dose radiotherapy (Zietman *et al.* 2010). Dose escalation can be safely achieved with proton boost, as protons can attenuate adverse reactions. This is proven by the observation that the combined proton-photon radiation of the high-dose arm in the above mentioned trial was not associated with increased late effects after a median follow-up of 9.4 years (Talcott *et al.* 2010).

A currently recruiting trial has defined as primary objective the feasibility study of proton radiation therapy using standard fractionation for low-risk adenocarcinoma of the prostate, aiming to deliver one fraction of proton radiotherapy once daily, 5 days a week for approximately 9 weeks unless limited by unacceptable normal tissue toxicity (Clinical Trials identifier NCT01045226). Secondary endpoints include freedom from failure, incidence of grade 2 gastrointestinal and genitourinary toxicity after 6 months, 2 years and 3 years and also quality of life assessment.

The clinical evidence on the efficiency of proton radiotherapy relies mainly on non-controlled studies, therefore is associate with low-level of evidence according to evidence based medicine criteria (Olsen *et al.*

2007). However, the number of successful studies on proton therapy should stimulate further research and the implementation of well-designed controlled clinical trials in order to validate the efficacy of particle treatment in the management of cancer. On the other hand, a Harvard Medical School team (Suit *et al.* 2008) has sought to demonstrate that a wider use of proton beams in radiotherapy should not necessarily be preceded by costly and time consuming phase III trials as the major biophysical properties of protons beams (such as (1) the Bragg peak, (2) the finite range which is exclusively dependent on the initial energy and density distribution along the path and (3) the uniform tumour coverage achievable through an appropriate energy distribution with the spread out Bragg peak) and also the smaller dose to the surrounding normal tissue talk for themselves. Perhaps indeed the time and efforts to conduct phase III clinical trials on protons versus photons would be more efficiently spent if employed into other clinical investigations which could lead to increased therapeutic gain (i.e. dose fractionation, suitability of combined treatment methods for certain tumour entities, etc).

13.5 PROTONS VERSUS INTENSITY MODULATED RADIOTHERAPY (IMRT)

Intensity modulated radiotherapy has been described in Chapter 8. In this section we review the performance characteristics of these two modern therapeutic modalities.

The ideal cancer treatment should be efficacious, safe and painless. There should be few adverse events to impact on quality of life. The therapeutic modality should be easy to use, have minimal disruption to patients and be at a reasonable cost. As both modalities are designed for local therapy of tumours, the importance of achieving local control is the key goal of cancer therapy.

There is increasing evidence for dose escalation leading to better control of micrometastatic disease. However, such effects are not significant if the cancer cells have already escaped from the primary tumour.

The strengths of radiotherapy are that it is minimally invasive, an out-patient procedure and is neither painful nor dangerous. Local control is increasingly important as patients live longer with systemic treatment. Radiotherapy is easily combined with other modalities.

Problems for radiotherapy include: the expectation that cancer will soon be cured, the high initial capital and that patients are reluctant to pay for essential treatments.

The ideal radiotherapy beam should have good physical dose distribution, predictable radiobiology for acute and late effects and be practical in its set-up and dose delivery. The ideal dose distribution should be as high as needed in the tumour and as low as possible in normal tissue. The tumour dose should not have cold spots and there should be an adequate margin for microscopic spread, organ movement and set-up variation. These comments apply to all external beam therapeutic modalities.

The key advantage of proton therapy is the Bragg peak in dose deposition. But even if this is broadened out for larger target volumes, as shown in Figure 13.2, the tumour to skin dose is still very much lower than for any other radiation therapy, as is the cutoff dose beyond the Bragg peak.

While the depth dose curves are very encouraging, therapeutic comparisons should be made with actual treatment dose distributions available with photon radiotherapy, as shown in Figure 13.10. Here the relative dose distributions for four orthogonal fields of 190 MeV protons are compared with photons from a 15 MV linac. Results are rather similar, except that the protons have a 20% higher peak dose to background. However, in terms of avoidance of sensitive normal tissue, as shown in Figure 13.11 on p. 220, the protons give a much greater tissue sparing in this plan.

13.5.1 Dose distributions

Photons and non-charged particles have an exponential fall-off of dose with depth in tissue and the slope and presence of build-up region varies. Charged particles have Bragg peak and very steep distal fall-off, markedly superior to photons and neutrons.

The ideal depth-dose distribution is that for protons. The range depends on energy: 5 cm at 70 MeV, 30 cm at 250 MeV. Even under the worst conditions for large tumours and spreadout Bragg peak, protons still have the superior dose-depth distribution.

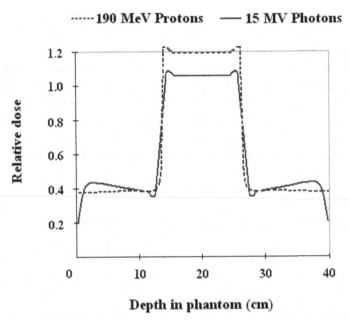

Figure 13.10. Comparative peak dose to background distributions of four orthogonal fields of 190 MeV protons and photons from a 15 MV linac.

While protons are clearly a superior single beam, most treatments involve multiple dose fractions and fields, as is the case for IMRT. The relative performance must be determined for avoidance of critical structures. The examples given above show the superior performance of protons. Further, dose to normal tissues is much higher for IMRT, but how important is this, not in terms of deterministic effects for much higher doses, but for stochastic effects, i.e. the incidence of secondary cancers? The incidence of secondary cancer in radiotherapy is only a few percent and is not regarded as an imperative issue.

The potential gains from protons include a 10% improvement in physical dose, a 20% improvement in biological effect, and avoidance of vital structures. There is reduced second malignancy, reduced general damage and less effect on growth in children. Improvements in delivered dose are most important when local control determines survival or quality of life.

The capital cost of a proton therapy facility is ~$140 million for a large facility with four treatment rooms, reducing to ~$50 million for a minimal facility. The cost per patient treatment is ~$20–25 000.

Standard radiotherapy is exceptionally cheap and perhaps should not be used for comparative purposes. One benchmark is $50 000 per life year saved, but it is

difficult to show that proton therapy actually saves lives. Costs for other therapeutic modalities are for surgery ~$15 000, chemotherapy ~$30 000 and bone marrow transplant ~$70 000. However, these modalities are not associated with high capital costs.

Summary of proton benefits:

- well defined beam edge, especially distally
- low integral dose with marked reduction of low dose volume or 'dose-bath'
- predictable radiobiology
- reasonable patient costs
- proven reliability in a hospital setting.

The major advantage of IMRT is its low capital and running costs. While patient charges are not so much of an issue for a well insured patient, there is a major health issue relating to the availability of radiotherapy to cancer patients. Does western society need many more IMRT units or just one proton therapy facility?

13.6   HEAVY ION THERAPY (HIT)

First investigation into the use of heavy ion therapy was conducted in the Lawrence Berkeley Laboratory, USA in 1957 when the Heavy Ion Linear Accelerator (HILAC) was built. Clinical trials with Ne-20 and

C-12 beams ran from 1975–1992. These studies provided the first clinical evidence that these ion beams were very effective at treating some cancers (e.g. cancers of the head & neck) that were not responsive to conventional therapies. The clinical trial results showed that the improved outcomes could be attributed to precise physical dose distributions, and also to high relative biological effectiveness. More interestingly, the results also showed that even heavier ions (e.g. silicon and argon) were not as beneficial as neon and carbon beams. This is because heavier ions break up into smaller fragments as they pass through tissue and that will carry energy beyond the Bragg peak, spoiling the sharp distal dose fall-off.

The Particle Therapy Co-Operative Group continuously lists treatment centers in operation and in the planning or construction stage (http://ptcog.web.psi.ch/). At present there are five centres using carbon ions in operation, in Japan, Germany and China (Figure 13.12). New facilities are being built in Austria, Italy as well as in China and Germany. All facilities use C-12 ion beams produced by synchrotrons. Techniques for delivery of heavy ions are similar to those used for protons but are more expensive because much

stronger magnetic fields are required to direct and focus the beam into the target volume.

Heavy ions combine the dose distribution advantages of protons and the biological advantages of neutrons (i.e. high LET advantage). The RBE increases in the Bragg peak, as shown in Figure 13.13.

13.7 CLINICAL STUDIES OF CARBON ION RADIOTHERAPY

The superior biophysical and radiobiological properties of heavy ions over conventional radiotherapy make them highly suitable for the management of complex anatomical structures and also radioresistant tumours without added normal tissue complications. Carbon ion therapy has been shown to be effective on unresectable bone and soft tissue sarcomas (Kamada *et al.* 2002; Serizawa *et al.* 2009). The small number of early trials has reported promising results regarding therapeutic gain. Unresectable osteosarcomas are good candidates for proton/carbon ion treatment as the dose necessary for curative radiotherapy is too large to be deliverable with photon therapy. Also, these tumours are often located in close proximity to radiosensitive organs such

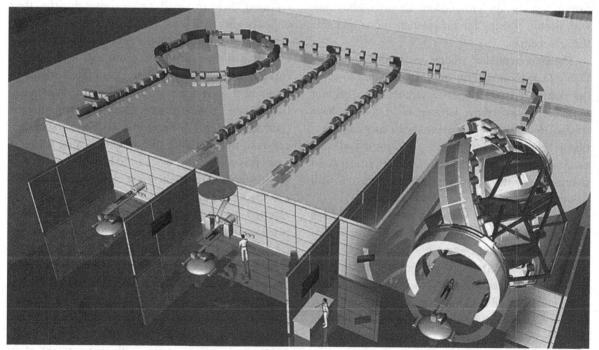

Figure 13.12. Heavy ion facility at the Heidelberg Ion-Beam Therapy Center – interior view of HIT with accelerator facility, gantry and treatment rooms. (Courtesy Heidelberg University Hospital)

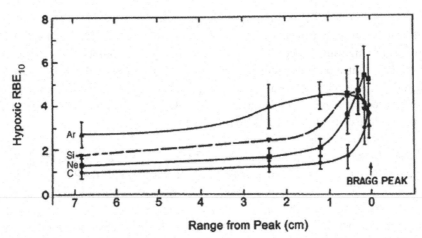

Figure 13.13. Variation of heavy ion RBE with depth in tissue relative to the depth of the Bragg peak. (Reprinted from Kraft 2000. Copyright (2000), with permission from Elsevier)

as brain, spinal cord or pelvis, therefore conventional treatment is not suitable for the management of unresectable bone cancers (Blattmann *et al.* 2010). The radiobiological advantage of protons and carbon ions due to the sharp dose falloff following the Bragg peak, meaning good tumour conformality and effective sparing of adjacent organs at risk, might constitute a step towards long-term survival of this patient category.

Table 13.3 is a compilation of early phase trials on carbon ion therapy either alone or in combination with proton therapy for unresectable bone and soft tissue sarcomas.

The aforementioned studies on carbon ion therapy (Table 13.3) show superior results compared to clinical results reported on bone sarcoma patients not receiving radiotherapy. Grimer *et al.* (1999) have treated 36 osteosarcoma patients with surgical resection +/- chemotherapy reporting a 5-year overall survival rate of 18% (for patients treated with surgery and chemotherapy the 5 year survival rate was 41%, still below the outcome of radiotherapy patients).

Noteworthy results with carbon ion therapy have been obtained for locally advanced head & neck cancers with a 75% local control at 5 years, out of which the patients treated for malignant melanomas, tumours of the ears and salivary glands achieved 100% local control at the maximum follow-up period (Mizoe *et al.* 2004). This study employed two different dose fractionation methods (dose escalation study): (1) of 70.2 GyE delivered in 18 fractions for 6 weeks

and (2) 64.0 GyE delivered in 16 fractions over 4 weeks with both schedules showing equal clinical outcome in terms of local control and normal tissue reaction.

One way to validate the efficiency of carbon ion therapy is to design two-arm randomised trials to enable the comparison of treatment endpoints for the two different arms (heavy ion therapy versus other treatment type). While results of phase III randomised trials on carbon ion therapy are yet to be reported, there are small studies comparing the effect of heavy ions with other therapeutic techniques such as surgery. In this respect, a retrospective study has evaluated the treatment outcome (either surgery or carbon ion therapy) of sacral chordoma patients in terms of disease-specific survival, local recurrence-free survival, complications, and functional outcome (Nishida *et al.* 2010). Regarding local recurrence-free survival, the results of the study indicated that at 5 years this endpoint was achieved by 62.5% of the surgery group and by 100% of the carbon ion radiotherapy group. Furthermore, carbon ion treatment resulted in less normal tissue toxicity and better functional outcome (preservation of urinary-anorectal function) than surgery.

A treatment planning intercomparison for spinal chordomas was undertaken using photon IMRT and carbon ions with the aim of investigating the potential physical advantage of combined IMRT-carbon ion therapy compared to IMRT-alone (Schulz-Ertner *et al.* 2003). For a representative patient, treatment plans

Table 13.3. Heavy ion therapy trials for unresectable bone and soft tissue sarcomas.

Trial/study	Radiation dose	Endpoints	Observations
Phase I/II non-randomised (single arm) monocentre trial trial registration no: NCT01005043 20 patients (*Blattmann* et al. *2010*)	Desired dose: 60-66 Cobalt Gray Equivalent (GyE) with 45 Gy proton therapy and a carbon ion boost of 15–21 GyE 5 × 2 Gy protons per week and 5–6 × 3 GyE heavy ions per week	Primary objective: the determination of feasibility and toxicity of heavy ion therapy. Secondary endpoints: tumour response, disease free survival and overall survival.	Trial not yet open for patient recruitment
Phase I/II feasibility study of carbon ion therapy for unresectable retroperitoneal sarcomas 24 patients (*Serizawa* et al. *2009*)	52.8 to 73.6 GyE in 16 fixed fractions over 4 weeks	Local control rates: 77% at 2 years 69% at 5 years Overall survival rates: 75% at 2 years 50% at 5 years Normal tissue effects: no toxicity greater than grade 2.	Unresectable retroperitoneal sarcomas are good candidates for carbon ion therapy with good local control and minimum normal tissue toxicity.
Retrospective Phase I-II and Phase II carbon ion radiotherapy trials for sacral chordomas 38 patients (*Imai* et al. *2009*)	52.8 to 73.6 GyE in 16 fractions over 4 weeks	Local control rate: 89% at 5-years Overall survival rate: 86% at 5-years Normal tissue toxicity: 2 patients – severe skin/soft tissue complication requiring skin grafts.	Carbon ion therapy is effective and presents a promising alternative to surgery.
Phase I/II dose escalation study of carbon ion radiotherapy 57 patients (*Kamada* et al. *2002*)	52.8 to 73.6 GyE administered in 16 fractions over 4 weeks (3.3 to 4.6 GyE/fraction)	Overall local control rates: 88% at 1 year 73% at 3 years follow-up Median survival time – 31 months Normal tissue effects: 12% – grade 3 acute skin reaction (group treated with highest dose). No severe acute reactions in rest.	Carbon ions seem safe and effective for unresectable sarcomas.

have been generated for carbon ion therapy, photon IMRT and combined plans of carbon ion–photon IMRT. It was concluded that the best target coverage was given by carbon ions alone, followed by the combined radiation therapy plan with a significant reduction of dose delivered to the non-target tissue compared to IMRT alone.

The Japanese research group from the Research Center for Charged Particle Therapy National Institute of Radiological Sciences, Chiba, have demonstrated the efficiency of carbon ion radiotherapy on several tumour sites and types (Tsujii *et al.* 2004; Mizoe *et al.* 2007; Kano *et al.* 2009):

- locally advanced head & neck tumours (mainly those with non-squamous cell histology) including adenocarcinoma, adenoid cystic carcinoma, and malignant melanoma
- early stage NSCLC and locally advanced NSCLC
- unresectable locally advanced bone and soft tissue sarcomas
- locally advanced hepatocellular carcinomas
- locally advanced prostate carcinomas, in particular for high-risk patients
- chordoma and chondrosarcoma of the skull base and cervical spine
- post-operative pelvic recurrence of rectal cancer

- malignant gliomas
- esophageal cancer (carbon ion combined with radio-sensitising agents).

Besides the improved treatment outcome, an added advantage of carbon ion radiotherapy over conventional photon treatment is the shorter overall treatment time which contributes towards increased quality of life of certain groups of cancer patients.

13.6   CONCLUSIONS

The encouraging results obtained with proton beam therapy and, to a lesser extent, with fast neutron therapy have encouraged interest in the further application of both protons and heavy ions.

As of 2010, there are 31 active proton therapy centres, 2 heavy ion facilities and approximately 12 neutron therapy centres in operation. There are as many as 22 new planned or proposed proton therapy centres, some of which are already under construction. In some of these new centres it is proposed to combine both proton and heavy ion therapy facilities. It is anticipated that in the next 10 years hadron therapy will become a much more familiar tool in the armamentarium for cancer therapy.

Radiotherapy is thought to be useful for ~50% of cancer patients. Of these, in some 50% of cases radiotherapy has a curative role and a fraction of these cases might be indicated for local treatment by external beam hadron therapy. The remaining applications are for palliation, i.e. pain management and improvement in quality of life.

Often local control by radiotherapy is indicated with systemic control by chemotherapy. How important is local control compared with systemic control? Obviously, if the primary tumour cannot be controlled then prognosis is very poor. Glioblastoma multiforme (GBM) is the prime example of this. Head & neck cancers can also be intractable. However, there is little evidence to suggest that hadron therapy changes outcome in these diseases. In the case of proton therapy for prostate cancer within the capsule, radiotherapy, hadron therapy, brachytherapy and surgery have similar efficacy and adverse events, yet have major differences in capital and patient costs.

In general, radiotherapy achieves local control for most cancers, and complete control is being approached asymptotically as new technologies are introduced. However, it is systemic disease that ultimately determines prognosis. What is the cost-benefit of radio-therapies for local control when the elephant in the room is the lack of systemic control of metastatic disease? This is the topic for Chapter 15 where internal, targeted, high LET radiation is reviewed.

13.7   REFERENCES

Amaldi U and Kraft G (2005) Radiotherapy with beams of carbon ions. *Reports on Progress in Physics* **68**: 1861–1882.

Ares C, Hug EB, Lomax AJ, Bolsi A *et al.* (2009) Effectiveness and safety of spot scanning proton radiation therapy for chordomas and chondrosarcomas of the skull base: first long-term report. *International Journal of Radiation Oncology Biology Physics* **75**: 1111–1118.

Blattmann C, Oertel S, Schulz-Ertner D, Rieken S *et al.* (2010) Non-randomized therapy trial to determine the safety and efficacy of heavy ion radiotherapy in patients with non-resectable osteosarcoma. *BMC Cancer* **10**: 96.

Chan AW and Liebsch NJ (2008) Proton radiation therapy for head & neck cancer. *Journal of Surgical Oncology* **97**(8): 697–700.

Frank SJ and Selek U (2010) Proton beam radiation therapy for head & neck malignancies. *Current Oncology Reports* **12**(3): 202–207.

Fuss M, Hug EB, Schaefer RA, Nevinny-Stickel M *et al.* (1999) Proton radiation therapy (PRT) for pediatric optic pathway gliomas: comparison with 3D planned conventional photons and a standard photon technique. *International Journal of Radiation Oncology Biology Physics* **45**(5): 1117–1126.

Georg D, Georg P, Hillbrand M, Pötter R *et al.* (2008) Assessment of improved organ at risk sparing for advanced cervix carcinoma utilizing precision radiotherapy techniques. *Strahlentherapie und Onkologie* **184**(11): 586–591.

Grimer RJ, Carter SR, Tillman RM, Spooner D *et al.* (1999) Osteosarcoma of the pelvis. *Journal of Bone and Joint Surgery, British Volume* **81**(5): 796–802.

Imai R, Kamada T, Tsuji H, Sugawara S *et al.* (2009) Effect of carbon ion radiotherapy for sacral chordoma: results of Phase I-II and Phase II clinical trials. *International Journal of Radiation Oncology Biology Physics* Nov 23 (in press).

Jäkel O (2007) State of the art in hadron therapy. *AIP Conference Proceedings* **958**(1): 70–77.

Kagei K, Tokuuye K, Okumura T, Ohara K *et al.* (2003) Long-term results of proton beam therapy for carcinoma of the uterine cervix. *International Journal of Radiation Oncology Biology Physics* **55**(5): 1265–1271.

Kamada T, Tsujii H, Tsuji H, Yanagi T *et al.* (2002) Efficacy and safety of carbon ion radiotherapy in bone and soft tissue sarcomas. *Journal of Clinical Oncology* **20**(22): 4466–4471.

Kano M, Yamada S, Hoshino I, Murakami K *et al.* (2009) Effects of carbon-ion radiotherapy combined with a novel histone deacetylase inhibitor, cyclic hydroxamic-acid-containing peptide 31 in human esophageal squamous cell carcinoma. *Anticancer Research* **29**(11): 4433–4438.

Kraft G (2000) Tumor therapy with heavy charged particles. *Progress in Particle and Nuclear Physics* **45**: S473–S544.

Lin R, Hug EB, Schaefer RA, Miller DW *et al.* (2000) Conformal proton radiation therapy of the posterior fossa: a study comparing protons with three-dimensional planned photons in limiting dose to auditory structures. *International Journal of Radiation Oncology Biology Physics* **48**(4): 1219–1226.

Lomax AJ, Bortfeld T, Goitein G, Debus J, Dykstra C, Tercier PA, Coucke PA and Mirimanof RO (1999) A treatment planning inter-comparison of proton and intensity modulated photon radiotherapy. *Radiotherapy and Oncology* **51**: 257–271.

Mizoe JE, Tsujii H, Kamada T, Matsuoka Y *et al.* (2004) Dose escalation study of carbon ion radiotherapy for locally advanced head-and-neck cancer. *International Journal of Radiation Oncology Biology Physics* **60**(2): 358–364.

Mizoe JE, Tsujii H, Hasegawa A, Yanagi T *et al.* (2007) Phase I/II clinical trial of carbon ion radiotherapy for malignant gliomas: combined X-ray radiotherapy, chemotherapy, and carbon ion radiotherapy.

International Journal of Radiation Oncology Biology Physics **69**(2): 390–396.

Nishida Y, Kamada T, Imai R, Tsukushi S *et al.* (2010) Clinical outcome of sacral chordoma with carbon ion radiotherapy compared with surgery. *International Journal of Radiation Oncology Biology Physics* Apr 16 (in press).

Nishimura H, Ogino T, Kawashima M, Nihei K *et al.* (2007) Proton-beam therapy for olfactory neuroblastoma. *International Journal of Radiation Oncology Biology Physics* **68**: 758–762.

Noel G, Boisserie G, Dessard-Diana B, Ferrand R *et al.* (2002) Comparison of dose-volume histograms of two-conformal irradiation techniques used for treatment of T2N0M0 nasopharyngeal cancer, one with association of photons and protons with photons alone. *Cancer Radiotherapy* **6**: 337–348.

Olsen DR, Bruland OS, Frykholm G and Norderhaug IN (2007) Proton therapy – a systematic review of clinical effectiveness. *Radiotherapy and Oncology* **83**(2): 123–132.

Pommier P, Liebsch NJ, Deschler DG, Lin DT *et al.* (2006) Proton beam radiation therapy for skull base adenoid cystic carcinoma. *Archives of Otolaryngology–Head & Neck Surgery* **132**: 1242–1249.

Schulz-Ertner D, Nikoghosyan A, Didinger B, Karger CP *et al.* (2003) Treatment planning intercomparison for spinal chordomas using intensity-modulated photon radiation therapy (IMRT) and carbon ions. *Physics in Medicine and Biology* **48**(16): 2617–2631.

Serizawa I, Kagei K, Kamada T, Imai R *et al.* (2009) Carbon ion radiotherapy for unresectable retroperitoneal sarcomas. *International Journal of Radiation Oncology Biology Physics* **75**(4): 1105–1110.

Slater JD, Yonemoto LT, Mantik DW, Bush DA *et al.* (2005) Proton radiation for treatment of cancer of the oropharynx: early experience at Loma Linda University Medical Center using a concomitant boost technique. *International Journal of Radiation Oncology Biology Physics* **62**: 494–500.

Suit H, Kooy H, Trofimov A, Farr J, Munzenrider J *et al.* (2008) Should positive phase III clinical trial data be required before proton beam therapy is more widely adopted? No. *Radiotherapy and Oncology* **86**(2): 148–153.

Talcott JA, Rossi C, Shipley WU, Clark JA *et al.* (2010) Patient-reported long-term outcomes after conventional and high-dose combined proton and photon radiation for early prostate cancer. *Journal of the American Medical Association* **303**(11): 1046–1053.

Tsujii H, Mizoe JE, Kamada T, Baba M *et al.* (2004) Overview of clinical experiences on carbon ion radiotherapy at NIRS. *Radiotherapy and Oncology* **73** (Suppl 2): S41–9.

Widesott L, Pierelli A, Fiorino C, Dell'oca I *et al.* (2008) Intensity-modulated proton therapy versus helical tomotherapy in nasopharynx cancer: planning comparison and NTCP evaluation. *International Journal of Radiation Oncology Biology Physics* **72**: 589–596.

Wilson R (1946) Radiological use of fast protons. *Radiology* **47**: 487.

Zietman AL, Bae K, Slater JD, Shipley WU *et al.* (2010) Randomized trial comparing conventional-dose with high-dose conformal radiation therapy in early-stage adenocarcinoma of the prostate: long-term results from proton radiation oncology group/american college of radiology 95-09. *Journal of Clinical Oncology* **28**(7): 1106–1111.

http://clinicaltrialsfeeds.org/clinical-trials/show/NCT01045226, accessed on the 27/04/2010.

http://clinicaltrialsfeeds.org/clinical-trials/show/NCT01005043, accessed on the 28/04/2010.

14 Fast neutron therapy

14.1 INTRODUCTION

Soon after the discovery of the neutron by Chadwick in 1932, neutrons were applied to radiobiological studies by L Lawrence at Berkeley and L H Gray in England. The Berkeley research led to the proposal by EO Lawrence to use fast neutrons for the therapy of cancer, using his brother's world first cyclotron. Between 1938 and 1939 over 200 patients were treated by Stone and Larkin (1942) at the Berkeley cyclotron. Unfortunately, the benefits of the treatment were overshadowed by severe complications, bringing the overall efficacy of the therapy into doubt. We now know that the neutron doses were too high because of the higher RBE for late effects for neutrons.

Detailed research at Hammersmith Hospital in England led to a new understanding of neutron effects and to its higher effectiveness for hypoxic cells (Giles et al. 1952). A 16 MeV cyclotron was used to accelerate deuterons onto a beryllium target to generate high neutron fluxes suitable for detailed biological studies and the determination of optimal doses regimes. Subsequently, a new clinical trial of fast neutrons therapy (FNT) for advanced tumours was begun (Morgan 1967). The degree of local control was found to be superior to that for the earlier treatments but with minimal complications. Pain and ulceration were nearly always resolved.

The first randomised trials began in 1971, with the comparison of fast neutrons and photon therapies (Catterall 1974a,b, 1976, 1977; Catterall and Bewley 1980). Of 102 patients with advanced head & neck cancer, 52 were treated with neutrons the rest with standard photon therapy. First results gave 70% remission rate for neutrons, well in advance of the 30% remission for photons. Further, there were no local recurrences with neutrons, whereas there was a 50% recurrence rate for photons. Death rates were similar because of the advanced nature of the disease. Local therapies would not be expected to change this parameter. These encouraging results led to new interest in the FNT modality and more clinical trials. However, results became controversial (Allen 1983).

There are two therapeutic modalities for neutrons. These are Neutron Capture Therapy (NCT) and Fast Neutron Therapy (FNT). NCT is discussed in Chapter 15 as a targeted modality. Even though an external epithermal neutron beam is used, its efficacy depends on the uptake of the neutron absorbing isotopes boron-10 or gadolinium-157 by the cancer cells and tumours. Thus it is primarily targeted internally. FNT,

L. Marcu et al., *Biomedical Physics in Radiotherapy for Cancer*,
DOI 10.1007/978-0-85729-733-4_14, © CSIRO 2012

however, is an external hadron modality, which relies on nuclear scattering reactions with hydrogen to impart secondary high LET radiation to the tumour.

14.2 RADIOBIOLOGY

As discussed in Chapter 2, the biological response to radiation exposure is determined by absorbed dose and the relative biological effect (RBE) is defined as the ratio of absorbed doses for the standard radiation (250 keV X-rays) and the test radiation for the same endpoint or biological effect.

The RBE for stochastic (probabilistic) effects such as causing cancer or hereditary defects is called the radiation weighting factor (w_R). According to the International Commission on Radiation Protection (ICRP) Report No. 103, the neutron w_R is defined as a continuous function of the incident neutron energy and can be written as:

$$w_R(E_n) = \begin{cases} 2.5 + 18.2 \exp\left[-\dfrac{(\ln E_n)^2}{6}\right] & E_n < 1\,\text{MeV} \\[2mm] 5.0 + 17.0 \exp\left\{-\dfrac{[\ln(2E_n)]^2}{6}\right\} & 1\,\text{MeV} \leq E_n \leq 50\,\text{MeV} \\[2mm] 2.5 + 3.25 \exp\left\{-\dfrac{[\ln(0.04E_n)]^2}{6}\right\} & E_n > 50\,\text{MeV} \end{cases}$$

where E_n is the neutron energy in MeV.

Table 14.1 shows neutron w_R values as a function of incident neutron energy (E_n). It can be noticed that w_R values for thermal neutrons ($E_n < 0.5\,\text{eV}$) ($w_R \approx 2.5$) are about 8 times smaller than those for fast neutrons ($E_n > 0.5\,\text{MeV}$) ($w_R \approx 20$).

The high weighting factor relates to the difficulty in high fidelity repair of non-lethal radiation damage by high LET radiation.

The RBE for deterministic effects above a given threshold is very much less and very dependent on the chosen biological endpoint. It is often the D_0 or 37% survival dose for in vitro studies or 2 Gy for in vivo or clinical measurements (see Chapter 2). There is a broad maximum in the neutron RBE in the 200–400 keV neutron energy range, peaking at values of RBE = 2–3, depending on the endpoint.

Neutrons transfer energy by elastic collisions with the abundant hydrogen atoms, creating high LET radiation in the form of protons. Thermalised neu-

trons are then captured by nitrogen, causing the emission of 630 keV protons. These high LET properties on neutrons impact on their biological effect.

In order to identify photon resistant tumours which are sensitive to neutrons the radiobiological effectiveness of fast neutrons (66 MeV) versus photons (60-Co) has been assessed using the micronucleus assay technique (Akudugu et al. 2003). The micronucleus assay has been evaluated in human glioblastoma (known for their radioresistance) and neuroblastoma cell lines after exposing the cell lines to either photon or neutron beams. The experimental results have shown that neutrons are 1.43–5.29 times more effective per unit dose in inducing micronuclei than photons. RBE values determined by micronucleus yield were strongly correlated to RBE values based on surviving fractions, suggesting that the micronucleus endpoint is a potential parameter in detecting photon/low LET-resistant tumours which exhibit increased radiosensitivity to neutron beams. It would, therefore, be useful to develop a predictive assay to facilitate the selection of those tumours which are potentially responsive to neutron irradiation (Britten et al. 1992).

14.2.1 Hypoxia

Hypoxia in tumours arises because of the lack of oxygen diffusing to cancer cells at more than 100 μm from the capillaries. At greater distances cells can become necrotic (see also Chapter 4). Fractionation in radiotherapy is designed to overcome this effect by allowing time between fractions for re-oxygenation of cancer cells.

The oxygen enhancement ratio (OER) is measured in vitro to determine D_0 values with and without oxygenation. Typically with photons, the OER is approximately 3. However, with neutron exposure, the OER decreases to about 1.6–1.7. Thus neutrons can be twice as toxic to hypoxic cancer cells as photons for the same absorbed dose. Still, the supporting experimental evidence for superior efficiency of neutrons as compared to photons on hypoxic tumours is inconclusive. The influence of hypoxia on the relative sensitivity of various tumour cell lines to 62.5 MeV fast neutrons and 4 MV photons has been investigated, by determining the **hypoxic gain factor** (the ratio of OERs for fast neutrons compared to photons) (Warenius et al. 2000).

Table 14.1. Variation of radiation weighting factor with neutron energy.

Incident neutron energy (E$_n$) in MeV	Radiation weighting factor (w$_R$)	Incident neutron energy (E$_n$) in MeV	Radiation weighting factor (w$_R$)
1.0E–06	2.5	0.4	18.3
1.0E–05	2.5	0.5	19.3
1.0E–04	2.5	1.0	20.7
1.0E–03	2.5	2.0	17.3
5.0E–03	2.7	4.0	13.3
1.0E–02	3.0	6.0	11.1
5.0E–02	6.6	8.0	9.7
0.1	10.0	10.0	8.8
0.2	14.3	20.0	6.8
0.3	16.8	40.0	5.7

The experiments resulted in hypoxic gain factor values within the range of 1.31–1.63. However, when comparing surviving fractions at clinically delivered doses (i.e. 1.6 Gy neutrons and 2 Gy photons) the advantage of neutrons by means of cell kill was not significantly superior to photons, suggesting that there might not be a radiobiological advantage of neutrons for hypoxic tumours in clinical settings as initially anticipated.

14.2.2 Cell cycle effects

The radiosensitivity of a cell varies with both cell type and phase of the cell cycle and is larger for photons than for neutrons. Qualitatively, the variation in radiosensitivity as a function of cell cycle phase was found to be similar for photons and neutrons, meaning that cells in and close to mitosis are the most sensitive, while maximum radioresistance is characteristic to cells situated in late S phase (Figure 14.1). The RBE for neutron irradiation of Chinese hamster ovary cells can vary from 1.75 to 5.1 for zero to 100% of cells in the radioresistant phases. This results in major changes in the therapeutic gain factor (TGF) for neutrons for different combinations of cell cycle phase and RBE values for normal and cancer cells:

$$TGF = \frac{RBE_{tumour}}{RBE_{tissue}} = 0.57 - 1.05$$

Under certain conditions, e.g. $TGF < 1$, neutrons could be less effective than photons. Thus the normal tissue response must always be considered.

14.2.3 Repair of Potentially Lethal Damage (PLD)

PLD is that component of damage influenced by post-irradiation environmental conditions (Hall and Cox 1994). It has no role in well nourished, proliferating cells but in cells presumed to be outside the growth fraction in a tumour, i.e. the hypoxic cells. There is no evidence of PLD for neutrons so a therapeutic gain over photons is suggested. However, it is always the ratio of effect for normal and tumour cells that determines the ultimate advantage or otherwise (Withers and Peters 1980).

14.2.4 RBE effects

The neutron RBE is energy dependent, exhibiting a broad peak from 200–400 keV. However, dose effects can be more important. The RBE decreases exponentially from ~5 at 1 Gy to 2.5 at 100 Gy for human and pig skin erythema, as shown in Figure 14.2 (Allen 1983). Single dose neutron damage is much greater than that for photons for low absorbed doses. This is because of repair of sublethal damage that can occur with photons at low doses. It is the variability of photon response that is responsible for the rapid changes in RBE with absorbed dose.

In vitro and in vivo animal studies allow the determination of neutron RBE values for specific endpoints. These results, while useful guides, cannot be directly translated to RBE values in patient treatments. Thus patient models are an invaluable source of practical and clinically applicable data.

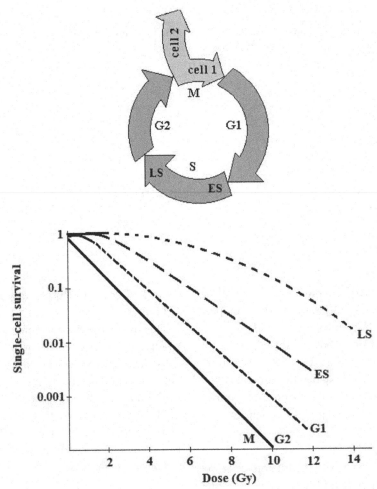

Figure 14.1. Changes in response to X-rays with cell cycle phase; showing early and late S phases (ES, LS); G1 and G2 are the gap phases and M represents mitosis.

One such example is the lung coin lesion study where doubling times and growth delays of pulmonary metastases were investigated for different grades of primary tumour using 14 MeV neutrons or Co-60 gamma irradiations (Battermann *et al.* 1981). Coin like lesions in the lung, readily observed by X-rays, show volume reduction, growth delay but regrow after a growth delay period. The neutron RBE for these parameters can be readily determined relative to the Co-60 results. The neutron RBE was found to be exponentially related to the doubling time (Figure 14.3) and was only greater than the normal tissue value (RBE = 3) for doubling times >80–100 days. Such tumours are mostly well differentiated, i.e. low grade with few mitoses. It is only for these cases that

the TGF >1. A successful application of FNT is for therapy of salivary gland tumours, which are slow growing and highly differentiated (Laramore 1993b). On the other hand, glioblastoma multiforme (GBM) has proven to be retractable to both neutrons and photons. An early study did not reveal a significant difference in survival time (11 months) and 2 year survival rates for fast neutrons, photons or mixed modality schedules (Geraci 1981).

A major problem associated with early fast neutron clinical studies was the higher incidence of complications. These were due in part to the poor beam penumbra and tissue penetration, with beam characteristics inferior to that of gamma rays from a Co-60 source. However, the high incidence of fibrosis was

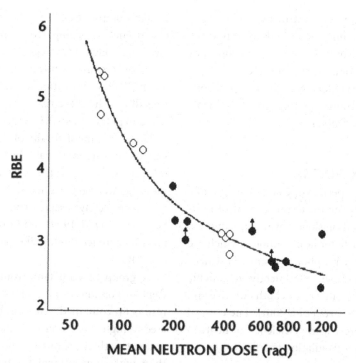

Figure 14.2. Neutron dose dependence of RBE for human (o) and pig (•) erythema. The data fall on the same curve indicating equivalent responses to photon and neutron radiation for both tissue types (reproduced after Allen 1983, with permission from the author).

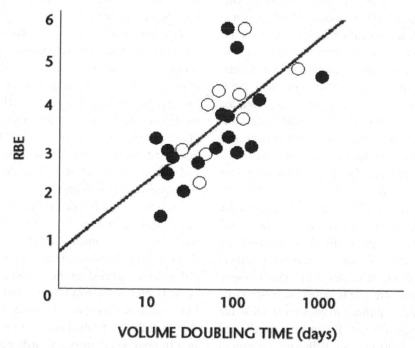

Figure 14.3. The doubling time is exponentially related to the RBE. Tumour RBE is only greater than the normal tissue value (RBE=3) for doubling times >80–100 days. (Reprinted from Battermann *et al.* 1981. Copyright (1981), with permission from Elsevier)

offset by improved tumour control rates compared with photons. For example, in a study of 401 cases from four clinics, the control and complication rates for epidermoid carcinoma of the head & neck were 60% and 18% respectively for FNT, giving a probability of uncomplicated control of 49%, compared with 34% for photons (Cohen 1982).

14.3   CLINICAL RESULTS

The radiobiological properties of fast neutrons make them a valuable candidate for the treatment of radioresistant, hypoxic and/or slowly growing tumours. Also, FNT is appropriate for large tumours which are not treated efficiently with photon beams. Fast neutron radiotherapy was shown to be effective in patients with high risk of local recurrence in both curative and palliative settings (Schwartz et al. 2001). The clinical studies/trials below present the efficiency of neutron radiotherapy over other irradiation techniques.

14.3.1   Soft tissue sarcoma

Clinical results for FNT of soft tissue carcinoma achieved 70–94% control rates after surgery (Wambersie 1982) with no residual tumour. However, similar results were achieved with photons. This was not the case for radioresistant tumours such as soft tissue sarcoma, osteogenic sarcoma and chondrosarcoma. A review of the published data (Laramore et al. 1989) showed that there was a therapeutic advantage for FNT compared with photons or electrons. Local control rates for soft tissue sarcoma were found to be 53% for neutrons versus 38% for photons; for osteosarcomas 55% versus 21% and for chondrosarcomas 49% versus 33% respectively.

A case report on extensive osteogenic sarcoma of the maxilla (10.5×9.0 cm in greatest diameter as measured on the CT scan) has been published by Smoron et al. (1999) underlining the efficiency of fast neutron therapy on large, unresectable tumours. Furthermore, osteogenic sarcomas are rare tumours for which satisfactory treatments are difficult to implement due to the involvement of organs at risk. Treatment was delivered using a 66 MeV neutron beam delivering an overall dose of 20.4 Gy in 13 fractions over 35 days. At 3-years follow up the patient has been well without treatment-

related complications. Besides higher radiobiological effectiveness as compared to photons, fast neutrons have the added advantage of reduced normal tissue sequelae. The low neutron kerma in bone reduces by about 25% the absorption of radiation in bony cavities, thus diminishing the risk of late tissue injury as compared to photons (Bewley 1989).

Good treatment results of fast neutron therapy in soft tissue sarcomas have been achieved by several other groups showing superior efficacy of neutron radiotherapy versus photon therapy particularly in the incompletely resected tumours (Prott et al. 1999; Schönekaes et al. 1999) and tumours with high risk of local recurrence (Steingräber et al. 1996; Schwartz et al. 2001).

A group of clinicians from the Detroit Medical Centre (Fontanesi et al. 2005) have published their results on combined neutron/photon treatment delivered to high-grade non-metastatic soft tissue sarcoma patients with the aim to achieve better local control than with conventional treatments. The group has achieved a combined dose equivalent to about 70–80 Gy delivered in 6 weeks, with an estimated RBE of 4.5. The reported local progression free survival at 3-years was 91% with an 87% overall survival. Normal tissue complication in terms of delayed wound healing was characteristic to three patients (out of 23 treated patients). The study reported an overall good tolerance of combined neutron-photon therapy (grade 1–2 skin toxicity). Since it has been suggested that the irradiated treatment volume may play an important role in complication development, the use of neutron beams as a boost in delivering radiation to the site of the tumour bed with a limited margin are a good treatment choice (Schwartz et al. 2001; Fontanesi et al. 2005).

Treatment with fast neutrons involves certain risks as well (Schwartz et al. 2001). As with other radiation modalities too, a major concern with fast neutron therapy is the risk of second cancers. MacDougall et al. (2006) have reported on the incidence of sarcomas in patients previously treated with fast neutrons. They have conducted a systematic review of long-term follow-up of clinical trials of fast neutron therapy for various tumour sites, involving 620 patients and have observed three cases of soft tissue sarcoma developed within the treated site. This incidence is considered to be significant, as it is 15 times the incidence of a comparable photon-treated group of patients. A case of post-irradiation sarcoma in a prostate cancer patient treated with a mixed beam of 18 MV photons and 65 MeV fast neutrons has been published (Prevost *et al.* 2004). The patient has developed soft tissue sarcoma 8 years after the external beam therapy for prostate adenocarcinoma. Although post-irradiation sarcomas are considered to be rare incidences after prostate radiotherapy, the combined beam therapy should require more attention in regards to risk of second cancer.

14.3.2   Prostate cancer

As indicated by the low α/β ratio, prostate cancers are slowly growing, being good responders to fast neutron radiotherapy. In a randomised study of 91 patients with locally advanced prostate cancer, 36 received photons and 55 mixed neutron (40%) and photon (60%) protocols (Laramore *et al.* 1985). Local control was significantly higher for the mixed beam than for photons, being 93% versus 78%), as was the 5 year survival (62% versus 35%). However, toxicity and severe adverse events were not significantly different. At 10 years local control was significantly superior for the mixed schedule (70% versus 58% for photons, with significance P = 0.03). These results indicate that a fast neutron component is quite advantageous in the treatment of locally advanced prostate cancer.

A review of the progress made with fast neutron therapy at Wayne State University involving around 700 patients in clinical trials has incorporated the results of three Phase II studies and one Phase III study (Forman *et al.* 2002). The escalations studies undertaken via Phase II trials have established the standard radiation dose which was later used in the Phase III trial. The results showed that the highest therapeutic ratio is achieved with mixed radiation beams delivering 10 Gy neutrons and 40 Gy photons underpinning the importance of radiation sequencing. Therefore, the disease-free survival was 93% for patients treated with neutrons first versus 73% for patients treated with neutrons last, without difference in the incidence of acute or late normal tissue toxicity.

A pioneering work has been undertaken by Santanam *et al.* (2007) on prostate adenocarcinoma by the employment of intensity modulated neutron radio-

therapy (IMNRT) using an in-house algorithm for segment optimisation. Treatment plans have been normalised such that IMNRT DVHs for prostate and seminal vesicles were identical to those for conventional fast neutron therapy. A major benefit from IMNRT consisted of substantial reduction in dose to normal tissue (10% reductions in rectum V(95) and 13% in V(80), respectively and reductions in bladder V(95) and V(80) of 12% and 4%, respectively).

14.3.3   Head & neck cancer

The role of fast neutron therapy in the management of head & neck cancers is presently limited to salivary gland tumours and radioresistant sarcomas (Laramore 2009). Conventional photon therapy for locally advanced or recurrent salivary gland tumours has demonstrated poor locoregional tumour control necessitating the implementation of high LET radiotherapy.

A combined RTOG randomised clinical trial of neutrons versus photons for non-resectable or recurrent salivary gland tumours has included only 25 subjects, with 13 patients in the neutron arm and 12 in the photon arm (Laramore *et al.* 1993). The protocol was 12 fractions of neutrons to 16.5 to 22 Gy and 70 Gy for 37 fractions or 55 Gy for 20 fractions of photons. The superiority of FNT was clearly apparent at 2 years, when local control and survival were 67% and 62% for neutrons versus 17% and 25% for photons. Control of lymph node metastases was also superior for neutrons. Local control at 10 years was 56% for neutrons compared with 17% for photons, all results being significant. This study was terminated on the grounds that to continue with the photon arm would be unethical.

A report on a larger group of patients (279) treated with curative intent for salivary gland cancer has been published by the University of Washington Cancer Centre team (Douglas *et al.* 2003). Patients have been treated with a 50.5 MeV neutron beam with fraction sizes ranging from 1.05 neutron Gy (nGy) to 1.7 nGy delivered 3–4 times a week (with total doses between 17.4 nGy and 20.7 nGy). The 6-year actuarial overall survival achieved was 59%, the same percent of patients presenting loco-regional control at 6-years follow-up. These results demonstrate again the superiority of neutrons in treating salivary gland carcinomas these tumours being by far the most successful application of FNT.

A retrospective analysis into radiotherapy of advanced adenoid cystic carcinoma of the head & neck has been undertaken to compare treatment outcome of three different irradiation modalities: neutrons, photons and mixed beam (neutrons + photons) radiotherapy (Huber *et al.* 2001). Median radiation doses used were as follows: 16 nGy for fast neutron therapy, 64 Gy for photon treatment and 8 nGy + 32 Gy photon dose for the mixed beam therapy. Although the actuarial 5-year local control was 75% for neutrons and 32% for both mixed beam and photons, this advantage of neutrons was not found in patient survival, endpoint which was mainly dictated by the occurrence of distant metastases. Fast neutron therapy can still be recommended in patients with bad prognosis or those with unresectable tumours.

14.3.4   Conclusions

Randomised phase III clinical trials employing fast neutron therapy versus conventional photon radiotherapy for various tumour sites showed very different results, depending on the treated lesion. In the early days of neutron therapy the largest number of patients randomised for neutron versus photon therapy have been those diagnosed with head & neck squamous cell carcinomas, non-small cell lung cancers and adenocarciomas of the prostate. Majority of these early trials have employed fast neutron beams originating from physics laboratory-based generators, fact that might have biased the outcome. Consequently, while for head & neck cancer patients neutrons showed no convincing advantage over photons, adenocarcinomas of the prostate responded well to neutron therapy, trials reporting superior outcome compared to photon therapy (Koh *et al.* 1994) (Table 14.2).

Mixed beams of fast neutrons and photons have also been trialled in randomised studies noticing a reduced normal tissue complication compared with neutron-only treated patients. The TAMVEC trial conducted at MD Anderson on 95 head & neck cancer patients has delivered a mixed beam of 70 Gy equivalent with 2 neutron and 3 photon fractions/week in one arm and a conventional 70 Gy with 2 Gy per fraction over 7 weeks of photons in the second arm (Maor *et al.* 1983). Severe normal tissue complication was

found to be the same in both arms, with 7% of the patients being affected. Neither loco-regional control (44% mixed arm versus 41% photons arm) nor overall survival (20% mixed arm versus 17% photons arm) have lead to significantly different outcome. Moreover, the slight advantage in survival of patients treated with mixed beam lasted for the first 2 years only, leaving the question about the effectiveness of neutron therapy on head & neck cancers unrequited.

On the other hand, mixed beams (neutron/photon) for the treatment of prostate adenocarcinoma have proven to be highly effective as shown by a randomised RTOG trial (Laramore *et al.* 1985), with a 5-year overall survival rate of 62% in the mixed treatment arm and only 35% survival rate in the photon arm.

Several trials have reported on high incidence of normal tissue toxicity resulting after FNT, fact that cautions upon careful beam collimation and treatment planning (Duncan *et al.* 1984, 1987; Laramore *et al.* 1986; Koh *et al.* 1994). However, over the last few decades, patients have been treated with performant, hospital-based, isocentric-treatment capable cyclotrons, excluding therefore planning and delivery difficulties which happened to arise with old generation research equipment.

14.4   NEUTRON SOURCES

The success of FNT depends to a large extent on the beam parameters and dose-depth distributions of the fast neutrons. The high radiation fields and neutron backgrounds arising place increased emphasis of radiation protection considerations. At the same time as the clinical niche for FNT was being defined, the quality of photon beams from linear accelerators continued to improve (see Chapters 6 and 8). Research has shown that state-of-the-art hospital-based facilities are necessary to deliver effective neutron treatments. The number of FNT centres has fallen from a peak of about 25 to between 10 and 15. Yet superior efficacy has been demonstrated in the treatment of slow growing tumors (e.g. prostate) and the treatment of large hypoxic tumours (salivary gland tumours, soft tissue sarcomas, osteosarcomas and chondrosarcomas).

The standard geometry for FNT is shown in Figure 14.4, where the cyclotron is located in a heavily

CYCLOTRON VAULT   TREATMENT ROOM

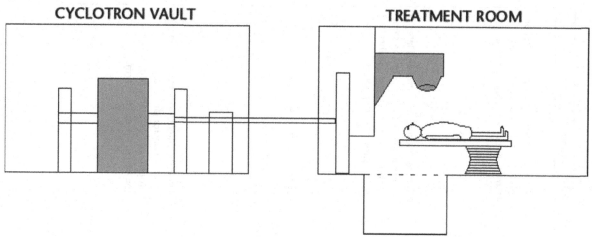

Figure 14.4. FNT facility comprising the cyclotron in a separate shielded room and the bending magnet and collimator in the therapy room.

shielded room. A large electromagnet is needed to focus the proton beam onto the neutron producing target (Be) in the irradiation room. The neutron beam so produced must be collimated to direct the neutrons to the target volume. Modern facilities produce neutron radiation by employing cyclotrons to accelerate deuterons or protons to energies larger than 48 MeV. To collimate the emergent neutron beam to the desired treatment shape multirod or multileaf collimators are used. Neutrons are much harder to collimate than photons so this is no easy task. Consequently, a FNT facility is rather more expensive and larger than a photon facility.

Super-cooled electromagnets can cut the cost and size requirements substantially, as demonstrated in the ground breaking FNT facility at the Karmanos Cancer Center, Wayne State University in Detroit, USA (the irradiation room is shown in Figure 14.5). This facility produces neutron beams by accelerating 48.5 MeV deuterons onto a beryllium target. The resulting neutron beam has a maximum energy of 52.5 MeV and a mean energy of approximately 20 MeV, presenting similar depth dose characteristics to 4 MV photons.

Superior beam shaping to define the target volume is provided by a 120-leaf computer controlled collimator built with a vision system for quality assurance of leaf position (Figures 14.6 and 14.7). This fully automatic neutron collimator enables delivery of intensity modulated neutron radiation, thus improving dose

conformality (Farr *et al.* 2006). Given that photons and neutrons have similar dosimetric behaviour, intensity modulation of neutron beams is expected to increase the efficiency of fast neutron therapy in the same way as intensity modulated photon radiotherapy overcomes, to a certain extent, the dosimetric deficiencies of photons.

14.5 NEUTRON BRACHYTHERAPY

Photon brachytherapy is now an accepted modality for the treatment of in capsule prostate and other cancers (see Chapter 9). However, brachytherapy is also possible with neutrons using californium-252 (Cf-252) as it decays by the fission process. Cf-252 is produced in a high flux nuclear reactor. It has a half life of 2.645 years and a specific activity of 536.3 Ci/g. The alpha emission branching ratio is 96.908%, with spontaneous fission accounting for the remainder. Neutrons are produced in the fission process with a mean energy of 2.14 MeV and a flux of 2.31×10^{12} n/s/g. The average gamma ray energy is 0.8 MeV.

The biological advantages of Cf-252 FNT relate to the low OER, even cell cycle sensitivity and the absence of repair of sublethal damage (Maruyama 1984). These factors could enhance local control of recurrent tumours.

Several clinical studies have investigated the effect of combined external beam radiotherapy and Cf-252 brachytherapy on various tumour types.

Table 14.2. Early randomised clinical trial results on fast neutron therapy for various tumour sites.

Clinical trial	Treatments compared	Outcome/endpoint	Observation
Head & neck			
Hammersmith hospital trial 161 patients (*Catterall et al. 1977*)	Neutrons: 15.6 nGy in 12 fractions over 4 weeks Photons: 45.4–68.4 Gy over 4–6 weeks	Loco-regional control at 2 years: 76% (neutrons) versus 19% (photons) Overall survival at 2 years: 28% (neutrons) versus 15% (photons) Normal tissue toxicity: 14% (neutrons) versus 3% (photons)	The superior loco-regional control of neutrons did not translate into the same advantage regarding overall survival.
Multicentre European trial 195 patients (*Duncan et al. 1984*)	Neutrons: 15.6–18 nGy in 20 fractions over 4 weeks Photons: 54–70 Gy in 20–35 fractions over 4–7 weeks	Loco-regional control at 2 years: 34% (neutrons) versus 39% (photons) Overall survival at 2 years: 33% (neutrons) versus 39% (photons) Normal tissue toxicity: similar overall complications	Both local tumour control and late morbidity were found to be the same for the two arms. Larynx patients had better survival with photons.
RTOG 76-10A trial 40 patients (*Griffin et al. 1984*)	Neutrons: 20.4–25 nGy over 7–8 weeks Photons: 66–74 Gy over 7–8 weeks	Loco-regional control at 2 years: 42% (neutrons) versus 13% (photons) Overall survival at 2 years: 25% (neutrons) versus 0% (photons) Normal tissue toxicity: 18% (neutrons) versus 33% (photons)	Superior outcome for the neutron arm.
Edinburgh trial 165 patients (*Duncan et al. 1987*)	Neutrons: 15.6–16.7 nGy in 20 fractions over 4 weeks Photons: 54–56 Gy in 20 fractions over 4 weeks	Loco-regional control at 2 years: 45% (neutrons) versus 45% (photons) Overall survival at 2 years: 29% (neutrons) versus 41% (photons) Normal tissue toxicity: 24% (neutrons) versus 13% (photons)	Superior outcome for the photon arm (particularly for larynx and oropharynx patients). More severe toxicity in the neutron arm.

Clinical trial	Treatments compared	Outcome/endpoint	Observation
Prostate			
Neutron Therapy Collaborative Working Group trial 172 patients (*Russell et al. 1994*)	Neutrons: 20.4 nGy in 12 fractions over 4 weeks Photons: 70 Gy with 1.8–2 Gy/fraction over 7–8 weeks	Loco-regional control at 5 years: 89% (neutrons) versus 68% (photons) Overall survival at 5 years: 68% (neutrons) versus 59% (photons) Normal tissue toxicity: 11% (neutrons) versus 3% (photons)	Fast neutron therapy is significantly superior to conventional photon radiotherapy
Non-small cell lung cancer			
RTOG 3 arm trial 102 patients (*Laramore et al. 1986*)	Neutrons: 60 Gy photon equivalent Mixed beam: neutrons + photons to a 60 Gy photon equivalent Photons: 60 Gy	Expected survival at 3 years: 37% mixed beam 25% neutrons 12% photons	Similar overall local response rates for the 3 arms with a trend towards increased long-term survival for neutron and mixed beam arms. Higher incidence of severe toxicity in the neutron and mixed beam arms.
Multicentre randomised trial 193 patients (*Koh et al. 1993*)	Neutrons: 20.4 nGy in 12 fractions over 4 weeks Photons: 66 Gy with 2 Gy/fraction over 7 weeks	Overall median survival: 9.7 months (neutrons) versus 8.9 months (photons) Overall survival at 2 years: 14% (neutrons) versus 10% (photons) Normal tissue toxicity: similar overall toxicity	No difference in overall survival was observed, however patients with squamous cell cancer did benefit from neutrons (16% versus 3% at 2 years).

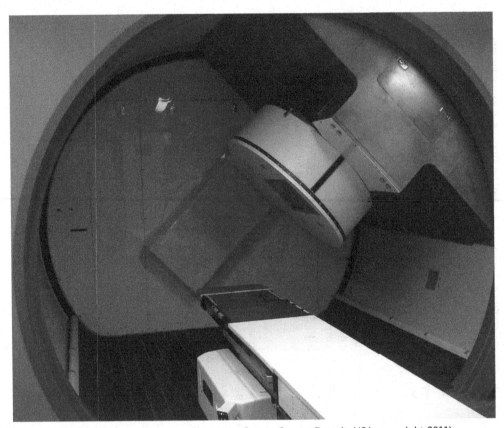

Figure 14.5. Irradiation room for FNT. (Courtesy Karmanos Cancer Center, Detroit, USA, copyright 2011)

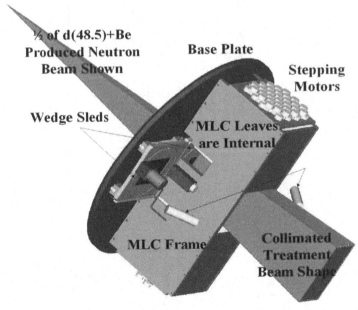

Figure 14.6. Neutron beam shaping with the automated MLC. (Courtesy Karmanos Cancer Center, Detroit, USA, copyright 2011)

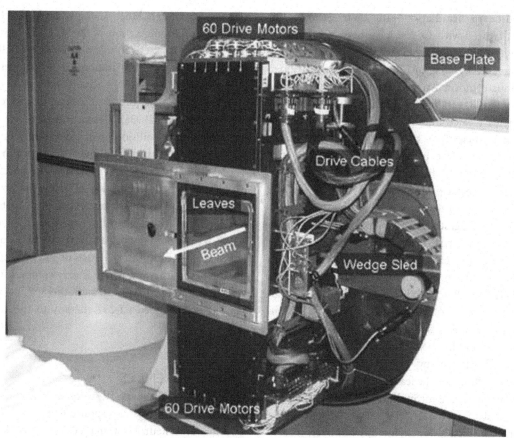

Figure 14.7. 120-leaf computer controlled MLC. (Courtesy Karmanos Cancer Center, Detroit, USA, copyright 2011)

Some of these studies have pointed out the importance of Cf-252 scheduling and sequencing for higher therapeutic ratio. Maruyama *et al.* (1993b) have reported the results of a Phase II trial on normal tissue complication after delayed Cf-252 brachytherapy for **cervical cancer.** They delivered 35 GyE (Gray-Equivalent) neutron brachytherapy (Cf-252) in 1 to 4 radiotherapy sessions and 40–45 Gy external beam irradiation, with excellent compliance. However, for patients receiving delayed implants the severe complication rates were highly superior to those who have received treatment without delay (40% rate of complications versus 3%). It was, therefore, postulated, that neutrons were greatly effective in initiating rapid tumour regression thus subsequent neutron doses have affected the surrounding organs with excessive doses.

Long term results of californium brachytherapy versus conventional gamma radiation brachytherapy trialled in a randomised study for advanced cervical carcinoma have been reported confirming the efficacy of neutron source in short-distanced radiotherapy (Tacev *et al.* 2003). Patients have been treated with either (1) 40 GyE of Cf-252 (in the first week of treatment) followed by 16 Gy of Ra-226 or Cs-137 in the 5th week or (2) by gamma radiation from Ra-226 or Cs-137 delivering a dose of 56 Gy in two fractions – weeks 3 and 5, followed by 40 Gy external radiation for both groups. The 5-years overall survival was better by 18.9% for the Cf-252 group due to reduced local relapses as compared to the conventionally treated group. The superior results obtained with neutron brachytherapy are probably due to higher radio-responsiveness of tumour subpopulations to high LET radiation. The same group (Tacev *et al.* 2005) has investigated the protective role of hypoxy-radiotherapy in dose escalation for cervical cancer patients treated with neutron brachytherapy and external-beam irradiation. In their study, 307 patients treated with Cf-252 have been randomised to receive either (1) 60 Gy external dose under conditions of acute hypoxia or (2) 40 Gy delivered under conditions of normal oxygenation. Overall survival after 5 years has indicated superior outcome by 7% for patients treated under hypoxic conditions and a better metastases-free survival rate (97.4% versus 85.7%) for the same patient group, validating the protective effect of hypoxy-radiotherapy for dose escalation in cervical cancer patients.

The potential of neutrons to cure high grade gliomas has been suggested in the 1970s. However, the first studies using external beam fast neutron therapy to cure gliomas have caused severe radiation necrosis to the brain despite good tumour response (Parker *et al.* 1976; Laramore *et al.* 1978). The aim, therefore, is not to investigate the efficiency of fast neutrons for brain tumours but a way to spare the organs at risk. Consequently, well localised, short-distanced irradiation by means of brachytherapy was found to be a suitable treatment technique. The feasibility of neutron brachytherapy using Cf-252 for **malignant gliomas** has been investigated in a Phase I trial (Patchell *et al.* 1997). Californium implant brachytherapy has been studied as a sole radiation technique within the dose escalation trial starting from 9 Gy neutron dose (equivalent to 54 Gy conventional photon dose, considering neutron RBE = 6) to 13 Gy neutron dose, which was shown to be the upper limit for normal tissue tolerance. Accordingly, the maximum tolerable dose used in a Phase II trial was set to be 12 Gy neutron dose (equivalent to 72 Gy conventional photon dose). The median survival time achieved with neutron brachytherapy was 10.9 months, comparable to conventional radiotherapy treatment endpoint. However, this outcome is the result of a dose escalation trial, in which patients receiving minimal dose have most likely been under-dosed, while patients receiving the upper dose limits had the adjacent normal tissue excessively exposed. Nevertheless, one great advantage of Cf-252 brachytherapy is the relatively short treatment time of 48 h (or less) as compared to several weeks required for conventional external photon irradiation.

In clinical studies of 19 cancer patients over 2 years, the relative biological efficiency, relative to radium implants, was found to be RBE = 6.5 (Oliver 1971). The efficacy of Cf-252 brachytherapy could be further enhanced by augmentation of the high LET dose with B-10 or Gd-157, selectively taken up by cancer cells after systemic or local administration. Cf-252 plaques could be used for radio-resistant superficial carcinomas as found in melanoma, breast and head & neck cancers (Maruyama *et al.* 1993a). The fast neutrons are slowed down by elastic collisions with hydrogen atoms and develop a thermal peak at about 5 cm depth in tissue. These thermal neutrons can provide additional cytotoxicity if selective tumour uptake of boron compounds is issued via boron neutron capture therapy (Chapter 15).

Given the limited world production of ~0.4 g per year, Cf-252 would not be practical for use as an external beam. Advances in the use of radioisotopes for photon brachytherapy, which is very competitive with surgical and external beam radiotherapy modalities, may have consigned Cf-252 therapy to the research laboratory.

14.6 REFERENCES

Akudugu JM, Slabbert JP, Roos WP and Böhm L (2003) Micronucleus response of human glioblastoma and neuroblastoma cells toward low-LET photon and high-LET p(66)/Be neutron irradiation. *American Journal of Clinical Oncology* **26**(3): 1–6.

Allen BJ (1983) Neutron therapy. *Austral Radiology* **28**(2): 195–214.

Battermann JJ, Breur K, Hart GA and van Peperzeel HA (1981) Observations on pulmonary metastases in patients after single doses and multiple fractions of fast neutrons and cobalt-60 gamma rays. European Journal of Cancer 17: 539–548.

Bewley DK (1989) *The Physics and Radiobiology of Fast Neutron Beams*. Adam Hilger, Bristol and New York.

Britten RA, Warenius HM, Parkins C and Peacock JH (1992) The inherent cellular sensitivity to 62.5 MeV(p----Be+) neutrons of human cells differing in photon sensitivity. *International Journal of Radiation Biology* **61**(6): 805–812.

Catterall M (1974a) The results of fast neutron therapy from the Medical Research Council's cyclotron at Hammersmith hospital, London, with particular reference to tumours of the head & neck. *Strahlentherapie und Onkologie* **148**: 447.

Catterall M (1974b) The treatment of advanced cancer by fast neutrons from the Medical Research Council's cyclotron at Hammersmith Hospital, London. European Journal of Cancer **10**: 343.

Catterall M (1976) Radiology now. Fast neutrons-clinical requirements. *British Journal of Radiology* **49**: 203.

Catterall M (1977) The results of randomised and other clinical trials of fast neutrons from the Medical Research Council cyclotron, London. *International Journal of Radiation Oncology Biology Physics* **3**: 247.

Catterall M, Bewley DK and Sutherland I (1977) Second report on results of a randomised trial of fast neutrons compared with x- or gamma rays in treatment of advanced tumours of head & neck. *British Medical Journal* **I**: 1642.

Catterall M and Bewley DK (1980) *Fast Neutrons in the Treatment of Cancer.* Academic Press, London; Grune & Stratton, New York.

Cohen LJ (1982) Expanding options in radiation oncology: neutron beam therapy. *Royal Society of Medicine* **75**: 394.

Douglas JG, Koh WJ, Austin-Seymour M and Laramore GE (2003) Treatment of salivary gland neoplasms with fast neutron radiotherapy. *Archives of Otolaryngology – Head & Neck Surgery* **129**(9): 944–948.

Duncan W, Arnott SJ, Battermann JJ, Orr JA *et al.* (1984) Fast neutrons in the treatment of head & neck cancers: the results of a multi-centre randomly controlled trial. *Radiotherapy and Oncology* **2**(4): 293–300.

Duncan W, Orr JA, Arnott SJ, Jack WJ *et al.* (1987) Fast neutron therapy for squamous cell carcinoma in the head & neck region: results of a randomized trial. *International Journal of Radiation Oncology Biology Physics* **13**(2): 171–178.

Farr JB, Maughan RL, Yudelev M, Blosser E, Brandon J and Horste T (2006) Compact multileaf collimator for conformal and intensity modulated fast neutron therapy: electromechanical design and validation. *Medical Physics* **33**(9): 3313–3320.

Fontanesi J, Mott MP, Kraut MJ, Lucas DR *et al.* (2005) A unique radiation scheme for the treatment of high-grade non-metastatic soft tissue sarcoma: the Detroit Medical Center experience. *Sarcoma* **9**(3–4): 141–145.

Forman JD, Yudelev M, Bolton S, Tekyi-Mensah S *et al.* (2002) Fast neutron irradiation for prostate cancer. *Cancer and Metastasis Reviews* **21**(2): 131–135.

Geraci JP (1981) Efficacy of neutrons in radiotherapy. *Health Physics* **40**: 41.

Giles NA, Beatty AV and Riley HP (1952) The effect of oxygen on the production of fast neutrons of chromosomal aberrations in tradescantia microspores. *Genetics* **37**: 641.

Griffin TW, Davis R, Hendrickson FR, Maor MH *et al.* (1984) Fast neutron radiation therapy for unresectable squamous cell carcinomas of the head & neck: the results of a randomized RTOG study. *International Journal of Radiation Oncology Biology Physics* **10**(12): 2217–2221.

Hall EJ and Cox JD (1994) Physical and biologic basis of radiation therapy. In: *Moss' Radiation Oncology.* 7th edn. (Ed. JD Cox) pp. 3–66. Mosby, St Louis.

Huber PE, Debus J, Latz D, Zierhut D *et al.* (2001) Radiotherapy for advanced adenoid cystic carcinoma: neutrons, photons or mixed beam? *Radiotherapy and Oncology* **59**(2): 161–167.

Koh WJ, Krall JM, Peters LJ, Maor MH *et al.* (1993) Neutron vs. photon radiation therapy for inoperable regional non-small cell lung cancer: results of a multicenter randomized trial. *International Journal of Radiation Oncology Biology Physics* **27**(3): 499–505.

Koh WJ, Griffin T, Laramore G, Stelzer K *et al.* (1994) Fast neutron radiation therapy: results of phase III randomized trials in head & neck, lung, and prostate cancers. *Acta Oncologica* **33**(3): 293–298.

Laramore GE (2009) Role of particle radiotherapy in the management of head & neck cancer. *Current Opinion in Oncology* **21**(3): 224–231.

Laramore GE, Griffin TW, Gerdes AJ and Parker RG (1978) Fast neutron and mixed (neutron/photon) beam teletherapy for grades III and IV astrocytomas. *Cancer* **42**(1): 96–103.

Laramore GE, Krall JM, Thomas FJ, Griffin TW *et al.* (1985) Fast neutron radiotherapy for locally advanced prostate cancer: results of an RTOG randomized study. *International Journal of Radiation Oncology Biology Physics* **11**(9): 1621–1627.

Laramore GE, Bauer M, Griffin TW, Thomas FJ *et al.* (1986) Fast neutron and mixed beam radiotherapy for inoperable non-small cell carcinoma of the lung. Results of an RTOG randomized study. *American Journal of Clinical Oncology* 9(3): 233–243.

Laramore GE, Griffith JT, Boespflug M, Pelton JG *et al.* (1989) Fast neutron radiotherapy for sarcomas of soft tissue, bone, and cartilage. *American Journal of Clinical Oncology* (CCT) 12: 320–326.

Laramore GE, Krall JM, Thomas FJ, Russell K *et al.* (1993a) Fast neutron radiotherapy for locally advanced prostate cancer. Final report of a RTOG randomized trial. *American Journal of Clinical Oncology* (CCT) 16: 164–167.

Laramore GE, Krall JM, Griffin TW *et al.* (1993b) Neutron vs photon irradiation for unresectable salivary gland tumours; final report of a RTOG randomized trial. *International Journal of Radiation Oncology Biology Physics* 27: 2235–2240.

Lawrence JH, Aebersold PC and Lawrence EO (1936) The biological action of neutron rays. *Proceedings of the National Academy of Sciences (USA)* 22: 543.

Lawrence EO (1937) The biological action of neutron rays. *Radiology* 29: 313.

Maor MH, Hussey DH, Barkley HT Jr and Peters LJ (1983) Neutron therapy for head & neck cancer: II Further follow-up on the M. D. Anderson TAMVEC randomized clinical trial. *International Journal of Radiation Oncology Biology Physics* 9: 1261–1265.

Maruyama Y (1984) Cf-252 brachytherapy an advance for bulky localized cancer therapy. *Nuclear Science Applications* 1: 677–748.

Maruyama Y, Wierzbicki J and Feola JM (1993a) Cf-252 for the treatment of superficial carcinomas. In: *Advances in Neutron Capture Therapy.* (Eds AH Soloway *et al.*) pp. 135–137. Plenum Press, New York.

Maruyama Y, van Nagell JR, Yoneda J, Gallion HH *et al.* (1993b) Schedule in Cf-252 neutron brachytherapy: complications after delayed implant therapy for cervical cancer in a phase II trial. *American Journal of Clinical Oncology* 16(2): 168–174.

MacDougall RH, Kerr GR and Duncan W (2006) Incidence of sarcoma in patients treated with fast neutrons. *International Journal of Radiation Oncology Biology Physics* 66(3): 842–844.

Morgan RL (1967) *Modern Trends in Radiotherapy.* Beely & Wood, Butterwortks London.

Oliver GD, Wright PR and Almond PR (1971) Experience in treatment dose calculations of Cf-252 patients. *Proceedings of the American Nuclear Society, Atlanta* 2: 16–221.

Parker RG, Berry HC, Gerdes AJ, Soronen MD *et al.* (1976) Fast neutron beam radiotherapy of glioblastoma multiforme. *American Journal of Roentgenology* 127(2): 331–335.

Patchell RA, Yaes RJ, Beach L, Kryscio RJ *et al.* (1997) A phase I trial of neutron brachytherapy for the treatment of malignant gliomas. *British Journal of Radiology* 70(839): 1162–1168.

Prevost JB, Bossi A, Sciot R and Debiec-Rychter M (2004) Post-irradiation sarcoma after external beam radiation therapy for localized adenocarcinoma of the prostate. *Tumori* 90(6): 618–621.

Prott FJ, Micke O, Haverkamp U, Pötter R *et al.* (1999) Treatment results of fast neutron irradiation in soft tissue sarcomas. *Strahlentherapie und Onkologie* 175 (Suppl 2): 76–78.

Russell KJ, Caplan RJ, Laramore GE, Burnison CM *et al.* (1994) Photon versus fast neutron external beam radiotherapy in the treatment of locally advanced prostate cancer: results of a randomized prospective trial. *International Journal of Radiation Oncology Biology Physics* 28(1): 47–54.

Santanam L, He T, Yudelev M, Forman JD *et al.* (2007) Intensity modulated neutron radiotherapy for the treatment of adenocarcinoma of the prostate. *International Journal of Radiation Oncology Biology Physics* 68(5): 1546–1556.

Schönekaes KG, Prott FJ, Micke O, Willich N *et al.* (1999) Radiotherapy on adult patients with soft tissue sarcoma with fast neutrons or photons. *Anticancer Research* 19(3B): 2355–2359.

Schwartz DL, Einck J, Bellon J and Laramore G (2001) Fast neutron radiotherapy for soft tissue and cartilaginous sarcomas at high risk for local recurrence. *International Journal of Radiation Oncology Biology Physics* 50(2): 449–456.

Smoron GL, Lennox AJ and McGee JL (1999) Osteogenic sarcoma of the maxilla: neutron therapy for unresectable disease. *Sarcoma* 3(2): 141–144.

Stone RS and Larkin JC (1942) The treatment of cancer with fast neutrons. *Radiology* **138**: 602.

Steingräber M, Lessel A and Jahn U (1996) Fast neutron therapy in treatment of soft tissue sarcoma – the Berlin-Buch study. *Bull Cancer Radiotherapy* **83** (Suppl): 122s–4s.

Tacev T, Ptácková B and Strnad V (2003) Californium-252 (252Cf) versus conventional gamma radiation in the brachytherapy of advanced cervical carcinoma long-term treatment results of a randomized study. *Strahlentherapie und Onkologie* **179**(6): 377–384.

Tacev T, Vacek A, Ptácková B and Strnad V (2005) Hypoxic versus normoxic external-beam irradiation of cervical carcinoma combined with californium-252 neutron brachytherapy. Comparative treatment results of a 5-year randomized study. *Strahlentherapie und Onkologie* **181**(5): 273–284.

Wambersie A (1982) The European experience in neutron radiotherapy at the end of 1981. *International Journal of Radiation Oncology Biology Physics* **8**: 2145–2152.

Warenius HM, White R, Peacock JH, Hanson J *et al.* (2000) The influence of hypoxia on the relative sensitivity of human tumor cells to 62.5 MeV (p-->Be) fast neutrons and 4 MeV photons. *Radiation Research* **154**(1): 54–63.

Withers HR and Peters LJ (1980) Radiobiology of high LET irradiation (neutrons). In: *Progress in Radiooncology: International Symposium, Baden, Austria.* (Eds KH Kärcher, HD Kogelnic and HJ Meyer) pp. 1–7. Georg Thiem Verlag, Stuttgart.

15 Targeted radiotherapy for cancer

15.1 INTRODUCTION

Linear energy transfer (LET) relates to the energy loss per unit length of any type of radiation, and ranges from 0.1 keV/um for photons to several hundred keV/um for heavy ions. High LET radiation increases the rate of double strand breaks (dsb) compared with that for low LET radiation, as shown in Figure 15.1. While the single strand breaks (ssb) still dominate, the higher the LET the smaller the ratio of ssb/dsb, being asymptotic to about 2.5. The increased rate of dsd has value in causing increased cell death, as the RBE increases for the same absorbed dose. There is a downside though, and this relates to the increased rate of imperfect dsb repairs, which increases the rate of somatic (genetic) mutation and the incidence of secondary cancers. As a result, the radiation weighting factors for alpha rays is 20, whereas it is 1 for photons (Valentin 2003).

Low LET radiation therapy has been the mainstay of external beam radiotherapy for a century, beginning with the use of X-rays and gamma radiation in the early 1900s. The first accelerator-produced radiation was, however, fast neutrons from the Ernest O Lawrence cyclotron, applied by his brother John H Lawrence, an early radiation oncologist, for brain tumour treatment (Svensson and Andberg 1994). This series of patient treatments were marked by serious late effects, arising from biological effects unknown at the time. With the development of the nuclear reactor, Co-60 sources became available and provided the next expansion phase for low LET external beam radiotherapy (XRT), with improved dose depth curves over that for X-rays. Radiofrequency linear accelerators with increasing energy began to replace aging Co-60 sources, such that there are barely an operating Co-60 source in the west. Yet Co-60 may find a new function in developing countries for palliative and simple curative radiotherapy applications (Allen and Rahman 2008).

The Bragg peak in heavy ions offers a high and localised dose with increased RBE at the end of the dose depth track. The first suggestion that energetic protons could be an effective treatment method was made by Robert R Wilson in a paper published in 1946 while he was involved in the design of the Harvard Cyclotron Laboratory (HCL). The first treatments were performed at particle accelerators built for physics research, notably Berkeley Radiation Laboratory in 1954 and at Uppsala in Sweden in 1957, with emphasis on therapy of eye cancers for as this treatment requires only a relatively low energy of about 70 MeV.

Much higher energies are required for deep body penetration and were achieved with a proton synchrotron. Proton therapy is now commercially available

L. Marcu et al., *Biomedical Physics in Radiotherapy for Cancer*,
DOI 10.1007/978-0-85729-733-4_15, © CSIRO 2012

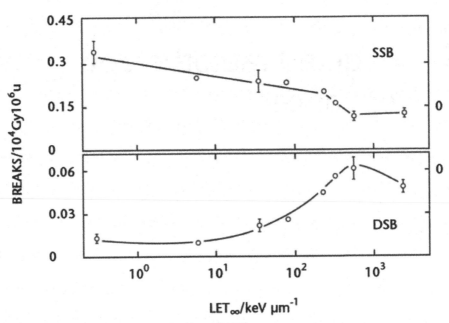

Figure 15.1. Variation of single and double strand breaks with LET.

but requires rapid patient throughput with good health insurance for commercial viability. It is highly doubtful that the excellent resolution of dose deposition, coming at a very high capital cost, is really in the interest of public health. It is important to realise that XRT is approaching asymptotic efficacy with developments in dose deposition for both low and high LET radiation. There are always cases where such high technology will give a better local result, but survival for most cancers has become long since independent of ever higher levels of local control.

Beta radiation from radioisotopes has found application in cancer therapy, beginning with I-131 for thyroid cancer. I-131, and more recently Lu and Y isotopes have been used to label targeting vectors such as monoclonal antibodies (MAbs) and peptides for the systemic management of many cancers. The recent development of new MAbs has led to an increase in therapeutic applications. However, the range of betas is both a strength and a weakness in therapeutic applications. It's a strength because of the crossfire effect, when long range electrons give rise to an average dose to a tumour, even though there may be a markedly heterogeneous uptake of radioisotope in the tumour. The weakness arises from the same, long range, low LET property of the beta radiation. Under reasonable assumptions of

maximum tolerance dose, it is very difficult to deliver a lethal dose to a targeted single cancer cell with a beta emitting radioisotope.

In this chapter we examine a range of targeted low and high LET therapies, both for external and internal targeting, and seek to determine their role in the armamentarium of cancer therapies.

15.2 BINARY THERAPIES

A binary therapy is one that involves two separate steps, either of which by itself might be incapable of regressing cancer. However, when administered in the correct sequence, the two steps have a synergetic effect, causing cancer regression.

An example is boron neutron capture therapy (BNCT), where a non-therapeutic Boron-10 compound is selectively taken up by a tumour. The B-10 is activated in situ by an external beam of epithermal neutrons that thermalise in the tumour and are absorbed by the B-10 nucleus, leading to the emission of He-4 and Li-7 ions in opposite directions. The short range and high LET ensure the high cytotoxicity of this combined two step process. Another example is the avidin-biotin effect, where targeted cells are first selected by biotin in a long time frame. Then the second component, which is labelled with a cytotoxic compound, targets the biotin receptor now attached to the cancer cell. This second reaction can be fast and limits dose to non-targeted cancer cells.

Some of the most common binary therapies are described in the following paragraphs.

15.2.1 Photodynamic therapy (PDT)

While the therapeutic potential of PDT was first suggested in 1900 by Raab, significant advances in this area occurred more than half a century later when it was demonstrated that certain photosensitising agents (hematoporphyrin derivatives) can accumulate in tumours (Lipson *et al.* 1961).

Photodynamic therapy is a two step process whereby a photosensitive molecule, e.g. a porphyrin derivative, is preferentially taken up by cancer and certain pre-cancerous cells with high metabolism. The photosensitising agent will therefore accumulate in higher percentages and for longer time periods in malignant cells than in healthy tissue. The compound is then activated in situ by monochromatic laser light. First, the photosensitiser is excited by light absorption in a short-lived state which afterwards changes into a more stable state. The action mechanism of PDT in tissues is via the O_2 pathway. It was shown that the oxygen dependency of PDT and ionising radiation are similar, therefore limitation in cellular oxygen supply can reduce the efficiency of photodynamic therapy. Furthermore, fractionated PDT improves the effect of the treatment, as is the case for radiation fractionation (Dougherty *et al.* 1979). One limitation of PDT consists of the short range in tissue of the laser beam used to activate the photosensitising agent, reason why the method is employed for treating superficial tumours or lesions on the lining of internal organs.

A potential application of PDT is for the treatment of glioblastoma multiforme (GBM). After promising results of a phase II malignant glioma trial with PDT and Photofrin as sensitising agent, two randomised prospective trials were initiated to determine the efficacy of PDT as an addition to standard therapies and also do evaluate the advantage of high light dose PDT (120 J/cm^2) over low light dose PDT (40 J/cm^2) in patients with recurrent malignant gliomas. The group showed that PDT is a successful palliative treatment for recurrent gliomas that have failed

radiotherapy and also that increasing light doses leads to increased survival (Muller and Wilson 2006). Similarly promising results, such as prolongation of time to tumour progression, reduced local recurrence and prolongation of overall survival of patient treated with PDT and Photofrin and/or ALA (5-aminolevulinic acid) for malignant gliomas have been reported by others (Eljamel 2004; Eljamel *et al.* 2008; Stepp *et al.* 2007).

A common clinical application is for the treatment of skin cancers in non-surgical applications. A recent prospective study conducted at eight dermatological clinics for the treatment of basal cell carcinoma (BCC), the most common form of skin cancer, reported an 89% complete response after PDT using methyl aminolevulinate (Caekelbergh *et al.* 2009). There are many treatment methods available for BCC and randomised controlled trials have confirmed the efficacy of PDT regarding both clinical and health economic outcomes and also patients' preference for the PDT technique (Annemans *et al.* 2008; Lehmann 2007; Ortiz-Policarpio and Lui 2009).

The success of PDT as a sole treatment was demonstrated by several trials. Furthermore, PDT has proven efficacy in combination with other treatment methods such as chemotherapy. It is known that drug resistance, which is induced by a tumour-created molecule called P-glycoprotein, limits the effectiveness of several anticancer drugs. An *in vitro* study on the combined effect of PDT using methylene blue and chemotherapy has shown that the photosensitising agent increases the cytotoxicity of doxorubicin by overcoming resistance mechanisms in drug resistant cells (Khdair *et al.* 2009). Improvement in cytotoxicity was correlated with increased intracellular delivery of the drugs (chemo and photosensitising) and also elevated levels of reactive oxygen species. Another recent study undertaken on hepatocellular carcinomas has confirmed the ability of PDT to inhibit multidrug resistance by down-regulating the expression of P-glycoprotein when pheophorbide is used as a photosensitiser and is combined with cytotoxic drugs (Tang *et al.* 2009). Recent studies confirm the prospect of PDT in overcoming multiple drug resistance and there is an increasing number of publications which prove the P-glycoprotein-inhibitive power of some photosensitising agents (Capella and Capella 2003).

Clinical trials are underway to assess the effectiveness of PDT on other cancers such as prostate, cervix, pancreas and intraperitoneal cavity, breast and head & neck (Dolmans *et al.* 2003). Porfimer sodium has been approved by FDA as a photosensitising agent to be used for esophageal and non-small lung cancer treatment. The future development and clinical approval of new photosensitisers such as second generation porphyrin derivatives with better light absorption from diode lasers or pulsed dye lasers will allow treatment for deeper seated tumours.

Kahl and Koo (1992) pioneered the development of a water soluble boronated porphryin (BOPP) containing 40 boron atoms for boron neutron capture therapy (BNCT). Promising in vivo studies were followed by an encouraging toxicity study of BOPP in GBM patients (Rosenthal *et al.* 2001). These authors were able to determine intra-tumour BOPP concentrations in biopsy samples taken at surgery (approximately 24 hours after administration). The intra-tumour concentration was associated with dose, and at 4.0 mg/kg, significant intra-tumour concentrations of 8.2 ± 3.7 mcg BOPP/g tumour (wet weight) were achieved, suggesting that, on the basis of rodent studies, selective tumour kill with sparing of normal brain could be achieved after activation with 630 nm light.

A relatively consistent tumour:plasma BOPP concentration was achieved at 24 h with a ratio of 0.21 at the 4.0 mg/kg dose level. In contrast, tumour:blood ratios at 24 hours in mice administered BOPP at doses of 10 and 100 mg/kg were 15 and 6.5, respectively, and in rats administered a dose of 35 mg/kg, the ratio was 6:1. The much lower value found in this study in humans undoubtedly reflects the much slower clearance of the drug from the blood and may suggest that future studies be designed with a longer time between drug administration and activation, which may allow more selective photosensitisation of tumour tissue, while minimising any potential normal brain phototoxicity mediated by elevated levels of BOPP in the bloodstream.

The elucidation of tumour BOPP levels was a critical finding. The substantial intra-tumour BOPP concentrations achieved at this dose suggests that an optimal biologic dose may be achieved at a lower BOPP dose than the MTD, thus further reducing the risk of toxicities such as thrombocytopenia and skin

sensitivity. Furthermore, the reported detection of BOPP (Hill *et al.* 1992) in the invasive glioma cells is significant because these cells are the targets of PDT as they are not surgically resectable and are responsible for tumour recurrence.

15.2.2 Photoactivation therapy (PAT)

Photoactivation therapy is a relatively novel treatment technique which consists in selectively introducing a high-Z atom into the nuclei of cancer cells which are then light-activated for an enhanced photoelectric effect on the high-Z atom. Photoactivation therapy utilises the K or L shell edges in atoms such as I. The isotope is absorbed by the cancer cells and activated by an external laser beam set at the K shell edge to maximise attenuation and toxicity from the photo-ejection of K shell electrons in the cell with subsequent Auger and Coster-Kronig electron transitions so as to minimise attenuation in normal tissue. While the electron energies are ~keV, the number is high so a high LET effect is observed. However, the short range of the electrons means that the high Z atoms must be located in the cell nucleus to have an impact on the cellular DNA.

As a monochromatic radiation beam would optimise this physical effect, synchrotron radiation would be the optimal tool for irradiation. The X-ray fluence is two orders of magnitude brighter than conventional X-ray sources and allows the beam to be tuned to a convenient wavelength while keeping a sufficient flux to allow radiotherapy applications. Experiments on F98 rat glioma (Biston *et al.* 2004) demonstrated that synchrotron irradiation of cisplatin, a widely-used chemotherapy drug, at the platinum absorption K-edge results in an increased toxicity, most likely due to an enhanced photoelectric effect on the platinum atoms.

15.2.3 Boron neutron capture therapy (BNCT)

Four years after Chadwick's discovery of neutrons in 1932, G. Locher described the principles of neutron capture therapy (Locher 1936). The neutron capture reaction by boron-10, $^{10}B(n, alpha)$ ^7Li, results in the emission of high energy alpha particle and Li-7 ions with high RBE (Figure 15.2), allowing localised energy release due to the short range of these ions in tissue. The neutrons are captured by the B-10 nucleus with a

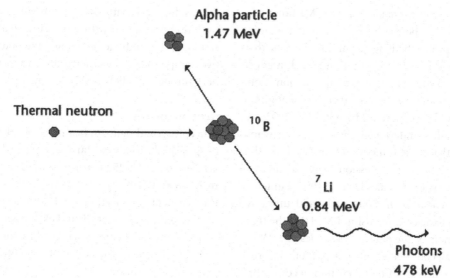

Figure 15.2. Schematic representation of Boron-10 neutron capture therapy.

very high cross section (3837 barn), resulting in the emission in opposite directions of two high-energy heavy ions (He-4 and Li-7) with high linear energy transfer >100 keV/μm. Due to the short range of the alpha (9 μm) and Li-7 (5 μm) ions and the high cross-section of boron neutron capture reaction, the cancer cells receive a much higher radiation dose that the surrounding normal tissue (Allen 2006).

The principle of BNCT is to administer the patient a boron-based agent which preferentially attaches to and is absorbed by malignant cancer cells in a tumour. The tumour is then exposed to an epithermal (~5 keV) beam for deep seated lesions or a thermal neutron beam (0.025 eV) for superficial lesions.

Some of the main advantages offered by neutron capture reaction in the presence of boron-10 include:

- the high cross-section of B-10 neutron capture reaction leads to selective targeting of boron to the tumour
- boron is available as a non-radioactive chemical element
- the known chemistry of boron allows its incorporation into various chemical compounds
- through the interaction with low energy neutrons, B-10 emits high LET, short ranged alpha and Li7 ions.

While this binary therapy has been tested in clinical trials in many countries, the success of the method

depends on the selective uptake of boronated compounds by cancer cells. The most commonly treated tumour with BNCT is glioblastoma multiforme. However, trials with melanoma and head & neck cancer have shown more promising results. The development of epithermal neutron beams and new boron carriers led to the progress in BNCT clinical trials.

Clinical studies

BNCT began with the pioneering treatments by W Sweet and G Brownell at the Brookhaven Graphite Reactor using B-10 sodium tetraborate and B-10 sodium pentaborate and later at the Medical Research reactor and the MIT reactor. With disappointing results, these compounds gave way to sodium mercapto-undecahydrododecaborate, called BSH, developed by A Soloway. A second phase of BNCT began when Hiroshi Hatanaka used BSH and a thermal neutron beam in intra-operative therapy, achieving some long term results (Hatanaka *et al.* 1992). Following earlier tumour debulking, a 30–60 min intra-carotid infusion of BSH is followed by a thermal neutron exposure of ~10^{13} neutrons cm^{-2} to achieve an absorbed dose to the distal tumour of at least 10 Gy. Heavy water replacement was also used to increase the neutron penetration into the tumour. For an average boron-10 concentration of 26 μg/g and a neutron fluence of 2.5 10^{12} neutrons cm^{-2}, the absorbed dose is ~10 Gy or 30RBE.Gy.

The Kobe group in Japan, led by Y Mishima, pioneered the use of boronophenylalanine for thermal neutron therapy of subcutaneous melanoma. The thermal ebam is ideal for this application and skin effects are limited to erythema and dry desquamation. Complete local eradication of subungual or acral lentiginous melanoma could be achieved (Mishima *et al.* 1992).

Clinical studies undertaken on malignant melanomas indicate that these tumours respond well to BPA-NCT, complete tumour regression being achieved in 60–80% of the patients (Fukuda *et al.* 1994; Fukuda *et al.* 2003; Menéndez *et al.* 2009). To avoid unwanted normal tissue toxicity while using BNCT for the treatment of melanomas, the pharmacokinetics of BPA and radiobiological considerations of the total absorbed dose to the skin have to be taken into account. In a phase I/II melanoma BNCT clinical trial, reported by Menéndez *et al.* (2009) on patients with multiple subcutaneous skin metastases of melanoma, the dose received by normal tissue ranged from 15.8 to 27.5 Gy-Eq. These doses led to acceptable side effects resulting in 30% grade 3 toxicity.

Boronophenylalanine (^{10}BPA) was developed for the treatment of melanoma, but found application for GBM as well. Epithermal neutron beams were installed at several clinical centres (Capala *et al.* 2003; Diaz 2003; Joensuu *et al.* 2003; Nakagawa *et al.* 2003; Henriksson *et al.* 2008). A special focus of the studies was on the dosage of BPA and infusion time showing that an increase in both parameters leads to an increase in median survival time. Henriksson *et al.* (2008) reported a 3 times increase in infusion time of BPA (from a 'conventional' 2 hours to 6 hours) and a dose amplification from an average of 300 mg/kg reported by other trials (Diaz 2003; Barth and Joensuu 2007) to 900 mg/kg, increasing the median survival time by 23%. The BNCT protocol was well tolerated in majority of the glioblastoma trials. An added advantage of the boron-based treatment is the relatively short treatment time (4–5 days) compared to conventional radiotherapy which can require up to 50 days.

While the past decades focused on the efficacy of BNCT for brain tumours and melanomas, lately attention has been on the exploitation of boron compounds for the treatment of other cancers. The most recent EORTC translational research/phase I trial investigated the possibility of treating squamous cell carcinomas of the head & neck with BNCT with either BPA or BSH (sodium borocaptate) infusion (Wittig *et al.* 2009). The results of the study demonstrated the potential for the two compounds to be efficient B-10 carriers to head & neck tumours to allow BNCT treatment.

Neutron sources

The epithermal neutron beam, essential for BNCT of deep seated tumours, can be obtained by reactor, accelerator or Cf-252 neutron sources (see references in Allen *et al.* 1992; Larsson *et al.* 1997). In each case the fast neutrons need to be slowed down to a Maxwellian temperature of ~1–10 keV for optimum depth penetration. This can be achieved by the use of various filters that down scatter the neutrons without excessive absorption.

A Monte Carlo study showed that epithermal BNCT with two fields could deliver adequate neutron fluence to treat metastatic cancer in the liver (Allen 1997). A Boron distribution study in colorectal liver metastases patients has been undertaken to investigate the feasibility of BNCT for multifocal unresectable liver metastases (Cardoso *et al.* 2009). Based on the BPA concentrations in the tumour, liver and blood and also on dose considerations, the study was confirmed to be feasible for the management of such lesions.

Although the number of clinical trials on BNCT increases slowly but steadily, there is a need for more conclusive studies to solve some of the major challenges of boron-related treatments such as estimation of tumour boron content before treatment and the development of more selective boron carriers (Barth *et al.* 2005). There is also need for randomised clinical trials to demonstrate the therapeutic efficacy of BNCT.

15.2.4 Gadolinium neutron capture therapy (GdNCT)

Gadolinium neutron capture therapy is a variant of Boron neutron capture therapy when the B-10 is replaced by Gd-157, which has the largest thermal neutron capture cross section of all stable isotopes (254 000 barn). The gadolinium neutron capture reaction ^{157}Gd(n, γ)^{158}Gd generates gamma emissions up to 7.8 MeV and also Auger electrons up to 40 keV. While the high energy photon emission and beta decay are not high LET radiation, the multiple X-rays emitted in inter and intra-orbit transitions do amount to high LET radiation. Further, the conversion of electrons and photons can deliver a 1/r2 dose response to eradicate established tumours by external epithermal neutron beams.

The use of gadolinium in neutron capture therapy was first suggested in the 1980s. However, due to the lack of evidence that Gd compounds could preferentially target cancer cells, further research was needed to warrant pre-clinical studies. Twenty years later, studies have accumulated on Gd compounds and their *in vitro* efficacy on tumour cells when bombarded with epithermal neutron beams. Complexes such as Gd-DTPA and Gd-DOTA have been developed in order to assess their efficacy to target cell nuclei and bind to DNA (De Stasio *et al.* 2001). While Gd-DTPA was shown to preferentially target 84% of cancer cells in culture, Gd-DOTA was observed to be less efficient, only targeting about half the cancer cells, which is not satisfactory for tumour control (De Stasio *et al.* 2005).

The affinity of gadolinium towards brain tumours is known from MRI studies, as several gadolinium compounds are used in magnetic resonance imaging technique as tumour contrast enhancing agents (Runge *et al.* 1985). However, the *in vitro* success of Gd-DTPA on human cultured glioblastoma multiforme could not be confirmed *in vivo*. Human GBM tumours injected with Gd-DPTA analyzed using synchrotron X-ray spectromicroscopy showed that only 6.1% of tumour cell nuclei contained Gd (De Stasio *et al.* 2005). While it is hypothesised that multiple injections with Gd-DTPA might induce infiltration of Gd in a larger number of tumour cells, new Gd-compounds with higher nuclear affinity are needed in order to proceed with clinical trials.

A Japanese research group has undertaken a study on a novel Gd compound for neutron capture therapy, investigating the uptake of Gd-BOPTA by tumour cells, as compared to Gd-DPTA (Matsumura *et al.* 2003). Their results have shown that tumours injected with Gd-BOPTA presented with more pronounced tumour growth delay as compared to tumours infiltrated with Gd-DPTA.

A clinical application of GdNCT was found in intravascular brachytherapy for the treatment of stenosis (Enger *et al.* 2006). The Gd-containing stent activated with neutrons led to a non-uniform dose distribution of gamma and beta radiation both inside and at the ends of the stent. Therefore, the doses to the surrounding tissues were high enough to prevent in-stent restenosis. The non-radioactive gadolinium stent offers an added advantage to personnel by reducing the radiation hazard.

Gadolinium neutron capture therapy is still an experimental cancer treatment modality which needs to undergo animal studies and clinical trials to be validated as an effective anticancer technique.

15.2.5 The avidin-biotin effect

The avidin-biotin effect is a binary technique employed by radioimmunotherapy (RIT), which is a promising cancer treatment based on radiolabelled antibodies. Monoclonal antibodies (MAbs) are able to recognise specific tumour antigens making them ideal radiation-carriers to cancer cells. The development of radioimmunotherapy has been slowed down because of the challenge of 'dispersed antibodies', the term used for radiolabelled proteins which do not succeed in reaching the cancer cell. The pharmacokinetics of MAbs often leads to an unfavourable distribution of radiolabelled antibodies when binding to non-specific tissues. A solution to this problem came from Paganelli *et al.* (1991) who proposed a binary technique consisting of the injection of non-labelled monoclonal antibodies into the patient then radiolabelling the tumour-bonded antibodies. The idea was based on the method described by Hsu *et al.* (1981) who made use of the covalent and irreversible binding between avidin and biotin. A system of these two naturally affinic molecules – *avidin* (a protein found in egg whites) and *biotin* (vitamin B-7, also known as vitamin H) – has been designed to be implemented into a three step therapeutic process against cancer (Paganelli *et al.* 1991):

1. administration of endovenous injection of biotin-bonded monoclonal antibodies which accumulate inside the tumour for the following couple of days (Figure 15.3.I);

2. administration of endovenous injection of avidin which bonds to the biotin present in the tumour (Figure 15.3.II);

3. administration of radiolabelled-biotin injection; the radioactive biotin seeks interaction with the tumour-bond avidin, reaching the target in a few minutes (avidin has affinity for four biotin molecules) (Figure 15.3.III).

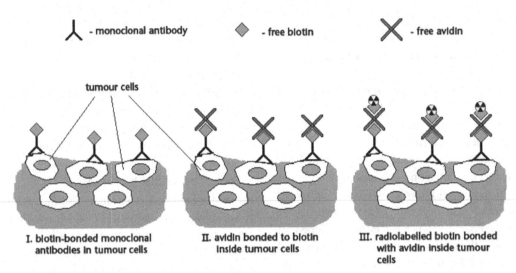

Figure 15.3. Diagram of avidin-biotin complex step-like effect on tumour cells.

This three-step avidin-biotin pretargeting technique was used for the management of recurrent high grade gliomas (Grana *et al.* 2002). The aim of the study was to evaluate the time to relapse and overall survival after the administration of ^{90}Y-labelled biotin. The low toxicity of high dose ^{90}Y-biotin constitutes a significant advantage over radiolabelled monoclonal antibodies used in radioimmunotherapy before the 1990s (Paganelli *et al.* 1988). Therefore, the treatment was well-tolerated, without notable side effects. Regarding tumour control, the results indicated an estimated median survival for grade III gliomas of 33.5 months which, considering the very poor prognosis of this disease, fully justifies the design of a randomised clinical trial. A study designed by the same group on recurrent glioblastoma combined the three-step avidin-^{90}Y-labelled-biotin approach with temozolomide, showing that the addition of the drug further increases treatment outcome without additional toxicities to normal tissue (Bartolomei *et al.* 2004). A controlled prospective, randomised trial is underway to further assess the efficacy of the combined method.

The therapeutic efficacy of radioimmunotherapy with ^{90}Y-labelled biotin was investigated also in ovarian cancers since these tumours remain the leading cause of death among gynecological malignancies (Grana *et al.* 2004). Although the highest efficacy with the avidin-biotin system was achieved by patients with minimal residual disease, the results showed a poten-

tial therapeutic role in advanced ovarian cancers which warrants further investigations. Besides ^{90}Y, there are other radionuclides pre-clinically assessed for RIT: ^{211}At (Lindegren *et al.* 2003), ^{99m}Tc, ^{153}Sm (Correa-Gonzalez *et al.* 2003), ^{166}Di/^{166}Ho (Ferro-Flores *et al.* 2003) just to name a few. While some of these chelated radionuclides underwent further clinical studies, others remained in the experimental phase.

The most common tumour sites approached so far with the avidin-biotin binary therapy due to their responsiveness are brain tumours (mainly GBM) ovarian cancers and lymphomas. There are, however, studies investigating the efficacy of the technique on other cancers. An animal model bearing human colon carcinoma was used to investigate multistep radioimmunotherapy with the ^{153}Sm-labelled avidin-biotin system (Li *et al.* 2005). Nuclear characteristics of ^{153}Sm such as low energy gamma radiation (103 keV), intermediate energy beta radiation (640 keV–810 keV) with a 2.5 mm peak path length in tissue and a half life of 1.95 days, make this radio-lanthanide a suitable candidate for RIT. This is proven by the obtained results which provide evidence for clinical implementation of pretargeting RIT with ^{153}Sm-biotin, especially for residual tumours. The study has also compared the efficacy of the multiple-step avidin-biotin technique with the administration of directly radiolabelled monoclonal antibodies, confirming previous clinical findings such as higher tumour to non-tumour ratio, decreased blood background levels (more rapid clearance of radioisotopes) and increased tumour radioactivity for the avidin-biotin treated group.

Results of a phase II study with ^{90}Y-labelled biotin RIT as a radiotherapy boost for breast cancer were recently published showing the clinical advantage of the combined RIT with external beam radiotherapy over external beam. The combination of the two radiation techniques led to accelerated irradiation without added normal tissue toxicity (Paganelli *et al.* 2010).

The avidin-biotin system is a promising binary technique for the management of certain cancers. Pre-clinical and clinical results indicate that beside gliomas which generally respond well to the multi-step technique of RIT, mainly residual cancers achieve good tumour control under this treatment. There is a need for further clinical trials to validate the role of the avidin-biotin complex in radiotherapy.

15.3 TARGETED ALPHA THERAPY (TAT)
15.3.1 Background

The use of gamma emitting radioisotopes for imaging is well established in Nuclear Medicine. Various radioisotopes such as I-131, I-123, Ga-69, Tl-205, and especially Tc99m, are used to label targeting vectors to allow the pharmacokinetics of radio-conjugates to be determined in human patients via single photon emission computer tomography (SPECT). Positron emission tomography (PET) is developing rapidly as an important diagnostic tool, with F-18 labelled FDG being the main workhorse with PET imaging machines. While most Nuclear Medicine procedures relate to imaging, a small proportion use I-131 and Y-90 for therapy of cancer. However, the therapeutic efficacy of beta emitting radioisotopes has been found to be limited, and applications are more successful in a palliative setting. In recent years, alpha emitting radioisotopes have been used in phase I and II clinical trials for various cancers. Results generally indicate substantial efficacy well below the maximum tolerance dose. It is these studies that are reviewed here.

A new high LET therapeutic approach was slowly developing late last century and gathered pace in the 1990s. This approach, called targeted alpha therapy (TAT), incorporates the essential elements for cancer

therapy: a targeting molecule that fixes to membrane bound molecules on the surface of cancer cells, and a toxic radiation that deposits a large fraction of energy into the targeted cell. There has been a slow but steady rate of alpha publications through the late 20th century, which clearly demonstrated the superiority of this therapeutic approach. One paper that stands out was the *in vivo* mouse study for mice with peritoneal ascites, which showed that only alpha radiation could lead to regression of the ascites, whereas beta emitters could not (Bloomer *et al.* 1984). This and other papers in the 1980s and 1990s were the foundations for extensive alpha research studies using different alpha emitting radioisotopes.

The essence of TAT is the construct of the targeting vector, the bifunctional chelator and radioisotope to form the alpha-immunoconjugate. The targeting vector may be a monoclonal antibody against a membrane bound antigen expressed by the targeted cancer cells. The bifunctional chelator is covalently bound to the antibody at one end and has an 'open hand' cage at its other end to enclose the radioisotope. The radioisotope is an alpha emitter with appropriate energy and half-life (Table 15.1).

Bi-213 is a popular radioisotope that emits alpha radiation with 98% 8.35 MeV and 2% 5.43 MeV, as well as beta radiation and a 4.4 MeV gamma ray. The alpha radiation has a short range (80 µm) and is highly toxic to targeted cells, causing single and double strand breaks, the latter being very difficult to repair. Cancer cells undergo apoptosis and if sufficient cells are killed, then the tumour regresses or the micrometastases are eliminated.

TAT was initially indicated for single cell cancer kill, being one to two orders of magnitude more efficacious than beta radiation. However, the short range of alpha radiation suggests that the heterogeneous radiation in a tumour would lead to hot and cold spots, the latter being the source of new tumour growth. The first clinical trials were for acute myelogenous leukaemia, where it was demonstrated that uptake by the leukaemia cells could occur within 5 minutes of systemic injection of the AIC (Jurcic *et al.* 2002). This is not expected to occur with solid tumours where the positive internal pressure in a tumour can delay infusion by 24 h or more.

Table 15.1. Alpha emitting radioisotopes.

Source $t_{1/2}$ or reaction	Generator $t_{1/2}$	Daughter $t_{1/2}$	No and $E\alpha$ MeV
Th-228 1.91 y	Ra-224 3.66 d	Bi-212 60 m	$1\alpha,1\beta$ 6
Th-229 7340 y	Ra-225 14.8 d	Ac-225 10.0 d	$4\alpha,2\beta$ 6–8
	Ac-225 10.0 d	Bi-213 45.6 m	$1\alpha,2\beta$ 8
Ac-227 22 y	Th-227 18.7 d	Ra-223 11.4 d	$4\alpha,2\beta$ 6–7
	Es-255 40 d	Fm-256 20.1 h	
Bi-209 (α,2n)	accelerator	At-211 7.21 h	1α 6
Th-232 (p, spallation)	Rn-211	At-211 7.21 h	1α 6
Th-232 (p, spallation)	accelerator	Tb-149 4.13 h	1α 4
		Pb-212 10.6 h	$1\alpha,2\beta$ 7.8

A number of workshops on alpha emitting radio-nuclides in therapy have been held. The principles and practices of targeted alpha therapy (TAT) have been reported elsewhere, most recently by Allen (2006) and Zalutsky (2005). The detailed development of the Bi alpha emitting radioisotopes for therapy has been reviewed by Hassfjell and Brechbiel (2001).

15.3.2 Alpha emitting radioisotopes

The most commonly used alpha emitting radioiso-topes used in targeted alpha therapy are presented in Table 15.1. The main physical properties of alpha and beta radiation as well as of chemical toxins are illus-trated in Table 15.2.

Radio-immunoconjugates

The radioisotope alone is usually ineffective for tar-geting cancers as, with the exception of I-131 for thy-roid cancer and bone seeking elements such as Ra-223 for bone metastases, it lacks affinity for the cancer. This problem is readily resolved by specific targeting vectors such as monoclonal antibodies against anti-gens over-expressed on cancer cell membranes. While labeling with Iodine is readily achieved by replacing hydrogen atoms in the MAbr, most other RIs cannot

be so used. Instead, a bispecific chelator is used where one end is covalently bound to the MAb, the other end forms a cage in which the RI can be sequestered (Has-sfjell and Brechbiel 2001). The more arms in he cage, the tighter the binding.

With the development of Bi radioisotopes for alpha therapy, chelating agents for Bi(III) radionuclides were developed, beginning with DTPA which has high thermodynamic stability constants for a variety of metal ions. However, lack of in vivo stability led to a C-functionalised DTPA ligand with a methyl group. However, stability was still inadequate. Merging the trans-cyclohexyl-EDTA complex with the DTPA led to the family of CHX-DTPA ligands. The solid state structure of the cyclohexl DTPA gave a coordination number of 8 and, in general, shorter Bi-ligand bond distances. Concurrent with the development of the acyclic bifunctional chealting agent for Bi(III) radio-sotopes, the inherent potential of macrocyclic poly-aminocarboxylates ligands such as NOTA, DOTA and TETA became apparent. The macrocyclic nature of these agents confers a high degree of preorganisa-tion and limits conformational disorder. While DOTA[BiIII)] was very stable, it has slow complex formation rates. However, DOTA was found to be

Table 15.2. Properties of radiation and chemical toxins.

Properties	Alphas	Betas	Toxins
Range (µm)	20–80	400–4000	zero*
Lifetime	~hours	~days	~weeks
Energy loss (keV/ µm)	~100	~0.3	n/a

* bystander effect can extend this range.

stable Pb(II), allowing conjugation and delivery of the longer lived Pb-212, the precursor of Bi-212. The CHX-DTPA ligands fulfill the requirements for rapid complex formation with Bi radioisotopes and for in vivo stability for conjugation with proteins.

Organs most at risk of radiation damage arising from free Bi-213 are the kidneys and bone marrow. Excessive toxicity in these organs arising from alpha versus beta radiation indicates an RBE ~1 (Behr *et al.* 1999).

Requirements for curative therapy

There are three major requirements for a curative therapeutic modality. These are the ability to:

1. *Kill isolated cells* in transit and so prevent the development of lethal cancer.
2. *Kill contiguous non-targeted cancer cells*, which may not express the targeted antigen with sufficient intensity to lead to lethal alpha hits.
3. *Spare* dose limiting cells, such as *stem cells*, for which severe complications may arise.

Isolated cells

Only alphas can achieve this at tolerable dose limits. The efficacy of alpha is 10 to 100 times that for betas. Thus the total injected dose would have to be that much higher to eliminate cancer cells in transit, with major implications for serious adverse events.

Contiguous non-targeted cancer cells

Variability of antigenic expression is a major limitation in immunotherapy. Both betas and toxins are unable to kill nearby cancer cells with low or zero antigenic expression. Alphas have sufficient energy to pass through several cells, causing high linear energy transfer double strand breaks that are difficult to repair and cell death.

Sparing stem cells

The ability to spare these cells requires a very short range of interaction, as is the case for alphas and even more so for toxins. Targeted therapy means that most of the dose is delivered to the targeted cancer cells or lost in the vascular system. This is not the case for long range betas (Table 15.3).

15.3.3 Preclinical studies

In vitro

Stable alpha-conjugates can be formed with MAbs and smaller proteins, that are highly selective of and cytotoxic to targeted cancer cells. In vitro cytotoxicity of alpha-conjugates is very much greater than beta conjugates, non-specific alpha-conjugates and free alpha isotope. The lethal pathway for alpha therapy is apoptosis.

In summary:

1. Stable alpha-conjugates can be formed with MAbs and PAI-2.
2. Alpha-conjugates are highly selective of targeted cancer cells.
3. In vitro cytotoxicity of alpha-conjugates is >> beta conjugates, non-specific alpha-conjugates and free alpha isotope.
4. Lethal pathway is by apoptosis.

In vivo

Activity tolerances are in the region of 24–36 mCi/kg for systemic injections. However, long term toxicity,

Table 15.3. Comparative performance of alphas, betas and toxins.

Parameter	Alpha	Beta	Toxin
Isolated cells	Yes x100	No	Yes
Adjacent non-targeted cells	Yes x100	No	No*
Spare stem cells	Yes x10	No	Yes
Antigenic expression	Yes x 250	No	No
DNA localisation	No	No	Yes
Tumours	No	Yes	No
Antivascular	Yes	No	No

* ignoring the possible bystander effect.

Table 15.4. Targeting vectors for TAT of cancer.

Targeting vector	Receptor or antigen	Cancer	Human
HuM195	CD33	leukaemia	Phase 1 & 2
81C6	Anti-tenascin	glioblastoma multiforme	Phase 1
9.2.27	MCSP	melanoma	Phase1
		pericytes	
		glioblastoma multiforme	staining
WM53		leukaemia	
		acute myeloid leukaemia	
C30.6		colorectal	
herceptin	HER2	breast	
		ovarian	
J591	PMSA	prostate	
		tumour capillary endothelial cells	
C595	MUC1	prostate	
		pancreatic	
		breast	
PAI2	uPA	prostate	
		pancreatic	
		breast	
		ovarian	

in the form of delayed radiation nephritis, reduces the MTD to approximately 9 mCi/kg in mice and between 3 and 9 mCi in rabbits. Local TAT with 75–100 µCi gives complete inhibition of tumourigenesis for all cancers at 2 days post-inoculation, i.e. at the preangiogenic stage. Intralesional TAT of melanoma with 300 µCi gives complete regression of melanoma xenografts in nude mice, but is less successful in breast and prostate tumours.

A single, systemic injection of AC causes all tumours to experience growth delay. The 2 day xenograft comprises individual cells and cell clusters, but no vasculature, and simulates micrometastases and preangiogenic lesions. Complete inhibition of in vivo tumourigenesis is achieved for local TAT at 2 days post-cancer cell inoculation, and tumour growth delay for systemic TAT, showing that TAT is indicated for the control of subclinical disease. However, efficacy decreases for longer growth times and larger tumours, but can be partially offset by multiple dosing.

While kinetics and biodistribution will depend on the type of vector used, the melanoma trial provides the basic data to determine specific organ Equivalent Doses for comparison with threshold dose levels and the probability of induced secondary cancer. These data will be of considerable value in ensuring patient safety in further systemic phase 1 clinical trials.

In summary:

1. Activity tolerances: 8 mCi/kg for intra-peritoneal injection; 10 mCi/kg for intra-lesional injections (melanoma).
2. Local TAT: complete inhibition of tumourigenesis for all cancers.
3. Intralesional TAT: 100 µCi gives complete regression of melanomas.

4. Systemic single dose TAT: all tumours experience growth delay.

15.3.4 Clinical trial protocols

The *in vitro* and *in vivo* preclinical studies show a consistent trend of targeted cancer cell toxicity. The *in vitro* cell survival data reveal the enhanced cytotoxicity of the ACs compared with non-targeted alpha radiation and targeted beta radiation.

The advantage of internal alpha radiation has been known for several decades now, but only in recent years has targeted alpha therapy achieved clinical trial status. Even so, there are only four current trials, one phase 2 for post-chemotherapy of acute myeloid leukaemia at Memorial Sloan Kettering Cancer Center (Allen *et al.* 2007), phase I trials for intralesional (Allen *et al.* 2005) and systemic (Raja *et al.* 2007) melanoma at SGH, glioblastoma at Duke University (Zalutsky 2005) and lymphoma at Dusseldorf (Schmidt *et al.* 2004). Solid tumours have never been envisaged as suitable targets for TAT, in contrast with liquid cancers and micrometastases, because of the short range of the alpha radiation and heterogeneous uptake of the targeting vector.

Intralesional TAT for melanoma in human patients was found to be safe and effective to 1350 μCi, and regresses the injected melanoma. Equivalent doses to organs are 0.05 cSv/μCi for the kidneys and for red marrow the estimated dose is 0.004 cSv/μCi. It is apparent that intralesional TAT for ocular melanoma and brain metastases is indicated.

The development of anti-angiogenic therapies opens up the possibility of inhibiting or regressing tumour growth. In the case of the Duke GBM trial (Zalutsky 2005), the vector tenescin targets endothelial receptors to achieve endothelial cell kill with alpha radiation from At-211.

The objective of these phase I trials with stage 4 cancer patients was to determine the safety of the AIC, and so far complications of any type or level have not been observed up to 25 mCi. However, unexpected tumour regressions have been observed at quite low doses. We introduce a new concept to explain the clinical responses observed after systemic alpha therapy, called tumour anti-vascular alpha therapy (TAVAT) (Allen *et al.* 2007). Some general considerations are given below for the conduct of clinical trials.

Ethics approval

The systemic trial must be approved by the relevant Human Ethics Committee. As well, approval by a Radiation Safety Council of the Environmental Protection Agency may be required.

Enrolment process

Clinical investigators invite eligible patients with required cancer and stage to participate in the trial. For a phase I dose escalation trial to determine safety:

Inclusion criteria may include:

- stage IV cancer.
- age $\geq$ 18 years
- adequate haematological function (ANC$\geq$ 1.5×10^9/l), plt$\geq$ 100×10^9/l)
- adequate renal function (calculated creatinine clearance $\leq$ 60 ml/min)
- adequate liver function (bilirubin WNL, transaminases $\leq$2.5 × ULN)
- ECOG Performance Status 0–2
- ability to provide informed consent

Exclusion criteria may include:

- untreated brain metastasis
- active infection or serious medical condition
- pregnancy or lactation
- known mouse product allergy
- chemotherapy, radiotherapy or immunotherapy within 4 weeks of enrolment. Corticosteroids are permitted.

Dose escalation monitoring

The AIC may be administered by bolus intravenous injection through a cannula, maximum of half a milliliter over a period of few seconds. The vital signs temperature, BP, heart rate and pulse will be monitored every 15 minutes for 2–3 hours. Patients will be kept hydrated with monitored intake of fluids after TAT. Urine is collected every 30 minutes and monitored for radiation over a 1 hour post-injection period. Subjects are scanned to determine the pharmacokinetics of the AIC over the kidneys, bladder, lungs, and any subcutaneous tumour every 30 minutes for up to 2–3 hours.

The patients receive a full physical examination with 24 h urine, full blood count, serum electrolyte levels and liver tests, HAMA assay at 0, 2, 4 and 8 weeks. Central and peripheral neurotoxicity are assessed clinically at each visit according to CTC criteria. It is considered sufficient observation at 6 weeks to permit dose escalation if no specified toxicity is observed. CT scans at 0 and 8 weeks identify measurable melanomas and the response to SMELT is assessed using standard RECIST criteria (New Guidelines 2000). The serum markers are also to be assessed. Follow-up clinic visits include history and physical examination, including neurological examination.

Cohort dose escalation

A classical '3&3' phase I design can be used. Dose limiting toxicities (DLT) are defined as G4 hematological toxicity, febrile neutropenia or G3 non-hematological toxicity occurring in the first six weeks after AIC administration, using NCI CTC V3 toxicity criteria. The maximum tolerated dose (MTD) is defined as the lowest dose at which ≥ 2 patients experience DLT. Three patients are accrued per dose level, starting at the lowest dose level, escalating to the next dose level if 0/3 experiences DLT, and expanding to 6 patients if 1/3 patients experiences DLT. Once the MTD is reached, the previous dose level will be expanded to a maximum of six evaluable patients. The recommended phase II dose (RPTD) will be defined as the highest dose level at which <2/6 patients experience DLT. Additional treatments may be made at this dose level to make a preliminary efficacy assessment to a maximum of 12 patients.

The AIC may be given as a single intravenous administration. The dose range chosen is expected to be completely safe at the entry point and likely to reach the expected tolerance limits at the high dose end.

The maximum organ doses should be well below the tolerance doses for the specified organs. However, alpha therapy requires microscopic dosimetry, and while these macroscopic limits are useful guidelines, they may not be applicable and a conservative approach in dose escalation is warranted.

Primary endpoint: toxicity monitoring

Patients can be monitored for toxicity for 12 weeks, although accrual to the next dose level will be permitted if no DLT has been observed when the third patient at a dose level has been observed for six weeks, to facilitate completion of the study in a timely manner.

Secondary endpoints

Clinical efficacy is not the endpoint of this study. However, where possible, response is evaluated according to RECIST criteria. Full body CT scans at 0 and 8 weeks are taken for each patient, which will identify measurable lesions and the response to TAT using standard RECIST criteria. Serum markers should be monitored when practicable.

Alpha therapy may be molecular or physiological in its targeting. Alpha emitting radioisotopes such as Bi-212, Bi-213, At-211 and Ac-225 are used to label monoclonal antibodies or proteins that target specific cancer cells. Alternatively, radium-233 is used for palliative therapy of breast and prostate cancers as it is a bone seeking element.

Progress in the development of clinical trials of alpha therapy is examined for leukaemia, lymphoma, melanoma, glioblastoma multiforme, bone metastases, ovarian cancer, pancreatic cancer and other cancers. Results of past and current trials are reviewed, and the bases of some proposed trials are presented.

A great deal of preclinical work paved the way for the advance to clinical trials in recent years. The Sloan Kettering Memorial Cancer Center has led the way, first with the application of Bi-213 immunotherapy and more recently with Ac-225. Other laboratories have concentrated on Bi-212 and At-211. The advantages of the Bi radioisotopes are that they can be generated from long lived parents, Ac-225 with 10 d and Th-228 with 1.91 y half lives, which can be imported from overseas. The Ac-Bi generator has an additional advantage in that it decays in house and does not need long term waste disposal. At-211, with a 7 h half life, needs to be used at or near the production site.

While the half lives of Bi-213 (46 minutes) and Bi-212 (61 minutes) are rather short, there is sufficient time for synthesis of the alpha-immuno-conjugates, and for vascular distribution throughout the body. However, there is inadequate time for infusion into tumours, which can take 24–48 hours. This is one reason for the development of the Ac-225 alpha-conjugate, as the 10 d half life allows plenty of time for infusion through the target tumours. On the other hand, the short range of the alpha products requires a high degree of uptake homogeneity if all tumour cells are to be neutralised.

Targeting vectors must be specific for the cancers to be treated. As such, a number of vectors are being used or are to be introduced into the clinic. The following monoclonal antibodies (MAb) are in use: humanised HuM195 targets acute myelogenous leukaemia; the murine 9.2.27 targets the MCSP antigen on melanoma cells and GBM cells; the anti-CD20 for lymphoma; MX35 F(ab')2 for ovarian cancer; and the human-mouse chimeric anti-tenascin 81C6 for glioblastoma multiforme (GBM). In the case of bone cancer, $RaCl_2$ has a natural affinity for bone. Other proposed vectors are PAI2 against uPA, which is widely expressed by many cancers at their most malignant stage, and C595 a murine MAB against MUC-1, also of generic nature. The polysaccharide capsule binding MAb 18 B7 is proposed for fungal infection.

Seven clinical trials were reported at the Aachen workshop in 2007. Bi-213 was used for studies in acute myelogenous leukaemia (AML), melanoma and lymphoma; Ac225 for AML; Ra-223 for bone cancer and At-211 for GBM and ovarian cancer. The original Bi-213 AML trial has been completed and the current trial is phase II with chemotherapy pre-treatment. The intralesional melanoma trial with Bi-213 has also been completed, being followed by a systemic trial with the same alpha conjugate. The following sections review the results of past and current clinical trials, and the objectives of proposed trials.

15.3.5   Clinical trials

Acute myelogenous leukaemia (AML)

The feasibility, safety and anti-leukaemic activity of the alpha-immunoconjugate (AIC), ^{213}Bi-CHX-A'-HuM195, was demonstrated in stage 4 subjects with AML (Jurcic *et al.* 2002). Eighteen patients with relapsed and refractory acute myelogenous leukaemia or chronic myelomonocytic leukaemia were treated with 10.36 to 37 MBq/kg of AIC. No significant extramedullary cytotoxicity was observed, but all 17 evaluable subjects developed myelosuppression, with 22 d median recovery time. The AIC localised rapidly

within 10 minutes and was retained in areas of leukaemic involvement, including the bone marrow and liver, as shown in Figure 15.4.

Absorbed dose ratios for these sites compared to normal tissue were 1000 times greater than for beta-emitting conjugates. 93% of subjects experienced reductions in circulating blasts, and 78% had reductions in bone marrow blasts. This first alpha therapy trial in humans showed that the approach was safe, feasible and efficacious.

Intralesional metastatic melanoma

The aim was to develop and implement intralesional targeted alpha therapy (ITAT) for metastatic melanoma, being the first part of a program to establish a new systemic therapy. Labelling the benign targeting vector 9.2.27 with ^{213}Bi forms the alpha-immunoconjugate ^{213}Bi-cDTPA-9.2.27 (AIC), which is highly cytotoxic to targeted melanoma cells (Allen *et al.* 2001).

The safety and efficacy of intralesional AIC in patients with metastatic skin melanoma was investigated in 16 melanoma patients, all with melanomas that were positive to the monoclonal antibody 9.2.27 (Allen *et al.* 2005). AIC doses from 50 to 450 µCi were injected into lesions of different sizes, causing massive tumour cell death as observed by the presence of tumour debris. The AIC was very effective in delivering a high dose to the tumour while sparing other tissues. There were no significant changes in blood proteins and electrolytes. There was no evidence of a human-antimouse-antibody reaction. Evidence of significant decline in serum marker melanoma-inhibitory-activity protein (MIA) at 2 weeks post-TAT was observed.

Intralesional TAT for melanoma was found to be quite safe up to 1350 µCi, and efficacious at a dose of 600 µCi. Melanoma inhibiting activity, apoptosis and ki67 proliferation marker tests all indicated that TAT is a promising therapy for the control of inoperable secondary melanoma or primary ocular melanoma.

Systemic metastatic melanoma – stage I

This phase I trial assessed toxicity and response of systemic alpha therapy for metastatic melanoma. This was an open-labelled Phase I dose escalation study to

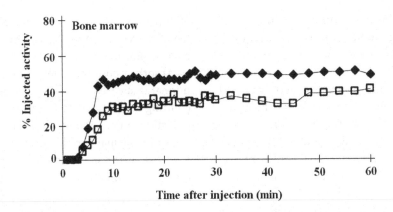

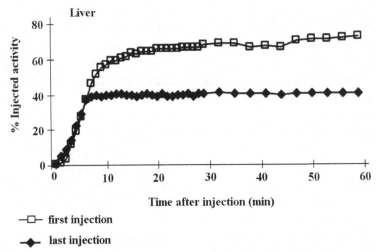

—□— first injection

—◆— last injection

Figure 15.4. Uptake of the AIC as a function of time in bone marrow and liver. Saturation occurs within 10 minutes post-injection. (Blood by American Society of Hematology. Copyright 2002 Reproduced with permission of American Society of Hematology (ASH) in the format Textbook via Copyright Clearance Center)

establish the effective dose of the alpha-immunoconjugate ^{213}Bi-cDTPA-9.2.27 (Raja *et al.* 2007). Tools used to investigate the effects were physical examination; imaging of tumours; pathology comparisons over 12 weeks; GFR; CT comparisons and changes in tumour marker over 8 weeks. Responses are based on RECIST criteria. 40 patients with stage IV melanoma/in-transit metastasis were treated with activities of 55–947 MBq. Using RECIST criteria 50% of subjects experienced stable disease and 12% showed partial response. One patient showed near complete response after a 5 mCi iv injection of the AIC, causing 20/21 lesions to completely disappear. This patient was retreated at 12 months because of this excellent

response to the initial treatment. Another patient showed complete regression of chest lesions and reduction in lung lesions. 30% of patients experienced progressive disease over 8 weeks, and all subjects eventually progressed and succumbed to the disease. The tumour marker melanoma inhibitory activity protein (MIA) reduced over 8 weeks in most patients. However, there was a disparity of dose with responders. Toxicity at any level was not observed over the range of administered activities.

The observation of tumour responses without any toxicity indicates that targeted alpha therapy has the potential to be a safe and effective therapeutic approach for metastatic melanoma. These unexpected responses are explained by the TAVAT principle. TAVAT depends on the following observations:

1. Neogenic tumour capillaries have leaky endothelial junctions (Baluk *et al.* 2005).
2. Capillaries are enclosed by pericytes which express the MCSP receptor (Bumol and Reisfeld 1982).
3. Cancer cells are contiguous with these capillaries.
4. As a consequence, the alpha-immunoconjugate (AIC) can extravasate and append to the contiguous pericyte and cancer cell receptors.
5. Alpha emission from the AIC can readily reach the endothelial cells, causing cell death and leading to capillary closure and interruption of nutritional support to the tumour (Figure 15.5 on p. 221). If enough capillaries are closed down, the tumour can regress and completely disappear.

In the case of melanoma, both targeted cancer cells and pericytes express the same MCSP receptor, enhancing the TAVAT effect. Further, selective uptake occurs because only tumour capillaries have leaky fenestrations. Thus complications are not expected to arise from damage to capillaries in normal tissue.

Only alpha radiation can kill endothelial cells in this manner. Auger electrons, while having high LET, do not have the range to reach contiguous endothelial cells. Internal conversion electrons have too great a range and would lose only a few % of their energy in nearest neighbour cells. Hundreds or thousands of hits would be needed to kill the endothelial cells, for which very high injected activities would be required. Toxins, e.g. ricin, have no direct range of interaction, and would spare contiguous cells, save for the bystander effect (Mothersill 2001).

These regressions of sc and internal lesions have been achieved at quite low activities, i.e. 4 and 7 mCi. These activities can be compared with 200 to 300 mCi for I-131 therapy. It is important to note that only a small fraction of our melanoma patients have shown such good responses, and that there is no evidence as yet of a dose dependence. Variations of the vascular structures and size of tumours, size and frequency of fenestrations and expression of targeted receptors

may all contribute to the observed variable efficacy of TAVAT.

Bone metastases from breast and prostate cancers- phase I trial

^{223}Ra is a bone seeking alpha emitter with potential for palliating breast and prostate cancer metastases to the bone. A phase I trial has been reported for 15 hormone refractory prostate cancer patients and 10 breast cancer patients, all with metastatic bone disease (Nilsson *et al.* 2005). Activities of 50 to 250 kBq/kg were well tolerated; 2/25 subjects experienced grade 3 leucopenia; there was no grade 2+ thrombocytopenia and no dose limiting toxicity. 10/25 subjects suffered diarrhoea.

Evidence of efficacy was found with substantial reductions in serum alkaline phosphatase (ALP) and improved pain control, but was not dose dependent.

Bone metastases from prostate cancers – phase II trial

A randomised, double blind, placebo controlled, multi-centre phase II study investigated the effect of multiple doses of Ra-223 in subjects with symptomatic hormone-refractory prostate cancer (Nilsson *et al.* 2007). Efficacy endpoints were the reduction in bone-specific ALP concentration and time to occurrence of skeletal-related events (SRE).

Patients due to receive external beam radiotherapy for pain relief were randomly assigned to 4 monthly Ra-223 injections or saline injections, in parallel with external beam radiotherapy. Subjects were monitored for survival and long term toxicity out to 24 months. Confirmed PSA response was defined as a 50% reduction from baseline; PSA progression a 25% increase from the nadir and 50% increase for those with a confirmed PSA response. 64 patients were recruited into the trial, 33 being assigned to XBRT plus Ra-233. Baseline values for both groups were not significantly different, nor were adverse events. However, the Ra-223 group had significant reductions in all five markers, i.e. bone-ALP, total-ALP, PINP, CTX-1 and ICTP. Significant differences were observed with changes in PSA from baseline to 4 weeks, PSA decreasing by 24% in the Ra-223 group and increasing by 45% in the placebo group. Median time to progression of

PSA and survival was 26 weeks and 65 weeks for Ra-223, compared with 8 weeks and 46 weeks for placebo (P=0.04 and 0.07).

Glioblastoma Multiforme (GBM)

The first clinical trial application of At-211 in humans involved the injection into the resection cavity of escalating doses of [211]At-human antimouse chimeric anti-tenascin MAb 81C6 (Zalutsky 2005). Injected activities ranged from 2 to 10 mCi, but the MTD was not reached. However, 6 of 17 subjects experienced grade 2 neurotoxicity at 6 weeks, which fully resolved in all but one case. Radionecrosis was not observed. The median delivered dose was 2800 Gy, giving a median survival for GBM subjects (N=14) of 52 weeks and 116 weeks for anaplastic oligodendroglioma (AO) (N=3). These results compare favourably with 36 weeks median survival after diagnosis for standard therapy. Serial MRI images are shown in figure 15.6 for an AO patient. Regional administration of [211]At-ch81C6 was found to be feasible, safe and efficacious.

Gliomas

The diffusible peptidic vector 1,4,7,10-tetraazacyclo-dodecane-1-glutaric acid-4,7,10-triacetic acid-substance P is being used in targeted radionuclide therapy of gliomas and GBM at the University of Basel, Switzerland. The neurokinin type-1 receptor (NK1R) is consistently over expressed in primary malignant gliomas (Hennig *et al.* 1995).

An earlier clinical study (Kneifel *et al.* 2006) used the DOTAGA chelator (Maecke 2005) conjugated to Arg[1] of the linear 11-mer peptide SP to generate a radiopharmaceutical with MW=1806 Da. A clinical pilot study was reported for 20 patients with gliomas grade 2–4 to assess biodistribution and short and long-term toxicity, as well as clinical and radiological responses. Radio-conjugates were prepared with [90]Y (high energy beta emitter), [177]Lu (very low energy beta emitter) and [213]Bi (high energy alpha emitter). Injections used an implanted catheter system either into the tumour or into the resection cavity. Injected activities were in the range 2250–7500 MBq for ^{90}Y,

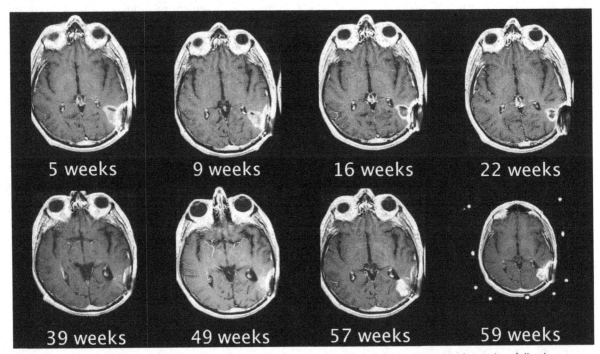

Figure 15.6. Serial MRI (gadolinium-enhanced T1-weighted images, axial plane) of a representative patient following administration of 104 MBq of [211]At-ch81C6. Following gross total resection, the surgically-created resection cavity (SCRC) rim minimally enhances. After [211]At-ch81C6 administration, the rim enhancement gradually becomes more prominent as the SCRC retracts. Focal nodular enhancement was noted 57 weeks following [211]At-ch81C6 administration. The lesion was subsequently confirmed to be recurrent anaplastic oligodendroglioma. (Reprinted by permission of the Society of Nuclear Medicine from Zalutsky *et al.* 2008.)

1125–6375 MBq for ^{177}Lu and 375–825 MBq for ^{213}Bi. In virtually all cases, positive results were obtained without significant toxicity.

However, ^{90}Y beta radiation has a maximum range of 12 mm, and could produce collateral damage to normal tissues. This effect could be reduced by the use of ^{177}Lu (beta range 1.5 mm) and ^{213}Bi (alpha range 80 μm).

Two patients were treated with alpha activities of 375 and 825 MBq for progressive GBM and low grade oligodendroglioma respectively. The GBM case was difficult to assess because of bulky residual tumour. However, the course of oligodendroglioma case has been excellent; a resection at 33 months showed radiation necrosis and absence of vital cancer cells, with no signs of tumour recurrence out to a further 34 months. An alpha therapy trial is now ongoing.

AML phase 1/2

The phase I study reported in the above section showed that while massive cell kill could be achieved with TAT, the tumour load (~1 kg) was far too high for control to be achieved. A phase 1/2 trial at MSK was implemented that uses partial cyto-reduction with cytarabine (200 mg/m^2/day for 5 days) followed by 0.5 to 1.25 mCi/kg of AIC. The MTD was 1 mCi/kg, the dose limiting toxicity being myelosupression. 6 of 25 subjects (24%) responded at >=1.0 mCi/kg, with 2 CRs lasting 9 and 12 months, 2 CRp lasting 2 and 5 months, and 2 PRs lasting 4 and 7 months (Jurcic et al. 2007).

AML phase I with Ac225

Longer lasting activity can be achieved using Ac-225 with a 10 d half life. Ac-225 emits 4 alpha particles and is 1000 times more cytotoxic in vitro than Bi-213. A phase I trial is in progress using ^{225}Ac-HuM195. Four patients have been treated with activities of 0.5 and 1.0 μCi/kg without significant toxicity (Jurcic et al. 2007). Peripheral blasts were eliminated in three patients, and reductions in marrow blasts were reported in two patients. Accrual continues in this trial.

Lymphoma

Twelve subjects with relapsed or refractory non-Hodgkins lymphoma have been treated so far with 28, 33, 39 and 44 MBq/kg of ^{213}Bi-anti-CD20, without evidence of short term toxicity. Delayed toxicity was experienced by 5 subjects with myelosuppression and one subject with fever. The dose limiting organ is bone marrow, which received 3.3 to 7.2 mGy/MBq (Schmidt et al. 2004).

Ovarian cancer

Seven subjects have been treated to 2007 in a phase 1 trial for women in remission after second line chemotherapy for recurrent Ovarian cancer. The MAb MX35(ab')$_2$ was labelled with 500 MBq of At-211. Patients were infused by peritoneal catheter with 50, 100 and 200 MBq of AIC, with a specific activity of 150 MBq/mg. No adverse effects were observed. Dose to the bone marrow was 0.08 mGy/MBq, to unblocked thyroid 15 mGy/MBq and to the peritoneal surface 8 mGy/MBq (Hultborn et al. 2007).

15.3.6 Conclusions

Alpha therapy for AML is very effective in reducing AML cancer cell load. When used with prior chemotherapy at the MTD level, some important complete and partial responses have been observed. Patient data for NHL are not as encouraging, and it is not yet clear if responses will be observed at the MTD.

In the case of intralesional TAT with Bi-213, quite low injected activities (0.6 mCi) can bring about tumour regression. Even with systemic therapy, and contrary to expectations, melanomas have been completely regressed without recurrence with systemic administration of <10 mCi of AIC. Yet there is no evidence of any adverse events up to 25 mCi. The ability to regress solid tumours was unexpected, and is explained by tumour anti-vascular alpha therapy (TAVAT), as hypothesised by Allen et al. (2007). The diffusion of AIC by leaky tumour capillaries into the peri-capillary space allows antigens of pericytes and contiguous cancer cells to be targeted, from which alpha rays can kill endothelial cells, leading to closure of the capillaries. If enough capillaries are closed down, then the tumour may regress.

Intra-cavity administration of the AIC for GBM showed improved survival of 52 weeks without serious adverse events. This approach holds great promise for improving prognosis of this fatal disease. The use of peptides for targeting is also under investigation.

Palliative therapy with Ra-223 appears promising for breast and prostate cancer metastatic to the bone.

When used as therapy adjunctive to external beam radiotherapy, marked reductions in PSA are seen for prostate cancer.

Intraperitoneal administration of the AIC for ovarian cancer may also be effective, and so far has not induced any adverse events.

A number of preclinical studies are leading to new clinical trials. Among these is the use of PAI2 as a targeting vector for pancreatic cancer. Being a small molecule (MW=47 kD), alpha-PAI2 may more easily diffuse through tumour capillary fenestrations to target cancer cells, and set up a TAVAT effect. On the down side is the higher renal uptake arising from the lower MW. PAI2 targets uPA, a generic receptor expressed by many cancers. Also generic in nature is the MUC-1 receptor, targeted by the MAb c595. The alpha-PAI2 trial is expected to commence in 2008, the alpha-c595 trial in early 2009.

Of major potential importance is the use of TAT for the control of microbial disease and for AIDS. Dadachova *et al.* (2006) have explored the potential role of alpha therapy against fungal disease, the human pathogens Cryptococcus neoformans and Histoplasma capsulatum, and pneumococcal infection and viral disease. Yet to be explored is the impact of secondary cancer, which, because of the high radiation weighting factors for alpha particles, could limit TAT to end stage cancers.

Alpha therapy is still a work in progress, but gains are being made in translating from preclinical studies to clinical trials. Ideally suited to leukaemia, alpha therapy is demonstrating efficacy, but at the MTD. GBM results from intra-cavity administration are very promising, with 52 week median survival. However, the promise of targeted alpha therapy is greatly extended by the development of TAVAT for solid tumours. Metastatic melanoma results show surprising tumour regressions at doses very much below the MTD, and if further research is successful, could change the prognosis for end-stage cancers.

15.4 REFERENCES

Allen BJ, Moore DE and Harrington BV (Eds) (1992) *Progress in Neutron Capture Therapy for Cancer.* Plenum Press, New York.

Allen BJ, Wallace SA and Carolan MG (1997) Can epithermal boron neutron capture therapy tret primary and metastatic liver cancer? In: *Advances in Neutron Capture Therapy.* (Ed. B Larson, J Crawford and R Weinreich) pp. 118–121. Elsevier, Amsterdam.

Allen BJ (1997) Can alpha-immunotherapy succeed where other systemic modalities have failed? *Nuclear Medicine Communications* **20**: 205–207.

Allen BJ, Rizvi SM and Tian Z (2001) Preclinical targeted alpha therapy for subcutaneous melanoma. *Melanoma Research* **11**: 175–182.

Allen BJ (2004) Antigenic expression of human prostate cancer cell lines and primary prostate cancer sections for in vitro multiple targeted alpha therapy with Bi-213 conjugates. *International Journal of Radiation Oncology Biology Physics* **60**(3): 896–908.

Allen BJ (2006) Internal high LET targeted radiotherapy for cancer. *Physics in Medicine and Biology* **51**: R327–R341.

Allen BJ, Raja C, Rizvi SMA *et al.* (2005) Intralesional targeted alpha therapy for metastatic melanoma. *Cancer Biology Therapy* **4**: 1318–1324.

Allen BJ, Raja C, Rizvi SMA, Song EY and Graham P (2007) Tumour anti-vascular alpha therapy: a mechanism for the regression of solid tumours in metastatic cancer. *Physics in Medicine and Biology* **52**: L15–L19.

Allen BJ and Rahman O (2008) Workshop on palliative radiotherapy for cancer in developing countries, Ho Chi Minh City. *Biomedical Imaging and Intervention Journal*, http://www.biij.org/2008/4/e50/e50.pdf

Annemans L, Caekelbergh K, Roelandts R, Boonen H *et al.* (2008) Real-life practice study of the clinical outcome and cost-effectiveness of photodynamic therapy using methyl aminolevulinate (MAL-PDT) in the management of actinic keratosis and basal cell carcinoma. *European Journal of Dermatology* **18**(5): 539–546.

Baluk P, Hashizume H and McDonald DM (2005) Cellular abnormalities of blood vessels as targets in cancer. *Current Opinion in Genetics and Development* **15**: 102–111.

Barth RF, Solloway AH and Fairchild RG (1990) Boron neutron capture therapy of cancer. *Cancer Research* **50**: 1061–1070.

Barth RF and Joensuu H (2007) Boron neutron capture therapy for the treatment of glioblastomas and extracranial tumours: as effective, more effective or less effective than photon irradiation? *Radiotherapy and Oncology* **82**(2): 119–122.

Barth RF, Coderre JA, Vicente MG and Blue TE (2005) Boron neutron capture therapy of cancer: current status and future prospects. *Clinical Cancer Research* **11**(11): 3987–4002.

Bartolomei M, Mazzetta C, Handkiewicz-Junak D, Bodei L *et al.* (2004) Combined treatment of glioblastoma patients with locoregional pre-targeted 90Y-biotin radioimmunotherapy and temozolomide. *Quarterly Journal of Nuclear Medicine and Molecular Imaging* **48**(3): 220–228.

Behr TM, Bene M, Stabin MG, Wehrmann E *et al.* (1999) High-linear energy transfer (LET) alpha versus low-LET beta emitters in radioimmunotherapy of solid tumors: therapeutic efficacy and dose-limiting toxicity of 213Bi- versus 90Y-labeled CO17-1A Fab' fragments in a human colonic cancer model. *Cancer Research* **59**(11): 2635–2643.

Biston MC, Joubert A, Adam JF, Elleaume H *et al.* (2004) Cure of Fisher rats bearing radioresistant F98 glioma treated with cis-platinum and irradiated with monochromatic synchrotron X-rays. *Cancer Research* **64**: 2317–2323.

Bloomer WD, McLaughlin WH, Lambrecht RM, Atcher RW *et al.* (1984) [211]At radiocolloid therapy: further observations and comparison with radiocolloids of ^{32}P, [163]Dy and [90]Y. *International Journal of Radiation Oncology Biology Physics* **10**(3): 341–348.

Bumol TF and Reisfeld RA (1982) Unique glycoprotein-proteoglycan complex defined by MAb on human melanoma cells. *Proceedings of the National Academy of Sciences (USA)* **79**: 1245–1249.

Caekelbergh K, Nikkels AF, Leroy B, Verhaeghe E *et al.* (2009) Photodynamic therapy using methyl aminolevulinate in the management of primary superficial basal cell carcinoma: clinical and health economic outcomes. *Journal of Drugs in Dermatology* **8**(11): 992–996.

Capala J, Stenstam BH, Sköld K, Munck af Rosenschöld P *et al.* (2003) Boron neutron capture therapy for glioblastoma multiforme: clinical studies in Sweden. *Journal of Neurooncology* **62**(1–2): 135–144.

Capella MA and Capella LS (2003) A light in multidrug resistance: photodynamic treatment of multidrug-resistant tumors. *Journal of Biomedical Science* **10**(4): 361–366.

Cardoso J, Nievas S, Pereira M and Schwint A (2009) Boron biodistribution study in colorectal liver metastases patients in Argentina. *Applied Radiation and Isotopes* **67**(7–8 Suppl): S76–9.

Correa-Gonzalez L, Arteaga de Murphy C, Ferro-Flores G, Pedraza-Lopez M *et al.* (2003) Uptake of 153Sm-DTPA-bis-biotin and 99mTc-DTPA-bis-biotin in rat as-30Dhepatoma cells. *Nuclear Medicine and Biology* **30**: 135–140.

Dadachova E, Patel MC, Toussi S *et al.* (2006) Targeted killing of virally infected cells by radiolabelled antibodies to viral proteins. *PLoS Medicine* **2**(11) e427.

De Stasio G, Casalbore P, Pallini R *et al.* (2001) Gadolinium in human glioblastoma cells for gadolinium neutron capture therapy. *Cancer Research* **61**: 4272–4277.

De Stasio G, Rajesh D, Casalbore P, Daniels MJ *et al.* (2005) Are gadolinium contrast agents suitable for gadolinium neutron capture therapy? *Neurological Research* **27**(4): 387–398.

Diaz AZ (2003) Assessment of the results from the phase I/II boron neutron capture therapy trials at the Brookhaven National Laboratory from a clinician's point of view. *Journal of Neurooncology* **62**(1–2): 101–109.

Dolmans DE, Fukumura D and Jain RK (2003) Photodynamic therapy for cancer. *Nature Reviews Cancer* **3**(5): 380–387.

Dougherty T, Lawrence G, Kaufman J, Boyle D *et al.* (1979) Photoradiation in the treatment of recurrent breast carcinoma. *Journal of the National Cancer Institute* **62**: 231–237.

Eljamel M (2004) Brain PDD and PDT unlocking the mystery of malignant gliomas. *Photodiagnosis and Photodynamic Therapy* **1**(4): 303–310.

Eljamel M, Goodman C and Moseley H (2008) ALA and Photofrin® Fluorescence-guided resection and repetitive PDT in glioblastoma multiforme: a single centre Phase III randomised controlled trial. *Lasers in Medical Science* **23**: 361–367.

Enger S, Rezaei A, Rosenschold P and Lundqvist H (2006) Gadolinium neutron capture brachytherapy (GdNCB), a new treatment method for intravascular brachytherapy. *Medical Physics* 33(1): 46–51.

Ferro-Flores G, Arteaga de Murphy C, Pedraza-Lopez M, Monroy-Guzman F *et al.* (2003) Labeling of biotin with 166Dy/166Ho as a stable in vivo generator system. *International Journal of Pharmaceutics* 255: 129–138.

Fukuda H, Hiratsuka J, Honda C, Kobayashi T *et al.* (1994) Boron neutron capture therapy of malignant melanoma using 10B-paraboronophenylalanine with special reference to evaluation of radiation dose and damage to the normal skin. *Radiation Research* 138(3): 435–442.

Fukuda H, Hiratsuka J, Kobayashi T, Sakurai Y *et al.* (2003) Boron neutron capture therapy (BNCT) for malignant melanoma with special reference to absorbed doses to the normal skin and tumor. *Australasian Physical and Engineering Sciences in Medicine* 26(3): 97–103.

Gendler S, Taylor-Papadimitriou J, Duhig T, Rothbard J and Burchell J (1988) A highly immunogenic region of a human polymorphic epithelial mucin expressed by carcinomas is made of tandem repeats. *Journal of Biological Chemistry* 263: 12820–12823.

Grana C, Chinol M, Robertson C, Mazzetta C *et al.* (2002) Pretargeted adjuvant radioimmunotherapy with Yttrium-90-biotin in malignant glioma patients: a pilot study. *British Journal of Cancer* 86: 207–212.

Grana C, Bartolomei M, Handkiewicz D, Rocca P *et al.* (2004) Radioimmunotherapy in advanced ovarian cancer: is there a role for pre-targeting with (90) Y-biotin? *Gynecologic Oncology* 93(3): 691–698.

Hassfjell S and Brechbiel MW (2001) The development of the alpha-particle emitting radionuclides ^{212}Bi and ^{213}Bi, and their decay chain related radionuclides, for therapeutic applications. *Chemical Reviews* 101: 2019–2036.

Hatanaka H, Sano K and Yasukochi H (1992) Clinical results on boron neutron capture therapy. In: *Progress in Neutron Capture Therapy for Cancer.* (Eds BJ Allen, DE Moore and B Harrington) pp. 561–568. Plenum Press, New York.

Hennig IM, Laissue JA, Horisberger U and Reubi JC (1995) Substance –P receptors inn human primary neoploasms: tumoral and vascular localization. *International Journal of Cancer* 61: 786–792.

Henriksson R, Capala J, Michanek A, Lindahl SA *et al.* (2008) Boron neutron capture therapy (BNCT) for glioblastoma multiforme: a phase II study evaluating a prolonged high-dose of boronophenylalanine (BPA). *Radiotherapy and Oncology* 88(2): 183–191.

Hill JS, Kahl SB, Kaye AH *et al.* (1992) Selective tumor uptake of a boronated porphyrin in an animal model of cerebral glioma. *Proceedings of the National Academy of Sciences (USA)* 89: 1785–1789.

Hsu S-M, Raine L and Fanger H (1981) Use of avidin-biotin-peroxidase complex (ABC) in immunoperoxidase techniques: a comparison between ABC and unlabeled antibody (PAP) procedures. *Journal of Histochemistry and Cytochemistry* 29: 577–580.

Hultborn R, Andersson H, Back T *et al.* (2007) Pharmacokinetics and dosimetry of 211At-MX35 F9ab)2 in therapy of ovarian cancer – preliminary results from on-going phase 1 study. In: *Workshop on Alpha Emitting Radionuclides in Therapy,* Achen, Germany 28–29 April.

Joensuu H, Kankaanranta L, Seppälä T, Auterinen I *et al.* (2003) Boron neutron capture therapy of brain tumors: clinical trials at the Finnish facility using boronophenylalanine. *Journal of Neurooncology* 62(1–2): 123–134.

Jurcic GJ, Larson SM, Sgouros G *et al.* (2002) Targeted alpha-particle immunotherapy for myeloid leukaemia. *Blood* 100: 1233–1239.

Jurcic JG, McDevitt MR, Pandit-Tasker N *et al.* (2007) Alpha particle immunotherapy for acute myeloid leukaemia (AML) with Bismuth-213 and Actinium-225. In: *Workshop on Alpha Emitting Radionuclides in Therapy,* Achen, Germany 28–29 April.

Kahl SB and Koo MS (1992) Synthesis and properties of tetrakis-cArborane-carboxylateters of 2,4-Bis-(α,β-dihydroxyethyl) deuteroporphyrin IX. In: *Progress in Neutron Capture Therapy.* (Ed. BJ Allen, DE Moore and BV Harrington) pp. 223–226. Plenum Press, New York.

Kampf G and Eichhorn K (1983) DNA strand breakage by different radiation qualities and relations to cell killing: further results after the influence of α-particles and carbon ions. *Studia Biophysica* 93(1), 17–26.

Khdair A, Handa H, Mao G and Panyam J (2009) Nanoparticle-mediated combination chemotherapy and photodynamic therapy overcomes tumor drug resistance in vitro. *European Journal of Pharmaceutics and Biopharmaceutics* **71**(2): 214–222.

Kneifel S, Corsier D, Good S, Ionescu MCS *et al.* (2006) Local targeting of malignant gliomas by the diffusible peptidic vector 1,4,7,10-tetra-azacyclododecane-1-glutaric acid-4,7,10-triacetic acid-substance P. *Clinical Cancer Research* **12**: 3843–3850.

Larsson B, Crawford J and Weinreich R (Eds) (1997) *Advances in Neutron Capture Therapy.* Elsevier, Amsterdam.

Lehmann P (2007) Methyl aminolaevulinate-photodynamic therapy: a review of clinical trials in the treatment of actinic keratoses and nonmelanoma skin cancer. *British Journal of Dermatology* **156**(5): 793–801.

Li G, Zhang H, Zhu C, Zhang J and Jiang X (2005) Avidin-biotin system pretargeting radioimmunoimaging and radioimmunotherapy and its application in mouse model of human colon carcinoma. *World Journal of Gastroenterology* **11**(40): 6288–6294.

Li Y, Rizvi SMA, Brown J, Cozzi PJ *et al.* (2004) Antigenic expression of human prostate cancer cell lines and primary prostate cancer sections for in vitro multiple targeted alpha therapy with Bi-213 conjugates. *International Journal of Radiation Oncology Biology Physics* **60**(3): 896–908.

Lindegren S, Karlsson B, Jacobsson L, Andersson H *et al.* (2003) 211At-labeled and biotinylated effector molecules for pretargeted radioimmunotherapy using poly-L- and poly-D-Lysine as multicarriers. *Clinical Cancer Research* 9: 3873S–3879S.

Lipson R, Baldes E and Olson A (1961) The use of a derivative of hematoporphyrin in tumor detection. *Journal of the National Cancer Institute* **267**: 1–8.

Locher GL (1936) Biological effects and therapeutic possibilities of neutrons. *American Journal of Roentgenology, Radium Therapy* **36**: 1–13.

Maecke HR (2005) 'Radiolabeled peptides in nuclear oncology: influence of pepide structure and labeling strategy on pharmacology'. Ernst Schering Research Foundation Workshop 43–72.

Matsumura A, Zhang T, Yamamoto T, Yoshida F *et al.* (2003) In vivo gadolinium neutron capture therapy using a potentially effective compound (Gd-BOPTA). *Anticancer Research* **23**(3B): 2451–2456.

Menéndez PR, Roth BM, Pereira MD, Casal MR *et al.* (2009) BNCT for skin melanoma in extremities: updated Argentine clinical results. *Applied Radiation and Isotopes* **67**(7–8 Suppl): S50–3.

Mishima Y, Ichihashi M, Honda C *et al.* (1992) Advances in the control of human cutaneous primary and metastatic melanoma by thermal neutron capture therapy. In: *Progress in Neutron Capture Therapy for Cancer.* (Eds BJ Allen, DE Moore and BV Harrington) pp. 577–584. Plenum Press, New York.

Mothersill C (2001) Radiation induced bystander effects: past history and future directions. *Radiation Research* **155**: 759–767.

Muller P and Wilson B (2006) Photodynamic therapy for recurrent supratentorial gliomas. *Seminars in Surgical Oncology* **11**: 346–354.

Nakagawa Y, Pooh K, Kobayashi T, Kageji T *et al.* (2003) Clinical review of the Japanese experience with boron neutron capture therapy and a proposed strategy using epithermal neutron beams. *Journal of Neurooncology* **62**(1–2): 87–99.

Nilsson S, Larsen RH, Fosså SD, Balteskard L *et al.* (2005) First clinical experience with alpha-emitting Radium-223 in the treatment of skeletal metastases. *Clinical Cancer Research* **11**: 4451–4459.

Nilsson S, Tranzen L, Parker C *et al.* (2007) Bone-targeted radium-233 in symptomatic, hormone refractory prostate cancer: a randomised, multicentre, placebo-controlled phase II study. *Lancet Oncology* **8**: 587–594.

Ortiz-Policarpio B and Lui H (2009) Methyl aminolevulinate-PDT for actinic keratoses and superficial nonmelanoma skin cancers. *Skin Therapy Letter* **14**(6): 1–3.

Paganelli G, Malcovati M and Fazio F (1991) Monoclonal antibody pretargetting techniques for tumour localization: the avidin-biotin system. *International Workshop on Techniques for Amplification of Tumour Targetting, Nuclear Medicine Communications* **12**(3): 211–234.

Paganelli G, Riva P, Deleide G, Clivio A *et al.* (1988) In vivo labelling of biotinylated monoclonal antibodies by radioactive avidin: a strategy to increase tumour radiolocalisation. *International Journal of Cancer* **2**: 121–125.

Paganelli G, De Cicco C, Ferrari ME, Carbone G *et al.* (2010) Intraoperative avidination for radionuclide treatment as a radiotherapy boost in breast cancer: results of a phase II study with (90)Y-labeled biotin. *European Journal of Nuclear Medicine and Molecular Imaging* **37**(2): 203–211.

Price MR, Pugh JA, Hudecz F, Griffiths W *et al.* (1990) C595-A monoclonal antibody against the protein core of the humanurinary epithelial mucin commonly expressed in breast carcinomas. *British Journal of Cancer* **61**: 681–686.

Qu Chang F, Song EY, Li Y, Rizvi SMA *et al.* (2005) Preclinical study of ^{213}Bi labeled PAI2 for the control of micrometastatic pancreatic cancer. *Clinical and Experimental Metastasis* **22**: 575–586.

Qu Chang F, Li Y, Song E, Rizvi SMA *et al.* (2004) MUC1 expression in primary and metastatic pancreatic cancer cells for in vitro treatment by ^{213}Bi-C595 radioimmunoconjugate. *British Journal of Cancer* **91**: 2086–2093.

Raja C, Graham P, Rizvi SMA, Song E *et al.* (2007) Interim analysis of toxicity and response in Phase 1 trial of systemic targeted alpha therapy for metastatic melanoma. *Cancer Biology Therapy* **6**: 846–852.

Rosenthal MA, Kavar B, Hill JS, Morgan DJ *et al.* (2001) Phase I and pharmacokinetic study of photodynamic therapy for high-grade gliomas using a novel boronated porphyrin. *Journal of Clinical Oncology* **19**(2): 519–524.

Runge VM, Clanton JA, Price AC, Wehr CJ *et al.* (1985) The use of Gd-DTPA as a perfusion agent and marker of blood-brain barrier disruption. *Magnetic Resonance Imaging* **3**: 43–55.

Schmidt D, Neumann F, Antke C *et al.* (2004) Phase 1 clinical study on alpha-therapy for non-Hodgkin Lymphoma. In: *4th Alpha-Immunotherapy Symposium.* (Ed. A Morgenstern) p. 12. ITU: Dusseldorf, Germany.

Song EY, Rizvi SMA, Qu CF, Raja C *et al.* (2007) Pharmacokinetics and toxicity of 213Bi-labelled PAI2 in preclinical targeted alpha therapy for cancer. *Cancer Biology and Therapy* **6**(6): 898–904.

Song EY, Rizvi SMA, Raja C, Qu Changfa *et al.* (2008) The cytokinesis–block assay as a biological dosimeter for targeted alpha therapy. *Physics in Medicine and Biology* **53**: 319–328.

Stepp H, Beck T, Pongratz T, Meinel T *et al.* (2007) ALA and malignant glioma: fluorescence-guided resection and photodynamic treatment. *Journal of Environmental Pathology, Toxicology and Oncology* **26**(2): 157–164.

Svensson H and Andberg T (1994) Neutron therapy – the historical background. *Acta Oncologica* **33**(3): 227–231.

Tang PM, Zhang DM, Xuan NH, Tsui SK *et al.* (2009) Photodynamic therapy inhibits P-glycoprotein mediated multidrug resistance via JNK activation in human hepatocellular carcinoma using the photosensitizer pheophorbide a. *Molecular Cancer* **8**: 56.

Tolnay M, Apostolidis C, Waser B, Arnold M *et al.* (2006) Local targeting of malignant gliomas by the diffusible peptidic vector 1,4,7,10-tetraazacyclododecane-1-glutaric acid-4,7,10-triacetic acid-substance P. *Clinical Cancer Research* **12**(12): 3843–3850.

Valentin J (2003) Relative biological effectiveness (RBE), quality factor (Q), and radiation weighting factor (w_R). *Annals of the ICRP Publication 92* **33**(4): 1–121.

Wilson RR (1946) Radiological use of fast protons radiology. *Radiology* **47**: 487–491.

Wittig A, Collette L, Appelman K, Bührmann S *et al.* (2009) EORTC trial 11001: distribution of two (10) B-compounds in patients with squamous cell carcinoma of head & neck, a translational research/phase 1 trial. *Journal of Cellular and Molecular Medicine* **13**(8B):1653–1665.

Zalutsky MR (2005) Current status of therapy of solid tumours: brain tumour therapy. *Journal of Nuclear Medicine* **46**: 151S–156S.

Zalutsky MR, Reardon DA, Akabani G, Coleman RE, Friedman AH, Friedman HS *et al.* (2008) Clinical experience with α-Particle-Emitting ^{211}At: treatment of recurrent brain tumor patients with ^{211}At-Labeled Chimeric Antitenascin Monoclonal Antibody 81C6. *Journal of Nuclear Medicine* **49**(1): 30–38.

16 Palliative radiotherapy

16.1 INTRODUCTION

The International Agency for Research on Cancer (IARC) predicts that cancer incidence in developing countries will increase dramatically in the first two decades of this millennium. Already some 80% of cancer patients in developing countries present with incurable disease. In many cases pain is a severe problem and palliation is needed to improve quality of life as well as extending survival.

WHO (1990) adopted the following definition for pain relief treatment: 'Palliative medicine is active total care of the patient, whose disease is not responsive to curative treatment. The control of pain and other symptoms and care of psychological problems are paramount. The goal is achievement of best quality of life'.

The need for provincial radiotherapy centres is profound, but whether they should specialise in palliative care only is the centre of discussion. The potential benefits of a dedicated palliative centre include lower cost (due to more basic equipment and the lower level of required expertise) and therefore more centres, enabling more patients to be able to reach palliative care. Arguments against dedicated palliative centres included potential lack of progression of quality of care, as well as the concern that these centres may be perceived simply as 'places to die'. Whilst there is an obvious need for palliative radiotherapy, simple curative treatments could also be managed.

It is usually assumed that Co-60 units are more appropriate for radiotherapy in developing countries, due to the higher initial cost of a linear accelerator, as well as the need for reliable power supply and the level of skill required by linac technicians and physicists. The beam characteristics of both Co-60 units and low energy linacs are compared in this chapter and both were deemed acceptable for palliation.

This chapter will cover the physical and clinical aspects of palliative radiotherapy (PRT), choice of radiation modality, alternative approaches to imaging and therapy and cost-benefit considerations. The concept of telemedicine is also discussed, using mobile phones and internet communication to allow rural clinics to receive support from specialists based in the cities, as well as to send images for remote diagnosis.

16.2 PRINCIPLES OF PALLIATIVE RADIOTHERAPY (PRT)

The intention of giving radiotherapy for palliation of symptoms is to improve the quality of life by decreasing or eradicating painful or restrictive symptoms.

L. Marcu et al., *Biomedical Physics in Radiotherapy for Cancer*,
DOI 10.1007/978-0-85729-733-4_16, © CSIRO 2012

370   Biomedical Physics in Radiotherapy for Cancer

Patients with metastatic cancer have a reduced life span and the treatment itself should not consume a major portion of that time. The major benefit of radiotherapy is the speed with which symptom improvement develops and the certainty of response. Sufficient radiation dose must be given to ensure that the symptom response will last for the rest of the patient's life. Too low a dose means retreatment at some later time may be required.

The guiding principles are (Drummond 2010):

1. Accurate anatomical localisation of the symptomatic tumour deposit.
2. Simple treatment techniques and field arrangements.
3. Short hypo-fractionated treatment regimes.
4. Moderate dose treatment to achieve a good predictable response and to keep treatment toxicity to a minimum.
5. Consider the patient's overall life expectancy when determining the treatment aims and the treatment duration.

As an example, some common cancers in Vietnam, their symptoms and effectiveness of symptom control with palliative radiation are presented in Table 16.1.

Key targets for PRT are bone metastasis and bone pain, cerebral metastases, bleeding and fungating tumour and obstruction/pressure symptoms (Drummond 2010).

16.2.1 Bone pain and bone metastasis

The skeleton is one of the commonest sites for metastatic cancer of any type. Whilst cancer in the bones is not usually directly life threatening it is frequently a source of pain which is a major debility. On occasions the more disabling complication of pathological fracture, spinal cord compression and hypercalcaemia may also occur. Local irradiation of one or more painful bone deposits is associated with a high probability of pain relief.

The probability of pain relief over time is shown in Figure 16.1 for both multi-fraction and single fraction regimes. The onset of pain relief may take 2–3 weeks to occur and a single fraction of 8 Gy is as effective as 30 Gy in 10 fractions for achieving pain relief.

Other studies show that longer term pain relief, greater tumour shrinkage, and fewer episodes of retreatment are achieved by a multifraction treatment program. The choice of dose and fraction number therefore needs to be tailored to the patient's general condition, expected survival and convenience of access. While single dose treatment may be adequate for pain relief, when tumour shrinkage is the goal this may not be adequate. An example is spinal cord compression, where extension of soft tissue tumour from the vertebral bone into the spinal canal causes the spinal cord to be compressed with neurological impairment, or in a weight bearing bone, where sufficient bone destruction has occurred to reduce the

Table 16.1. Symptoms and efficacy of palliative radiation for some common cancers in Vietnam (Hanna *et al.* 2010).

Common cancers in Vietnam	Common indications for palliative treatment	Symptom control with radiation (PRT)	
		RT usually effective	RT usually not effective
Lung	Shortness of breath, hemoptysis (mediastinal mass), pain (bone metastasis), anorexia, brain metastasis, malaise	Hemoptysis, pain, (equivocal: shortness of breath, brain metastasis)	Anorexia, malaise
Liver	Nausea, pain, anorexia, malaise	No established indications	Nausea, pain, anorexia, malaise
Colorectal	Rectal bleeding, pain, mass, bowel obstruction	Bleeding, pain, rectal mass	Other mass (lung, liver), bowel obstruction
Cervix	Bleeding, pelvic mass, pain, ureteric obstruction, edema	Bleeding, pelvic mass, pain	Ureteric obstruction, edema
Nasopharynx	Neck mass, painful bone metastases, lung, liver metastases	Mass, pain	Lung, liver metastases

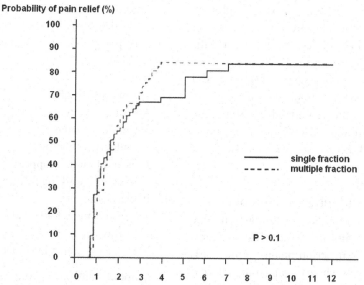

Figure 16.1. Probability of pain relief for single and fractionated treatments. (Reproduced from Workshop on Palliative Radiotherapy for Developing Countries, Workshop Proceedings, November 2008, editors B. Allen and M. Rahman with permission)

mechanical strength of the bone. In these situations, when significant tumour shrinkage is required to relieve symptoms, short course fractionated treatment is preferred either 30 Gy in 10 fractions or 20 Gy in five fractions at five fractions per week.

In weight bearing bones (e.g. femur), bone metastases may cause enough bone destruction to reduce the mechanical strength of the bone, which can only be restored if the bone can heal and repair. Fractionated radiotherapy causes the tumour to shrink relatively rapidly and bone healing proceeds a lot more slowly by the normal bone healing processes. It may take 3 months or more for the mechanical strength of a bone to be restored after radiotherapy, so the bone remains at risk of facture for this time. Radiotherapy is still essential to shrink the tumour at the site to allow bone healing but the mechanical weakness and fracture risk can be remedied by the surgery.

When there are multiple sites of pain arising from widespread bone metastases, wide field irradiation is a useful technique for palliating pain. This is referred to as hemi-body radiotherapy, in which a single dose of radiotherapy is given to one half of the body. An RTOG study of 168 patients reported an overall response rate of 73%. The onset of pain relief may be within 24 hours, but the full effect may take up to 6 weeks to develop. The duration of response is usually measured in months but significant tumour regression is not observed. It is possible to treat one half of the body and six or more weeks later treat the other half to achieve whole body pain relief. This treatment has little toxicity when the patient is pre-medicated with corticosteroids and antiemetics prior to treatment. As the main toxicity is bone marrow depression which can be quite prolonged, it is important to check the blood count prior to each treatment.

16.2.2 Cerebral metastases

Brain metastases are a major cause of symptoms and neurological disability. In general, patients present with multiple tumour deposits in the brain in the setting of widespread metastatic disease elsewhere. The brain is protected by the blood brain barrier from chemotherapy, so brain metastases may be the first site of metastatic disease. The treatment program can be tailored to the patient's general condition and expected survival. Single, 5 or 10 fractions can be used with effect. The median survival for patients with brain metastases varies from 1 month to several years depending on the primary cancer. Survival is related to the extent of neurological deficit at diagnosis and the extent of metastatic disease outside the brain.

Corticosteroids can palliate symptoms in a proportion of cases but the beneficial effect diminishes with time. Palliative cerebral irradiation, because it kills the cancer cells and causes tumour shrinkage, consolidates and augments the steroid response and maintains the response for a prolonged time.

Palliative brain irradiation is aimed at maintaining and improving neurological function and performance status until death occurs from metastases at other sites.

16.2.3   Bleeding and fungating tumour

Bleeding, ulcerating and fungating tumours are one of the most disabling and unpleasant sequelae for a patient, with a major impact on quality of life. This may occur on the skin or where the mucosal surface is breached. In order to achieve any meaningful palliation, significant tumour regression must be achieved.

Radiotherapy has a major role in controlling bleeding and ulceration. Only slight tumour shrinkage is needed to stop bleeding but higher doses of palliative radiotherapy result in cancer shrinkage, which allows the surface to heal.

16.2.4   Obstruction/compression symptoms

A range of symptoms are produced from a cancer mass developing within or around a normal structure and obstructing a hollow organ such as the bronchus or oesophagus or compressing adjacent normal tissues causing pain and functional disturbance, for example spinal cord compression or brachial plexus entrapment.

Irradiation of these cancer masses can relieve the obstruction or pressure and thus relieve the symptoms. Short courses of irradiation can achieve this e.g. bronchogenic carcinoma causing bronchial obstruction and collapse of distal lung.

16.2.5   Control of physical symptoms

Radiotherapy is one of the main tools used for the control of physical symptoms arising from cancer. Other tools used in addition to radiotherapy include:

1. Symptom controlling drugs
   - Analgesics – Aspirin, Panadol, NSAIDS, opiates, Morphine, Codeine
   - Antiemetics – Stemetil, Maxalon, Ondansetron
   - Corticosteroids
   - Bisphosphonates – alendronate, zolendronate, chlodronate
   - Aperients
   - Antispasmodics
2. Anticancer systemic therapy
   - Cytotoxic drugs
   - Endocrine therapy
3. Aids and physical supports
   - Crutches, walking frames, slings
4. Palliative surgery
   - Laminectomy for spinal cord compression
   - Orthopaedic operations to prevent fractures
   - Stents for ureter, bile duct or bronchus.

Symptom controlling drugs essentially suppress the symptoms while anticancer therapy is implemented. If it is possible to remove the cause of the symptoms, e.g. with palliative radiotherapy, much more effective palliation is achieved.

The effective treatment of physical symptoms requires:

1. Accurate diagnosis
2. Good clinical judgement
3. Patient focused and tailored treatment
4. Comprehensive knowledge of cancer and its available treatment
5. Appropriate follow up and reassessment

In summary the Palliative Management Plan elements follow:

1. Recognition of the symptoms and its significance. Any symptom which interferes with or has the potential to interfere with the patients' functional state deserves attention.
2. Specific treatment for the cause of that symptom
3. Systemic treatment for the cancer
4. Non specific symptom suppression
5. Review and reassessment

16.3   EXTERNAL BEAM RADIOTHERAPY WITH COBALT-60 AND 6 MV LINAC

External beam radiotherapy is the modality most commonly applied for PRT. The traditional source has been Co-60, but this has been displaced in the West by linacs. While linacs are much preferred for curative therapy, this is not necessarily the case for PRT. In this section the comparative performance of Co-60 sources and 6 MV linacs is examined, with reference to:

- radiation beam characteristics (e.g., beam edge sharpness, beam penetration, scatter/dose uniformity, contour and inhomogeneity corrections, dose to bone)
- machine characteristics (e.g., dose rate, patient to collimator distance, isocentre height, gamma rays vs X-rays)
- service/maintenance issues
- safety considerations
- cost considerations.

Considering that palliative radiation therapy can generally be performed with simple techniques and simple technology, Cobalt-60 provides a strong option for improving the quality of life of cancer patients.

Indeed, its low cost, easy maintenance and relative ease of availability may provide a viable treatment option versus no treatment at all in rural regions of developing countries.

Central ray dose profiles for parallel-opposed beams for Cobalt-60, 6 MV and 25 MV linac photons for a large patient with thickness of 25 cm and a large field size of 25×25 cm^2 are shown in Figure 16.2 (van Dyk 2010). The inset shows the ratios of maximum to mid-plane dose as well as the depth at which the dose near the surface reaches 95% of the dose at 12.5 cm, indicative of entry dose skin sparing effects. In principal the higher skin dose would be a dose limiting factor in curative therapy, but may not be significant in palliative therapy.

Dose plans for nasopharangeal and prostate cancers are shown in Figures 16.3 and 16.4 (pp. 222 and 223) for Co-60 and 6 MV linac sources (Hu and Wu 2010). The plans are very similar and are not indicative of serious limitations for either therapy.

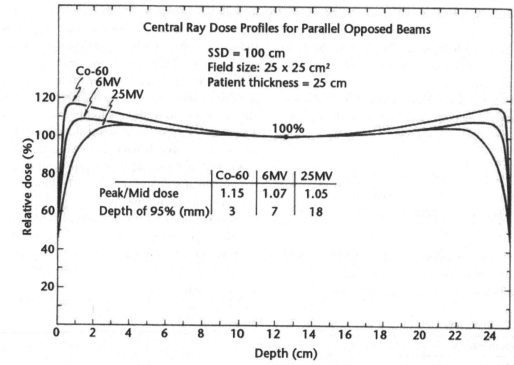

Figure 16.2. Central ray dose profiles for parallel-opposed beams for Cobalt-60, 6 MV and 25 MV linacs for a large patient with thickness of 25 cm and a large field size of 25×25 cm^2. The inset shows the ratios of maximum to mid-plane dose as well as the depth at which the dose near the surface reaches 95%. (Reproduced from Workshop on Palliative Radiotherapy for Developing Countries, Workshop Proceedings, November 2008, editors B. Allen and M. Rahman with permission)

Table 16.2. Comparative performances for Co-60 and 6 MV linac photon beams.

Parameter \ Unit	Co-60	6 MV Linac
Energy (MeV)	1.33 1.17	6 MV X-ray
Source diameter (mm)	~20	~2 × 3
D_{max} (cm)	0.5	1.5
Dose rate (cGy/min)	≤200	~600
PDD at 10cm	55%	67%
Minimum field size (cm)	≥5 × 5	0.5 × 0.5
Penumbra (mm)	≥10	≤7
Source replacement (wave guide)	~Every 7 years	Depends on patient load ~2–3 years (1500 HT hrs)

The Cobalt-60 therapy unit provides gamma rays with energy ideally suited for treatment of head & neck cancers and other superficially located tumours like breast cancers and soft tissue sarcomas of extremities. A modern Cobalt-60 therapy unit equipped with Multi Leaf Collimator (MLC) is suitable for treatment of more deep seated tumours like lung and liver cancers, though the plans are more complicated. The Cobalt-60 source emits mono-energetic gamma rays that are very suitable for using the compensator technique for advanced treatment with beam intensity modulation (IMRT).

The beam characteristics of the Co-60, 4 MV and 6 MV photon beams to be compared, with emphasis on palliative care, are:

- surface dose
- dose build-up depth
- penetration – depth dose at 5 cm and 10 cm
- beam flatness and symmetry
- stability of dose-rates

Dose distributions for some simple clinical cases, Lung, Breast, Maxillary Sinus, Oesophagus and Cervix, generated using beam data for both Co-60 and 4

or 6 MV are compared, showing that the Co-60 treatments are satisfactory for the most part. The differences are small when multiple beams are used, even though the single beam characteristics show a slight advantage for use of the 4 or 6 MV beams.

The differences in the surface dose and build-up region, between Co-60 and 6 MV beams, show an advantage in using the Co-60 beams in treating breast and head & neck cancers. Good skin sparing is achieved and adequate dose is delivered to the superficial tissues, which are part of the clinical target volumes.

For larger depths and different field sizes (FS), the percentage depth dose for Co-60 decreases more rapidly compared to 6 MV photon beams as shown in Figure 16.5 on p. 224 (Suntharalingam 2010). The percent depth dose differences between Co-60, 4 MV and 6 MV, at 5 cm and 10 cm depth, for a 10 cm × 10 cm field at a Source to Surface Distance (SSD) of 100 cm are listed in Table 16.3.

Most palliative treatments are delivered with two parallel opposed beams, for a total dose of 30 Gy in 10 fractions. When treating thin body sections, about 10 cm thick, the Co-60 beams are preferable to ensure adequate dose delivery even at shallow

Table 16.3. Depth doses for each source.

Radiation therapy	5 cm	10 cm
Cobalt-60	80	59
4 MV photon beam	85	65
6 MV photon beam	87	67

Table 16.4. Annual operational costs for Cobalt and Linacs (normalised to Co-60).

	Cobalt	Low Energy Linac	High Energy Linac
Rawlinson 1989	$38.1 K	$122.8 K	$181.8 K
	1.0	3.2	4.8
Glasgow *et al.* 1996	$62 K		$100 K
	1.0		1.6
Van der Giessen 1991	$23.3 k	$48.1 k	$61.8 K
	1.0	2.1	2.7
Van der Giessen 2002 Old machines	$31.5 K	$70.7 k	$64.4 k
	1.0	2.2	2.0
Van der Giessen 2002 New machines	$49.0 K	$116.9 k	$111.3 k
	1.0	2.4	2.3
Average costs	1.0	2.5 ± 0.4	2.7 ± 1.2

depths. The build-up zone of higher energy beams can be a disadvantage. If one considers thick body sections, like in the pelvic region, as for example cervix, then there is a gradual improvement in the dose to subcutaneous tissues when one treats with the higher energy beams. However, a more used technique for such situations is the use of multiple beams, 3-field or 4-field 'box', and the dose distributions between these different beams are very similar, recognising that more normal tissue is being irradiated with slightly higher doses with Co-60 beams. Overall, for palliative treatment Co-60 beams are more than adequate.

16.4 COMPARATIVE COSTS FOR C0-60 AND LINACS

Relative to linacs, the following statistics apply (van der Giessen *et al.* 2004) (see also Table 16.4):

- Capital costs ~4 times lower for Co 60.
- Running costs are ~10 times lower.
- Down time ~8 times lower.
- Maintenance and QA ~7 times lower.
- Cost per dose fraction 2–3 times lower.
- Power costs ~10 times lower.

These factors may not represent the situation in the Western city hospitals or in rural locations in developing countries, but are based on median values. Power costs are not an important consideration in the West, but this may not be the case in the Provincial

hospitals serving rural communities. Down-time from equipment failure may be much worse than stated above, depending on available funds for repairs and availability of replacements and engineers.

The availability of trained radiation oncologists, medical physicists, radiologists and engineers will be quite poor in rural centres, such that a balance between expertise, on site skills and training and telemedicine must be achieved. Telemedicine may provide an important element in spanning the knowledge gap between the city specialist and rural radiotherapist.

16.4.1 Comparative radiotherapy technical costs in USA

Four types of external beam radiation therapy (XBRT) are available in the United States of America (USA) (Hayman *et al.* 2000):

- Palliative simple: 10 fractions, 1 field
- Palliative complex: 10 fractions, 2 fields
- Curative: 30 fractions, 1 field + β boost for breast cancer treatment
- Curative: 35 fractions, 4 fields for prostate cancer treatment.

Using the average of Medicare cost to charge ratios (CCR) and cost accounting systems (CAS) that includes labour, capital equipment, overheads, the technical costs for each type of radiotherapy is indicated in Table 16.5. Palliative radiotherapy costs are 3.5 to 7 times lower than curative costs in the US. The

Table 16.5.   Technical costs per patient for cancer treatment.

XBRT Type	Cost (US $)	Ratio
Palliative simple	1250	1
Palliative complex	2000	2
Curative breast	5800	5
Curative prostate	8500	7

costs of treatment per patient in developing countries are generally much lower with Co-60 teletherapy than with a Linac (Table 16.6).

16.5   PALLIATIVE TREATMENT BY UNSEALED SOURCES OF RADIOPHARMACEUTICALS FOR BONE METASTASES OF CANCER

Systemic radiotherapy can be delivered more selectively to the site of multiple bone metastases by a single intravenous injection of bone seeking radioisotopes (An 2010). The bone seeking radioisotopes of Strontium or Samarium are selectively taken up at sites of osteoblastic bone metastasis, where they are retained enabling the delivery of significant doses of β irradiation to the metastases. More recently the alpha emitting radioisotope Radium (Ra-223) has been used with good effect. Systemic palliative radiotherapy (SPRT) is primarily suitable for cancers which produce osteoblastic metastasis, such as prostate and some breast cancers.

Intravenous bone seeking radio-isotopes appear to give similar response rates to hemi-body radiotherapy but there have been no trials comparing the two. The toxicity is primarily bone marrow depression, particularly with repeat treatments.

Almost all primary malignancies can result in bone metastases. Bone metastasis is very common in patients with carcinomas of prostate, breast, lung and myelomas. The proportion and prediction of bone metastases percentage rate in a survey time duration for different cancerous patients are shown in Table 16.7. There is often increased bone destruction (osteolytic), increased bone formation (osteosclerotic) or both. Pain is one of the commonest symptoms, fractures and vertebral compression are not rare, and hypercalcemia occurs in 5–10% of patients with later stages of disease. Bone metastases result is a worse quality of life and even death.

Sometimes bone metastases can be the first symptom of cancer. The application of nuclear medicine techniques such as bone scan can help to detect early metastasis and to diagnose disease stage earlier than other diagnostic imaging at 6–12 months.

Many opioid or non-opioid medicaments are not efficacious in reducing pain and drugs can be habit-forming or cause severe complications. In those cases bone seeking radiopharmaceuticals with beta radiation nuclides such as P-32, Sr-89, Sm-53, Re-188 and more recently Ra-223 will be an appropriate treatment to reduce pain and to improve the quality of the patient's life.

Local bone metastasis increased bone destruction (osteolytic) and formation (osteosclerotic) – macroscopically no qualitative difference, in most cases new bone formation takes place along side destruction.

Table 16.6.   Costs of radiotherapy per treatment course (the costs incorporate local labour costs and are based on an IAEA study. Costs are in US dollars at 2002 prices, and are intended for comparison purposes only.).

Country	Palliative radiotherapy (single fraction)		Radical radiotherapy (30 fractions)	
	60Co unit	6 MV linac	60Co unit	6 MV linac
India	3	11	90	330
Indonesia	10	17	300	510
Netherlands	34	32	1020	960

Table 16.7. Proportion and prediction of bone metastasis.

Cancer type	Proportion (%)	Median of survey (months)	Survival % of 5 years
Myeloma	95–100	20	10
Breast	65–75	24	20
Prostate	65–75	40	25
Lung	30–40	<6	<5
Kidney	20–25	6	10
Thyroid	60	48	40
Melanoma	14–45	<6	<5

Radiologic and scintigraphic appearance merely reflects the process that predominates. 50–60% of patients with bone tumour experience bone pain. The other causes for bone pain are tumour infiltration, expansion of periosteal membranes (richly innervated nociceptors), stimulation of endothelial nerve ending by prostaglandin, mechanical instability (resulting from osteolytic tumour, weakened bones) including bone pathological fractures, spread of tumour bone to contiguous neurological structures (spinal cord, nerve roots etc).

Overall pathological bone fractures (BF) occurs in about 8% of cases, especially in osteolytic lesions. BF can occur in breast 53%, kidney 11%, lung 8%, thyroid 5%, lymphoma 5% and prostate 3%. Hypercalcemia occurs in 5–10% of patients with bone metastasis, commonly in breast (30%), multiple myeloma, non-small cell lung carcinoma (NSCLC).

Bone metastases can be detected by X ray, CT Scanner, MRI, Gamma camera, SPECT, SPECT/CT, PET, PET/CT. Skeletal scintigraphy is also used for its simple performance, economical examination, whole skeletal scan and early detection of micrometastases. The main radiopharmaceutical for skeletal scintigraphy is Tc-99m labelled MDP. Other radiopharmaceuticals are Gallium (Ga-67), Thallium (Tl-201) or Tc-99m-MIBI.

There are three phases of skeletal scintigraphy. Phase 1 is known as the vascular phase, which is the early dynamic phase commonly used for arthritic and soft tissue inflammations. Phase 2 is the early static phase and Phase 3 is the later static phase, which is the standard static phase (2–3 h after injection) for the status of bone metabolism. All detected hot radioactive uptakes are suspicious.

Although skeletal scintigraphy is not a specific method it is the preferred one for evaluation of metabolic status of the skeletal system. It has high sensitivity (>95%) and can detect early bone metastases, 3–6 months earlier than X-rays. It is standardised for the diagnosis of Osteosarcoma, Ewing Sarcoma and Chondrosarcoma. It can better differentiate the lesions of infections (arthritis, osteochondritis), rheumatism and others. It is very valuable for assessment of osteochondrodystrophy, algodystrophy, bone infarct and trauma.

Positron emission tomography (PET) is used for cancer imaging because of:

- whole body imaging
- high resolution
- high sensitivity
- quantitative measurement abilities with Standardised Uptake Value (SUV)
- early detection of tumours
- staging of cancer
- distinction of residual active tumour from scar
- detection of recurrence
- assessment of therapeutic response
- monitoring post-therapy.

PET is useful in decision making in 89–96% of cancer treatments, the treatment method being changed in 45–60% patients based on PET images. Doctors can predict treatment outcome and response i.e. after 1 cycle of chemotherapy, PET (+) means 90% relapse and PET (-) means 85% remission (Kostakoglu

Table 16.8. Sensitivity (Accuracy) and specificity of skeletal scintigraphy by SPECT vs [18]FDG- PET in detection of bone metastasis.

	SPECT		[18]FDG - PET	
	Accuracy	Specificity	Accuracy	Specificity
Vertebra	84%	29%	87%	82%
Ribs	80%	12%	85%	77%
Pelvis	100%	13%	100%	88%
Others	91%	60%	89%	50%
Total	87%	21%	90%	77%

et al. 2002). A comparison of the sensitivity and specificity of skeletal scintigraphy by SPECT and [18]FDG-PET in detection of bone metastasis is given in Table 16.8.

The strategies of cancer treatment are primary prevention, early diagnosis, curative therapy and palliative care (pain relief). Palliative care includes chemotherapy, surgery, analgesics, external beam radiotherapy, and systemic radiotherapy. Overall anti-cancer treatment adopted for each type of primary cancer is always the first step in the management of metastatic bone pain. The key objectives are to relieve or remove pain and improve quality of life. External beam radiotherapy is highly effective in reduction of tumour size or removal of the entire gross tumour burden. It is also effective in pain relief by providing better quality of life and enhancing functional performance. Biphosphonate (BP) is used to treat bone fractures, bone compression and hypercalcemia and impacts on skeletal-related events.

The World Health Organization (WHO) has a 3 step pain relief method for medicaments:

1. Non-opioid drugs, e.g. aspirin and paracetamol.
2. Non-opioid and opioid drugs e.g. codeine, cyclizine and amitriptyline, benzodiazepines.
3. Opioid drugs e.g. morphine, hydromorphine and pethidine for moderate and severe pain.

Bone seeking radionuclide therapy relies on the uptake of Ca and P during the osseous metabolism, so they and their analogues can incorporate into the DNA of rapidly proliferating cells of the bone marrow as well as in the trabecular and the cortical structures of the bone. Therefore, the beta emitter radioisotopes can be used to treat bone metastasis of cancers (Table 16.9).

The advantages of bone seeking radionuclide therapy are its simplicity, effectiveness in ameliorating bone pain over a few months to years depending on radionuclide, especially for multifocal metastasis.

Table 16.9. Properties of radiopharmaceuticals used in therapy.

Radioisotope	$T_{1/2}$ (hours)	Energy β MeV	Energy γ keV	Compound
Arsenic – 76	26.3	2.97	559 (43)	Phosphonate
Holmium – 166	26.8	1.84	806 (6)	Chelate
Iodine – 131	193	0.61	365 (81)	NaI
Phosphorus – 32	343	1.71	–	Phosphates
Rhenium – 186	90.6	1.07	137 (9)	Phosphonate
Rhenium – 188	17.0	2.12	155 (10)	Phosphonate
Samarium – 153	46.7	0.8	103 (28)	Chelate
Tin – 117m	327	–	159 (86)	Chelate
Strontium – 89	1212	1.46	–	Ionic
Yttrium – 90	64	2.27	–	Citrate

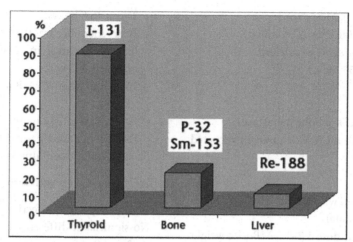

Figure 16.6. Use of radioisotopes in cancer therapy.

However, this treatment is not readily accessible in many developing countries because of high cost and non-availability of radionuclide. The pain may be increased after receiving the dose but the effect of pain relief can appear after 1 week. The side effects may appear in the hemopoietic system but this is not severe and can ameliorate and recover in weeks.

The most used unsealed sources of radiopharmaceuticals are I-131, P-32, Sr-89, Sm-153-EDTMP, Re-188-HEDP and Zn-117m-DTPA. Most applications are for I-131 for thyroid cancer; 20% of applications for bone palliation with the radioisotopes P-32 and Sm-153; 5% of applications for liver cancer with Re-188. Figure 16.6 shows this relative use of radioisotope applications in therapy.

16.5.1   Clinical practice

Entry criteria for patients with palliative treatment by unsealed sources of radiopharmaceuticals (Phan 2010) are as follows:

- Positive bones scan. Abnormalities corresponding to sites of bones pain.
- Require analgesics for control of pain.
- WBC >3500 cells/mL.
- Platelet counts >100 000/mL.
- Absolute granulocytes >1500.
- Serum creatinine <1.5 mg/dL.
- Patient is on stable hormone regime for not less than 3 months.
- No external RT within the past 6 weeks.

- No chemotherapy within the past 6 weeks.
- No treatment with inactive phosphorates during past 6 weeks.
- No signs of spinal compression.
- Patient can return to clinic for follow-up.
- Life expectancy greater than 6 weeks.
- Not pregnant or nursing, if the patient is female.
- Patient is not in another clinical trial.
- Informed consent is obtained.

16.5.2   Therapeutic procedure

Radiopharmaceuticals for the treatment of pain relief for bone metastasis are:

1. Phosphorus – 32 (^{32}P):
   - ^{32}P solution: $Na_2H_32(PO_4)$.
   - $T_{1/2}$ is 14.3 days.
   - Average beta energy is 0.695 MeV.
   - 3 to 5 times more uptake in the metastatic lesion than in normal tissue.
   - Patients should be treated with parathyroid hormone.
   - Dose: 37–250 MBq (1–6.75 mCi) for one oral dose or four consecutive doses, each dose of 111 MBq (3 mCi) for each day. The total dose may reach to 444 MBq (11.89 mCi).
   - The toxic effect in blood appears from 4–5 weeks after given dose.
   - The haematological components can recover without intervention at 6–7 weeks post-treatment with ^{32}P.

2. Strontium – 89 (^{89}Sr), Metastron:
   - Strontium Chloride (^{89}SrCl$_2$ solution).
   - Metabolism is the same as calcium.
   - Beta energy is 1.53 MeV.
   - T$_{1/2}$ is 50.5 days.
   - Vein Injection.
   - Indication: multifocal bone metastases.
   - Dose: 150 MBq (4 mCi) which may be repeated after 3 months.

   Metastron:
   - Often is associated with HEDP (Hydroxy ethylidene diphosphonate)
   - Dosage: The total dose 1.2–1.5 MBq/kg weight (0.3–0.4 mCi/kg weight) can be up to 150 MBq (4.05 mCi).
   - Slow intravenous injection.
   - Efficacious in 80% of patients. A good response in 60%–70% of cases.
   - Complications: temporary reduction of platelets, recovery after 3–6 weeks. Toxic effects for disappear at 7–8 weeks post-therapy.
   - Many scientific papers found that ^{89}Sr is less toxic than ^{32}P.
   - Pain may increase temporarily in 10% of the treated patients.
   - The average effect time is 4 months.

3. Rhenium – 186 (^{186}Re)
   - β energy 1.07 MeV, γ energy 137 keV.
   - Scintigraphic images to detect metastasis by the gamma rays.
   - T$_{1/2}$ is 89.3 hours.
   - The ratio of radioactive concentrations between metastatic and normal tissue is 20:1.

4. Rhenium – 188 (^{188}Re)
   - Generator ^{188}W/^{188}Re
   - T$_{1/2}$ of ^{188}W is 69.4 days and T$_{1/2}$ of ^{188}Re is 16.9 hours.
   - Strong β rays (2.1 MeV) is attached to EDTMP (ethylene diamine tetra methylene phosphonate) or DTPA (diethylene triamine penta acetic acid) for treatment.
   - The average dose 1147 ± 222 MBq (31± 6 mCi).
   - Results are very good.
   - Less toxic for bone marrow.

5. Samarium – 153 (^{153}Sm)
   - T$_{1/2}$ is 46.8 hours.
   - Beta energies are 0.64 Mev, 0.71 Mev and 0.81 MeV, range in tissue 3–4 mm. Gamma energy is 103 keV.
   - Injection dose 37 MBq/kg weight (1 mCi/kg weight).
   - Can repeat after 2 months.
   - Results: reduced pain in 70% patients after 1 week and is maintained to 4 months.

IAEA conclusions with respect to P-32 and Sr-89

- Both isotopes give effective pain relief.
- No significant difference between the efficacy of P-32 and Sr-89.
- Overall 60–75% responded to radionuclide therapy.
- If a patient responded, duration of response was dependent of given dose.
- With respect to safety of treatment (in haematological parameters) P-32 was worse in comparison with Sr-89 as the proportion of patients who showed a fall in WBC and platelet counts was greater in P-32 treated patients. But none of treated patients needed any medical intervention as result of fall in blood cells.

Thus P-32 should be accepted as an effective alternative to Sr-89 for bone pain palliation in situations where Sr-89 is not readily available and cost is a consideration. This is an important factor in the choice of radiopharmaceuticals.

16.5.3 Conclusions

Palliative treatment by unsealed sources of radiopharmaceuticals for bone metastases of cancer is a promising method because of its low cost, convenient use and suitability. It can overcome the limitations of other methods of analgesia for advanced cancer patients.

16.6 MULTIDISCIPLINARY CARE AND TELEMEDICINE

The care of the patient with metastatic cancer is just as much a multidisciplinary team activity as curative cancer treatment. However, the multidisciplinary team do not need to be physically all at the one location. Teleconferencing, video conferencing and computer links enable the specialist to liaise with the local medical community and provide expert advice. A doctor locally would need to take the history from the patient, complete a physical examination and assessment to relay the information to the specialist at the central site, as well as be able to implement the planned treatment. Images can be transmitted for viewing and specialist diagnosis by computer links to allow treatment planning and field marking for radiotherapy to be done remotely.

One specialist radiation oncologist could thus support several radiotherapy treatment facilities delivering treatment to patients close to their home and assist the local medical and paramedical team care for the patient.

Telemedicine could allow a small number of specialists at a central location to assist non-specialists to deliver effective palliative patient care at the local level.

The cost of palliative therapy was found to be 10–30% less than that of curative therapy. Professional staff requirements for palliative therapy were 60% lower than for curative therapy and palliative radiotherapy with Co-60 costs 20% of that for the equivalent Linac. The same curative therapy facilities are not cost-effective for palliative therapy.

16.7 CONSENSUS AND RECOMMENDATIONS

The 2008 workshop on palliative radiotherapy for cancer in Ho Chi Minh City, Vietnam arrived at the following consensus (Allen and Rahman 2010):

- Some 80% of cancer patients in the developing world present with incurable stage 4 cancer. However, the fraction of cancer patients that do not present is unknown.
- Opiates are not generally available for pain relief in developing countries.
- Radiotherapy is a cost-effective means of reducing pain and improving quality of life.
- The availability of palliative therapy is grossly inadequate in developing countries.
- Co-60 and 6 MV linac photon sources provide similar and adequate dose-depth distributions for palliative radiotherapy.

- Co-60 has important operational and cost saving advantages for developing countries.
- The annual running costs for low complexity palliative radiotherapy are a small fraction of those for complex curative radiotherapy.
- Palliative care centres can be upgraded for curative applications.

Recommendations:

- Provincial hospitals should set up palliative care centres.
- These centres should offer multidisciplinary support and opiates as required.
- Telemedicine should be introduced between provincial and city hospitals first, then with district hospitals and health stations.
- Low complexity radiotherapy should be offered initially to the palliative care centres.
- Co-60 sources are the preferred modality for palliative radiotherapy in rural areas.
- The palliative care centres should also become centres for breast and cervical cancer screening.
- The palliative care centres should also screen for curative cancer patients, for whom treatment would be indicated at the city hospitals.
- In the longer run, palliative care centres should evolve to provide curative treatment care closer to home.
- Research into the further development of telemedicine and low cost bioimpedance tomography should be encouraged.

16.8 REFERENCES

Allen BJ (2010) Comparative cost analyses for Co-60 and linacs in developing countries. In: *Workshop on Palliative Radiotherapy for Developing Countries, November 1, 2008, Vietnam.* (Eds BJ Allen and O Rahman) pp. 125–127.

Allen BJ and Rahman O (2010) Workshop on Palliative Radiotherapy for Developing Countries, November 1, 2008, Ho Chi Minh City, Vietnam.

An PS (2010) Palliative treatment by unsealed sources of radiopharmaceuticals for bone metastases of cancers. In: *Workshop on Palliative Radiotherapy for Developing Countries, November 1, 2008*. (Eds BJ Allen and O Rahman) pp. 81–88.

Drummond R (2010) The role of radiotherapy in palliative care. In: *Workshop on Palliative Radiotherapy for Developing Countries, November 1, 2008*. (Eds BJ Allen and O Rahman) pp. 14–21.

Enrique O, Zhonyun P, Prma EP, Pusuwan P *et al.* (2002) Efficacy and toxicity of Sm-153 EDTMP in the palliative treatment of painful bone metastases. *World Journal of Nuclear Medicine* 1(1): 21.

Friedman AM (1987) *Radionuclides in Therapy*. CRC Press, Boca Raton, Florida.

Glasgow GL, Kurup RG, Leybovich L, Wang S *et al.* (1996) Dosimetry and use of 60Co 100 cm source-to-axis distance teletherapy units. *Current Oncology* 3: 17–25.

Hanna TP, Schreiner LJ, Dunscombe P and Wu JS (2010) Considerations in developing a regionalized palliative oncology program in a low- or middle-income country: a radiation oncology perspective. In: *Workshop on Palliative Radiotherapy for Developing Countries, November 1, 2008, Vietnam*. (Eds BJ Allen and O Rahman) pp. 22–31.

Hayman JA, Lash KA, Tao ML and Halman MA (2000) Comparison of two methods for estimating the technical costs of external beam radiation therapy. *International Journal of Radiation Oncology Biology Physics* 47: 461–467.

Hu Y and Wu H (2010) Is Cobalt 60 therapy still needed for developing countries? In: *Workshop on Palliative Radiotherapy for Developing Countries, November 1, 2008*. (Eds BJ Allen and O Rahman) pp. 35–42.

Kostakoglu L, Coleman M, Leonard JP, Kuji I *et al.* (2002) PET predicts prognosis after 1 cycle of chemotherapy in aggressive lymphoma and Hodgkin's disease. *Journal of Nuclear Medicine* 43(8): 1018–1027.

Petelenz B (1999) International seminar on therapeutic applications of radiopharmaceuticals. Hyderabad, India 18–22 January. IAEA, Book of Extended Synopses, Synopsis no. *IAEA*-SR-209, p. 182.

Phan Sy An (2010) Palliative treatment by unsealed sources of radiopharmaceuticals for bone metastases of cancer. In: *Workshop on Palliative Radiotherapy for Developing Countries, November 1, 2008, Vietnam*. (Eds BJ Allen and O Rahman) pp. 80–87.

Rawlinson JA (1989) The choice of equipment for external beam radiotherapy. *Proceedings of the IAEA Seminar on Organization and Training of Radiotherapy in Africa, Cairo, 11–15 December*.

Suntharalingam N (2010) Radiation therapy with Cobalt-60 Vs 6 MV photons for palliative care: comparison of beam characteristics. In: *Workshop on Palliative Radiotherapy for Developing Countries, November 1, 2008*. (Eds BJ Allen and O Rahman) pp. 43–46.

Tuner JH (2003) A report on the 5th International Radiopharmaceutical Therapy Colloquium and The Final Planning Meeting of the Radiopharmaceutical Therapy Council, Santiago, Chile, 29 September 2002. *World Journal of Nuclear Medicine* 2(1): 67.

van der Giessen P (1991) A comparison of maintenance costs of cobalt machines and linear accelerators. *Radiotherapy and Oncology* 20(1): 64–65.

van der Giessen P (2002) Maintenance costs for cobalt machines and linear accelerators: new machines versus old. *Radiotherapy and Oncology* 62(3): 349–350.

Van der Giessen PH, Alert J, Badri C, Bistrovic M *et al.* (2004) Multinational assessment of some operational costs of teletherapy. *Radiotherapy Oncology* 71: 347–355.

Van Dyk (2010) Cobalt-60 versus linear accelerators: a review. In: *Workshop on Palliative Radiotherapy for Developing Countries, November 1, 2008, Vietnam*. (Eds BJ Allen and O Rahman) pp. 46–53.

WHO (1990) Definition of Palliative Care. http://www.who.int/dsa/justpub/cpl.htm

World Journal of Nuclear Medicine, Abstract of the 8th Congress of the World Federation of Nuclear Medicine & Biology, Santiago, Chile, 29 September–2 October, Vol.1 (Suppl. 2), 2002.

www.iupesm.org. HTTG reports.

17 Predictive assays

17.1 INTRODUCTION

The aim of predictive assays is to enable an individual treatment protocol that is optimal for a particular patient to be chosen. Individualised treatment planning is the trend in cancer therapy because there is very large inter-patient variability of tumour response as well as normal tissue toxicity for the same treatment of the same malignant disease. Therefore, pre-treatment assessment of tumour response would provide an important indication of likely treatment outcome. Predictive assays for biological assessment of tumour response are based on the individual characteristics of each tumour. Consequently, they can be expected to reliably predict tumour response to treatment. As discussed in the sections below, some problems still need to be overcome with these assays before they can be efficiently implemented in routine clinical practice at the present time. Although a variety of predictive assays proposed have proved to be disappointing when trialled, a number of assays under investigation offer promise in predicting treatment outcome.

Though predictive assays based on biological evaluation of tumour properties would be expected to be the best indicators of tumour response to treatment, other useful methods such as assessment of the treatment plan and delivery as well as the post-treatment response of the tumour are also useful. While these alternative methods are not designed with tumour kinetics and composition in mind, they still provide an objective basis for treatment appraisal.

17.2 PREDICTIVE ASSAYS

Tumour radioresponsiveness depends strongly on the kinetics of its constituent cells, since cell proliferation is indicative of tumour behaviour during and after treatment. Tumours with high proliferative potential are more responsive to radiotherapy due to their high cell turnover, but these tumours also have the ability to successfully repopulate during treatment. The oxygenation level of the tumour is another crucial factor which dictates the response of the cancer to radiotherapy. It is well known that hypoxic cells are up to three times more resistant to radiation than well oxygenated tumours. Therefore, the oxygenation level of the tumour as a whole, and also the proportion of hypoxic cells within it provide a good indication of tumour response during treatment. There is also information clinically to suggest that the cells of some tumours have intrinsically higher radiosensitivity than others. These characteristics of the tumour in a

L. Marcu et al., *Biomedical Physics in Radiotherapy for Cancer*,
DOI 10.1007/978-0-85729-733-4_17, © CSIRO 2012

particular patient determine the treatment modality and schedule most beneficial to the patient.

Thus, the three main assays used to predict the response to radiation of a tumour are based on the following characteristics of the constituent cells:

- oxygenation status
- proliferative potential
- intrinsic radiosensitivity.

Apart from the above mentioned tumour characteristics, other factors that determine the success (or failure) rate of the treatment include: the size (volume) of the tumour at the start of the treatment and its metastatic potential. Large tumours are more difficult to control than small ones, mainly because larger radiation doses are required to achieve cell kill.

Assays can be designed to predict the response of normal tissue to radiotherapy. Similarly to differences occurring in tumour response among a group of patients who are given the same radiation treatment, there are variations in normal tissue reaction. The response of normal tissue to radiation varies as a function of:

- dosimetry (differences in distribution of dose delivered arising from differences in patient anatomy and/or technical factors)
- treatment volume (arising from the need to encompass different tumour size)
- physiology (inter-patient differences in tissue blood flow and biology including proliferation rate)
- genetics (rare syndromes involving genes which predispose to radiation damage).

17.2.1 Predictive assays for tumour response

I. Oxygen status

The presence of oxygen in tumour cells is crucial for a good response to radiotherapy. It has been shown that hypoxia leads to poor response to radiation, due to the ability of hypoxic cells to repair the radiation-induced damage. Hypoxia also plays an essential role in the promotion of angiogenesis and metastasis, both of which result in tumour progression. Over the last decade, it has become apparent that hypoxia changes the patterns of gene expression in numerous ways result-

ing in alteration of the malignant potential of tumours and therefore more aggressive behaviour.

The major goal in the assessment of oxygenation status of tumour cells in a patient is to select the likelihood of benefit from the addition of radiosensitisers. Hypoxia is a characteristic that limits the effectiveness of both radiotherapy and chemotherapy. Moreover, several cancer patients continue to smoke whilst undergoing radiotherapy, which makes the treatment less efficacious because of restriction of blood flow and therefore poor oxygenation. Besides radio- and chemotherapy, there is evidence that hypoxia limits the effectiveness of surgery as well (Isa *et al.* 2006). Studies found that the median partial oxygen pressure (pO_2) is the strongest independent prognostic factor of disease-free and overall survival in patients with squamous cell carcinoma, irrespective of treatment modality. Therefore, assessment of the extent of tumour hypoxia in individuals would be critical for improvement in tumour control.

In a review paper of the importance of hypoxia in treatment outcomes of radioresistant cancers, Isa *et al.* (2006) stated that 'there is an unmet need for biological parameters to individualise treatments'. Developing and implementing a tool for measuring hypoxia would allow clinicians to choose treatment based on an individualised, scientific basis rather than by clinical protocol.

Several methods are currently employed to determine the oxygenation status of tumours. Although intratumour variability in oxygenation level may confound assessment, this is small in comparison to inter-patient variability (Hockel and Vaupel 2001). The most common methods involve the use of electrodes inserted into tumours, or the injection of radionuclides used as markers for hypoxic cells as well as tumour biopsies (comet assay). To date, none of these have been implemented into clinical practice, because of problems with each of them.

The first clinical method used to characterise tumour hypoxia was the measurement of oxygen tension (pO_2). Using ***polarographic electrode*** measurements Gatenby *et al.* (1988) showed that hypoxia was associated with a poor prognosis after radiotherapy in advanced head & neck tumours. Oxygen distribution was measured in 31 fixed lymph node metastases from squamous cell carcinoma of the head & neck through a needle electrode inserted under CT guidance. Thirteen tumours were found to have uniform oxygen distribution, all of which had a pO_2 under 10 mmHg, whilst six tumours had uniform oxygen distribution characterised by a pO_2 above 10 mmHg, with the remaining 12 tumours showing variable oxygen distribution with pO_2 higher in the periphery than in the centre of the tumour. Response to radiation therapy was assessed by changes in tumour volume 90 days following completion of therapy compared to pre-therapy volume of 12 tumours with greater than 26% of their volume with a pO_2 less than 8 mmHg. Eleven were assessed to be non-responders to treatment. Several later studies have confirmed the association between oxygenation status and clinical outcome. In one recent study based on 397 head & neck cancer patients, Nordsmark et al. (2005) concluded that tumours with pO_2 values ≤ 2.5 mmHg showed the worst results in tumour control.

Within a prostate carcinoma study, polarographic electrode measurements were undertaken on patients with localised disease before radiotherapy (Parker et al. 2004). Among the 55 patients investigated for tumour hypoxia, the median pO_2 ranged from 0.2 to 57.3 mmHg, leading to the conclusion that localised prostate cancers are characterised by marked hypoxia and significantly heterogeneous oxygenation. Furthermore, the extent of hypoxia in prostate carcinomas correlates with pretreatment characteristics and prognostic factors. Over 10 000 individual measurements for pO_2 were undertaken by Movsas et al using custom made Eppendorf microelectrodes. They observed that the extent of tumour hypoxia in localised prostate carcinoma increases with patient age and clinical stage (Movsas et al. 2000) indicating the need for further correlations between pretreatment characteristics and tumour hypoxia.

While polarographic measurements of oxygen tension were able to predict tumour behaviour and treatment outcome for certain cancers, there are studies showing no correlation between tumour hypoxia (quantified by the median tumour oxygen tension) and clinical endpoint. Such a result was reported by a study investigating the impact of hypoxia on high grade glioma patients' survival (Lally et al. 2006). The patients were divided into groups as a function of median tumour oxygen tension as follows: $pO_2 \leq$ 2 mmHg; 2 mmHg $< pO_2 \leq 5$ mmHg or 5.1 mmHg $<$ $pO_2 \leq 10$ mmHg. While histological grade had prognostic value for survival, the oxygen tension measurement results showed no significant difference in overall survival, and therefore could not be used as an independent prognostic indicator.

An indirect method of ascertaining tumour oxygenation involves evaluating its **vascular density**. Poor vascularisation of tumours is thought to imply poor delivery of oxygen, leading to the presence of chronically hypoxic tumour cells. Therefore, measurements of the density of tumour vasculature are indicative of the extent of hypoxia in tumours. These measurements are achieved through tumour biopsies. Cryospectrophotometric studies of intra-capillary oxyhemoglobin saturation have shown that poorly vascularised tumours have high levels of hypoxia (Mueller-Klieser et al. 1981). While vascular density measurements give no indication of the acutely hypoxic cell population inside the tumour, these experiments demonstrate that chronically hypoxic cells are an important component of the total tumour hypoxic fraction influencing treatment outcome.

The **comet assay**, based on evaluating individual tumour cells derived from needle biopsies, is a sensible method of quantifying the fraction of radiation-resistant hypoxic cells found in solid tumours (Olive et al. 1999). The comet assay measures DNA strand breaks after exposure to single doses of radiation of 3.5–10 Gy. The method is based on the observation that ionising radiation produces up to 3 times more damage to well oxygenated cells compared with the hypoxic cell population. The advantage of this method is that only hypoxic and not necrotic cells are measured. A limitation, however, is that the hypoxic fraction cannot be measured in clinical samples given a dose of less than 3.5 Gy per fraction since the DNA damage produced by conventional doses (2 Gy) is not sufficient for assessment with the comet assay.

All methods presented so far share the common disadvantage of being invasive assays. Beside the invasiveness, assays based on biopsies are unreliable (tumour oxygenation varies within the tumour), unless several tissue samples are taken from the patient thus increasing the invasiveness of the procedure. A non-invasive way of determining tumour oxygenation is through imaging techniques. Positron emission tomography (PET) and Blood Oxygen Level-Dependent Magnetic Resonance Imaging (**BOLD MRI**) are two diagnostic imaging methods widely used in oncology. These two techniques characterised by robustness, ease of use and reliability are able to heterogeneously assess hypoxia status (Padhani 2005). While PET requires the injection of radioactive contrast material for imaging, BOLD MRI uses paramagnetic deoxyhaemoglobin as contrast agent. One of the drawbacks of the MRI technique is that it does not allow direct measurement of tissue pO_2. Furthermore, while BOLD MRI seems to be a more sensitive measure of oxygen levels adjoining perfused vessels (acute hypoxia), its sensitivity to more distant hypoxic regions within the tumour (diffusion-dependent or chronic hypoxia) is unknown (Padhani et al. 2007).

Positron emission tomography (PET) is a functional imaging technique which measures the *in vivo* distribution of radiolabelled isotopes. The positron emitted by the radioisotope annihilates inside the body with a free electron, resulting in the release of two photons in opposite directions detectable by PET gamma cameras. For hypoxia imaging, PET uses radiolabelled nitroimidazole because nitroimidazoles are known to bind selectively to hypoxic cells where they are reduced (Nunn et al. 1995). Since reoxygenation is hindered in hypoxic cells, the result is intracellular accumulation of nitroimidazole. The first labelled nitroimidazole compound developed for PET detection was FMISO ([18F] Fluoromisonidazole) (Rasey et al. 1987). PET has the ability to noninvasively quantify regional hypoxia and furthermore, pretreatment FMISO uptake has been shown to be an independent prognostic indicator following treatment of hypoxic tumours (Rajendran et al. 2006).

Gagel et al. (2007) have undertaken a comparative study on patients with head & neck cancer where they determined tumour oxygenation either with direct, invasive measurements of tissue oxygenation by pO_2 polarography (the 'gold standard' in hypoxia measurement) and non-invasive [18F] Fluoromisonidazole (FMISO) and [18F] Fluorodeoxyglucose (FDG) PET. They concluded that the noninvasive techniques were valid and highly feasible methods for determining

radiotherapeutically relevant hypoxia. A similar study comparing the clinical potential of FDG, FMISO and pO_2 polarography in detecting hypoxic regions in metastatic head & neck cancers was undertaken on 24 patients (Zimny et al. 2006). The uptake of FMISO in hypoxic tumours was significantly higher than in normoxic ones, the results being in good correlation with pO_2 measurements. However, the maximum standardised uptake value of FDG was similar in hypoxic and normoxic tumours, making FGD PET a less reliable radiotracer regarding hypoxia evaluation in tumours.

With the limitations presented by FGD PET in assessing hypoxia extent in tumours, research was underway to find more selective and unfailing radiotracers. The last decade of investigations has revealed a most promising hypoxia-specific radiotracer in the form of a copper complex: Cu-ATSM. *In vivo* studies on hepatic tumour cell lines implanted in white rabbits have compared the intra-tumoral distribution of 64Cu-ATSM and FDG showing that while 64Cu-ATSM has accumulated around the outer rim of the tumour mainly consisting of actively hypoxic cells, FDG was largely distributed in the inner region of the tumour, populated by pre-necrotic cells (Obata et al. 2003). The results suggest an advantage of the copper complex over FDG in evaluating the hypoxic extent of tumours *in vivo*.

Pretreatment tumour hypoxia with 60Cu-ATSM assessed in cervical cancer patients was predictive of tumour behaviour and response to subsequent treatment, showing again a lack of correlation between FDG and Cu-ATSM uptake (Dehdashti 2003a). The same research group has investigated the feasibility of clinical imaging and the clinical potential of Cu-ATSM in predicting treatment outcome in patients with non-small-cell-lung cancer (Dehdashti 2003b) and rectal cancer (Dietz et al. 2008). The effectiveness of Cu-ATSM on non-small-cell-lung cancer was proven to be notable in revealing unique clinical information. Furthermore, the rectal study results are promising and they warrant further investigations.

Whereas hypoxic evaluation of high grade gliomas with polarographic electrode measurements did not correlate with clinical endpoints in several studies, the results obtained with FAZA-PET, another hypoxia-specific radiotracer, are encouraging. A recent clinical study has evaluated the biodistribution

Table 17.1. Hypoxia-specific radiotracers for PET imaging.

Radiotracer	Observation	References
[18F]FDG	still considered the 'queen' of radiotracers for its clinical advantages and widespread use; some novel radiotracers show the potential to replace FDG due to conflicting results when correlating tracer uptake and hypoxia content of the tumour	Rajendran *et al.* 2004 Oswald *et al.* 2007 Dierckx and Van de Wiele 2008
[18F]MISO	nitroimidazoles bind selectively to hypoxic cells; offers advantage over FDG in hypoxia evaluation	Kubota *et al.* 1999 Zimny *et al.* 2006 Lee and Scott 2007
Cu-ATSM	very promising radiotracer; able to distinguish between actively hypoxic and necrotic tumour regions	Chao *et al.* 2001 Dehdashti *et al.* 2003a,b Obata *et al.* 2003 Anderson and Ferdani 2009
[18F]FAZA	good accumulation in tumours; encouraging results for high grade gliomas	Souvatzoglou *et al.* 2007 Postema *et al.* 2009

pattern of [18F]FAZA (fluoroazomycin-arabinoside) in a range of hypoxic tumours such as: small and non-small-cell lung cancer, squamous cell carcinoma of head & neck, high grade glioma and malignant lymphoma (Postema *et al.* 2009). While all tumour types accumulated FAZA in their hypoxic regions, the high uptake of the radiotracer by hypoxic glioma cells was especially encouraging.

Head & neck cancers are known for their high hypoxic content, therefore there is an imperative need to determine the most efficient radiotracer for hypoxia imaging in these cancers. FAZA was shown to be a feasible radiotracer because of the good tumour uptake which resulted in an adequate PET image quality (Souvatzoglou *et al.* 2007), though comparative studies of FAZA and FMISO show only minor advantages of the former, consisting of higher tumour to background and tumour to blood ratios, due to more rapid clearance from blood and non-target tissues (Sorger *et al.* 2003).

The number of studies investigating feasible hypoxia-specific radiotracers is increasing, together with the number of compounds trialled. Table 17.1 presents a short list of the most commonly used radiotracers in today's clinics for imaging hypoxic regions in tumours.

II. Proliferative potential

Tumour proliferation and repopulation are evidenced by the higher doses of radiation required to control a tumour when overall treatment time is prolonged, or if the treatment is interrupted for a certain period of time. Accelerated repopulation during radiotherapy was first observed in head & neck cancers when the efficacy of treatment decreased with increasing overall treatment time of fractionated radiotherapy. It was suggested that the dose necessary for local tumour control increases by about 0.6 Gy/day after 4 weeks of fractionated irradiation (Withers *et al.* 1988).

Some clinical trials have shown that accelerated fractionation overcomes, to a certain extent, tumour repopulation during treatment for highly proliferating tumours, by shortening the overall treatment time and also the time between fractions (usually, accelerated treatment involves delivery of the radiation dose on 6 out of 7 days a week, with the overall treatment duration no longer than 5 weeks).

Other clinical trials employing altered fractionation schedules for rapidly proliferating tumours (see Chapter 5) did not show significant improvement regarding loco-regional control or overall survival compared to conventional radiotherapy. For example, the RTOG 9003 reported a 2 year endpoint for locoregional control of 54.4% after hyperfractionated radiotherapy and 47.5% after accelerated irradiation with split, results which are not significantly better than the 2 years loco-regional survival after standard fractionation (46%) (Fu *et al.* 2000).

An explanation of the discrepancies between some clinical trial results and the expected superior outcome after altered fractionation radiotherapy was given by Bentzen (2003) stating that 'this is most likely the result of a wide variability in biological factors affecting the outcome of therapy causing the beneficial effect of any therapeutic modification in a hypothetical subset of patients to be counterbalanced by a lack of effect or even a detrimental effect in other cases.' Monte Carlo modelling work undertaken by Marcu and Bezak (2009) has shown the superiority in tumour control of either hyperfractionated or accelerated radiotherapy compared to conventionally fractionated treatment when the radiobiological aspects of tumour repopulation are taken into consideration. The authors have simulated the RTOG trial schedules for two of the three clinical arms: hyperfractionated and accelerated radiotherapy with split, on a virtual head & neck tumour undergoing accelerated repopulation (Figure 17.1).

An obvious conclusion from the above results is the need to select those patients who could benefit from altered radiotherapy schedules, therefore from individualised treatment planning. In clinical settings this aim is achievable through *image-guided radiotherapy*. Functional imaging techniques, such as PET, are gaining importance due to the superior outcome of PET-guided radiotherapy as compared to radiotherapy alone, as indicated by recent trials. The results

obtained by Vernon *et al.* (2008) in regards to locoregional control and overall survival after 2 years with PET/CT guided radiotherapy are far superior to the outcome of altered fractionation therapy employed by RTOG (Table 17.2).

The inclusion of PET/CT imaging in radiotherapy planning is also justified by the good correlation between clinical outcome and the maximum standard uptake value of the radiotracer obtained on a PET scan.

From an accelerated repopulation point of view, PET can be of great assistance as it provides a three-dimensional map of cellular proliferation in tumours. While [18F]FDG is still the most used radionuclide in PET imaging, there is a continuous search for proliferation kinetics-specific radiotracers. PET scanning with 3'-deoxy-3'-[18F]fluorothymidine (FLT) was shown to correlate with tumour proliferation (Barthel *et al.* 2003). Furthermore, the investigation group has demonstrated that FLT is a more powerful marker of tumour proliferation than FDG. Research is underway to assess the tracer's efficacy in predicting tumour response to anti-proliferative treatment *in vivo*. The effect of cisplatin on a fibrosarcoma tumour model *in*

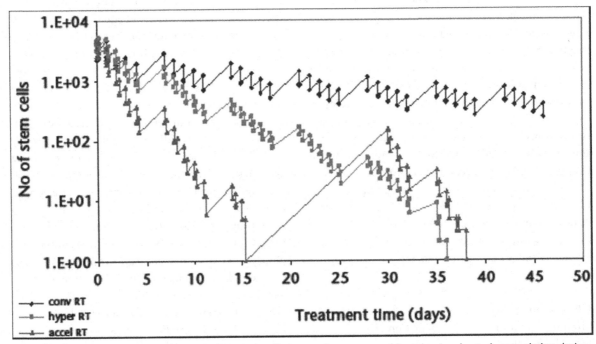

Figure 17.1. Conventional versus altered fractionated radiotherapy for tumours undergoing accelerated repopulation during treatment.

Table 17.2. RTOG 9003 endpoints versus PET/CT guided radiotherapy endpoints.

2–year endpoints	Accelerated fractionation with split	Hyperfractionation	PET/CT guided RT
Loco-regional control	47.5%	54.4%	71%
Overall survival	46.2%	54.5%	82.8%

vivo was evaluated using 3'-deoxy-3'-[^{18}F]fluorothymidine (FLT) PET. Leyton *et al.* (2005) have assessed the potential of FLT-PET to measure early cytotoxicity induced by cisplatin in fibrosarcoma tumour-bearing mice. For the quantitative measurement of tumour cell proliferation FLT-PET was, once again, proven to be more effective than FGD-PET. All of the above results indicate that further clinical studies with 3'-deoxy-3'-[^{18}F]fluorothymidine (FLT) are warranted.

Sigma receptors are membrane-bound proteins which were shown to play a role in a multitude of cellular functions, one of them being the inhibition of tumour proliferation (Brent and Pang 1995). A number of studies have reported an overexpression of sigma receptors both in human and rodent tumours (Bem *et al.* 1991; John *et al.* 1995; Vilner *et al.* 1995). *In vitro* study results have proven that the expression of sigma-2 receptors is up to 10 times higher in proliferative tumour cells than in quiescent tumour cells. Furthermore, it was observed that sigma-2 receptors followed the population growth kinetics when quiescent cells were recruited into the mitotic cycle (Wheeler *et al.* 2000). Therefore, the initiative of using the expression of sigma-2 receptors as a biomarker of tumour cell proliferation followed as an obvious measure. Breast cancer is characterised by a proliferative potential that has a considerable inter-patient variability. The rate of cell proliferation in these tumours is predictive of tumour response to both radio- and chemotherapy. Consequently, carbon-11 labelled sigma-2 receptor ligands were developed for breast cancer imaging showing a similar or even better tumour uptake than [^{18}F]FLT (Tu *et al.* 2005). An imaging study of various tumour sites with 2 sigma receptor ligands ([^{18}F]-labelled compound and a [^{11}C]-labelled drug) was conducted in order to evaluate the clinical potential of the two compounds in tumour-bearing nude rats (van Waarde *et al.* 2004). While both radioligands demonstrated specific binding to sigma-receptors *in vivo*, the [^{18}F]-labelled compound showed a better correlation with tumour staging than the [^{11}C]-labelled drug. A similar study evaluating two [^{11}C]-labelled compounds for PET imaging of sigma receptors in animal tumours showed good tumour uptake and feasibility of carbon-labelled ligands for *in vivo* use (Kawamura *et al.* 2005).

A new radiotracer in the form of [^{18}F]ISO-1 (FISO PET/CT) is aimed to be trialled by Washington University School of Medicine in a study which is currently recruiting patients with one of the following three conditions: breast cancer, head & neck cancer and diffuse large B-cell lymphoma (ClinicalTrials.gov Identifier: NCT00968656). The primary goal of the study 'Assessment of Cellular Proliferation in Tumors by Positron Emission Tomography (PET) Using [^{18}F]ISO-1 (FISO PET/CT)' is to evaluate the diagnostic quality of [^{18}F]ISO-1-PET/CT images at the proposed 8 mCi dose. As secondary outcome measures, the trial intends to quantitatively determine the relationship between tumour [^{18}F]ISO-1 uptake and Ki-67 (cellular marker for proliferation), S-phase, mitotic index and sigma-2 receptors content of the tumour.

While the current number of radionuclides for the assessment of cellular proliferation within tumours via PET imaging is relatively small, the interest in the development of proliferation kinetics-specific radiotracers is continuously growing (Table 17.3).

The purpose of assessing the tumour's proliferative potential is to distinguish between rapidly and slowly proliferating cells within the tumour. Common methods to achieve this goal include measurements of cell kinetic parameters before treatment such as potential doubling time (Tpot) and the length of S phase (T_S) to correlate with the treatment outcome. Measurement of kick-off time (T_K), which represents the time period from the start of radiotherapy until the initiation of accelerated repopulation, can provide an indication of the need to adjust

Table 17.3.   Proliferation kinetics-specific radiotracers for PET imaging.

Radiotracer	Observation	References
[18F]FDG	not the most performant anymore; still the most commonly used	Barthel *et al.* 2003 Leyton *et al.* 2005 Dierckx and Van de Wiele 2008
[18F](FLT)	promising results; better correlation between uptake and proliferation than FDG	Barthel *et al.* 2003 Leyton *et al.* 2005 Ullrich *et al.* 2008
11C	effective for imaging of sigma receptor-rich tumours; promising results in breast cancer	Wheeler *et al.* 2000 Tu *et al.* 2005
[18F]ISO-1	under trial	trial currently recruiting

the treatment schedule, e.g. hyperfractionation, accelerated fractionation or a combination of the two altered schedules.

Flow cytometric methods are common techniques used in the study of the predictive values of various pretreatment parameters. Several studies have been undertaken to assess cell kinetic parameters and their relationships with treatment outcome (Corvo *et al.* 1993; Bourhis *et al.* 1996; Eschwege *et al.* 1997; Begg *et al.* 1999). The cytometry measurements have been based on tumour biopsies obtained after intravenous injection of **bromodeoxyuridine**, which is a thymidine analogue incorporated in DNA-synthesising cells. Preliminary results obtained by Corvo *et al.* (1993) have suggested that Tpot could be a prognostic factor influencing radiotherapy outcome in head & neck cancer patients. Although the initial results were promising, very few further studies have confirmed the efficacy of Tpot as a predictor of treatment outcome. Tpot was not the only parameter poorly associated with outcome, since the majority of the studies have also shown that other parameters such as the length of S phase, and the labelling index had poor predictive power. On the other hand, the classic clinical prognostic factors (tumour stage and nodal status) were strongly associated with clinical outcome. Begg *et al.* (1999) have established that the only pretreatment kinetic parameter with some evidence of an association with local control in head & neck patients was labelling index (LI), therefore concluding that pretreatment cell kinetic measurements determined by flow cytometry techniques provide a relatively weak overall prediction of radiotherapy outcome.

The **proliferation-associated nuclear antigen, p105**, an antigen which identifies only proliferating cells has been reported to be a potentially useful predictor for loco-regional control and survival of treated head & neck cancer patients (Fu *et al.* 1994). The method is also based on flow cytometry measurements, but instead of pretreatment injections with thymidine analogues, nuclei suspensions from paraffin blocks obtained from pretreatment biopsies are prepared and processed for p105 antibody and DNA staining. Subsequent flow cytometric quantification of p105 labelling indices and DNA content are undertaken and correlated with radiotherapy outcome. Later studies (Hammond *et al.* 2003) however, showed no association between p105 labelling indices, DNA ploidy and treatment outcome. Among head & neck cancers, no significant differences in proliferation parameters with respect to site of origin have been reported (Struikmans *et al.* 2001).

To date, cell kinetic measurements have not conclusively established a correlation between pretreatment parameters and treatment outcome. While several studies have shown weak or no relationship between kinetic parameters and radiotherapy end points, other studies suggest good association between the classic clinical prognostic factors (TNM staging classification) or tumour volume (Kurek *et al.* 2003) and treatment outcome. Therefore, there is great need for developing more powerful kinetic parameters which more accurately reflect the proliferative ability of tumours.

Nowadays, the role of PET/CT within image-guided radiotherapy becomes remarkable together with the development of new proliferation kinetics-specific radiotracers. The focus should be on identifying reliable biomarkers of neoplastic proliferation to facilitate the non-invasive assessment of tumour proliferation status using PET imaging techniques.

III. Intrinsic cellular radiosensitivity

Intrinsic radiosensitivity depends on the susceptibility to cellular damage induced by a certain radiation dose and the extent of cell repair. Both damage induction and repair can be measured at the DNA or chromosome level. Cell survival is also an indication of cell damage and repair, and determining cell survival is the final endpoint of this predictive assay. For a reliable predictive assay, the ultimate goal would be to correlate the *in vitro* radiosensitivity of human cell lines with the clinical responsiveness of tumours.

Besides determining hypoxic levels in tumours, the **comet assay** is used to estimate DNA repair after irradiation. Terris *et al.* (2002) used the comet assay to evaluate DNA damage in fine-needle aspirates of lymph nodes containing metastatic squamous cell carcinoma in patients with head & neck cancer 1, 2, and 3 minutes after treatment with 5 Gy of irradiation. They concluded that the decrease in DNA damage corresponds to a repair half-life of 4.2 minutes. The comet assay has shown to be a promising tool for evaluating radiation sensitivity in individual cells.

A study conducted by Malaise *et al.* (1987) on 110 human tumour cell lines has shown that *in vitro* **survival curves** of cells derived from human tumours did vary from one cell line to another. They demonstrated that the level of survival of different tumour cell lines was dose dependent over the range 1 to 6 Gy. More precisely, the dose-response (cell survival) relationship was represented by a bell shaped curve, with a maximum peak at 1.5 Gy. Malaise's work has confirmed that intrinsic radiosensitivity is a determinant of tumour response to radiotherapy, suggesting therefore, that tissue cultures may be used as predictive assays.

One of the studies confirming the findings by which the initial slope of the survival curve correlates with clinical responsiveness (characterised by SF2) was undertaken by a Swedish group, on head & neck cancer patients (Bjork-Eriksson *et al.* 2000). It was shown that patients with *in vitro* sensitive tumour cells are better responders to radiation.

Although the above-mentioned pre-clinical studies have successfully demonstrated the association between *in vitro* tumour and clinical response, one of the main drawbacks of tissue culture methods limiting clinical utility is the time factor. Growing cell lines from human tumours (colony assays) is too time consuming for practical use. Several studies have implemented alternative assays to evaluate dose-response characteristics such as evaluation of mutations, gene expression, and gene function involved in the repair of radiation-induced damage (Steel 2002). The majority of the studies have shown poor correlation between intrinsic radiosensitivity and these cellular parameters. It can then be concluded that cell-based assays currently have limited potential as radiotherapy outcome predictors, and there is need to better understand the differences in gene expression profiles of tumours.

Table 17.4 summarises the major goals of the three predictive assays discussed above, and their clinical limitations.

17.2.2 Predictive assays for normal tissue response

The aim of radiotherapy is to achieve a high therapeutic ratio by delivering a dose to the tumour sufficiently large to control its growth, but small enough to limit damage to the surrounding normal tissue. Predictive assays would be ideal tools in attaining high therapeutic ratios. Similarly to tumour response after radiotherapy, one should consider the inter-patient variability of normal tissue reaction. The tolerance of patients with the most severe normal tissue reactions currently determine the dose level of the patient group as a whole for a given tumour site and type. The aim would be to develop a sufficiently robust predictive assay to enable individual dose adjustment, but this time with respect to normal tissue toxicity (Russell and Begg 2002).

There is clear evidence in the literature that the variation in radiation sensitivity is determined, at least in part, by genetic factors. Although several research groups have been focusing on determining an *in vitro* radiosensitivity parameter, there are several factors that would limit the clinical utility of such a parameter. The main factors that influence the correlation between an *in vitro* test and the clinical endpoint can

Table 17.4.   Summary of current predictive assays for tumour response and their main limitations.

Predictive assay	Aim	Methods	Limitations
Oxygen status	To select patients likely to benefit from radiosensitisers	electrodes biopsy (vascular density) hypoxic markers imaging techniques (PET with hypoxia-specific markers)	invasive (electrodes) unreliable (biopsy) unpredictable (imaging acute hypoxia only) some radiotracers cannot reliably differentiate between hypoxic and normoxic tumours
Proliferative potential	To distinguish between rapidly and slowly proliferating cells	to measure Tpot, T_S, LI and correlate with outcome to adjust treatment schedule as a function of Tk PET imaging with proliferation-specific radiotracers	no correlation between Tpot and radiotherapy outcome T_S shows weak correlation. new PET radiotracers are under investigation
Intrinsic cellular radiosensitivity	To correlate the in vitro radiosensitivity of human cell lines with the clinical responsiveness of tumours	– comet assay – cell survival curves – functional assays	growing cell lines from human tumours is too time consuming.

be classified in three major groups: biological factors (such as cell kill, vascular injury, fibrogenesis), clinical factors (such as total radiation dose, dose distribution, fractionation schedule, volume irradiated, the random-nature of radiation-induced cell killing, anatomical site, previous treatments (surgery, radiotherapy)) and life-style factors (such as diet, smoking, alcohol consumption). Finding a good predictor for normal tissue damage needs to consider the factors listed above.

Colony formation assays have been considered as the gold standard for cell kill assessment. However, the time consuming nature of these assays led to their substitution with other assays evaluating chromosomal and DNA damage.

The cytokinesis-block micronucleus assay developed by Michael Fenech is a reliable and precise method for assessing chromosome damage in lymphocytes (Fenech and Morley 1986). The micronucleus assay in human lymphocytes measures both whole chromosome loss and chromosomal breakage. **Micronuclei** (MN) derive from either chromosomal fragments or whole chromosomes lagging at anaphase. Micronuclei, though smaller, are morphologically identical to the main nuclei, and therefore easily identified. One of the main advantages of the MN assay is

the capability to differentiate between dividing and non-dividing cells, since a non-dividing cell is unable to express its chromosome damage as micronuclei. The cytokinesis-block micronucleus (CBMN) assay uses cytochalasin-B to stop cells from performing cytokinesis (the partitioning of the cytoplasm following nuclear division). As a result, cells that have completed one nuclear division after exposure to a toxic agent are recognised by their binucleate appearance.

The initial *in vitro* studies with CBMN (Fenech and Morley 1986) indicated that by knowing the baseline frequency of MN of an individual before exposure, it is possible to detect increments in MN induction after exposure (even as small as 0.05 Gy). This method was, later, implemented in clinics by measuring micronucleus induction in cancer patients undergoing fractionated radiotherapy (Fenech *et al.* 1990). Measurements during radiotherapy showed a dose-related increase in MN in all treated patients.

Some of the main applications of CBMN assay include: assessment of inter-individual variation in radiosensitivity and prediction of tumour response to radiation (Fenech 1993).

It was concluded that while the *in vitro* intrinsic radiosensitivity of normal cells may influence the degree of normal tissue response to radiation this is the only parameter that determines normal tissue response. To date, there are no sufficiently accurate predictive assays to be used in clinics and there is need for further research to develop methodologies with better predictive power than the existing ones.

17.3 DISEASE STAGING

Though not generally considered a predictive assay, the accurate staging of a tumour is crucial in the development of an appropriate treatment strategy which impacts on prognosis. Staging describes the severity of an individual's cancer based on the extent of the primary tumour and the degree of spread in the body (metastasis).

Depending on stage of disease, the patient may undergo any of the following treatment methods, either alone or in combination: surgery, radiotherapy, chemotherapy, gene therapy, hyperthermia, immunotherapy.

Staging of tumours are based on the following factors:

- location of the primary tumour
- tumour size and number of tumours
- lymph node involvement (spread of cancer into lymph nodes)
- cell type and their resemblance to the tissue of origin

- presence or absence of metastasis.

One of the most commonly used staging classifications is the TNM system. This system is based on the extent of the tumor (T), the extent of spread to the lymph nodes (N), and the presence or not of metastasis (M). The number added to the letter indicates the degree (extent) of the particular characteristic of the tumour (size, spread to lymph nodes, presence or not of metastasis) (see Table 17.5).

Based on the above factors staging can be defined as shown in Table 17.6.

The most common investigations performed to assist cancer staging include: physical examination, imaging studies (CT, MRI, PET, X-rays), and laboratory tests (blood, urine and tissue sample analysis, and specific tumour marker assays). Biopsy reports, as well as cytology and surgical reports complement the list of investigations for accurate disease staging.

17.4 TREATMENT ASSESSMENT

While predictive assays, being based on biological evaluation would be expected to be the best indicators of tumour response to treatment, there are other methods based on physical assessment of the treatment plan and delivery of the radiation dose as well as post-treatment analysis of tumour response which

Table 17.5.   The TNM system (www.cancer.org).

Primary tumour (T)	
TX	Primary tumour cannot be evaluated
T0	No evidence of primary tumour
Tis	Carcinoma in situ (early cancer in epithelial-lined surfaces that has not spread beyond the basement membrane)
T1, T2, T3, T4	Size and/or extent of the primary tumour
Regional lymph nodes	
NX	Regional lymph nodes cannot be evaluated
N0	No regional lymph node involvement (no cancer found in the lymph nodes)
N1, N2, N3	Involvement of regional lymph nodes (number and/or extent of spread)
Distant metastasis	
MX	Distant metastasis cannot be evaluated
M0	No distant metastasis (cancer has not spread to other parts of the body)
M1	Distant metastasis (cancer has spread to distant parts of the body)

Table 17.6. Staging of cancer.

Stage	Definition
Stage 0	Carcinoma in situ (early cancer that is present only in the epithelial cell layer of tissue from which it originated).
Stage I, Stage II and Stage III	Higher numbers indicate more extensive disease: greater tumour size, and/or spread of the cancer to nearby lymph nodes and/or organs adjacent to the primary tumour.
Stage IV	The cancer has spread to another organ.

have clinical utility. Some of these methods are presented in the sections below.

17.4.1 Dose volume histograms

A Dose Volume Histogram (DVH) is a plot of cumulative dose-volume frequency distribution, which graphically summarises the simulated radiation dose distribution within a volume of interest based on three dimensional (3D) treatment planning systems for radiotherapy.

Ideal DVHs and DVHs in practice

Though the two DVH diagrams in Figure 17.2 represent the ideal situation, in clinical radiotherapy the reality is that even in the most localised form of treatment such as brachytherapy or conformal external beam radiotherapy the choice of treatment plans is a compromise between the need for a DVH which shows high tumour control and low normal tissue toxicity (see Figure 17.3).

The following is one interpretation of the DVH curves in Figure 17.3:

DVH for the tumour (continuous curve):

- 100% Planning Target Volume (PTV) receives at least 40 Gy
- 95% PTV receives at least 50 Gy
- 83% PTV receives the maximum prescribed dose (60 Gy)

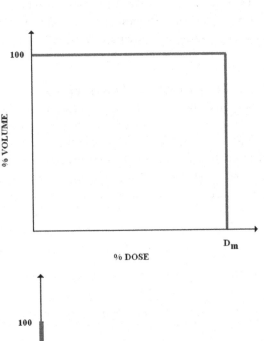

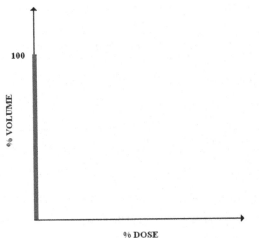

Figure 17.2. Ideal DVH curves for tumour control (top) and normal tissue complications (bottom).

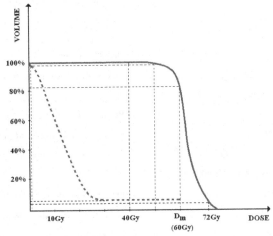

Figure 17.3. Typical DVH curves for tumour control and normal tissue complications.

- 4% PTV however, receives more than prescribed (72 Gy)

DVH for the normal tissue toxicity (dotted curve):

- nearly the whole volume of normal tissue receives a small dose (3 Gy)
- 6% of normal tissue receives almost the maximum prescribed dose.

In summary, DVHs are useful planning tools in order to:

- check dose levels and dose uniformity throughout the planning target volume for the tumour
- determine hot spots in the surrounding normal tissue
- select the most acceptable plan (allows for quantitative assessment of plans).

A major limitation of DVHs is the lack of information in regard to spatial dose distribution.

17.5 REFERENCES

Anderson C and Ferdani R (2009) Copper-64 radiopharmaceuticals for PET imaging of cancer: advances in preclinical and clinical research. *Cancer Biotherapy and Radiopharmaceuticals* **24**: 379–393.

Barthel H, Cleij MC, Collingridge DR, Hutchinson OC *et al.* (2003) 3'-deoxy-3'-[18F]fluorothymidine as a new marker for monitoring tumor response to antiproliferative therapy in vivo with positron emission tomography. *Cancer Research* **63**: 3791–3798.

Begg AC, Haustermans K, Hart AA, Dische S *et al.* (1999) The value of pretreatment cell kinetic parameters as predictors for radiotherapy outcome in head & neck cancer: a multicenter analysis. *Radiotherapy and Oncology* **50**: 13–23.

Bem WT, Thomas GE, Mamone JY *et al.* (1991) Overexpression of sigma receptors in nonneural human tumors. *Cancer Research* **51**: 6558–6562.

Bentzen SM (2003) Repopulation in radiation oncology: perspectives of clinical research. *International Journal of Radiation Oncology Biology Physics* **79**: 581–585.

Bjork-Eriksson T, West C, Karlsson E and Mercke C (2000) Tumour radiosensitivity (SF2) is a prognostic factor for local control in head & neck cancers. *International Journal of Radiation Oncology Biology Physics* **46**: 13–19.

Bourhis J, Dendale R, Hill C, Bosq J *et al.* (1996) Potential doubling time and clinical outcome in head & neck squamous cell carcinoma treated with 70 Gy in 7 weeks. *International Journal of Radiation Oncology Biology Physics* **35**: 471–476.

Brent PJ and Pang GT (1995) Sigma binding site ligands inhibit cell proliferation in mammary and colon carcinoma cell lines and melanoma cells in culture. *European Journal of Pharmacology* **278**: 151–160.

Chao K, Bosch WR, Mutic S, Lewis JS *et al.* (2001) A novel approach to overcome hypoxic tumor resistance: Cu-ATSM-guided intensity-modulated radiation therapy. *International Journal of Radiation Oncology Biology Physics* **49**: 1171–1182.

Corvo R, Giaretti W, Sanguineti G, Geido E *et al.* (1993) Potential doubling time in head & neck tumors treated by primary radiotherapy: preliminary evidence for a prognostic significance in local control. *International Journal of Radiation Oncology Biology Physics* **27**(5): 1165–1172.

Dehdashti F, Grigsby PW, Mintun MA, Lewis JS *et al.* (2003a) Assessing tumor hypoxia in cervical cancer by positron emission tomography with 60Cu-ATSM: relationship to therapeutic response – a preliminary report. *International Journal of Radiation Oncology Biology Physics* **55**: 1233–1238.

Dehdashti F, Mintun MA, Lewis JS, Bradley J *et al.* (2003b) In vivo assessment of tumor hypoxia in lung cancer with 60Cu-ATSM. *European Journal of Nuclear Medicine and Molecular Imaging* **30**: 844–850.

Dierckx RA and Van de Wiele C (2008) FDG uptake, a surrogate of tumour hypoxia? *European Journal of Nuclear Medicine and Molecular Imaging* **35**: 1544–1549.

Dietz D, Dehdashti F, Grigsby PW, Malyapa RS *et al.* (2008) Tumor hypoxia detected by positron emission tomography with 60Cu-ATSM as a predictor of response and survival in patients undergoing Neoadjuvant chemoradiotherapy for rectal carcinoma: a pilot study. *Diseases of the Colon and Rectum* **51**: 1641–1648.

Eschwege F, Bourhis J, Girinski T, Lartigau E *et al.* (1997) Predictive assays of radiation response in patients with head & neck squamous cell carcinoma: a review of the Institute Gustave Roussy experience. *International Journal of Radiation Oncology Biology Physics* 39: 849–853.

Fenech M (1993) The cytokinesis-block micronucleus technique and its application to genotoxicity studies in human populations. *Environmental Health Perspectives* 101(Suppl 3): 101–107.

Fenech M and Morley A (1986) Cytokinesis-block micronucleus method in human lymphocytes: effect of in vivo ageing and low-dose X-irradiation. *Mutation Research* 161: 193–198.

Fenech M, Denham J, Francis W and Morley A (1990) Micronuclei in cytokinesis-blocked lymphocytes of cancer patients following fractionated partial-body radiotherapy. *International Journal of Radiation Biology* 57: 373–383.

Fu K, Hammond E, Pajak TF, Clery M *et al.* (1994) Flow cytometric quantification of the proliferation-associated nuclear antigen p105 and DNA content in advanced head & neck cancers: results of RTOG 91-08. *International Journal of Radiation Oncology Biology Physics* 29(4): 661–671.

Fu KK, Pajak T, Trotti A *et al.* (2000) Radiation Therapy Oncology Group (RTOG) phase III randomized study to compare hyperfractionation and two variants of accelerated fractionation to standard fractionation radiotherapy for head & neck squamous cell carcinomas: first report of RTOG 9003. *International Journal of Radiation Oncology Biology Physics* 48: 7–16.

Gagel B, Piroth M, Pinkawa M, Reinartz P *et al.* (2007) pO polarography, contrast enhanced color duplex sonography (CDS), [18F] fluoromisonidazole and [18F] fluorodeoxyglucose positron emission tomography: validated methods for the evaluation of therapy-relevant tumor oxygenation or only bricks in the puzzle of tumor hypoxia? *BMC Cancer* 7: 113.

Gatenby RA, Kessler HB, Rosenblum JS, Coia LR *et al.* (1988) Oxygen distribution in squamous cell carcinoma metastases and its relationship to outcome of radiation therapy. *International Journal of Radiation Oncology Biology Physics* 14: 831–838.

Grosu AL, Souvatzoglou M, Röper B, Dobritz M *et al.* (2007) Hypoxia imaging with FAZA-PET and theoretical considerations with regard to dose painting for individualization of radiotherapy in patients with head & neck cancer. *International Journal of Radiation Oncology Biology Physics* 69: 541–551.

Hammond E, Berkey BA, Fu KK, Trotti A *et al.* (2003) P105 as a prognostic indicator in patients irradiated for locally advanced head-and-neck cancer: a clinical/laboratory correlative analysis of RTOG-9003. *International Journal of Radiation Oncology Biology Physics* 57: 683–692.

Hockel M and Vaupel P (2001) Tumour hypoxia: definitions and current clinical, biologic, and molecular aspects. *Journal of the National Cancer Institute* 93: 266–276.

Isa A, Ward T, West C, Slevin N *et al.* (2006) Hypoxia in head & neck cancer. *British Journal of Radiology* 79: 791–798.

John CS, Bowen WD, Varma VM, McAfee JG *et al.* (1995) Sigma receptors are expressed in human non-small cell lung carcinoma. *Life Sciences* 56: 2385–2392.

Kawamura K, Kubota K, Kobayashi T, Elsinga PH *et al.* (2005) Evaluation of [11C]SA5845 and [11C]SA4503 for imaging of sigma receptors in tumors by animal PET. *Annals of Nuclear Medicine* 19: 701–709.

Kubota K, Tada M, Yamada S, Hori K *et al.* (1999) Comparison of the distribution of fluorine-18 fluoromisonidazole, deoxyglucose and methionine in tumour tissue. *European Journal of Nuclear Medicine* 26: 750–757.

Kurek R, Kalogera-Fountzila A, Muskalla K, Dafni U *et al.* (2003) Usefulness of tumor volumetry as a prognostic factor of survival in head & neck cancer. *Strahlentherapie und Onkologie* 179: 292–297.

Lally B, Rockwell S, Fischer DB, Collingridge DR *et al.* (2006) The interactions of polarographic measurements of oxygen tension and histological grade in human glioma. *Cancer* 12: 461–466.

Lee ST and Scott AM (2007) Hypoxia positron emission tomography imaging with 18F-fluoromisonidazole. *Seminars in Nuclear Medicine* 37: 451–461.

Leyton J, Latigo JR, Perumal M, Dhaliwal H *et al.* (2005) Early detection of tumor response to chemotherapy by 3'-deoxy-3'-[18F]fluorothymidine positron emission tomography: the effect of cisplatin on a fibrosarcoma tumor model in vivo. *Cancer Research* 65: 4202–4210.

Malaise E, Fertil B, Deschavanne P, Chavaudra N and Brock W (1987) Initial slope of radiation survival curves is characteristic of the origin of primary and established cultures of human tumor cells and fibroblasts. *Radiation Research* 111: 319–333.

Marcu L and Bezak E (2009) Radiobiological modelling of the interplay between accelerated repopulation and altered fractionation schedules in head & neck cancer. *Journal of Medical Physics* 34: 206–211.

Movsas B, Chapman JD, Greenberg RE, Hanlon AL *et al.* (2000) Increasing levels of hypoxia in prostate carcinoma correlate significantly with increasing clinical stage and patient age: an Eppendorf pO(2) study. *Cancer* 89: 2018–2024.

Mueller-Klieser W, Vaupel P, Manz R and Schmidseder R (1981) Intracapillary oxyhemoglobin saturation of malignant tumors in humans. *International Journal of Radiation Oncology Biology Physics* 7: 1397–1404.

Nordsmark M, Bentzen S, Rudat V, Brizel D, Lartigau E *et al.* (2005) Prognostic value of tumor oxygenation in 397 head & neck tumors after primary radiation therapy. An international multi-center study. *Radiation Oncology* 77: 18–24.

Nunn A, Linder K and Strauss HW (1995) Nitroimidazoles and imaging hypoxia. European Journal of Nuclear Medicine 22: 265–280.

Obata A, Yoshimoto M, Kasamatsu S, Naiki H *et al.* (2003) Intra-tumoral distribution of ^{64}Cu-ATSM: a comparison study with FDG. Nuclear Medicine and Biology 30: 529–534.

Olive P, Durand R, Jackson S, Le Riche J *et al.* (1999) The comet assay in clinical practice. *Acta Oncologica* 38: 839–844.

Oswald J, Treite F, Haase C, Kampfrath T *et al.* (2007) Experimental hypoxia is a potent stimulus for radiotracer uptake in vitro: Comparison of different tumor cells and primary endothelial cells. Cancer Letters 254: 102–110.

Padhani AR (2005) Where are we with imaging oxygenation in human tumours. *Cancer Imaging* 5: 128–130.

Padhani A, Krohn K, Lewis J and Alber M (2007) Imaging oxygenation of human tumours. *European Radiology* 17: 861–872.

Parker C, Milosevic M, Toi A, Sweet J *et al.* (2004) Polarographic electrode study of tumor oxygenation in clinically localized prostate cancer. *International Journal of Radiation Oncology Biology Physics* 58: 750–757.

Postema EJ, McEwan AJ, Riauka TA, Kumar P *et al.* (2009) Initial results of hypoxia imaging using 1-alpha-D: -(5-deoxy-5-[18F]-fluoroarabinofuranosyl)-2-ni troimidazole (18F-FAZA). *European Journal of Nuclear Medicine and Molecular Imaging* 36: 1565–1573.

Rajendran JG, Mankoff D, O'Sullivan F, Peterson L *et al.* (2004) Hypoxia and glucose metabolism in malignant tumors: evaluation by [18F]Fluoromisonidazole and [18F]Fluorodeoxyglucose Positron Emission Tomography Imaging. *Clinical Cancer Research* 10: 2245–2252.

Rajendran JG, Schwartz DL, O'Sullivan J, Peterson LM *et al.* (2006) Tumor hypoxia imaging with [F-18] fluoromisonidazole positron emission tomography in head & neck cancer. *Clinical Cancer Research* 12: 5435–5441.

Rasey J, Grunbaum Z, Magee S, Nelson NJ *et al.* (1987) Characterization of radiolabelled fluoromisonidazole as a probe for hypoxic cells. *Radiation Research* 111: 292–304.

Russell N and Begg A (2002) Editorial radiotherapy and oncology 2002: predictive assays for normal tissue damage. *Radiotherapy and Oncology* 64: 125–129.

Sorger D, Patt M, Kumar P *et al.* (2003) [^{18}F]Fluoroazomycinarabinofuranoside (^{18}FAZA) and [^{18}F] fluoromisonidazole (^{18}FMISO): a comparative study of their selective uptake in hypoxic cells and PET imaging in experimental rat tumors. *Nuclear Medicine and Biology* 30: 317–326.

Souvatzoglou M, Grosu AL, Röper B, Krause BJ *et al.* (2007) Tumour hypoxia imaging with [18F]FAZA PET in head & neck cancer patients: a pilot study. *European Journal of Nuclear Medicine and Molecular Imaging* 34: 1566–1575.

Steel GG (2002) *Basic Clinical Radiobiology*. 3rd edn. Arnold Publishing, London.

Struikmans H, Kal HB, Hordijk GJ and van der Tweel I (2001) Proliferative capacity in head & neck cancer. *Head & Neck* 23: 484–491.

Terris D, Ho E, Ibrahim H, Dorie M *et al.* (2002) Estimating DNA repair by sequential evaluation of head & neck tumor radiation sensitivity using the comet assay. *Archives of Otolaryngology – Head & Neck Surgery* **128**: 698–702.

Tu Z, Dence CS, Ponde DE, Jones L *et al.* (2005) Carbon-11 labeled sigma2 receptor ligands for imaging breast cancer. *Nuclear Medicine and Biology* **32**: 423–430.

Ullrich R, Backes H, Li H, Kracht L *et al.* (2008) Glioma proliferation as assessed by 3'-fluoro-3'-deoxy-L-thymidine positron emission tomography in patients with newly diagnosed high-grade glioma. *Clinical Cancer Research* **14**: 2049–2055.

van Waarde A, Buursma AR, Hospers GA, Kawamura K *et al.* (2004) Tumor imaging with 2 sigma-receptor ligands, 18F-FE-SA5845 and 11C-SA4503: a feasibility study. *Journal of Nuclear Medicine* **45**: 1939–1945.

Vernon MR, Maheshwari M, Schultz CJ, Michel MA *et al.* (2008) Clinical outcomes of patients receiving integrated PET/CT-guided radiotherapy for head & neck carcinoma. *International Journal of Radiation Oncology Biology Physics* **70**(3): 678–684.

Vilner BJ, John CS and Bowen WD (1995) Sigma-1 and sigma-2 receptors are expressed in a wide variety of human and rodent tumor cell lines. *Cancer Research* **55**: 408–413.

Wheeler KT, Wang LM, Wallen CA, Childers SR *et al.* (2000) Sigma-2 receptors as a biomarker of proliferation in solid tumours. *British Journal of Cancer* **82**: 1223–1232.

Withers HR, Taylor JM and Maciejewski B (1988) The hazard of accelerated repopulation during radiotherapy. *Acta Oncologica* **27**: 131–146.

Zimny M, Gagel B, DiMartino E, Hamacher K *et al.* (2006) FDG – a marker of tumour hypoxia? A comparison with [18F]fluoromisonidazole and pO2-polarography in metastatic head & neck cancer. *European Journal of Nuclear Medicine and Molecular Imaging* **33**: 1426–1431.

http://www.cancer.org

18 Elements of health physics

18.1 RADIATION RESPONSE AND TOLERANCE OF NORMAL TISSUE

The first animal experiments that studied the effect of radiation on normal tissues were conducted in 1906 by Bergonié and Tribondeau. After irradiating rat testes they observed that rapidly dividing cells in the germinal layer were severely damaged, while non-dividing interstitial cells appeared unaffected. Based on these observations they stated that rapidly proliferating cells are radiosensitive, while slowly, or non-proliferating cells are radioresistant.

Today this statement is misleading since it is now known that radio-responsiveness does not depend on intrinsic cellular radiosensitivity. The response of normal tissues and organs to radiation is dependent upon their division rate (or length of mitotic cycle) of their constituent cells. This does not mean that an organ with an early response is more sensitive than one responding later. In rapidly proliferating tissues the radiation-induced damage becomes evident shortly after exposure (early effects of radiation), while the damage from slowly proliferating tissues is expressed much later (late effects) (see Table 18.1). The kinetics of cell division rather than the tissue type determines radio-responsiveness.

Early (acute) effects result from the death of a large number of cells and occur within a few days or weeks of irradiation. As already mentioned, early effects occur mainly in tissues with rapid cell turnover, e.g. skin, gastrointestinal epithelium, and bone marrow tissue. This is reflected in the first side effects a cancer patient treated with radiotherapy experiences. Nausea and vomiting are very common among cancer patients receiving abdomen irradiation because of damage sustained by the epithelial lining of the gastrointestinal tract. Patients receiving chemotherapy experience the same effects in addition to hair loss (hair follicles have short mitotic cycles as well) since chemotherapeutic agents affect mainly proliferating cells not only of the tumour but also of normal tissues. Acute damage may be completely reversible since it is repaired rapidly by the proliferation of the stem cells.

Late effects appear after a delay of months or years and occur mainly in slowly proliferating tissues, e.g. lung, heart, kidney, liver, central nervous system. Since these organs have long cell cycle times, it takes much longer time for the damage to be recognised by the cell. For the damage to be detected the cells have to go through the mitotic cycle, passing cell cycle check points for the abnormalities to be picked up and

L. Marcu et al., *Biomedical Physics in Radiotherapy for Cancer*,
DOI 10.1007/978-0-85729-733-4_18, © CSIRO 2012

Table 18.1.   Kinetic properties of cell populations of various tissues and organs.

No mitosis (no cell renewal)	Low mitotic index (little cell renewal)	High mitotic index (cell renewal)
Central nervous system	Liver	Epidermis
Muscle	Thyroid	Intestinal epithelium
Sense organs	Vascular endothelium	Bone marrow
Adrenal medulla	Connective tissue	Gonads

cell signals to be generated in response to damage. A latent period before the clinical appearance of the radiation-induced damage is characteristic for the tissues that are mainly constituted of quiescent cells. The recruitment of high proportions of quiescent cells in these tissues into the cell cycle results in the appearance of an 'avalanche' of late effects particularly as any late damage is never completely repaired.

Radiosensitivity of normal tissues is strongly influenced by genetic factors. The most convincing evidence linking genetic alterations to radiosensitivity originates from clinical studies involving patients with rare genetic conditions such as ataxia telangiectasia, Fanconi's anaemia, and Bloom's syndrome. These patients present with enhanced cellular radiosensitivity due to mutations in repair genes. Other host related factors that alter the susceptibility to radiation injury include age, smoking and co-morbidities such as primary malignancy, various infections, collagen vascular disease, diabetes mellitus, and hypertension (Bentzen and Overgaard 1994).

18.2   LOW LEVEL IRRADIATION

It is now known that biological effects of low-dose radiation are far more complex than predicted by the linear no-threshold model. The adaptive-response model and the bystander effect clearly illustrate this complexity. The adaptive-response model postulates that certain doses of low-dose radiation may be beneficial. Usually the adaptive response is induced with 1–100 mGy of γ-rays. It is important to note that a 1 mGy dose of γ-rays generates on average one track of clustered reactive oxygen species per nucleus and is therefore considered the lowest dose that can affect a whole cell culture or animal (Rothkamm and Lobrich 2003). With 1 mGy, approximately 3% of irradiated cells undergo a DNA double strand break. This model

was first proposed in 1984 to explain the finding that cultures of human lymphocytes growing in low concentrations of radioactive thymidine developed fewer chromosomal aberrations than cultures of non-radioactive lymphocytes when both were challenged with high-dose radiation (Olivieri *et al.* 1984). On the other hand, the bystander-effect model, postulates that low-dose radiation may be even more damaging than that predicted by the linear no-threshold model. It has been reported that 1% of cells in cell cultures directly irradiated with an α-particle, 'transmitted' the chromosomal damage to 30% of the total cell population (Nagasawa and Little 1992), via cell-to-cell communication.

Radiation-induced bystander effects are a subject of great interest both in radiation protection and, lately, in radiotherapy. It was concluded that bystander effects (radiation-induced effects detected in non-irradiated cells) predominate at low doses. The possible impact of bystander effects in radiotherapy has become a hotly debated topic, since normal tissue effects might be more pronounced than previously thought.

In contrast, studies have shown that low doses of radiation can induce an adaptive response in the exposed cells, making them resistant to subsequent doses. There is, therefore, evidence of conflicting phenomena at low doses: *bystander effects* which exaggerate the effect of radiation at low doses and *adaptive response* which confers resistance to subsequent fractions of radiation.

18.3   DETERMINISTIC AND STOCHASTIC EFFECTS OF RADIATION

Radiation can cause both cell loss and mutations. The two effects that can arise after exposing the living matter to ionising radiation are either deterministic or stochastic in nature.

18.3.1 Deterministic effects

Deterministic effects arise from lethally damaged cells which, depending on the amount of damage can, eventually, impair the function of the affected organ or tissue. A small radiation dose can lead to cell loss without affecting the exposed tissue or organ. However, if the dose is greater than a certain threshold dose, the probability of causing damage increases with the dose: higher dose implies more cell loss. Thus, not only is the incidence of an effect dose dependent but the severity of the damage as well.

18.3.2 Stochastic effects

Stochastic effects arise from non-lethally damaged clonogenic cells. Most clonogenic cells will be eliminated by the body's defence system however, the probability of one of the clones developing into a cancerous cell will depend on the initial number of mutated clones. Therefore, the probability of malignancy is dependent on the initial dose of radiation that led to mutation.

An irradiated cell which is still viable but undergoes mutation can lead to carcinogenesis or hereditary effects. If the effect (mutation) occurs in germ cells the damage can be genetic or hereditary. When somatic cells are exposed to radiation the interaction with the DNA can lead to damage which, if misrepaired, may result in transformation of the cell into a malignant clone. The probability of cancer increases with dose, however, the severity of cancer is not dose-related (cancer caused by a small dose of radiation is not better or worse than cancer produced by a larger dose).

The process of carcinogenesis appears to be random although some individuals might be more susceptible through genetic or environmental predisposition.

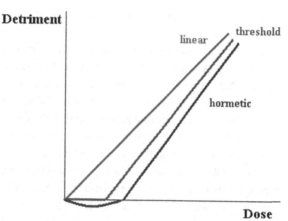

Figure 18.1. Detriment as a function of dose.

18.3.3 Detriment

Detriment is a measure of the total harm that will result after exposure to radiation. Generally, the detriment from radiation is considered to be caused by stochastic effects, since for deterministic effects the equivalent doses are below the threshold.

There are three possible models investigating the relationship between detriment and dose: the linear no-threshold, the threshold and the hormetic models (Figure 18.1).

The linear, no-threshold (LNT) theory of radiation was originated in the 1950s as a prudent operational guideline. In some opinions, the LNT theory was never more than a working hypothesis, which has acquired the appearance of fact even though no one has ever generated any evidence for it. The theory has been derived from direct extrapolation of the harm at high exposures of radiation to the very small doses to which all living cells are exposed to. It would, therefore, follow that even the natural background

Table 18.2. Characteristics of deterministic and stochastic effects of ionising radiation.

	Deterministic effects	Stochastic effects
Damage	Sufficient cells killed to impair function of organ	DNA damage in single cell
Severity	Dependent on dose	Independent of dose
Time delay	Prompt: days–months	Latent period: 5–30 years
Dose threshold	Yes	No
Incidence of an effect	Dependent on dose	Dependent on dose
Example	Cataract	Cancer

radiation with an average value of 2.4 mSv/year could lead to carcinogenesis.

The principal basis for the LNT is theoretical, and very simple. A single particle of radiation hitting a single DNA molecule in a single cell nucleus of a human body can initiate a cancer. The probability of a cancer initiation is therefore proportional to the number of such hits, which is proportional to the number of particles of radiation, therefore to the dose.

The problem with this simple argument is that factors other than initiating events affect the cancer risk. Our bodies have biological defence mechanisms which prevent the vast majority of initiating events from developing into a fatal cancer. For instance:

- Our bodies produce DNA repair enzymes, which repair the effects of initiating events with high efficiency.
- Cancer development is a multi-stage process, and consideration must be given to how radiation may affect stages other than initiation.
- Radiation can alter cell-cycle timing, which can affect cancer development. Damage repair is effective only until the next mitosis, so changing this available time can be important.
- There is fine evidence that the immune system plays an important role in preventing cancer development, and its potency can be altered by radiation.

A completely opposing theory to the linear no-threshold one is radiation hormesis. There are now substantial cellular and molecular investigations indicating that low-level exposures to radiation can cause adaptive responses, therefore enabling protection from subsequent irradiation. It was indicated that such defence mechanisms prevent and repair DNA damage, and reduce the number of surviving mutations.

18.4   RADIATION HORMESIS

The 'no threshold' hypothesis of the radiation effects on cells is a very controversial one since an obvious conclusion resulting from this theory is that even the natural background radiation is harmful. For estimating risk factors for radiation carcinogenesis, epidemiological studies of about 90 000 survivors of the

nuclear attack in Japan have been made (Jaworowski 1997). The studies indicated that cancers are induced by doses thousands of times higher than the annual dose from background radiation.

After the acceptance of a threshold dose for biological damage, studies have been undertaken for doses below the threshold value (very low dose radiation). While a few years ago the low dose radiation was considered harmful, now the other side of the coin is supposed to be true: very low dose radiation has beneficial effects. The positive effect of radiation on humans is called radiation hormesis. The word 'hormesis' is derived from the Greek word 'hormaein' which means 'to excite' and it was founded by Southam and Erlich in 1943. Hormesis is an effect where an agent given in a small dose acts like a stimulant but it is an inhibitor in large doses (examples of such agents: medication, alcohol, radiation from the Sun). In other words, low doses of various agents evoke a biopositive effect while large doses of the same agents produce a bionegative effect.

The first complete report on radiation hormesis was published in 1980 by Luckey. His work consists of an ample review of pro-hormesis reports (Luckey 1980). His message through the publication is that 'small and large doses induce opposite physiologic results'.

The main concern in radiation protection at molecular level is protection of DNA. It is a well-known fact that high doses of radiation are damaging to the DNA, suppressing the DNA-damage-control biosystem. It was shown that low dose radiation is able to stimulate and improve the DNA damage-control which results in a reduced number of misrepaired and non-repaired breaks within the double helix (Pollycove 1998). Several experiments have been conducted with invertebrates kept in radiation-deficient conditions. The general result was that their optimal development was unachieved, therefore the conclusion that small doses of radiation are vital for good health. Many biological mechanisms are stimulated by low dose radiation: protein synthesis, gene activation, detoxication of free radicals, stimulation of the immune system, etc. These mechanisms were observed in bacteria, plants, animals and also in humans (Table 18.3).

In dealing with hormesis there is no clear demarcation between a harmful and a harmless dose. Although

Table 18.3. Biological mechanisms stimulated by low dose radiation in plants, animals and humans.

Receptor	Biological effect
Bacteria Plants Animals	stimulation of protein synthesis
	gene activation
	detoxication of free radicals
	stimulation of the immune system
Humans Animals Plants	increased growth
	increased fertility
	increased longevity
	reduction in cancer frequency

the concept of radiation hormesis is usually applied to physiological benefits from low LET radiation in the range of 1–50 cGy, some other publications consider the level of background radiation as low dose. Whatever the exact dose range, there is a common agreement regarding the hormetic outcomes of low level exposure (Sagan 1987): increased longevity, increased growth and fertility of both plants and animals and a reduction in cancer frequency.

Even if hormesis, as a concept, was not recognised in unanimity and there are many controversial theories regarding the biopositive effect of low dose radiation, there is a strong logical support behind it: hormesis has an evolutionary basis. The actual radiation background is lower than hundreds of thousands of years ago when many species of plants and animals which disappeared along the centuries have grown and thrived in those conditions, and many of them were more developed than the common ones nowadays. Since background radiation was always present and it is part of our environment, each organism became adapted to these conditions, so humankind is living with radiation.

18.5 NATURAL BACKGROUND RADIATION

Naturally occurring radioactive materials are widely dispersed throughout the Earth's crust and also in the air. There are some very long lived radionuclides that have existed within the Earth since its formation and have not substantially decayed. The most important

are ^{40}K ($t_{1/2} = 1.28 \times 10^9$ y), ^{87}Rb (4.7×10^{10} y), ^{238}U (4.47×10^9 y), ^{232}Th (1.41×10^{10} y). Cosmic radiation varies with altitude while the dispersion of terrestrial radioactive materials depends on the local geological composition of the earth. Therefore, there are areas with higher natural background radiation, due to both higher altitude (compared to sea level) and geologically 'richer' soil.

The average annual dose of background radiation is calculated to be about 2.4 mSv. Obviously, regions around the world with higher-than-average altitudes and more radioactive soils would have several times higher background radiation levels.

There are a few regions in the world with a high natural radiation background. Common sources for the unusual radiation levels are coastal monazite sands and granite-rich locations. One high background radiation area is Kerala (India), where more than 100 000 people receive an annual dose of about 13 mSv. Brazil has a high radiation background region too, Guarapari, also a coastal area, where 30 000 people are exposed to 5 mSv/y, more than double the normal average. Similar values were found in Guangdong province in China (6.4 mSv/yr), since the monazite sands present in those regions are rich in thorium, uranium and also radium. In France, people from Burgundy are exposed to radiation (3.5 mSv/yr) higher than the average natural background, because of the abundance of granite rocks found there.

In some areas of Ramsar (Iran) the background radiation is exceptionally high, reaching up to 260 mSv/yr, which is 13 times higher than the 20 mSv/yr dose limit for radiation workers. This markedly high radiation level is due to the presence of very high amounts of ^{226}Ra and its decay products originated from hot springs and also the existence of large quantities of thorium in rocks and soil. Residents are using these hot springs as health spas, and the rocks as building materials. Mortazavi *et al.* (2001) and Ghiassi-nejad *et al.* (2002) have published preliminary results of the cytogenetical, immunological and hematological studies on residents of the high background radiation areas of Ramsar. They suggest that exposure to high levels of natural background radiation can induce radioadaptive response in human cells. Their studies showed that lymphocytes of

404

Ramsar residents when exposed to 1.5 Gy of gamma rays presented with fewer induced chromosome aberrations compared to residents in a nearby normal background control area whose lymphocytes were subjected to the same radiation dose.

No excess incidence of cancer have been observed in the high natural radiation background areas, however, higher number of chromosomal aberrations leading to Down's syndrome were detected, compared to regions with normal background radiation.

18.6 BYSTANDER EFFECTS AND ADAPTIVE RESPONSES TO RADIATION

For over half a century it has been accepted that radiation-induced damage required radiation interaction with the cellular DNA. This interaction could occur by either direct ionisation or by indirect ionisation, via hydroxyl radicals produced in water molecules close to the DNA. However, over the past few decades, several experimental studies have shown that there is no need for interaction between cellular DNA and radiation in order to produce damage characteristic to ionising radiation. The phenomenon by which unirradiated cells, in the vicinity of irradiated cells, present with radiation-specific injury is called the bystander effect.

Bystander effects are radiation-induced effects observed in non-irradiated cells in the proximity of irradiated cells (Figure 18.2a).

The most common experimental method to demonstrate the viability of bystander effects is the microbeam experiment ('single-cell microbeam') in which cells on a Petri dish are individually irradiated by a predefined number of α particles, allowing an individual assessment of the cells. Typically, the experiment shows a larger number of cells with radiation-induced damage than the cells traversed by the α particles. Several experimental groups have developed single-cell microbeams to evidence cellular changes through bystander effects (Geard *et al.* 1991; Nelson *et al.* 1996; Folkard *et al.* 1997).

Another method substantiating the existence of radiation-induced bystander effects is the use of growth medium harvested from irradiated cells (from exposed Petri dishes or flasks) on non-irradiated cells (Figure 18.2b). There is evidence for release of a survival controlling signal into the medium during irradiation (Mothersill and Seymour 1998), suggesting that cell-to-cell contact is not necessary to induce bystander effect when irradiated medium is transferred to the non-irradiated cells.

Therefore, bystander effects can be identified through:

- direct methods (direct cell-to-cell contact), when cells are irradiated and the biological effect of radiation observed in the neighbouring cells;
- indirect methods (irradiated cells are not in contact with the non-irradiated cells), when the growth

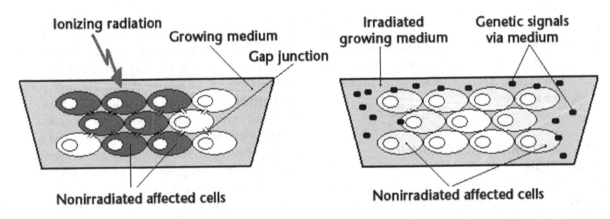

a) bystander effect via gap junction   b) bystander effect via irradiated medium

Figure 18.2. Illustration of the bystander effect by a) cell-to-cell communication via postulated gap junctions; b) via signals from medium transferred from irradiated cells.

medium is transferred from irradiated cells to non-irradiated cells and the biological effects observed on the non-irradiated cell population.

There is some indication that cell-to-cell communication via gap junctions may be more common for signals induced by high LET radiation while low LET radiation induces bystander signals that are transferred to unexposed cells through medium. However the evidence for a clear-cut difference is not strong (Lorimore and Wright 2003).

Possible mechanisms proposed to be involved in this phenomenon include endocytosis of toxic cell debris, apoptosis, exposure to soluble toxins, involvement of undefined immune responses, or blood vessel destruction (Mesnil *et al.* 1996).

In the 1960s Subak-Sharpe postulated that 'a cell in contact with a different cell may be capable – at least for some time – of a metabolic function for which it lacks genetic information (Subak-Sharpe *et al.* 1969). Thus, in a monolayer, an individual cell's metabolic capability would not be totally limited by the cell's own genotype, but rather by the total gene pool of all the cells with which it is directly or indirectly in contact'. It has now been scientifically proven that the damage to the non-irradiated cells is transmitted by intercellular signals through gap junctions, which are small channels that are formed between neighbouring cells and allow the sharing of small molecules and ions (Trosko *et al.* 1993; Krutovskikh *et al.* 2002). It has been reported that the bystander effect is of a much larger magnitude when cells are in such close proximity to allow gap junction communication, than that able to be demonstrated in medium transfer experiments (Hall 2003).

The exact type of the signals involved in the bystander effect is still under investigation. However, there is some evidence that oxidative stress may play a role in the damage inflicted to neighbouring cells. The evidence is based on the observation that reactive oxygen species are highly cytotoxic and could theoretically pass through the gap junctions directly, or their production induced by other signalling molecules. The notion that hypoxic cells present with reduced, or even absent bystander effects is therefore possible. It is also likely that normal, well oxygenated cells experience more pronounced bystander effects than hypoxic cells.

Some of the common bystander effects or biological end points which are evidenced after both low-dose and high-dose (radiotherapy) irradiation are: chromosomal instability, cell killing and delayed cell death, mutagenesis, micronucleus formation, gene and protein expression changes. Through these end points it is likely that bystander effects can be both detrimental and beneficial. By increasing mutation levels of cells bystander effects increase the likelihood of genetic defects and in turn cancer. On the other hand by removing damaged cells from the population and preventing the growth of cancer cells, bystander effects are beneficial. It is assumed that both beneficial and detrimental effects occur at the same time (Waldren 2004).

There is published evidence that bystander mechanisms following irradiation are possibly involved in adaptive responses. Published data for low dose, low LET radiation demonstrates that signals produced by irradiated cells can induce protection against higher doses of radiation (Mothersill and Seymour 2002). Although cell death is a common response following exposure to bystander signals, this can be considered a protective response, as damaged cells will be stoped from undergoing further divisions which ultimately lead to mutagenesis and carcinogenesis. In experiments simulating fractionated treatment, the first dose of radiation has proven to be more effective than subsequent doses. This observation was equally valid whether the first radiation dose was directly targeting the cells or the dose has derived from bystander medium (medium harvested from previously irradiated cells and used on non-irradiated culture). These experiments (Mothersill and Seymour 2002) conflict with the still accepted 'isoeffect per fraction' theory, since cell kill varied significantly between the first and subsequent doses.

Experiments on mouse embryonic fibroblast cell line cultures (C3H 10T1/2) have been conducted to assess the relative importance of the adaptive response and the bystander effect induced by radiation (Sawant *et al.* 2001a). Single-cell microbeam was delivered from 1 to 12 alpha particles through the nuclei of 10% of the cultured cells observing that more cells were inactivated than hit by alpha particles. It was noticed that the magnitude of this bystander effect increased with the number of particles per cell. To assess the extent of the adaptive response to radiation, the cells were irradiated beforehand with 2 cGy of γ rays, which has cancelled out around half of the bystander effect produced by the alpha particles. The results are in agreement with the data published by Azzam *et al.* (1994) on pre-exposure of C3H 10T1/2 cells to low-dose γ radiation showing a reduction in oncogenic transformation frequency after exposure to a 4 Gy challenge dose.

The cellular adaptive response to ionising radiation is manifested through: reduction in chromosome aberrations, reduction of mutation frequency and also reduction in micronucleus formation.

The two processes are conflicting in the sense that they operate in opposite directions (Table 18.4):

- the bystander effect, enhances the effect of low doses, and
- the adaptive response, confers resistance to a subsequent dose.

While the bystander effect can induce some biological endpoints (such as chromosomal instability, cell killing and delayed cell death, mutagenesis, micronucleus formation, gene and protein expression changes) which can be detrimental, these endpoints can be considered at the same time beneficial, through removal of damaged cells from the population and prevention of cell growth of mutated origin. Furthermore, signals produced by irradiated cells can induce protection against a subsequent (and also higher) dose of ionising radiation, conferring them adaptive response. The two mechanisms of bystander effects and adaptive response dominating at low doses are part of the cellular homeostatic response and there is little evidence that they translate into harm. This could, therefore, imply that low doses of radiation induce radiation hormesis.

18.7 BYSTANDER EFFECTS AND CLINICAL IMPLICATIONS

Bystander effects induced by various LET radiation have been experimentally demonstrated in both tumour and normal cells. Therefore, bystander effects could have clinical implications, influencing the whole process of treatment planning and delivery.

18.7.1 Bystander effects and implications for head & neck cancer

Bystander effects have been observed *in vivo* after partial organ irradiation. Khan *et al.* (1998) showed in rat experiments that when the base of the lung was irradiated, there was a marked increase in the frequency of micronuclei in the shielded lung apex. The same phenomenon occurred in the right lung when the left was exposed to radiation. These experiments suggest the presence of a bystander effect which has significant biological implications in radiotherapy.

The finding that gamma-ray-induced bystander effects affect *epithelial cells* and not fibroblasts, suggested that tissue architecture and also cell communication play a significant role in this process (Mothersill and Seymour 1997). Since squamous cell carcinomas originate from epithelial cells, the bystander effect becomes an important consideration in the treatment of head & neck tumours.

In normal tissues, gap junctions physiologically connect one cell to the one adjacent to it in order to facilitate the transmission of genetic signals between cells. Gap junctions are required for metabolic cooperation between cells and for regulation of normal tissue

Table 18.4. Consequences of bystander effect versus adaptive response.

Bystander effect	Adaptive response
chromosomal instability	reduction in chromosome aberrations
cell killing/delayed cell death	
mutagenesis	reduction of mutation frequency
micronucleus formation	reduction in micronucleus formation
changes in gene and protein expression	

homeostasis through the transfer of small molecules between neighbouring cells. This normal phenotype is usually lost during head & neck carcinogenesis.

Though the whole function of gap junctions in malignant head & neck tissues is not fully elucidated, experimental studies demonstrate that gap junctional intercellular communication (GJIC) could mediate apoptotic cell death in non-targeted squamous cell carcinoma adjacent to individually targeted squamous cell carcinomas of the head & neck (SCCHN) (Frank *et al.* 2005). While bystander effect (apoptosis) was observed in non-targeted cells after single-cell microinjection of cytochrome c (protein that mediates apoptosis), blocking GJIC activity with a specific pharmacologic inhibitor of gap junctions, (18-beta-glycerretinic acid) abolished the bystander effect in the experiment.

Novel therapeutic methods like gene therapy are widely used to investigate bystander effects in cancers including head & neck carcinomas. A number of viral vectors have been developed that are able to transfer genes to therapy of tumours known as gene transduction. The presence and requirements of a bystander effect after wild-type p53 gene transduction have been investigated for human squamous cell carcinomas of the head & neck (Frank *et al.* 1998). Wild-type p53 gene transduction for apoptosis-inducing molecular therapy has been shown capable of producing a bystander effect in SCCHN *in vitro,* and that this phenomenon requires intercellular contact between wild-type p53 transduced and bystander (non-transduced) cell populations. The study concluded that other therapies associated with apoptosis (like radiotherapy, chemotherapy) may also demonstrate bystander effects.

Despite encouraging *in vitro* studies in head & neck squamous cell carcinoma (Frank *et al.* 1998), initial clinical trials with adenovirus-mediated gene therapy have been disappointing. Although the adenovirus is a highly efficient vector, its effectiveness for *in vivo* transduction is still limited (Li *et al.* 1999).

Another gene, the E1A tumour suppressor, which was once thought to cause cancer when altered, has been shown to induce bystander effect by inhibiting angiogenesis and inducing apoptosis (Shao *et al.* 2000). Preclinical gene therapy studies have shown that complete growth suppression can be achieved by incomplete transfer of E1A into tumours, suggesting therefore an association of E1A with bystander effects.

Enhancing gap-junctional intercellular communication in squamous cell carcinomas of the head & neck and also understanding the other mechanisms by which cancer cells communicate with each other may, eventually lead to increased therapeutic efficacy. Furthermore, bystander effects might have a key role in the future development and implementation of gene therapy, as only a fraction of the tumour cells is transfected with the gene.

18.7.2 Bystander effects and implications for prostate cancer

While the most common method to evidence the viability of bystander effects is the use of alpha particle microbeam, the number of studies employing gamma rays for the same purpose is increasing. The LET dependence of the bystander effect was extensively studied and debated, the current literature results remaining inconclusive. Anzenberg *et al.* (2008) has conducted a study on DU-145 prostate cell lines investigating the LET dependence of the bystander effect. The group studied the ability of DU-145 human prostate carcinoma cells irradiated with either alpha particles or 250 kVp X-rays to cause medium-interceded bystander effects in two unirradiated populations (one prostate tumour cell line and one human fibroblast). Two of the monitored endpoints were micronucleus formation and surviving fraction. It was observed that the incidence of micronuclei increased 1.5–2.0-fold in both tumour and fibroblast bystander cells when co-cultured with directly irradiated cells with either alpha or X-rays. However, only the fibroblasts showed bystander effects for surviving fraction, specifically a decrease to 0.8, when co-cultured with cell directly exposed to X-rays. Consequently, the study concluded that there are LET-dependent differences in the signal released from DU-145 human prostate carcinoma.

Retinoic acid, a derivative of vitamin A, has been shown to have significant anticancer activity in both pre-clinical and clinical studies involving prostate cancer (Huss *et al.* 2004; Webber *et al.* 1999). There is experimental proof that all-trans retinoic acid (ATRA) has an inhibitive effect on malignant tumour growth by altering gap junctional intercellular communication. It was shown that alteration of gap junctional communication by ATRA may directly enhance the bystander effects of suicide gene therapy against prostate cancer, both *in vitro* and *in vivo* (Chen W *et al.* 2008).

18.7.3 Bystander effects and implications for lung cancer

The bystander effect of carbon ions (220 MeV) on human lung cancer cells was investigated using microbeam irradiation (Harada *et al.* 2009). The bystander effect was materialised through an increase in cell death by clonogenic assay, a response which was suppressed when cells were treated with an inhibitor of gap junctional intercellular communication and enhanced when a GJIC stimulator was added. These observations led to the conclusion that bystander effects induced by heavy ions are channelled via direct cell-to-cell communication. These results reinforce previous pre-clinical observations by which cell-to-cell communication via gap junctions are more common for signals induced by high LET radiation while low LET radiation induces medium-mediated bystander signals (Lorimore and Wright 2003).

In vitro studies on human lung cancer cell lines of different radiosensitivities involving I-125 seeds investigated the bystander effect of low dose rate irradiation (Chen H *et al.* 2008). Cells directly exposed to I-125 were co-cultured with unirradiated cells for 24 hours. Through the assessment of micronuclei and apoptosis it was concluded that low dose rate radiation has the potential to induce bystander effects, independent of tumour radioresistance, a result that could compensate for the non-uniform dose distribution of I-125 implant in clinical settings.

Similar to the above study, another investigation focused on the effect of *high dose radiation*-induced bystander signalling on two lung cell lines with different radiosensitivities (Shareef *et al.* 2007). While one cell line (A549) was found to be more resistant when co-cultured with the irradiated A549 cells, the other cell line (H460) presented with an increased bystander response after being co-cultured with the exposed H460 cells. The reduced bystander response in the A549 cell line was considered to be due to the significant release of tumour necrosis factor-alpha (TNF-

alpha), whereas the increased response of H460 cells was attributable to the release of TNF-related apoptosis-inducing ligand (TRAIL).

18.8 RADIATION INCIDENTS AND RADIATION ACCIDENTS IN MEDICAL ENVIRONMENT

A *radiation accident* is considered to be a deviation from normal operations of an apparatus that produces or uses radiation or radioactive materials, or activities associated with a hazard which has the potential to result in a radiation emergency. *Radiation incident* is caused by any deviation from normal operations of apparatus that produces or uses radiation or activities associated with a hazard which has the potential to result in a radiation emergency (radiation exposure to humans or environment), with lesser magnitude than a radiation accident.

The first radiation accident in a medical environment occurred in 1896 in Chicago, consisting of radiography overexposure, when a man with a broken ankle X-rayed by a doctor developed severe skin injuries after diagnosis, eventually requiring amputation of the foot (Berlin 2001).

The use of radiological apparatus became widespread in the second half of the 20th century, together with the acceptance of the benefits of both radiodiagnostic and radiotherapy. However, the mounting use of radiation for medical purposes led to an increase in accidents and incidents involving insufficiently experienced personnel. Overexposure during diagnosis or during source replacement, accidental exposure to Co-60 and mishandling of radioisotopes are some examples of the most common radiation accidents which have occurred in the past. Several accidents could have been prevented should the involved personnel have been suitably trained and compliant with basic radioprotection requirements.

Prevention is always better than dealing with the consequences, especially in a radiation environment: it is much easier preventing an accident than cleaning up a spill or managing the side effects of radiation exposure. The number of reported radiation incidents and accidents in medical environment has considerably dropped over the last decades. While in the 1970s and the 1980s the number of radiation accidents in

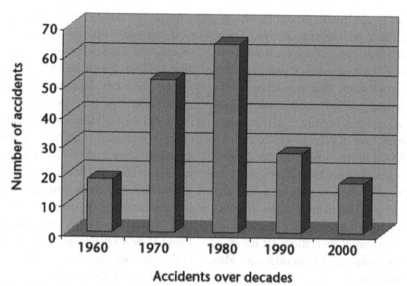

Figure 18.3. Medical radiation accidents over five decades which have produced radiation casualties.

medical environment reached its peak, in the 21st century the number of the reported accidents was considerably smaller (Figure 18.3) (Johnston 2010).

18.9 BIOLOGICAL DOSIMETRY

It is difficult to establish a prognosis for individuals irradiated above the threshold doses for acute effects solely from an estimate of the dose, because of the steepness and uncertainty in the dose-response curves, including uncertainty of the value of the LD50/60 for man.

Biological dosimetry (or biodosimetry) represents a useful tool in determining the radiation dose a person has been accidentally exposed to. By definition, biological dosimetry is a diagnostic method for the measurement of the individual dose absorbed in the case of accidental overexposure to ionising radiation. Scientists worldwide are focusing on the development of bioassays, in order to standardise the techniques that would assist biodosimetry. Some of the key elements in the process of developing a complete bioassay program are the following:

- to establish the conventional cytogenetic assay and also the blood cell (lymphocyte) depletion kinetic bioassay
- to develop a biodosimetry assay system that is based on chromosomal aberrations and permits

rapid, high-throughput radiation exposure assessment for large numbers of casualties
- to identify and validate radiation-responsive molecular biomarkers (gene expression, DNA mutations, encoded proteins).

After an accidental exposure, the most specific method to estimate the exposure dose is scoring of unstable chromosome aberrations (dicentrics, centric rings and acentrics) in peripheral blood lymphocytes. Chromosome analysis is largely based on the counting of uniformly stained dicentrics in metaphase preparations of peripheral lymphocytes. It is an accurate method for estimating absorbed doses within some weeks after acute, largely uniform whole-body exposures. Calibration curves for dicentric chromosomes have been established for gamma rays, x rays, 14-MeV neutrons, fission neutrons and tritium exposures. The method is capable of measuring acute doses from gamma rays as low as 150 mGy (ICRU report). This technique has been used for dose reconstruction following the Chernobyl nuclear power plant accident on some of the workers. For longer times after exposure, the yield of dicentrics in peripheral blood declines because of a decreasing chance of survival of cells carrying these unstable aberrations during mitotic divisions.

There were speculations whether past exposure to ionising radiation leaves a distinctive and permanent mark in the genome. Such a biomarker would definitely have a strong impact on epidemiologic studies on cancer causation and also on genetics. It was shown (Hande *et al.* 2003) that there is a long-lived, low-background and sensitive biomarker of past exposure to densely ionising radiation. This biomarker relates to the frequency of large, stable (transmissible to subsequent cell generation) intrachromosomal rearrangements (like inversion or deletion), which can be measured in the blood of irradiated individuals several years after exposure. This biomarker relates to high LET particles, since densely ionising radiations produce highly localised DNA damage at the chromosomal level, with multiple breaks within single chromosomes (*intrachromosomal* aberration) (Prise *et al.* 2001). X-rays, other mutagens (chemicals) and also aging, produce a more homogenous spatial distribution of DNA damage, therefore they are more likely to cause *interchromosomal* aberration (translocations). The method of detecting intrachromosomal aberrations is called 'mBAND' and consists of chromosome-painting techniques: a series of coloured bands are painted along the axis of the chromosomes, therefore any loss or change in the order of the coloured bands indicates an intrachromosomal rearrangement (Chudoba *et al.* 1999).

A disadvantage of the above described assay is that relatively high skill and a long time (4 to 5 days) is required for a precise analysis. An alternative method is the micronucleus (MN) test, which is less time consuming, having a great potential for automation. This test is based on the observation that dividing cells with chromatid[1] breaks display instabilities in the anaphase distribution of their chromatin.[2] After telophase the displaced chromatin can be excluded from the nuclei of the daughter cells. Micronuclei would then arise from the small chromatin fragments (or entire chromosomes) remaining in the cytoplasm during cell division. They resemble in most aspects the cell nucleus except for the size (therefore the name 'micronuclei'). Micronuclei are predominantly scored in peripheral lymphocytes. Dose reconstruction by

counting micronuclei in lymphocytes is mostly limited to the determination of average doses in population groups. The induction of micronuclei as a function of dose has been determined for gamma rays, x rays and 14-MeV neutrons. However, the disadvantage of the micronucleus test is a weak sensitivity at the low dose range of ionising radiation (doses as low as 300 mGy may be measured), resulting predominantly from a high individual variability of the spontaneous micronucleus frequency. There are currently studies on how to combine the classic micronucleus test with centromere detection (Wojcik *et al.* 2000).

A decline in absolute lymphocyte count has been found to be a reliable and practical method to assess radiation dose after an accidental exposure (within hours or days, depending on dose). It requires approximately 4 days for the lymphocyte count to decline into the abnormal range for individuals receiving a dose of 2 Gy, and approximately 2 days for individuals receiving a dose of 4 Gy.

Tests of the proliferative ability of the marrow may also be regarded as useful dosimetric indicators. A drop in the mitotic index, for example, is a sign of doses higher than 1 Gy. The migration of granulocytes into the bloodstream after the injection of ethiocholanolon suggests the active production of granulocytes by the bone marrow. Cultures of mixed-cell colonies and granulocyte/macrophage colonies give some indication of the concentration of precursor cells in the marrow, as a function of dose. By contrast, erythrocytes are relatively radioresistant and long-lived, and hence their concentration in the blood is a poor indicator of dose; however, marrow scans for erythropoiesis may be used to estimate marrow doses.

18.10   RADIOPROTECTORS

Radioprotectors are chemical agents able to reduce the biological effects of radiation. Radioprotectors are used in radiotherapy to increase the therapeutic ratio by decreasing normal tissue complications, and also in the field of radiation protection to ameliorate the effects of an accidental exposure to ionising radiation.

Under normoxic conditions radiation-damaged cells are prone to apoptotic death due to the irreparable damage resulting from the interaction of the

---

1   chromatid is the name given to each of the two strands of chromosomes while they are still attached to each other at the centromere after replication in the early phase of mitosis.
2   chromatin is a complex of eukaryotic DNA combined with proteins.

highly reactive free radical $RO_2\bullet$ with the cells (see also the oxygen effect):

$$R\bullet + O_2 \rightarrow RO_2\bullet \qquad (18.1)$$

In this way, cells become highly sensitised to radiation damage. Oxygen is by far the most effective radiosensitiser. This is evidenced by the results of clinical trials comparing the radiation response of normally oxygenated tumours with that of hypoxic tumours.

On the other hand, the most effective radioprotection is achieved in the absence of oxygen. In order to protect cells against radiation-induced damage, the free radicals (ionised molecules) should be restored to their normal state. Another way of achieving radioprotection is to use sulphydryl compounds, agents with a -SH bond which by virtue of being endogenous hydrogen donors compete with the oxygen molecule for the free radical:

$$R\bullet + -SH \rightarrow RH + -S \qquad (18.2)$$

Starting in 1959 in the US, several studies were conducted to identify and synthesise radio-protective drugs with minimal toxic effects on tissue. One breakthrough in this area was the realisation that sulphydryl compounds covered by a phosphate group are much less toxic than the original –SH compounds. Inside the cell, the phosphate group is stripped, and the sulphydryl group starts scavenging free radicals. The first developed sulphydryl compounds (cysteine, cysteamine) have proved toxic in the concentrations necessary to be effective in clinical situations. The next class of radioprotectors, the thiophosphates, have no toxic effect on normal tissue, but their protective potential is only realised after activation by enzymatic conversion inside the cell.

Sulphydryl compounds are naturally occurring radioprotectors, found in measurable amounts in cells, nevertheless in too small concentrations in order to compete with the oxygen molecule for the free radical ($R\bullet$).

Previously known as WR-2721, amifostine is an agent which is currently used in radiotherapy as a radio-protector. Amifostine is a prodrug meaning that it becomes active, inside the normal tissues only after dephosphorylation by the enzyme alkaline phosphatase, which is either not present in tumours or not active in the low pH environment found in tumours.

This drug has been originally developed by the U.S. Walter Reed Army Institute of Research in the 1950s as a radio-protective agent for military personnel in a classified nuclear warfare project. Following project declassification it was investigated as a cytoprotective drug against cisplatin and other cytotoxic agents including radiation therapy.

Protection of normal tissue to a greater extent than tumours is achieved through preferential uptake of amifostine by normal tissue and also by differences in the alkaline phosphatase concentrations of normal versus tumour tissues. The differential uptake of amifostine by normal tissue versus tumour tissue could be due to the differences in the membrane structure between normal and malignant cells, which slows penetration of the drug into tumours. Another cause of the slow penetration of the drug into tumours might be the poor (and abnormal) vascularisation of these tissues compared with the dense and normal vascularisation found in normal tissues.

For treatments involving total-body irradiation the drug is administered immediately before radiotherapy, at maximum tolerable concentrations. To express the effectiveness in protecting normal tissue, the Dose Reduction Factor (DRF) has been defined as:

$$DRF = \left| \frac{\textit{Dose of radiation in the presence of the drug}}{\textit{Dose of radiation in the absence of the drug}} \right|$$

for the same biologic effect

In other words, the dose reduction factor is an expression of the increase in radioresistance of the tissue under consideration.

Table 18.5 is a listing of normal tissues and their responsiveness to amifostine (DRF) (Hall 2000).

As evidenced by the dose reduction factors from Table 18.5, amifostine exerts a differential protection on the various normal tissues listed. The mechanism behind this preferential behaviour is, nevertheless, unknown. However, it is important to note that the brain and spinal cord are not protected by amifostine, probably because the drug does not cross the blood-brain barrier.

Preclinical animal studies have demonstrated that amifostine is able to reduce some of radiotherapy and chemotherapy-related toxicities (Thomas and Devi

Table 18.5. Normal tissues and their responsiveness to protection by amifostine.

Tissue	DRF
Bone marrow	2.4–3
Immune system	1.8–3.4
Skin	2–2.4
Small intestine	1.8–2
Colon	1.8
Lung	1.2–1.8
Esophagus	1.4
Kidney	1.5
Liver	2.7
Salivary gland	2.0
Oral mucosa	>1
Testes	2.1

1987; Capizzi et al. 1993; Cassatt et al. 2002). Clinical trials have confirmed the effectiveness of amifostine in diminishing certain treatment-related side effects, although some limitations of the drug delayed the introduction of amifostine into routine clinical practice. Despite the long list of preclinical normal tissues with demonstrable reduction of radiation-induced toxicities by amifostine, only few have been confirmed in the clinical settings (Lindegaard 2003).

One of the main issues regarding the clinical implementation of amifostine was the selective cytoprotection of the drug when it comes to normal and cancerous tissues. While this property of amifostine is still under clinical investigation, the findings up to now are encouraging. Based on a critical literature review Koukourakis (2003) has concluded that any experimental evidence suggesting tumour protection is weak.

18.11   RISK OF SECOND CANCER DEVELOPMENT FOLLOWING RADIATION THERAPY

Radiotherapy either alone or in combination with chemotherapy and/or surgery is an increasingly common therapeutic option for patients with cancer. However, unlike surgery, radiotherapy can poten-

tially contribute towards the development of second malignancies.

There has been some evidence that longer survival times for patients with cancer as a result of improvements in radiation therapy techniques and earlier diagnosis at younger ages contribute to an increased risk of radiation-induced carcinogenesis (Brenner et al. 2000). In general, second primary cancer is defined as a new tumor (neoplasm) which develops from normal tissue exposed to radiation and has histopathologic features different from the primary tumor ≥5 years after radiation treatment (Abdel-Wahab et al. 2008). The latent period between radiation exposure and the development of SPC is 5 to 15 years, which may be perceived as a negative long term consequence of the successful radiation therapy for cancer (Baxter et al. 2005).

In the United States, the 5-year relative survival rate of locally and regionally confined prostate cancer approaches 100% and the 5-year survival rate for all stages of prostate cancer combined has increased from 69% to almost 99% over the past 25 years (American Cancer Society 2008). The most recent data of 10-year relative survival of 91% and of 15-year relative survival of 76% has also been reported to result from earlier diagnosis and improved treatments. Hence, there is a distinct chance of the development of SPC among these long-term prostate cancer survivors after radiation therapy. However, the influence of radiation techniques on the risk of development of SPC has not been adequately studied. The need to compare radiotherapy plans in order to reduce if not avoid SPC induction is likely to increase in the future (Schneider et al. 2005).

Our knowledge about the risk of radiation-induced cancer was derived from survivors of atomic-bomb attacks on Japan. In addition, documentation of several radiation accidents worldwide and medical reports on incidence of second cancers following radiotherapy have also provided valuable insights into this area. Hall and Wuu (2003) pointed out that the malignancies observed in the Japanese A-bomb survivors' data were leukemias and cancers of the body lining cells (carcinomas) with no excess of sarcomas (cancers of the connective tissues including bone). The overall risk of fatal cancers was estimated to be 8% per Gy, with young children being 15 times more

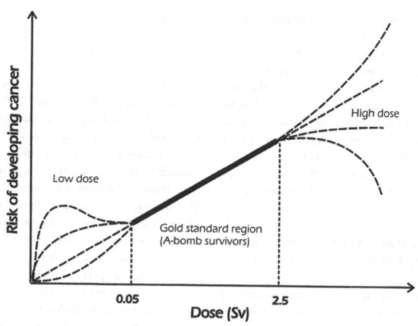

Figure 18.4. Dose-response relationship for radiation-induced carcinogenesis in humans including the dose range with the best quantitative data and the dose ranges where there is considerable uncertainty. (Reprinted from Hall 2006. Copyright (2006), with permission from Elsevier)

sensitive than middle-aged adults. In second cancers induced by radiation used to treat cancer, carcinomas were as prevalent as in A-bomb survivors, especially for the normal tissues which received lower radiation doses. However, in contrast to the observations in A-bomb survivors, sarcomas were reported in tissues exposed to high radiation doses. The best quantitative data or gold standard for radiation-induced carcinogenesis in humans is derived from epidemiological data obtained from Japanese A-bomb survivors which shows a clear dose-response relationship especially for the 0.1 to 2.5 Gy dose range (Figure 18.4).

Apart from the dose range where there is a clear dose-response relationship between radiation dose and carcinogenesis, major uncertainties exist in the relationship for the low dose and high dose regions (Figure 18.4). In radiotherapy the low dose region is represented by the tissues which are located remotely from the treatment fields. These tissues receive small but significant doses (especially from external beam therapy). The high dose region is represented by the tissues which are located in the vicinity of, if not within the radiation treatment fields where moder-

ately high doses of radiation are delivered for the tissues to survive the injury and be capable of continued proliferation. By measuring the doses which different tissues receive during therapeutic irradiation, the associated risks of Second Primary Cancer (SPC) can be calculated to provide information in the regions of uncertainty.

Improvements in radiotherapeutic techniques and earlier diagnosis have resulted in longer survival times for patients with treated prostate carcinoma. The longer survival times, particularly in younger patients are likely to result in increased risks of radiation-related second malignancy which will impact on decisions relating to choice of treatment (Brenner *et al.* 2000). Improvements in radiotherapy techniques, like Intensity Modulated Radiation Therapy (IMRT), have inadvertently increased the possibility for the induction of potentially fatal second cancers outside of the treatment field through secondary radiations (scatter and leakage). Assessment of the risk of second malignancy in association with the out-of-field secondary radiations resulting from different radiation treatment techniques is also needed to assist in treatment choice.

18.11.1   Evaluations of the second primary cancer risk

Generally, there are two main approaches to evaluate the risk of second primary cancers: *an epidemiologic study* and *model-based risk estimation*. In the first approach, two classic epidemiologic study designs using cohort and case-control methodologies have been used in most studies of therapy-related cancers (Travis 2006). Details of this approach will not be discussed here but results of several epidemiologic studies of second primary cancers after prostate cancer irradiation are summarised in Table 18.6.

18.11.2   Estimation of second primary cancer risks using radiation dosimetric data and risk models

Apart from epidemiologic studies, measurements of radiation doses in normal organs/tissues located close to or at a distance to the planning target volume (PTV) can be used to estimate the risk of second primary cancer using existing models (Takam *et al.* 2009). Radiation dosimetric data can be in the form of dose-volume histograms (DVHs) generated from the treatment plan of the particular radiation technique for organs/tissues located within or close to the PTV. Radiation dose data can also be obtained from direct measurement using various radiation dosimetry techniques. The appropriate risk estimation model is then applied to the dose data to determine the risk of second primary cancer.

As mentioned previously, the main sources of knowledge relating to the risks of radiation-induced cancer are derived from A-bomb survivors in Japan; from radiation accidents and from medically exposed individuals including exposure to radiation therapy (Hall and Wuu 2003). Although some data about induction of cancers has been collected from radiation accidents and medical exposures, the most recent Biological Effects of Ionizing Radiations (BEIR V) and The United Nations Scientific Committee on Effects of Atomic Radiation (UNSCEAR) reports base their risk estimates almost entirely on the data from survivors of the A-bomb attacks (Hall 2000).

The dose-response relationship for radiation-induced carcinogenesis for doses larger than 2 Gy is not clear, however, several estimates have been published. Schneider *et al.* (2007) confidently expects that the rela-

tionship which best represents the real situation lies between the extremes of a linear and a linear-exponential model. In practice, using the data from A-bomb survivors which covers a range of doses from 0.005 to 4 Gy, the excess incidence for solid tumors was found to be a linear function of dose (Hall 2000). This model can be applied by multiplying the average absorbed dose with a risk coefficient to calculate the risk of radiation-induced carcinogenesis, assuming that the cells mutated by the radiation exposure survive the irradiation. However, in clinical radiation therapy, the total dose delivered to patients is always larger than 2 Gy which could mean that the dose-response relationship for cancer induction is likely to be non-linear. In addition, the radiation dose is inhomogeneously distributed to organs at risk, parts of which will receive varying amounts of radiation dose. The concept of an average organ dose may not be applicable in this situation. Furthermore, when radiation doses larger than 2 Gy are delivered to the organs at risk, sterilisation of the mutated cells within the organs becomes an important consideration since this counteracts the effect of mutation and subsequently of cancer induction.

The simplest approach to estimate the risk of SPC after radiotherapy is to first calculate the average organ/tissue dose and then to apply a linear risk coefficient corrected for dose and dose rate level. For example, assuming that a half of the organ receives a dose of 1 Gy and the other half is irradiated to 19 Gy, the average dose in the organ is simply 10 Gy (Schneider *et al.* 2005). However, this method can lead to errors in the risk estimation as it does not take into account the heterogeneity of the dose distribution in the irradiated organ/tissue (Dasu and Toma-Dasu 2005). The estimated risk obtained using this method leads to an overestimate as the effect of cells sterilised by the dose of radiation is also not taken into account. Hence, this method is not applicable to clinical radiotherapy where the organs are usually exposed to radiation doses at both the low and high ends of the dose range.

Instead of using the simple average organ dose together with the linear risk coefficient to estimate the risk, the mean organ dose derived from the DVH in combination with a non-linear equation can be used which takes into account the competition between induction of mutations and cell survival (Dasu and Toma-Dasu 2005). Although such model allows for

Table 18.6. Examples of reports on the incidence and risks of second cancers after prostate cancer radiotherapy.

Reference	Radiotherapy Modality	No. of patients	Second cancer and status
Kleinerman et al. (1985)	Not stated	18 135	Except for salivary gland cancer and leukemia, 15% less for all other cancers compared with general population.
Osterlind et al. (1985)	Not stated	19 886	3% of patients developed second cancer with less than expected incidence of cancers of digestive organs and respiratory system.
Neugut et al. (1997)	Not stated	34 889	Risk of bladder but not rectal carcinoma increased. Risk of acute non-lymphocytic or chronic lymphocytic leukemia also not increased.
Pawlish et al. (1997)	Not stated	9794	Around 5.5% of patients developed bladder cancer but risk increased only for patients receiving radiotherapy as primary treatment.
Movsas et al. (1998)	Conformal and conventional 4-field	543	Overall, 5.7% of patients developed second cancers including lung, bladder, GI, and head & neck cancers.
Levi et al. (1999)	Not stated	4503	A total of 380 cases (8.4%) of second cancers reported. Incidence of lung and other tobacco-related cancers reduced.
Brenner et al. (2000)	Not stated	51 584	6.9% of prostate patients who received radiotherapy developed second cancers of the bladder, rectum, and lung as well as sarcomas.
Gershkevitsh et al. (1999)	Not stated	–	Non statistically significant increase in risk of leukemia.
Pickles and Phillips (2002)	Not stated	9890	Significantly increased risks for colo-rectal cancers and sarcoma. Overall risk of second cancers 1 in 220.
Thellenberg et al. (2003)	Not stated	135 713	Overall, second cancers found in 7.7% of patients with significantly increased risk of breast, small intestinal, renal and bladder cancers.
Abdel-Wahab et al. (2008)	EBRT, XRT and brachytherapy	228 235	Age-adjusted estimates of SPCs were higher with EBRT than brachytherapy and other treatments. Hazard ratio was constant with EBRT but increased with follow-up length in brachytherapy.
Bhojani et al. (2010)	EBRT	17 845	External beam radiotherapy may predispose patients to second cancers of the bladder, rectum and lung, with absolute differences in incident rates between surgery and EBRT ranging from 0.7 to 5.2%.
Huang et al. (2011)	Conventional, 3D-CRT, IMRT	4240	The risk of second cancers varies with the radiation technique: conventional radiotherapy presents the highest risk among current methods. Most common second cancers were found to be bladder carcinomas, sarcomas and lymphoproliferative malignancies.

the effect of sterilisation of cells from exposure to high radiation doses, it does not fully account for the inhomogeneity of the radiation dose distribution over the entire irradiated organ and therefore is subject to errors in the calculation of the estimated risk. An example of an approach based on the concept of Organ Equivalent Dose (OED) to account for inhomogeneity of dose in organs at risk in the estimation of radiation-induced second malignancy following radiotherapy was proposed by Schneider *et al.* (2005). Schneider *et al* used OED in the calculation of radiation-induced second primary cancer following 3D-CRT for Hodgkin's disease. Assuming that I_0^{org} is the low dose radiation-induced cancer incidence rate (absolute excess risk per 10 000 patients/year/Gy) of a fractionated radiotherapy schedule of a total dose D given in k fractions of dose d, the organ-specific cancer incidence rate after a single treatment session with a low dose is $I_0^{org} xd$. The number of mutated stem cells which result in the development of the malignant growth is proportionally related to the radiation-induced cancer incidence rate. However, following a single fraction of dose d, the total number of cells including the already mutated cells in the organ is, in a first approximation, reduced by $e^{-\alpha d}$ due to cells sterilisation. Providing that I_0^{org} is the organ-specific cancer incidence rate (absolute excess risk per 10 000 patients/year) after prescription of the total dose D in k fractions, accordingly the cancer incident rate of an organ/tissue as a result of fractionated irradiation is described by the following equation (Schneider *et al.* 2005):

$$I^{org} = I_0^{org} D e^{-\alpha_{org} D} \qquad (18.3)$$

where, I_0^{org} is the organ-specific cancer incidence rate for low dose irradiation as defined earlier and α_{org} is an organ-specific cell sterilisation parameter.

A dose-response curve for radiation-induced cancer of a specified organ can be derived from equation (18.3). The OED for radiation-induced cancer of the irradiated organ is then obtained from the equation as follows (Schneider *et al.* 2005):

$$OED_{org} = \frac{1}{N} \sum_{i=1}^{N} D_i e^{-\alpha_{org} D_i} \qquad (18.4)$$

where the sum is taken over N dose calculation points in the same constant volume of the organ. OED

is the dose (in Gy) distributed uniformly over the entire organ/tissue which causes the same radiation-induced cancer incidence as that if it was inhomogeneously distributed within the same organ.

In the risk estimation model described above, I_0^{org} and α_{org} are parameters which need to be known. The organ-specific cancer incidence rate at low radiation dose (I_0^{org}) can be obtained from the atomic bomb survivor data whilst the organ-specific cell sterilisation parameter (α_{org}) needs to be estimated from experiments. It has been suggested that the precision of the OED concept in the estimation of SPC risk is mainly dependent on the precision of the determination of α_{org} for the different organs (Schneider *et al.* 2005).

To fully take into consideration the inhomogeneity of the dose distribution across the entire volume of an irradiated organ as a result of radiotherapy, a non-linear competition model should be used to estimate risk at each dose interval of the DVH. Integration of these risks across the actual dose distribution over the entire organ volume would then yield the final result (Dasu and Toma-Dasu 2005). This is the basis of the competitive risk model used in estimation of the risk of radiation-induced SPC developed by Dasu and Toma-Dasu (2005) from the concept proposed by Gray (1965) (see Hall 2006). This model can be used to estimate the risk of second primary cancer in organs-at-risk following various techniques of radiation therapy for cancer.

In the UNSCEAR model of radiation-induced carcinogenesis, the general equation of which is based on the linear quadratic (LQ) model of radiation effects, the total radiation effect in terms of risk is the product between the probabilities of inducing DNA mutations and survival of the irradiated cells. This radiation effect is defined by Dasu and Toma-Dasu (2005) and Gray (1965) as:

$$\text{Effect} = \left(\alpha_1 D + \beta_1 D^2 \right) \times e^{-\left(\alpha_2 D + \beta_2 D^2 \right)} \quad (18.5)$$

where D is the dose delivered in a single exposure, α_1 and β_1 are the linear and quadratic coefficients for induction of DNA mutations, and α_2, β_2 are the linear and quadratic coefficients for cell kill (UNSCEAR 1993).

The first term of equation (18.5) represents the induction of DNA mutations whilst the second term represents the cell survival. The equation, therefore, describes risk of mutation of the irradiated surviving cells after a single radiation dose, D. It is notable that for very low doses, the quadratic component of the second term in equation 18.5 approaches unity and becomes negligible thus making the dose-effect relationship approximately linear with α_1, the slope of the curve. For this situation, the first term of the equation can be assumed to be equal to the risk coefficients derived from epidemiological population studies of low dose irradiation (Dasu and Toma-Dasu 2005).

In clinical radiotherapy, the organs-at-risk are usually exposed to a range of fractionated radiation doses as described earlier. Therefore, equation (18.5) needs to be modified to reflect this. Assuming firstly that the radiation dose fraction affects DNA mutation and cell killing of the organ/tissue equally, the effect on the risk of radiation-induced SPC can be expressed (Dasu and Toma-Dasu 2005) as:

$$\text{Effect} = \left(\alpha_1 D + \frac{\beta_1 D^2}{n}\right) \times \exp\left[-\left(\alpha_2 D + \frac{\beta_2 D^2}{n}\right)\right]$$

(18.6)

where D is the total dose given in n fractions. As discussed for equation (18.5) earlier, for very low doses the quadratic component of the second term in equation (18.6) becomes negligible and the risk approximates to a linear function of dose with α_1 the slope of the dose-effect curve.

The equation (18.4) is then applied for each dose interval in the DVH of the organ-at-risk and the total effect is obtained by integrating the effects on the dose intervals using the following equation (Dasu and Toma-Dasu 2005):

$$\text{Total effect} = \frac{\sum_i \left(v_i \times \text{Effect}(D_i)\right)}{\sum_i v_i}$$

(18.7)

where v_i is the volume of organ/tissue receiving dose D_i delivered in n individual fractions and $\text{Effect}(D_i)$ is the non-linear dose-response relationship of the competition model.

As discussed earlier, the main advantage of the competitive risk model is that it allows the DVH of the irradiated organ/tissue to be used without the need to transform all the dose intervals into a single uniform dose value which does not accurately reflect the actual clinical situation. Therefore, the model accounts for the effects of dose-distribution inhomogeneity in the risk estimation of SPC. It also allows for the two competitive processes of DNA mutation and cell kill as a result of the wide range of radiation doses the organ at risk is exposed to in clinical radiotherapy to be incorporated in the risk estimation. The competitive risk model is based on the hypothesis that the probability of second primary cancer increases with increasing radiation dose initially until a peak is reached and then decreases due to the predominance of cell kill effects (Harrison 2004). This reflects the skewed bell-shape dose-effect curve of the competitive risk model shown in Figure 18.5.

The report of Dörr and Herrmann (2002) provides support for the clinical applicability of the competitive risk model. They reported that the majority (58%) of SPCs occurred within the margin around the treatment volume where organs-at-risk received radiation doses of ≤6 Gy. The study involved 85 patients treated with radiotherapy for their primary tumours that met selection criteria for the spatial relation between a new tumour and the primary treatment field. Approximately 35% of the SPCs developed at doses between 10 and 30 Gy and only 7% were found within the volume of tissue of organ-at-risk receiving radiation doses larger than 30 Gy. The results of this study are consistent with the dose-response relationship in terms of radiation-induced carcinogenesis predicted by the competitive risk model. However, it has been previously reported that some SPCs occur in areas which received radiation doses as large as 65 Gy (Dörr and Herrmann 2002). Hall and Wuu (2003) have also reported that there was no significant change in the relative risk of bladder carcinogenesis when radiation doses of between 2 and 80 Gy were delivered to the organ-at-risk in the radiation treatment of cervical and prostate carcinoma. These reports are however consistent with the existence of a plateau in the probability of radiation-induced carcinogenesis at higher radiation doses. There has been no data over the wide range of fractionated doses the organs-at-risk are exposed to in clinical radiotherapy to support the contention of a plateau in risk of induction of SPC at higher radiation doses. The International Committee on Radiation Protection (ICRP) based implicitly on a linear dose response in relation to cancer induction probabilities is currently the most appropriate guide

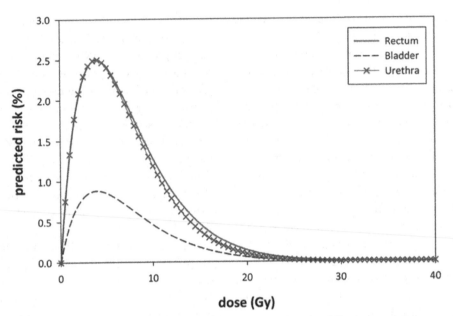

Figure 18.5. Predicted second primary cancer risks of rectum, bladder, and urethra following prostate cancer standard (2 Gy) fractionated 3D-Conformal Radiotherapy using the competitive risk model. The bell-shape dose-effect curve exhibits the result of two competing processes, with increasing dose induction of DNA mutation dominating at low doses and the predominance of cell kill at higher doses.

to permissible radiation dose limits for occupational exposure (Harrison 2004). However, the competitive risk model of SPC risk estimation for organs-a-risk may provide a more appropriate basis to compare the SPC risks corresponding to various radiotherapy techniques used in the treatment of cancer.

18.11.3 Peripheral photon and neutron doses from cancer external beam irradiation and the risk of second primary cancers

Organs lying in the high dose gradient, i.e. in the proximity to the target volume, are generally irradiated to high radiation doses leading to high probability of normal tissue complications and usually to a small risk of radiation-induced SPCs. However, with the current practice of external beam radiation therapy where high-energy (up to 25 MV) medical linear accelerators are used routinely to produce photon beams, there are leakage and scattered out-of-field radiations produced from the primary radiation beams. In addition, it is well known that high-energy photons (above 8 MeV) also produce neutrons by interacting with the constituents of accelerator structures and the treatment room as well as with the

patient (d'Errico *et al.* 1998). Neutron fluence spectra are produced from interactions between bremsstrahlung photons and materials of the linac head. The average neutron energy ranges from 0.4 MeV–1.2 MeV depending on the incident electron beam energy and the accelerator type.

These out-of-field radiations irradiate organs located within or around the targeted area as well as organs located distally from the treatment volume. As a result there is a need to evaluate the effects of radiation exposure in such organs also in terms of radiation-induced second primary cancers. In general, the out-of-field dose from photons was observed to be strongly dependent on the distance from the field edge (Howell *et al.* 2006) and the photon dose rate was the highest around the isocentre (Vanhavere *et al.* 2004). However, the neutron dose rate appeared to be more constant with some distance from the isocentre. Hence, at some point along the patient plane, the neutron doses are comparable or larger than the photon doses resulting in a larger neutron to photon absorbed dose ratio (Carinou *et al.* 2005).

Measuring neutrons is important as they have a higher radiation weighting factor (W_R) than photons,

$(W_R = 1)$ resulting in higher Relative Biological Effectiveness (RBE) (see section 14.2).

Taking into account that: (i) neutrons are produced from high-energy (>10 MV) accelerators, (ii) neutrons have significantly higher W_R than photons; and (iii) neutrons have a larger contribution to the dose delivered to distal normal organs/tissues during the external beam radiotherapy, it is therefore necessary to evaluate the dose from photons as well as neutrons in order to assess the risk of radiation-induced second malignancy resulted from radiotherapy using a high-energy linear accelerator.

Prior to 1970s, attention to scattered radiations and their potential to induce second cancers in patients was limited, but later on especially during the 1970s and 1980s a number of experimental and theoretical investigations on secondary photon and neutron exposures of patients as well as environment from widely used radiation therapy techniques were performed. As a result, understanding of dose distributions inside patients who undergo radiation treatments has been greatly improved.

In conclusion, localised cancer can be managed by surgery, radiation therapy, chemotherapy or others. Each management approach has its advantages and disadvantages. Following cancer radiation treatment, a small (≤5%) risk of normal tissue complications is accepted as a trade-off for control of the cancer. The level of risk of normal tissue complications depends on the dose received, treatment technique, and radiobiological response characteristics of normal tissue. It is now also acknowledged that cancer radiotherapy is associated with an increase in the risk of development of second malignancies compared to patients treated with surgery. This risk might be enhanced for prostate cancer patients because of earlier diagnosis and longer survivorship. Assessment of the risk of second malignancy following radiation treatment for prostate cancer is urgently needed because the increasing number of patients now diagnosed are faced with a wide choice of radiation treatment modalities such as 3D-Conformal Radiotherapy, Intensity Modulated Radiotherapy, Low Dose Rate Brachytherapy and High Dose Rate Brachytherapy either alone or in combination. The risk estimates are important in treatment decision making particularly for low risk cancers where the risk of developing a treatment related complication may exceed the risk of dying of that cancer.

18.12   REFERENCES

Abdel-Wahab M, Reis IM and Hamilton K (2008) Second primary cancer after radiotherapy for prostate cancer – a SEER analysis of brachytherapy versus external beam radiotherapy. *International Journal of Radiation Oncology Biology Physics* **72**: 58–68.

American Cancer Society (ACS) (2008) 'Cancer Facts & Figures 2008'. American Cancer Society, Inc., Atlanta.

Anzenberg V, Chandiramani S and Coderre JA (2008) LET-dependent bystander effects caused by irradiation of human prostate carcinoma cells with X rays or alpha particles. *Radiation Research* **170**: 467–476.

Azzam EI, Raaphorst GP and Mitchel RE (1994) Radiation-induced adaptive response for protection against micronucleus formation and neoplastic transformation in C3H 10T1/2 mouse embryo cells. *Radiation Research* **138**: S28–S31.

Baxter NN, Tepper JE, Durham SB *et al.* (2005) Increased risk of rectal cancer after prostate radiation: a population-based study. *Gastroenterology* **128**: 819–824.

Bentzen SM and Overgaard J (1994) Patient to patient variability in the expression of radiation induced normal tissue injury. *Seminars in Radiation Oncology* **4**: 68–80.

Berlin L (2001) Malpractice issues in radiology: radiation-induced skin injuries and fluoroscopy. *American Journal of Roentgenology* **177**: 21–25.

Bhojani N, Capitanio U, Suardi N, Jeldres C *et al.* (2010) The rate of secondary malignancies after radical prostatectomy versus external beam radiation therapy for localized prostate cancer: a population-based study on 17,845 patients. *International Journal of Radiation Oncology Biology and Physics* **76**(2): 342–348.

Brenner DJ, Curtis RE, Hall EJ *et al.* (2000) Second malignancies in prostate carcinoma patients after radiotherapy compared with surgery. *Cancer* **88**: 398–406.

Capizzi RL, Scheffler B and Scein PS (1993) Amifostine-mediated protection of normal bone marrow from cytotoxic chemotherapy. *Cancer* **72**: 3495–3501.

Carinou E, Stamatelatos IE, Kamenopoulou V *et al.* (2005) An MCNP-based model for the evaluation of the photoneutron dose in high energy medical electron accelerators. *Physica Medica* **21**: 95–99.

Cassatt DR, Fazenbaker CA, Kifle G and Bachy CM (2002) Preclinical studies on the radioprotective efficacy and pharmacokinetics of subcutaneously administered amifostine. *Seminars in Oncology* **29**: 2–8.

Chen H, Jia RF, Yu L, Zhao MJ *et al.* (2008) Bystander effects induced by continuous low-dose-rate 125I seeds potentiate the killing action of irradiation on human lung cancer cells in vitro. *International Journal of Radiation Oncology Biology Physics* **72**(5): 1560–1566.

Chen W, Yan K, Hou J, Pu, J *et al.* (2008) ATRA enhances bystander effect of suicide gene therapy in the treatment of prostate cancer. *Urologic Oncology* **26**: 397–405.

Chudoba I, Plesch A, Lorch T, Lemke J *et al.* (1999) High resolution multicolor-banding: a new technique for refined FISH analysis of human chromosomes. *Cytogenetics and Cell Genetics* **84**: 156–160.

Dasu A and Toma-Dasu I (2005) Dose-effect models for risk-relationship to cell survival parameters. *Acta Oncologica* **44**: 829–835.

d'Errico F, Nath R, Tana L *et al.* (1998) In-phantom dosimetry and spectrometry of photoneutrons from an 18 MV linear accelerator. *Medical Physics* **25**: 1717–1724.

Dörr W and Herrmann T (2002) Second primary tumours after radiotherapy for malignancies. *Strahlentherapie und Onkologie* **178**: 357–362.

Folkard M, Vojnovic B, Prise KM, Bowey AG *et al.* (1997) A charged-particle microbeam: I. Development of an experimental system for targeting cells individually with counted particles. *International Journal of Radiation Biology* **72**: 375–385.

Frank D, Frederick M, Liu T and Clayman G (1998) Bystander effect in the adenovirus-mediated Wild-Type p53 gene therapy model of human squamous cell carcinoma of the head & neck. *Clinical Cancer Research* **4**: 2521–2527.

Frank DK, Szymkowiak B, Josifovska-Chopra O, Nakashima T *et al.* (2005) Single-cell microinjection of cytochrome c can result in gap junction-mediated apoptotic cell death of bystander cells in head & neck cancer. *Head & Neck* **27**: 794–800.

Geard CR, Brenner DJ, Randers-Pehrson G and Marino SA (1991) Single-particle irradiation of mammalian cells at the Radiological Research Accelerator Facility: induction of chromosomal changes. *Nuclear Instrumentation Methods* **B54**: 411–416.

Gershkevitsh E, Rosenberg I, Dearnaley PD *et al.* (1999) Bone marrow doses and leukemia risk in radiotherapy of prostate cancer. *Radiotherapy and Oncology* **53**: 189–197.

Ghiassi-nejad M, Mortazavi SMJ, Cameron JR, Niroomand-rad A and Karam PA (2002) Very high background radiation areas of Ramsar, Iran: preliminary biological studies. *Health Physics* **82**: 87–93.

Gray LH (1965) Radiation biology and cancer. In: *Cellular Radiation Biology: A Symposium Considering Radiation Effects in the Cell and Possible Implications for Cancer Therapy*. pp. 8–25, 165. William & Wilkins, Baltimore.

Hall EJ (2000) *Radiobiology for the Radiologist*. 5th edn. Lippincott Williams & Wilkins, Philadelphia.

Hall EJ (2003) The bystander effect. *Health Physics* **85**: 31–35.

Hall EJ (2006) Intensity-modulated radiation therapy, protons, and the risk of second cancers, *International Journal of Radiation Oncology Biology Physics* **65**: 1–7.

Hall EJ and Wuu C-S (2003) Radiation-induced second cancers: the impact of 3D-CRT and IMRT. *International Journal of Radiation Oncology Biology Physics* **56**: 83–88.

Hande P, Azizova T, Geard C, Burak L *et al.* (2003) Past exposure to densely ionizing radiation leaves a unique permanent signature in the genome. *American Journal of Human Genetics* **72**: 1162–1170.

Harada K, Nonaka T, Hamada N, Sakurai H *et al.* (2009) Heavy-ion-induced bystander killing of human lung cancer cells: role of gap junctional intercellular communication. *Cancer Science* **100**: 684–688.

Harrison RM (2004) Second cancers following radio-therapy: a suggested common dosimetry framework for therapeutic and concomitant exposures. *The British Journal of Radiology* 77: 986–990.

Howell RM, Ferenci MS, Hertel NE *et al.* (2006) Calculation of effective dose from measurements of secondary neutron spectra and scattered photon dose from dynamic MLC IMRT for 6 MV, 15 MV, and 18 MV beam energies. *Medical Physics* 33: 360–368.

Huang J, Kestin LL, Ye H, Wallace M *et al.* (2011) Analysis of second malignancies after modern radiotherapy versus prostatectomy for localized prostate cancer. *Radiotherapy and Oncology* 98(1): 81–86.

Huss W, Lai L, Barrios RJ, Hirschi KK and Greenberg NM (2004) Retinoic acid slows progression and promotes apoptosis of spontaneous prostate cancer. *Prostate* 61: 142–152.

Jaworowski Z (1997) Beneficial effects of radiation and regulatory policy. *Australasian Physical* Engineering and *Sciences in* Medicine 20: 125–138.

Johnston WR (2010) Database of radiological incidents and related events. www.johnstonsarchive.net/nuclear/radevents/index.html (accessed on 21/07/2010).

Khan MA, Hill RP and Van Dyk J (1998) Partial volume rat lung irradiation: an evaluation of early DNA damage. *International Journal of Radiation Oncology Biology Physics* 40: 467–476.

Kleinerman RA, Liebermann JV and Li FP (1985) Second cancer following cancer of the male genital system in Connecticut, 1935–82. *National Cancer Institute Monograph* 68: 139–147.

Koukourakis MI (2003) Amifostine: is there evidence of tumour protection? *Seminars in Oncology* 30: 18–30.

Krutovskikh V, Piccoli C and Yamasaki H (2002) Gap junction intercellular communication propagates cell death in cancerous cells. *Oncogene* 21: 1989–1999.

Levi F, Randimbison L, Te V-C *et al.* (1999) Second primary tumors after prostate carcinoma. *Cancer* 86: 1567–1570.

Li D, Duan L, Freimuth P and O'Malley B (1999) Variability of adenovirus receptor density influences gene transfer efficiency and therapeutic response in head & neck cancer. *Clinical Cancer Research* 5: 4175–4181.

Lindegaard J (2003) Has the time come for routine use of amifostine in clinical radiotherapy practice? *Acta Oncologica* 42: 2–3.

Lorimore SA and Wright EG (2003) Radiation-induced genomic instability and bystander effects: related inflammatory-type responses to radiation-induced stress and injury? A review. *International Journal of Radiation Research* 79: 15–25.

Luckey TD (1980) Hormesis with ionizing radiation. CRC Press, Boca Raton, Florida.

Mesnil M, Piccoli C, Tiraby G, Willecke K and Yamasaki H (1996) Bystander killing of cancer cells by herpes simplex virus thymidine kinase gene is mediated by connexins. *Proceedings of the National Academic Sciences USA* 93: 1831–1835.

Mortazavi SMJ, Ghiassi-Nejad M and Beitollahi M (2001) Very high background radiation areas (VHBRAs) of Ramsar: do we need any regulations to protect the inhabitants? *Proceedings of the 34th midyear meeting, Radiation Safety and ALARA Considerations for the 21st Century*, California, USA, pp. 177–182.

Mothersill C and Seymour CB (1997) Medium from irradiated human epithelial cells but not human fibroblasts reduces the clonogenic survival of unir-radiated cells. *International Journal of Radiation Biology* 71: 421–427.

Mothersill C and Seymour CB (1998) Cell-cell contact during gamma irradiation is not required to induce a bystander effect in normal human keratinocytes: evidence for release during irradiation of a signal controlling survival into the medium. *Radiation Research* 149: 256–262.

Mothersill C and Seymour CB (2002) Bystander and delayed effects after fractionated radiation exposure. *Radiation Research* 158: 626–633.

Movsas B, Hanlon AL, Pinover W *et al.* (1998) Is there an increased risk of second primaries following prostate irradiation? *International Journal of Radiation Oncology Biology Physics* 41: 251–255.

Nagasawa H and Little JB (1992) Induction of sister chromatid exchanges by extremely low doses of alpha-particles. *Cancer Research* 52: 6394–6396.

Nelson JM, Brooks AL, Metting NF, Khan M *et al.* (1996) Clastogenic effects of defined numbers of 3.2 MeV alpha particles on individual CHO-K1 cells. *Radiation Research* **145**: 568–574.

Neugut AI, Ahsan H, Robinson E *et al.* (1997) Bladder carcinoma and other second malignancies after radiotherapy for prostate carcinoma. *Cancer* **79**: 1600–1604.

Olivieri G, Bodycote J and Wolff S (1984) Adaptive response of human lymphocytes to low concentrations of radioactive thymidine. *Science* **223**: 594–597.

Osterlind A, Rorth M and Prener A (1985) Second cancer following cancer of the male genital system in Denmark, 1943–80. *National Cancer Institute Monograph* **68**: 341–347.

Pawlish KS, Schottenfeld D, Severson R *et al.* (1997) Risk of multiple primary cancers in prostate cancer patients in the Detroit metropolitan area: a retrospective cohort study. *The Prostate* **33**: 75–86.

Pickles T and Phillips N (2002) The risk of second malignancy in men with prostate cancer treated with or without radiation in British Columbia, 1984–2000. *Radiotherapy and Oncology* **65**: 145–151.

Pollycove M (1998) Nonlinearity of radiation health effects. *Environmental Health Perspective* **101**: 363–368.

Prise KM, Pinto M, Newman HC and Michael BD (2001) A review of studies of ionizing radiation-induced double-strand break clustering. *Radiation Research* **156**: 572–576.

Rothkamm K and Lobrich M (2003) Evidence for a lack of DNA double-strand break repair in human cells exposed to very low x-ray doses. *Proceedings of the National Academic Sciences USA* **100**: 4973–4975.

Sagan LA (1987) What is hormesis and why haven't we heard about it before? *Health Physics* **52**: 521–525.

Sawant S, Randers-Pehrson G, Metting N and Hall E (2001a) Adaptive response and the bystander effect induced by radiation in C3H 10T1/2 cells in culture. *Radiation Research* **156**: 177–180.

Sawant S, Randers-Pehrson G, Geard C, Brenner D and Hall E (2001b) The bystander effect in radiation oncogenesis: I. Transformation in C3H 10T1/2 cells in vitro can be initiated in the unirradiated neighbours of irradiated cells. *Radiation Research* **155**: 397–401.

Schneider U, Zwahlen D, Ross D *et al.* (2005) Estimation of radiation-induced cancer from three-dimensional dose distributions: concept of organ equivalent dose. *International Journal of Radiation Oncology Biology Physics* **61**: 1510–1515.

Schneider U, Lomax A, Besserer J *et al.* (2007) The impact of dose escalation on secondary cancer risk after radiotherapy of prostate cancer. *International Journal of Radiation Oncology Biology Physics* **68**: 892–897.

Shao R, Xia W and Hung M (2000) Inhibition of angiogenesis and induction of apoptosis are involved in E1A-mediated bystander effect and tumor suppression. *Cancer Research* **60**: 3123–3126.

Shareef MM, Cui N, Burikhanov R, Gupta S *et al.* (2007) Role of tumor necrosis factor-alpha and TRAIL in high-dose radiation-induced bystander signaling in lung adenocarcinoma. *Cancer Research* **67**: 11811–11820.

Subak-Sharpe JE, Burk RR and Pitts JD (1969) Metabolic co-operation between biochemically marked mammalian cells in tissue culture. *Cell Science* **4**: 353–367.

Takam R, Bezak E and Yeoh EE (2009) Risk of second primary cancer following prostate cancer radiotherapy: DVH analysis using the competitive risk model. *Physics in Medicine and Biology* **54**: 611–625.

Thellenberg C, Malmer B, Tavelin B *et al.* (2003) Second primary cancers in men with prostate cancer: An increased risk of male breast cancer. *The Journal of Urology* **169**: 1345–1348.

Thomas B and Devi PU (1987) Chromosome protection by WR-2721 and MPG-single and combination treatments. *Strahlentherapie und Onkologie* **163**: 807–810.

Travis LB (2006) The epidemiology of second primary cancers. *Cancer Epidemiology, Biomarkers and Prevention* **15**(11): 2020–2026.

Trosko JE, Madhukar BV and Chang CC (1993) Endogenous and exogenous modulation of gap junctional intercellular communication: toxicological and pharmacological implications. *Life Science* **53**: 1–19.

UNSCEAR (1993) 'Sources and effects of ionizing radiation'. United Nations Scientific Committee on the Effects of Atomic Radiation, New York.

Vanhavere F, Huyskens D and Struelens L (2004) Peripheral neutron and gamma doses in radiotherapy with an 18 MV linear accelerator. *Radiation Protection Dosimetry* **110**: 607–612.

Waldren C (2004) Classical radiation biology dogma, bystander effects and paradigm shifts. *Human and Experimental Toxicology* **23**: 95–100.

Webber M, Bello-DeOcampo D, Quader S, Deocampo ND *et al.* (1999) Modulation of the malignant phenotype of human prostate cancer cells by N-(4-hydroxyphenyl)retinamide (4-HPR). *Clinical and Experimental Metastasis* **17**: 255–263.

Wojcik A, Kowalska M, Bouzyk E, Buraczewska I *et al.* (2000) Validation of the micronucleus-centromere assay for biological dosimetry. *Genetics and Molecular Biology* **23**: 1083–1085.

Index

L. Marcu et al., *Biomedical Physics in Radiotherapy for Cancer*,
DOI 10.1007/978-0-85729-733-4, © CSIRO 2012

Printed in the United States
By Bookmasters